SJ
ALLE ZEIT WACH
1842

The Cranial Nerves

Anatomy · Pathology · Pathophysiology
Diagnosis · Treatment

Edited by
M. Samii and P. J. Jannetta

With 410 Figures

Springer-Verlag Berlin Heidelberg New York 1981

Dr. med. M. SAMII
Professor and Chairman
Neurosurgical Clinic, Krankenhaus Nordstadt City of Hannover
Haltenhoffstraße 41, D-3000 Hannover, FRG

PETER J. JANNETTA, M.D.
Professor and Chairman
Department of Neurological Surgery, Presbyterian University Hospital
230 Lothrop Street, Pittsburgh, PA 15213, USA

ISBN-13:978-3-642-67982-7 e-ISBN-13:978-3-642-67980-3
DOI: 10.1007/978-3-642-67980-3

Library of Congress Cataloging in Publication Data. Main entry under title: The Cranial nerves. "Contributions ... [to] the International Symposium on Cranial Nerves held in Hanover, Federal Republic of Germany, from June 2nd to June 6th, 1980" — Foreword. Bibliography: p. Includes index. 1. Nerves, Cranial—Diseases—Congresses. 2. Nerves, Cranial—Congresses. I. Samii, Madjid. II. Jannetta, Peter J. III. International Symposium on Cranial Nerves (1980: Hannover, Germany) [DNLM: 1. Cranial nerves. WL 330 C891] RC410.C7 616.8 81-5617 ISBN-13:978-3-642-67982-7 AACR2

2122/3130-543210

List of Contributors

Arold, R.: Universitäts-Hals-Nasen-Ohrenklinik, Geiststraße 10, D-3400 Göttingen

Bennet, M. H.: Department of Neurological Surgery, University of Pittsburgh, School of Medicine, 230 Lothrop Street, Pittsburgh, PA 15213, USA

Berg, M.: Hals-Nasen-Ohren-Klinik der Universität Erlangen-Nürnberg, Waldstraße 1, D-8520 Erlangen

Brihaye, J.: Clinique Neurochirurgicale, Université Libre de Bruxelles, Rue Heger Bordet, 1, B-1000 Bruxelles

Brock, M.: Abteilung für Neurochirurgie, Neurochirurgische/Neurologische Klinik und Poliklinik, Universitätsklinikum Steglitz, Freie Universität Berlin, Hindenburgdamm 30, D-1000 Berlin 45

Cohen, N. L.: Department of Otolaryngology, New York University Medical Center, 550 First Avenue, New York, NY 10016, USA

Daniels, D. L.: Department of Neurosurgery, The Medical College of Wisconsin, 8700 West Wisconsin Avenue, Milwaukee, WI 53226, USA

Davis, J. P.: Department of Neurosurgery, The Medical College of Wisconsin, 8700 West Wisconsin Avenue, Milwaukee, WI 53226, USA

Denecke, H. J.: Moltkestraße 20, D-6900 Heidelberg

Dengler, R.: Neurologische Klinik und Poliklinik der Technischen Universität München, Möhlstraße 28, D-8000 München 80

Dietz, H.: Neurochirurgische Klinik, Medizinische Hochschule Hannover, Karl-Wiechert-Allee 9, D-3000 Hannover

Draf, W.: Klinik für Hals-Nasen-Ohren-Krankheiten und Plastische Gesichtschirurgie, Städtische Kliniken Fulda, Pacelliallee 4, D-6400 Fulda

Ehrenberger, K.: Universitäts-Hals-Nasen-Ohren-Klinik, Allgemeines Krankenhaus der Stadt Wien, 9, Alserstraße 4, A-1090 Wien

Erbel, F.: Neurologische Klinik der Technischen Universität München, Möhlstraße 28, D-8000 München 80

Fahlbusch, R.: Neurochirurgische Klinik im Klinikum Großhadern der Universität München, Ludwig-Maximilians-Universität, Marchionistraße 15, D-8000 München 70

Ferran, E.: Service of Neurosurgery, Ciudad Sanitaria Principes de Espana, Hospitalet, Barcelona, Spain

Fukado, Y.: Department of Ophtalmology, Showa University, School of Medicine, 1-5-8. Hatanodai, Shinagawa-ku, Tokyo, 142, Japan

Gager, W. M.: Department of Ophthalmology, The Medical Center of Wisconsin, 8700 West Wisconsin Avenue, Milwaukee, WI 53226, USA

Galic, M.: Hals-Nasen-Ohren-Klinik, Universität Tübingen, Silcherstraße 5, D-7400 Tübingen

Grau, H.: Abteilung Neuroradiologie im Zentrum Radiologie, J. W. Goethe-Universität, Schleusenweg 2–16, D-6000 Frankfurt am Main

Haid, T.: Klinik und Poliklinik für Hals-Nasen-Ohrenkranke der Universität Erlangen-Nürnberg, Waldstraße 1, D-8520 Erlangen

Hamer, J.: Neurochirurgische Abteilung des Chirurgischen Zentrums der Universität Heidelberg, Im Neuenheimer Feld 280, D-6900 Heidelberg 1

Haughton, V. M.: Department of Neurosurgery, The Medical College of Wisconsin, 8700 West Wisconsin Avenue, Milwaukee, WI 53226, USA

Helms, J.: Hals-Nasen-Ohrenklinik, Johannes-Gutenberg-Universität, Langenbeckstraße 1, D-6500 Mainz

Herberhold, C.: Klinik für Hals-, Nasen- und Ohrenkrankheiten, Universitätskrankenhaus Eppendorf, Universität Hamburg, Martinistaße 52, D-2000 Hamburg 20

Heuser, M.: Neurologische Klinik, Klinikum Großhadern, Ludwig-Maximilians-Universität München, Marchionistraße 15, D-8000 München 70
Hoffmann, K.: Augenklinik der Städtischen Kliniken Hannover, Haltenhoffstraße 41, D-3000 Hannover 1
Isamat, F.: Clinical Sagrada Familia Neurochirurgica, Torras y Pujalt, 1, Barcelona, 22, Spain
Ishikawa, J.-I.: Department of Neurosurgery, Fukui Red Cross Hospital, 2-4-1, Tsukimi, Fukui, Fukui, Japan
Jannetta, P. J.: Department of Neurological Surgery, University of Pittsburgh, School of Medicine, 230 Lothrop Street, Pittsburgh, PA 15213, USA
Jensen, H.-P.: Neurochirurgische Klinik, Universität Kiel, Weimarer Straße 8, D-2300 Kiel 1
Jongkees, L. B. W.: Keel-, neus- en oorheelkundige kliniek, Academish Ziekenhuis, Wilhelmina Gasthuis, BIJ de Universeiteit van Amsterdam, Eerste Helmersstraat 104, NE-1054 EG Amsterdam
Klinge, H.: Neurochirurgische Klinik, Universität Kiel, Weimarer Straße 8, D-2300 Kiel 1
Kluyskens, J.: Neurochirurgisch Centrum, Sint-Vincentiusziekenhuis, Sint-Vincentiusplein, 1, B-9000 Gent
Kondo, A.: Department of Neurosurgery, Fukui Red Cross Hospital, 2-4-1, Tsukimi, Fukui, Fukui, Japan
Konishi, T.: Department of Neurosurgery, Fukui Red Cross Hospital, 2-4-1, Tsukimi, Fukui, Fukui, Japan
Koos, W.: Neurochirurgische Universitätsklinik Wien, Alserstraße 4, A-1097 Wien
Kreutzberg, G. W.: Max-Planck-Institut für Psychiatrie, Kraepelinstaße 2, D-8000 München 40
Kruger, L.: Department of Anatomy, University of California, Center for Health Sciences, Los Angeles, California 90024, USA
Lang, J.: Anatomisches Institut, Universität Würzburg, Koellikerstraße 6, D-8700 Würzburg
Lasjaunias, P.: Departement de Radiologie, Centre Hospitalier et Universitaire de Bicetre, Hôpitaux de Paris, 78, Rue du General Leclerc, F-94270 Kremlin-Bicetre
Loew, F.: Neurochirurgische Klinik, Universitätsklinik Homburg, D-6650 Homburg/Saar
Manelfe, Cl.: Departement de Neuroradiologie, Hôpital St. Julien, 1, Rue Foller, F-54037 Nancy/Cedex
Marguth, F.: Neurochirurgische Klinik im Klinikum Großhadern, Ludwig-Maximilians-Universität München, Marchionistraße 15, D-8000 München 70
Meissl, G.: Ludwig-Boltzmann-Institut für Experimentelle Plastische Chirurgie, Alserstraße 4, A-1090 Wien
Menzel, J.: Neurochirurgische Abteilung im Chirurgischen Zentrum der Universität Heidelberg, Im Neuenheimer Feld 110, D-6900 Heidelberg
Meyer, G. A.: Department of Neurosurgery, The Medical College of Wisconsin, 8700 West Wisconsin Avenue, Milwaukee, Wisconsin 53226, USA
Miehlke, A.: Hals-Nasen-Ohren-Klinik der Universität Göttingen, Geiststraße 5–10, D-3400 Göttingen
Millesi, H.: Ludwig-Boltzmann-Institut für Experimentelle Plastische Chirurgie, Alserstraße 4, A-1090 Wien
Mingrino, S.: Istituto di Neurochirurgia, Universita Degli Studi di Padova, Via Giustiniani, 5, I-35100 Padova
Mizoi, K.: Division of Neurosurgery, Tohoku University School of Medicine, Institut of Brain Diseases, 5-13-1, Nagamachi, Sendai, Japan 982
Moret, J.: Departement de Neuroradiologie, Hôpital St. Julien, 1, Rue Foller, F-54037 Nancy/Cedex
Muhtaroglu, U.: Neurochirurgische Klinik, Universität Kiel, Weimarer Straße 8, D-2300 Kiel 1
Mulch, G.: Hals-Nasen-Ohrenklinik, Klinikum Charlottenburg der Freien Universität Berlin, Spandauer Damm 130, D-1000 Berlin 19
Mumenthaler, M.: Neurologische Universitätsklinik, Inselspital Bern, CH-3010 Bern
Naessens, P.: Neurochirurgisch Centrum, Sint-Vincentiusziekenhuis, Sint-Vincentiusplein, 1, B-9000 Gent
Ohlemutz, A.: Hals-Nasen-Ohren-Klinik im Krankenhaus Nordstadt der Landeshauptstadt Hannover, Ellernstraße 39, D-3000 Hannover 1

Oppel, F.: Abteilung für Neurochirurgie, Neurochirurgische/Neurologische Klinik und Poliklinik, Universitätsklinikum Steglitz, Freie Universität Berlin, Hindenburgdamm 30, D-1000 Berlin 45
Osterwald, L.: Hals-Nasen-Ohrenklinik, Städtische Kliniken Hannover, Ellernstraße 39, D-3000 Hannover 1
Penzholz, H.: Neurochirurgische Abteilung des Chirurgischen Zentrums der Universität Heidelberg, Im Neuenheimer Feld 110, D-6900 Heidelberg 1
Perneczky, A.: Neurochirurgische Universitätsklinik, Allgemeines Krankenhaus der Stadt Wien, 9, Alser Straße 4, A-1090 Wien
Perwein, J.: Psychiatrische Klinik der Technischen Universität München, Möhlstraße 28, D-8000 München 80
Picard, L.: Departement de Neuroradiologie, Hôpital St. Julien, 1, Rue Foller, F-54037 Nancy/Cedex
Plester, D.: Hals-Nasen-Ohren-Klinik, Universität Tübingen, D-7400 Tübingen
Poppendieck, J.: Hals-Nasen-Ohren-Klinik, Universität Tübingen, D-7400 Tübingen
Quaknine, G.-E.: Service of Neurosurgery, Hôpital Notre-Dame, Centre Hospitalier Affilié à l'Universite de Montreal, 1560, Rue Sherbrooke Est, Montreal, Quebec H2L 4K8, Canada
Ransohoff, J.: Department of Neurosurgery, New York University Medical Center, 550 First Avenue, New York, NY 10016, USA
Regli, F.: Service de Neurologie, Hôpital Kantonale, Universitaire Lausanne, Hôpital Beaumont, Ch-1011 Lausanne
Rettinger, G.: Hals-Nasen-Ohren-Klinik der Universität Erlangen-Nürnberg, Waldstraße 1, D-8520 Erlangen
Roland, J.: Departement de Neuroradiologie, Hôpital St. Julien, 1, Rue Foller, F-54037 Nancy/Cedex
Rommel, Th.: Neurochirurgische Abteilung im Chirurgischen Zentrum der Universität Heidelberg, Im Neuenheimer Feld 110, D-6900 Heidelberg 1
Sakurai, Y.: Division of Neurosurgery, Institute of Brain Diseases, Tohoku University School of Medicine, 5-13-1 Nagamachi, Sendai, Japan 982
Samii, M.: Neurochirurgische Klinik im Krankenhaus Nordstadt der Landeshauptstadt Hannover, Haltenhoffstraße 41, D-3000 Hannover 1
Sato, T.: Division of Neurosurgery, Institute of Brain Diseases, Tohoku University School of Medicine, 5-13-1 Nagamachi, Sendai, Japan 982
Schäfer, M.: Abteilung für Allgemeine Neurochirurgie, Zentrum der Neurologie und Neurochirurgie, Klinikum der Johann Wolfgang Goethe-Universität, Schleusenweg 2–16, D-6000 Frankfurt am Main 71
Schaupp, H.: Zentrum der Hals-Nasen-Ohrenheilkunde, Klinikum der Johann Wolfgang Goethe-Universität, Theodor-Stern-Kai 7, D-6000 Frankfurt am Main 70
Schröder, J. M.: Abteilung Neuropathologie, Johannes Gutenberg Universität Mainz, Langenbeckstraße 1, D-6500 Mainz
Schürmann, K.: Neurochirurgische Klinik, Johannes Gutenberg Universität Mainz, Langenbeckstraße 1, D-6500 Mainz
Schuster, H.: Neurochirurgische Universitätsklinik, Allgemeines Krankenhaus der Stadt Wien, 9, Alser Straße 4, A-1090 Wien
Siegfried, J.: Neurochirurgische Klinik, Universitätsspital Zürich, Rämistrasse 100, CH-8091 Zürich
Søgaard, I.: Grantoften 5, DK-9210 Aalborg SØ
Steinbach, E.: Hals-Nasen-Ohrenklinik, Universität Tübingen, Silcherstraße 5, D-7400 Tübingen
Stennert, E.: Hals-Nasen-Ohren-Klinik, Universität Göttingen, Geiststraße 5–10, D-3400 Göttingen
Sterkers, J.-M.: O.R.L. de l'Hôpital Cochin, 42, Rue Ampère, F-75017 Paris XVIIe
Steudel, W. I.: Abteilung für Allgemeine Neurochirurgie, Johann Wolfgang Goethe-Universität, Schleusenweg 2–16, D-6000 Frankfurt am Main 71
Struppler, A.: Neurologische Klinik der Technischen Universität München, Möhlstraße 28, D-8000 München 80
Sunderland, S.: Anatomy Department, Medical Centre, University of Melbourne, Parkville, Victoria, Australia, 3052

Suzuki, J.: Division of Neurosurgery, Tohoku University School of Medicine, Institute of Brain Diseases, 5-13-1 Nagamachi, Sendai, Japan 982
Thumfart, W.: Hals-Nasen-Ohrenklinik der Universität Erlangen-Nürnberg, Waldstraße 1, D-8520 Erlangen
Waele, L. F. de: Neurochirurgisch Centrum, Sint-Vincentiusziekenhuis, Sint-Vincentiusplein, 1, B-9000 Gent
Wigand, M. E.: Hals-Nasen-Ohrenklinik der Universität Erlangen-Nürnberg, Waldstraße 1, D-8520 Erlangen
Wild, K. von: Neurochirurgische Klinik der Städtischen Kliniken Hannover, Haltenhoffstraße 41, D-3000 Hannover 1
Yoshimoto, T.: Division of Neurosurgery, Institute of Brain Disease, Tohoku University School of Medicine, 5-13-1 Nagamachi, Sendai, Japan 982
Young, R. F.: Division of Neurosurgery, Harbor General Hospital, 1000 West Carson Street, USA-Torrance, California 90509
Zuccarello, M.: Istituto di Neurochirurgia, Universita Degli Studi di Padova, Via Giustiniani, 5, I-35100 Padova
Zühlke, D.: Abteilung für Neurochirurgie, Neurochirurgische/Neurologische Klinik und Poliklinik, Universitätsklinikum Steglitz, Freie Universität Berlin, Hindenburgdamm 30, D-1000 Berlin 45
Zülch, K. J.: Max-Planck-Institut für Hirnforschung, Ostmerheimer Straße 200, D-5000 Köln 91

Foreword

No special field of surgery dealing with the cranial nerves exists today. This is not surprising in view of the characteristics of this group of morphologically and topographically heterogenous nerves. Morphologically we must differentiate between central nerves (I, II and VIII) and the so-called peripheral nerves (nn. III to VII and IX to XII), in which post-lesion rgeneration is quite different. Anatomo-topographically we must consider an intracranial and an extracranial part of each cranial nerve. For practical reasons at operation, further subdivisions of the intracranial course of cranial nerves are to be distinguished in the anterior, middle and posterior cranial fossae as well as within the petrous bone. This underscores the extensive tasks awaiting surgeons operating in the ventral part of the brain and facial skull as well as in the more dorsal part of the skull and neck. This very wide field cannot be covered by a single surgical discipline alone. In our opinion, considerable progress has been made in surgery of the cranial nerves only in recent years. This may be explained by the increased mastery of microsurgical techniques by all surgeons interested in the surgery of the base of the skull as well as with the initiation of more interdisciplinary consultation and jointly performed operations. Possibilities of future development can be discerned in the text. The base of the skull separating the extra- and intracranial part of cranial nerves should not be a barrier but a connecting link.

This symposium brought together specialists from various fields who exchanged their experience and views. We hope to encourage a multidisciplinary approach to our problems and to prepare the next step forward.

This volume, therefore, contains articles from various experts (anatomists, physiologists, neurophysiologists, neuropathologists, neurologists, neuroradiologists, neurosurgeons, earsurgeons, plastic and reconstructive surgeons) who have made substantial experimental and clinical contributions in this field. The text proves the effectiveness of such an interdisciplinary team with an exchange of ideas on the part of colleagues approaching the same problem from different angles. It contains, in a condensed form, the most essential information on the topic of cranial nerves. This is otherwise available only through articles which are widely scattered throughout various journals. This volume constitutes an unusual survey of surgery of cranial nerves which was not previously available. We take great pleasure in thanking the initiators, Doctor Madjid Samii and Doctor Peter J. Jannetta for their ideas and their excellent organization of this symposium. We should also like to thank the authors and Springer Verlag for their good cooperation which has enabled this volume to be presented in such a short time.

Mainz K. Schürmann

Preface

This volume consists of contributions by a large group of distinguished experts who participated in the International Symposium on Cranial Nerves held in Hannover, Federal Republic of Germany, from June 2nd to June 6th, 1980. During this symposium it became clear to us that major new concepts in our understanding of cranial nerves, anatomy, physiology and pathology have recently been described, and further, that these concepts were evolving in many areas by investigators of diverse and even disparate disciplines. It seemed reasonable in our many discussions concerning this symposium, being the only potential one there is at present, that a platform consisting of leaders in various disciplines could share their knowledge and ideas with each other and with an audience composed of well informed investigators and that the result of this exchange could be advantageous in many ways.

Perhaps the most important single point demonstrated in the volume is that the sharing of our present knowledge in a true interdisciplinary approach to problems in science and medicine, as evidenced in the particular problems of the cranial nerves, might provide a basis for sharing information in a way that would be beneficial to physicians and basic investigators working in these areas and of course to patients with the various, often disabling problems that interfere with their lives. Each section of the volume is organized around one, or a logically organized group of cranial nerves and contains contributions concerning the anatomy, physiology, pathology and clinical diagnoses and treatment of the clinical disorders in that nerve or group of nerves. A discussion concerning the major problems of that nerve or nerves is then included.

In these discussions, as well as in the primary contribution by each author, recent developments in our knowledge of cranial nerves function and malfunction are evaluated. Since all disciplines came together for purposes of evaluation, a synthesis could usually be evolved, composed of multiple view points upon the same problem, so that the current state in many areas improved. In addition to this information, the exploration of new possibilities for basic investigation, clinical research and new methods of treatment have been presented and discussed during the symposium and are interpreted here for the reader.

We feel that this volume will be useful to physicians and students who are working with patients with clinical cranial nerve problems and also those investigating the basic function of cranial nerves.

Hannover and Pittsburgh — M. Samii and P. J. Jannetta

Contents

Cochleo-Vestibular Nerve

Caudal Cranial Nerves

History of Cranial Nerves Surgery. Introductory Lecture

F. LOEW, Homburg, Saar/FRG

One expects a real introduction to start with a historical review which leads from the earlier roots of knowledge of the topic in concern to the present situation, outlines the actual problems and finally gives some perspectives of future development. The earlier the historical starting point, the better an introduction.

To fulfill these requirements I travelled to Greece. You certainly remember that in prehistoric times neurosurgery started in this area and that the first major published neurosurgical operation was the delivery of the goddess Athena from the head of her godfather Zeus. Therefore I asked the delphic Sybilla whether she could give me some informations about the beginning of cranial nerve surgery. After appropriate opening of my mind by smoke and a lot of Greek wine, she told me that I was foolish to travel to Greece. I should have known myself that neurosurgery started with cranial nerve surgery, with other words, that cranial nerve surgery is the fundament of neurosurgery, a statement which clearly underlines the importance of this meeting. I needed some more rhezina, this strange but lovely resined wine, to understand the meaning of this very delphic information. Zeus, when pregnant with his daughter Athena in his forehead, suffered from a neuralgia of the first trigeminal branch, surely a symptomatic trigeminal neuralgia, and was cured by removal of the tumor-like girl.

The differentiation between idiopathic and symptomatic trigeminal neuralgia had been unknown in those prehistoric days and is an invention mainly of our last century. You will learn during this symposium, that we are going to return to the wisdom of old Greek goddesses and doctors and to abandon the idea of essential or idiopathic trigeminal neuralgia, detecting more and more real and treatable causes of seemingly idiopathic neuralgias. One of the pioneers in this field, Dr. Jannetta, is present at this course as one of its initiators and lecturers.

Also in more recent times surgical procedures for cranial nerve diseases and symptoms belong to the beginning of modern neurosurgery. The first major operations for *relief of optic nerve compression* by transcranial subfrontal or subtemporal approach were done as early as 1889 by Horsley, followed by Krause (1900), Kiliani (1904), Schloffer (1907), Halstead (1909), only to mention some pioneers in neurosurgery.

The first *intracranial operation for treatment of trigeminal neuralgia* was performed by Horsley in 1891, unfortunately with fatal outcome. It was Fedor Krause who in 1892 successfully sectioned the second and third branch of the trigeminal nerve by an intracranial approach and in 1893 removed the trigeminal ganglion in order to treat trigeminal neuralgia.

The next important steps were:

- the retrogasserian section of the trigeminal root, using a subtemporal approach, first published in 1901 by Spiller and Frazier,

- puncture and alcohol injection into the gasserian ganglion by Härtel in 1913,
- subtentorial approach and trigeminal root section by Dandy (1925),
- electrocoagulation of the trigeminal ganglion (Kirschner 1933),
- Sjöqvist's procedure of transsection of the descending spinal trigeminal tract (1937)
- and attempts to cure trigeminal neuralgia without neurological deficit by decompression procedures (Taarnhøj 1952, Stender 1953).

The last steps towards optimal treatment of trigeminal neuralgia have been the thermocontrolled selective trigeminal rhizotomy in the modification of Sweet, which tries to mainly destroy the poorly myelinated fibers for pain and thus to preserve the other functions of the trigeminal nerve, and the search for vessel loops and other mechanical factors which irritate the trigeminal root thus producing seemingly idiopathic trigeminal neuralgia, in order to treat the very causes of this disease without any function loss. Dandy was the first to perform this last mentioned way which nowadays is mainly propagated by Jannetta.

The long history of neurosurgical attempts to treat trigeminal neuralgia clearly shows two main tendencies:

- to improve our knowledge about the reasons of cranial nerve diseases in order to find causative treatment possibilities,
- or to treat the symptoms with a minimum of neurological deficit.
- Both trends are to be followed also in diseases of other cranial nerves.

Before leaving the trigeminal nerve I have to mention that neurosurgeons not only and always try to destroy this nerve but, in some special situations, to restore its function. To the best of my knowledge it was Samii, initiator, organizer and host of this course, who first described the reinnervation of the important first trigeminal branch by nerve graft.

Similar to the optic and trigeminal nerves also *lesions of the VIIth and VIIIth nerves* have been in the center of neurosurgical attention. The acoustic-vestibular nerve has the unfortunate tendency to produce neurinomas. The removal of these neurinomas confronted neurosurgeons with the problems of preserving the facial nerve or to restore its function when preservation failed. Improvement of operative technique improved not only the results of *acoustic neurinoma removal* regarding mortality and morbidity but also with regard to facial nerve preservation. The present state of operative technique recently has been described by Yaşargil (1977).

For *restoration of facial nerve function or compensation of its loss,* had the preservation of this nerve not been possible, four main ways have been used:

- plastic surgical methods for restoration of facial symmetry,
- anastomoses of the facial nerve with other nerves, mainly with the accessory, hypoglossal or phrenic nerves (for literature see Loew and Kivelitz 1973),
- anastomosis with the healthy facial nerve of the other side (Samii 1976, 1980),
- intracranial suture of the facial nerve or bridging or bypassing a facial nerve defect using a nerve graft. Prototype and starting point of this last mentioned possibility has been the Dott procedure (Dott 1958). Charles Drake as well as I myself tried the method of Norman Dott in the early 1960's – like Dott without having a microscope – with remarkable good results.

Indications, contraindications and results of the different possibilities have been reviewed by Loew and Kivelitz (1973). One of the results has been that in cases with simultaneous homolateral trigeminal lesions, it is useless to perform an anastomosis with other cranial nerves. The patients are unable to relearn using properly the re-innervated mimic muscles, because they have no sufficient feed-back.

Not only neurosurgery but also otology and plastic surgery have part in the progress of facial nerve and face restitution possibilities. The recent progress of micro-surgery of the temporal bone permits the safe approach to the whole intratemporal segment of the facial nerve from the internal auditory meatus to the stylomastoid foramen. Nearly all intratemporal facial nerve lesions are accessible to surgical repair. An excellent survey recently has been published by Fisch (1980). As demonstrated besides others by Miehlke and by Millesi, it is also possible to reconstruct the continuity of facial nerve branches within the face, when destroyed by accident or during tumor removal. By means of plastic surgery, for instance transplantation of innervated and vascularized muscles, the cosmetic results may be improved even more.

Hemifacial spasm is another good example of the before mentioned two different approaches to treatment: the operations for relief of symptoms, if possible with a minimum of neurological deficit, or the attempts to cure real causes. For symptomatic treatment I mention the different methods of partial dissection of facial nerve branches, especially the modifications published by Miehlke and by Fisch. Unfortunately, recurrencies after a few years in our experience are not uncommon. Jannetta (1975) also in hemifacial spasm propagates the causative treatment by exposure and decompression of the facial nerve within the cerebello-pontine angle and the internal auditory meatus. He surely will present his late results during this course and I wonder whether his patients remained recurrence-free.

Neuro-, oto- and plastic surgeons have learnt and can learn from each other and should closely cooperate in many individual cases for the benefit of our patients.

In my introduction I deliberately avoided giving a complete survey on cranial nerve surgery. I mentioned only some historical landmarks, dealt with some but not all cranial nerves, touched only some few principles, trends and aspects. So take my introduction as a kind of hors d'œuvre, offered to stimulate your appetite for eating the whole menu of this course, so well cooked by Dr. Samii and Dr. Jannetta and their coworkers. Good appetite!

References

Cushing H (1903) The surgical treatment of facial paralysis by nerve anastomosis. With the report of a successful case. Ann Surg 37:641–659

Dandy WE (1925) Section of the sensory root of the trigeminal nerve at the pons. Preliminary report of the operative procedure. Bull Johns Hopkins Hosp 36:105–106

Dandy WE (1934) Concerning the cause of trigeminal neuralgia. Am J Surg 24:447–455

Dott NM (1958) Facial paralysis restitution by extrapetrous nerve graft. Proc Soc Med 51:900–902

Drake CG (1960) Acoustic neurinoma – Repair of facial with autogenous graft. J Neurosurg 17:836–842

Fisch U (1976) Cross-face grafting in facial paralysis. Arch Otolaryng 102:453–457

Fisch U (1977) Facial nerve surgery. Kugler Medical Publ. B. V., Amstelveen

Fisch U (1980) Management of intratemporal facial nerve palsy. In: Advances and Technical Standards in Neurosurgery, vol 7, Springer, Wien New York

Härtel F (1913) Die Leitungsanästhesie und Injektionsbehandlung des Ganglion Gasseri und der Trigeminusstämme. Arch Klin Chir 100: 193–292

Härtel F (1914) Die Behandlung der Trigeminusneuralgie mit intrakraniellen Alkoholeinspritzungen. Dtsch Z Chir 126:429–552

Haines StJ, Martinez AJ, Jannetta PJ (1979) Arterial cross compression of the trigeminal nerve at the pons in trigeminal neuralgia. J Neurosurg 50:257–259

Halstead AE (1910) Remarks on the operative treatment of tumours of the hypophysis. With the report of two cases operated on by an oronasal method. Trans Am Soc Artif Intern Organs 28:73–93

Horsley V, Taylor J, Colman WS (1891) Remarks on the various surgical procedures devised for the relief or cure of trigeminal neuralgia (tic douloureux). Br Med J 2:1139–1143, 1191–1193, 1249–1252

Horsley (1906) On the technique of operations on the central nervous system. Br Med J 2:411–423

Jannetta PJ (1967) Arterial compression to the trigeminal nerve at the pons in patients with trigeminal neuralgia. J Neurosurg: 159–162

Jannetta PJ (1975) Trigeminal neuralgia and hemifacial spasm – Etiology and definite treatment. Trans Am Neurol Assoc 100:89–91

Jannetta PJ, Tew JW (1979) Treatment of trigeminal neuralgia. Neurosurgery 4:93–94

Kiliani OGT (1904) Some remarks on tumours of the chiasm with a proposal how to reach the same by operation. Ann Surg 40:35–43

Kirschner M (1933) Die Punktionstechnik und die Elektrokoagulation des Ganglion Gasseri; über „gezielte“ Operationen. Arch Klin Chir 176:581–620

Kivelitz R, Loew F, Hübner H (1974) Perspectives on the indications and contraindications of various nerve transplant techniques in cases of facial nerve paralysis after pontine angle tumour operations. Chir Plastica (Berl) 2:161–167

Kivelitz R, Loew F, Hübner H (1975) Gesichtspunkte für die Indikation und Kontraindikation verschiedener Methoden der Nerventransplantate bei Fazialislähmung nach der Operation von Brückenwinkeltumoren. Plastische und Wiederherstellungschirurgie. F. K. Schattauer, Stuttgart, New York, p 129–136

Krause F (1892) Resektion des Trigeminus innerhalb der Schädelhöhle. Verh Dtsch Ges Chir 21:199–210

Krause F (1893) Entfernung des Ganglion Gasseri und des zentral davon gelegenen Trigeminus-Stammes. Dtsch Med Wschr 19:341–344

Krause F (1896) Die Neuralgie des Trigeminus nebst der Anatomie und Physiologie des Nerven. F. C. W. Vogel, Leipzig

Krause F (1905) Hirnchirurgie. Die Deutsche Klinik am Eingange des zwanzigsten Jahrhunderts in akademischen Vorlesungen. 8:953–1024

Krause F (1908) Chirurgie des Gehirns und Rückenmarks, nach eigenen Erfahrungen. Freilegung der Hypophysis. Bd. 1:74–82. Urban und Schwarzenberg, Berlin Wien

Loew F (1962) Die kombinierte intrakranielle-extratemporale Fazialisplastik nach Dott. Langenbecks Arch Chir 298:934–935 und Saarl. Ärzteblatt 9

Loew F, Kivelitz R (1973) Surgical reconstruction of intracranial lesions of cranial nerves. Advances in Neurosurgery 1, Springer, Berlin Heidelberg New York, p 242–247

Miehlke A (1960) Die Chirurgie des Nervus facialis. Urban und Schwarzenberg, München Berlin

Miehlke A (1973) Surgery of the facial nerve. Urban und Schwarzenberg, München Berlin Wien

Millesi H, Samii M (1975) Erfahrungen mit verschiedenen Wiederherstellungsoperationen am Nervus facialis. In: Köhler H (Hrsg) Plastische Wiederherstellungschirurgie. New York

Millesi H. (1980) Extratemporal surgery of the facial nerve. Palliative surgery. In: Advances and Technical Standards in Neurosurgery, vol 7, Springer, Wien New York

Mingrino S (1980) Intracranial surgical repair of the facial nerve. In: Advances and Technical Standards in Neurosurgery, vol 7, Springer, Wien New York

Samii, M (1972) Autologe Nerventransplantion im Trigeminusbereich. Mels Med Mitteilungen 46:189–194

Topographical Anatomy of the Cranial Nerves *

J. LANG, Würzburg/FRG

Naturally, it is not possible in a short time to discuss in full detail even a gross topography of the twelve cranial nerves. Nevertheless, I will try to describe the most significant topographical relations and a few less known details.

As you all know, the olfactory nerve is not a cranial nerve – it is called also olfactory tract. This tract, having an average length of 25 mm and thickness of 3 mm, runs straight or slightly bowed outwards from the olfactory bulb towards the olfactory trigonum which is located rostral to the substantia perforata rostralis. The kidney-shaped or oval-formed olfactory bulb is vertically flattened, rostrally it is usually peaked and medially convexed (Fig. 1 a). On the average it is 10 (6–14) mm long, 4.5 (3–7) mm wide and 2.1–2.3 mm thick. From below through the lamina cribrosa about 30 bundles of fibers enter into the olfactory bulb. These fibers are central processes of the olfactory cells (Epitheliocyti neurosensorii). They are collected out of minute fibers into bundles which pass through the lower region of the lamina cribrosa. On this layer, there are on the average 43 foramina cribrosa to the right and 44 of them to the left, occasionally 60–70 on one side. The lamina cribrosa which has an average length of 20.78 (14.5–26.7) mm and, in posterior regions, a width of 5.17 (2.0–8.1) mm, is situated adjacent to the dura mater thus forming a dural olfactory fossa which has an average length of 15.87 (11.00–24.00) mm on the right side and width of 3.8 (2.00–5.00) mm in the middle part. From rostral and from dorsal aspects, it is covered by smaller dura folds. The anterior bundles from rostral, the posterior from dorsal, the central from below, reach the medial and lateral margins of the olfactory fossa, pierce through it and enter the olfactory bulb. The central processes of the olfactory cells, known presently as olfactory nerves pass through the dura portals accompanied by arachnoid sheaths. The olfactory bulb and tract are supplied from branches of the anterior cerebral artery, particularly, from the medial fronto-basal ramus; and from the long central artery which normally crosses the posterior region of the olfactory tract. The olfactory tract enters a small cistern. The blood outflow from this region takes place over orbital veins of the orbital frontal lobe to the anterior cerebral vein, then to the superior sagittal sinus as well as through the lamina cribrosa to the nasal cavity.

Today, in the afternoon session, I will cover in more detail the optic nerve, the optic canal, its postnatal size development, and its lining membranes. The optic nerve and the optic chiasma are clamped by both, the internal carotid artery and anterior cerebral artery. As you know, the optic nerve is also not really a nerve, rather it represents essentially the centripetal fibers of the stratum ganglionare retinae. Schaeffer (1924) has studied the position of the optic chiasma relative to the prechiasmatic sulcus, to the diaphragma sellae, and to the dorsum sellae. According to

* Supported by Deutsche Forschungsgemeinschaft

Samii M (1975) Modern aspects of peripheral and cranial nerve surgery. In: Advances and Technical Standards in Neurosurgery, vol 2:33–85, Springer, New York Wien

Samii M (1976) Faziofaziale Anastomose durch Nerventransplantation. Fortschritte d. Kiefer- und Gesichtschirurgie, vol 20, G. Thieme, Stuttgart

Samii M (1980) Nerves of the head and neck. In: Omer GE, Spinner M (Hrsg) Management of peripheral nerve problems, W. B. Saunders, Philadelphia London Toronto

Siegfried J (1975) Technique of the controlled thermocoagulation of trigeminal ganglion and spinal roots. In: Advances and Technical Standards in Neurosurgery, vol 2:199–209, Springer, Wien New York

Sjöqvist O (1937) Eine neue Operationsmethode bei Trigeminusneuralgie. Durchschneidung des Tractus spinalis trigemini. Zbl Neurochir 5:274–281

Spiller WG, Frazier CH (1901) The devision of the sensory root of the trigeminus for the relief of tic douloureux; an experimental, pathological and clinical study, with a preliminary report of one surgically successful case. Philadelphia Med. J 8:1039–1049 and Univ Pennsylvania Med Bull 24:341–352

Sweet WH (1969) Pain, vol I:167–197 and 607–609, Charles C. Thomas, Springfield/Ill

Sweet WH, Wespic JG (1970) Relation of fibers size in trigeminal posterior root condition of impulses for pain and touch: Production of analgesia without anaesthesia in the effective treatment of trigeminal neuralgia. Trans Am Neurol Assoc 95:134–137

Sweet WH, Wespic JG (1974) Controlled thermocoagulation of trigeminal ganglion and rootlets for differential destruction of pain fibers. Part 1: Trigeminal neuralgia. J Neurosurg 40:143–156

Schloffer H (1906) Zur Frage der Operation an der Hypophyse. Beitr Klin Chir 50:767–817

Stender A (1953) Die „Gangliolyse“ des Ganglion Gasseri (Ein neuer, vereinfachter Weg zur operativen Behandlung der Trigeminusneuralgie). Zbl Neurochir 13:321–326

Taarnhøj P (1952) Decompression of the trigeminal root and the posterior part of the ganglion as treatment in trigeminal neuralgia. J Neurosurg 9:288–290

White, JC, Sweet WH (1969) Pain and the neurosurgeon. A fourty year experience. Charles C. Thomas, Springfield/Ill

Yaşargil MG, Smith RD, Gasser JC (1977) Microsurgical approach to acoustic neurinomas. In: Advances and Technical Standards in Neurosurgery, vol 4. Springer, Wien New York, p 93–129

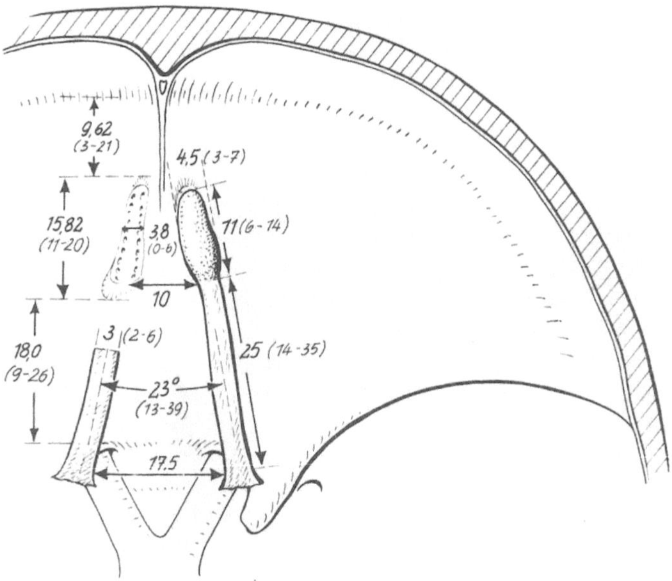

Fig. 1 a. Olfactory bulb and tract, measurements

him and on the basis of recent investigations, the chiasma in 75 to 96 percent of the cases lies totally or partially over the diaphragma sellae. In 12 percent, according to Schaeffer, it lies completely over the diaphragma sellae; in 5 to 10 percent, depending on the investigators, only the dorsal part of the chiasma lies over the diaphragma and the anterior part in the region of prechiasmatic sulcus, the so-called prefixed-chiasma. A backward displaced (postfixed) chiasma was found, by Schaeffer, in four percent of the cases; whereas by Bergland et al. (1968) in 11 percent, and Renn and Rhoton (1975) in 15 percent. The distance between the anterior margin of the prechiasmatic sulcus and tuberculum sellae according to our investigations, was found to be 6.8 (3.3–10.3) mm. The average distance from the intracranial apertura of optic canal up to the front end of the anterior cranial fossa was 42.45 (32.0 –52.0) mm and to the anterior part of the prechiasmatic sulcus about 45 (36–54) mm. According to Renn and Rhoton, the optic nerves form an intracranial angle (to their medial margins) of between 50 und 80 degree. The nerves which approach each other in an acute-angle form reduce the transfrontal access to hypophyse like a strongly developed tuberculum sellae. They found that the nerve has an average width of 5 (3.4–6.0) mm, heigth of 3 (2.0–5.0) mm and length of 12 (8–19) mm (Fig. 2).

The fibers of the third cranial nerve stem from the 5 mm long somatomotoric nucleus comprising of approximately 12,000 cells, which is almost of the same length as nucleus Westphal-Edinger; whereas the Perlia nucleus is, firstly, uneven and secondly, smaller. The recent views indicate that the fibers for the M. rectus inferior stem from dorso-lateral, for the M. rectus medialis from the dorso-medial and for the M. obliquus inferior from an underlying region. Basal from it are the nuclei

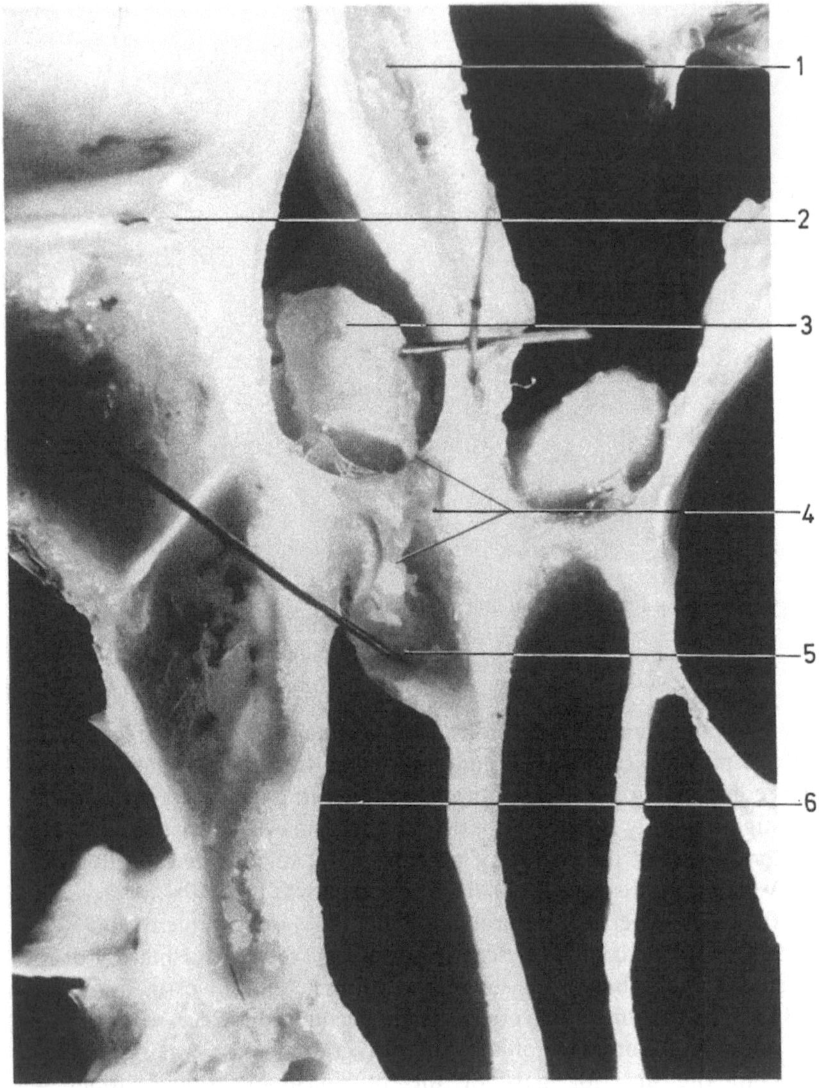

Fig. 1 b. Nervi olfactorii and arachnoid-pockets. *1* = Crista galli, *2* = A. ethm. ant., *3* = Bulbus olf. fixed upwards, *4* = Nervi olfactorii, below arachnoid pockets, *5* = Mucosa removed, *6* = lateral wall of nasal cavity

related to the M. rectus medialis and dorsocaudal for the M. levator palpebrae superioris; whereas the fibers of the Mm. levator palpebrae superioris et rectus superior exclusively, and of the M. rectus medialis to a large extent come from the equilateral nucleus; the fibers of the M. obliquus inferior and of the M. rectus inferior stem almost completely from the contralateral nucleus. The Perlia nucleus gives off its stem fibers in both sides.

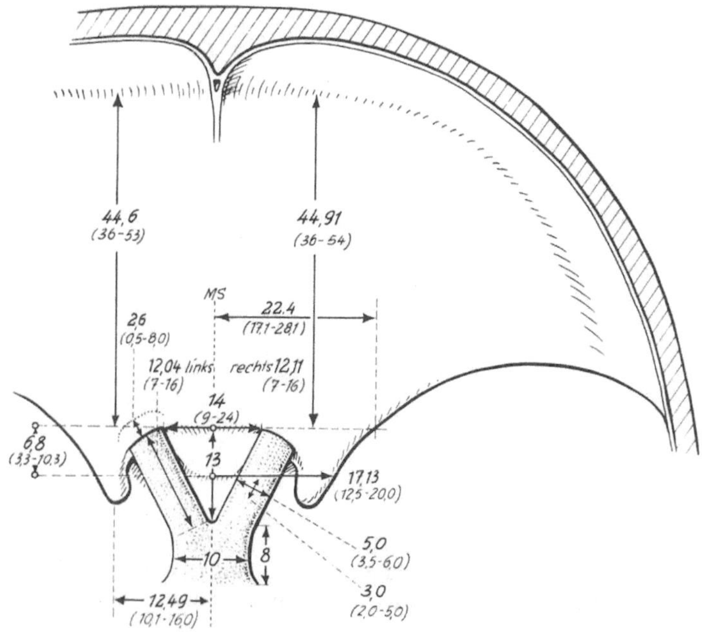

Fig. 2. Optic nerve, chiasma and anterior cranial fossa measurements (in mm)

The Westphal-Edinger nucleus joins the nucleus accessorius rostralis, the nucleus accessorius medianus (Panegrossi) and the nucleus accessorius caudalis. The fibers for the ciliary muscles stem from the nucleus accessorius caudalis and for the M. sphincter pupillae from the nucleus accessorius rostralis, a view which is not undisputed. The neurites of these nuclei regions run in a laterally convexed arch partially through the nucleus ruber towards basal and enter the interpeduncular fossa, mostly go through the sulcus medialis cruris cerebri in the form of a medial eight fibersbundle group; and leave in the form of a lateral group of the same strength behind and beside the sulcus. They merge into a flat or round intracranial nerve which passes between the superior cerebellar and posterior cerebral arteries and runs forward and laterally, and then reaching through the interpeduncular cisterna to the transversal plate of the cavernous sinus. Not seldom its initial path is interrupted by a vein, or an A. laminae tecti. The "perforating point" of the nerve into cavernous sinus is located lateral to the posterior clinoid process and always medial to the anterior petroclinoid plica. The distance between the anterior clinoid process and the anterior end of the porus n. oculomotorii in the transversal plate of the cavernous sinus is, on the average, 7.4 (3–13) mm (Fig. 3). The lateral distance from posterior clinoid process (measured diagonally) is 7.5 mm on the right and 7.8 (3–11) mm on the left. The anterior margin of the porus n. oculomotorii is located, on the average, 2.29 mm on the right, 2.38 mm on the left behind a transversal plane through the posterior clinoid process. The anterior margin of the porus can lie up to 2 mm before and up to 8 mm behind this plane. The nerve with a 6–8 mm long dura and

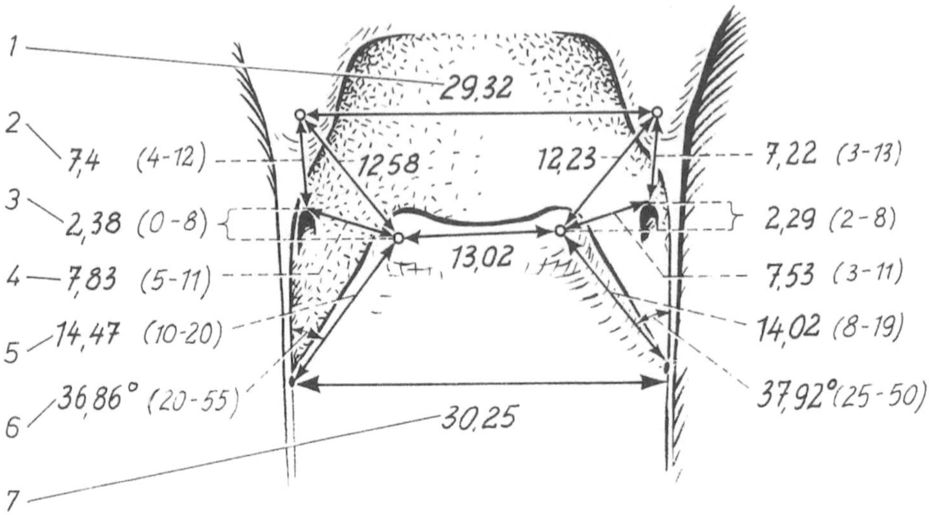

Fig. 3. Hypophysial region measurements (in mm). *1* = Distances Proc. clin. ant., *2* = Proc. clin. ant. Porus n. III, *3* = Proc. clin. post. Porus n. III (sagittal), *4* = Proc. clin. post. Porus n. III, *5* = Proc. clin. post. Porus n. IV, *6* = Plic. petroclin., angle in °, *7* = Incisura tentorii, width

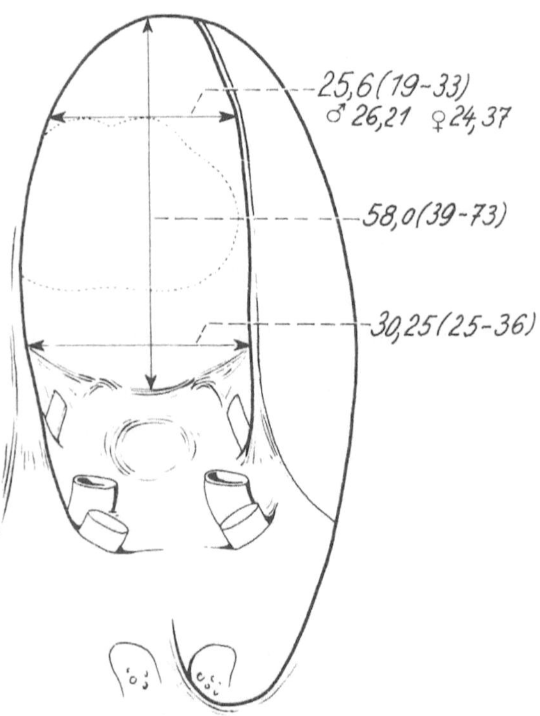

Fig. 4. Area 12.76 cm² (8.7–15.8)

arachnoid pouch traverses the cavernous sinus beneath the anterior clinoid process and then it unites with the dura and arachnoid. We call the superior wall of the cavernous sinus and of the diaphragma sellae the transversal plate which laterally and dorsally change over into a more or less deep tub. In this region, normally, the third and often also the fourth cranial nerve enter the cavernous sinus. The "tub" is confined by the anterior and posterior petroclinoid plicae which extend from the anterior branches of the tentorial notch and of the cerebellar tent. Between these two plicae, there is an angle of about 38 degree to the right and about 37 degree to the left. The limiting values lie by 20 degree and 55 degree. The angle reduces with increase of the skull width. No correlation is observed in general. The anterior petroclinoid plica in 71.67 percent is considerably thicker, in 20 percent somewhat thicker, and in 8.3 percent as thick as the posterior petroclinoid plica.

The nucleus of the fourth cranial nerve, situated in the recess between the medial lemnisci at the level of caudal colliculus contains about 3,000 cells. Its neurites pass backwards and downwards, surround the central gray matter and reach the border region, between mesencephalon and rhombencephalon on the dorsal surface. They cross the rostral region of the cranial medullary velum to reach the opposite side (some of the researches assume incompletly). The nerve leaves the velum in 60 percent with two radices, in 25 percent with one radix, and in 13.5 percent with three radices, seldom with up to six radices (Nathan and Goldhammer, 1973). The single fibers join each other either directly after leaving the velum or after traversing a distance up to 20 mm intercisternally. Then normally, the nerve enters, the arachnoid which covers the ambient cistern below the tentorium. After that, it sinks in the tub region of the cavernous sinus (in about 80 percent), and in about 47 percent directly on the top of the tub, in 20.34 percent the nerve enters (as normally given in Anatomy textbooks) the lower aspect of the tentorium cerebelli, exactly named, its incisural region. The average distance from the piercing of dura up to the posterior clinoid process is a little over 14 (8–20) mm (see Fig. 3). Also the trochlear nerve in its initial "intradural" segment is surrounded by an arachnoid sheath. It merges with the nerve before it contacts the oculomotor nerve. Also Pachioni granulations have been verified, in the intradural route of the fourth cranial nerve.

Since Meyer (1920) referred to the tentorial herniae, the Incisura tentorii as well as the neighbouring structures have gained significant medical importance. Sunderland and Hughs (1946) have indicated a certain concentration of the pupillary constrictive fibers in the upper segment of the third cranial nerve. Sunderland and Bradley (1952/53) investigated the third cranial nerve in more than 100 cadavers, and the cerebral dislocation by tentorial herniae in nine specimens. They described, as did others, the disposition of the brain, the strangulation of the nerves and vessels and the resulting outfall symptoms of the third cranial nerve and of the mesencephalon. They particularly emphasized that the third cranial nerve would be damaged in the region where it is depressed against the tentorial margin and not there, where it crosses the (great) ala of sphenoid bone or in the superior orbital fissure. According to Sunderland and Hughes (1948), the length of the tentorial notch varies between 44 and 75 mm, the largest width between 23 and 39 mm. In the region of the dorsum sellae, according to their findings (50 specimens) between 19 and 35 mm. On the basis of our examinations, the average width of the tentorium notch in the region where the anterior and posterior petroclinoid plicae diverge is 30.25

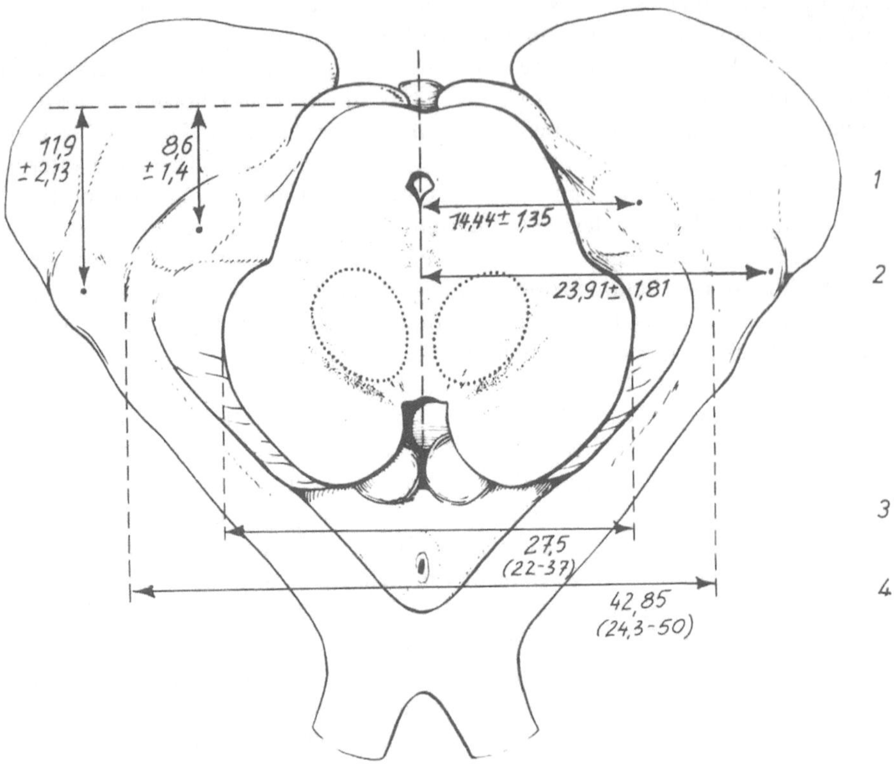

Fig. 5. Mesencephalon and Diencephalon, measurements. *1* = medial geniculate body, *2* = lateral geniculate body, *3* = Mesencephalon, width (level inferior colliculus), *4* = Mesencephalon, width on rostral level

(25–36) mm (Fig. 4). At the level of caudal colliculus, the average values were measured to be 25.60 (19–33) mm. In most of the specimens, the width of the notch at the level of caudal colliculus is narrower than in the rostral region. In two cadavers the distances were equally wide and in two other cases (from 57 specimens) 2 mm wider. It is emphasized that the average width of the notch at the colliculus level is in males 26.21 mm and in females 24.37 mm. At the rostral point of measurement the width in the male population is 30.40 and in female 29.95 mm. As to the length of the notch, our investigations yielded an average value of 46.58 for males and of 47.95 for females, with a total average of 47.05 (38.0–58.0) mm. In these cases, the measurements were performed from the middle of the posterior clinoid process (covered with dura) and the apex of the notch. The area bordered by the notch is, on the average, 12.67 (8.7–15.8) square cm. Also opposite to the sphenoid plane, the notch is quite variable. Figure 5 gives various dimensions of the mesencephalon. In addition to the possibility of lesions due to supratentorial space-occupying processes and descending herniation through tentorial notch strangulations of the posterior cerebral artery with loss of blood supply to the visual cortex, lesions of the posterior communicating artery, and of the superior cerebellar artery may ensue. We point out the possibility of lesions of the A. laminae tecti which in 57.6 percent arises from the pre-communicating part of the posterior cerebral artery. In 26.8 percent it gives off at the level of junction and in the rest distal to it. This vessel transverses around the crura cerebri and normally supplies, with two large branches, the arterial plexus of the cranial colliculus. In addition, it gives off interpeduncular rami, peduncular rami and several other more fine branches. Finally, the lesions can occur through strangulation of the tentorium notch in the thalmogeniculate rami arising from the posterior cerebral artery, which also gives off branches to the cerebral pedunculus, as well as to the thalamus and corpora geniculata.

The topographical and functional anatomy of the trigeminal nerve will be described by Kruger tomorrow, hence I mention only a few findings regarding the structure of trigeminal ganglion and a few nerve-vessel relationships.

The abducent nerve leaves the ponto-medullar sulcus (at the lateral margin of the pyramid and on the average 3.93 (2.0–6.5) mm lateral to the median plane with two to three, seldom with up to six radix fibers. In 7.5 percent arise, right after the emergence, two small nerve-stems which enter their own dural pori that may be separated from each other by 2 to 4.5 mm (Fig. 6). The distance from the inferior me-

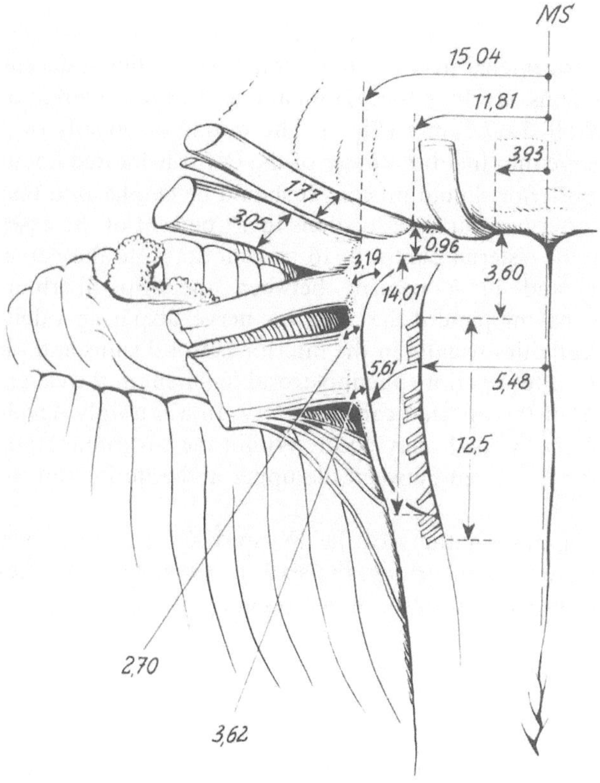

Fig. 6. Lower cranial nerves, measurements (in mm)

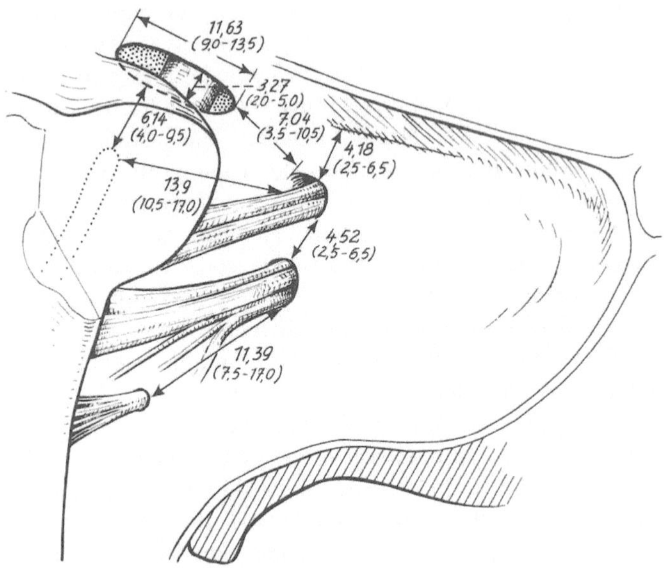

Fig. 7. Lower cranial nerves, distances of the nerve dural portals

dial labium of the porus of the trigemenal nerve to the dural porus of the abducens nerve, according to our investigations, is 6.14 (4.0–9.5) mm and to the lower margin of the internal acoustic porus 13.9 (10.5–17.0) mm (Fig 7). The mostly diagonally oval enterance of the sixth cranial nerve into the dura mater of the clivus is located about 20 (16–29) mm away from the posterior clinoid process. It should be emphasized that the anterior inferior cerebellar artery in our investigations in 79 percent of the cases runs basal to the nerve through the cisterna pontis, in 16 percent dorsal to the nerve, between pons and abducent, and in 5 percent between the two fiberbundle of the abducent nerve. After having pierced the dura, the nerve, acquiring a delicate dura and an arachnoid sheath, lies usually in the inferior petrosal sinus and on its lateral wall region, runs below the superior sphenopetrosal ligament in the cavernous sinus on the lateral aspect of the internal carotid artery. In a multiply developed nerve numerous variations in the path may occur. Within the cavernous sinus normally an autonomic ganglion is located between the upper and anterior carotid nerves and the abducent nerve.

The topographical and functional anatomy of the IX upto XII cranial nerves will be presented by Sir S. Sunderland on Friday, the sixth of June. Therefore regarding these nerves, I present only a few of our recent figures and findings.

Summary

Measurements and topographical relations are demonstrated on slides and diagrams.

References

Bergland RM, Bronson SR, Torack RM (1968) Anatomical Variations in the Pituitary Gland and Adjacent Structures in 225 Human Autopsy Cases. J Neurosurg 28:93–99

Meyer (1920) Arch Neurol Psychiat (Chicago) 4:387 (1920) zit. n. Sunderland, Herniation of the Brain. Arch Neurol Psychiat 4:387–400

Nathan H, Goldhammer Y (1973) The rootlets of the trochlear nerve. Anatomical observations in human brains. Acta Anat (Basel) 84:590–596

Renn, WH, Rhoton Jr AL (1975) Microsurgical anatomy of the sellar region. J Neurosurg 43:288–298

Schaeffer JP (1924) Some points in the regional anatomy of the optic pathway with especial reference to tumors of the hypophysis cerebri and resulting ocular changes. Anat Rec 28:243–279

Sunderland S, Bradley KC (1953) J Neurol Neurosurg Psychiat 16:35

Sunderland S, Hughes ESR (1946) The pupilloconstrictor pathway and the nerves to the ocular muscles in man. Brain 69:301–309

Cranial Nerve Injury. Structural and Pathophysiological Considerations and a Classification of Nerve Injury

S. SUNDERLAND, Melbourne/Australia

Any discussion on the pathophysiology of cranial nerve injury would be incomplete if it failed to direct attention to certain differences in the structure of the extra- and intracranial parts of a cranial nerve and to the manner in which these differences influence the damaging effects of stretch and compression on nerve fibres. This Chapter is devoted to this aspect of the subject.

The Extracranial Part of the Nerve

The extracranial part of the nerve has the same structure as any peripheral nerve in which the nerve fibres are collected into funiculi which repeatedly divide and unite along the nerve to form funicular plexuses (Fig. 1). These plexuses cause variations in the size and number of the funiculi from level to level and also bring about a funicular redistribution and rearrangement of the nerve fibres representing individual branches.

Two generalisations relating to funiculi are:

1. at any level the nerve may be composed of a single large funiculus or several smaller funiculi.
2. a funiculus may be composed of fibres representing one branch or of fibres from different branches in varying proportions and combinations.

Another structural feature worth noting is the undulating course pursued by the nerve trunk in its bed, by the funiculi in the nerve trunk, and by the nerve fibres inside the funiculi. These undulations protect nerve fibres from any traction deformation that might be introduced during movement of the parts.

Associated with the nerve fibres and funiculi are three types of supporting tissue.

The endoneurium is the delicate connective tissue which fills each funiculus and forms a fine endoneurial sheath about each nerve fibre. This sheath has some elasticity and maintains an endoneurial pressure.

The perineurium is the thin distinctive sheath surrounding each funiculus. It is composed of 3 to 20 concentric layers of flattened interlocking lamellar cells, the number of layers depending on the size of the funiculus. Collagen fibrils occupy the interlamellar clefts. This specialised sheath has the following important properties:

1. It maintains an intrafunicular pressure.
2. It constitutes an effective diffusion barrier.
3. It constitutes an effective barrier against the spread of infection.
4. It imparts tensile strength and elasticity to the nerve trunk and is the principal component protecting the nerve from traction deformation.

The sequence of events when a nerve is stretched to and beyond its elastic limits follows a characteristic pattern (Fig. 2). Traction on the nerve first eliminates the undulations in the nerve trunk and then those in the funiculi at which point the resistance to further stretching of the nerve is provided by the perineurium. Continued traction leads to further stretching of the nerve and its contained funiculi until the intrafunicular undulations in the nerve fibres are eliminated, the nerve fibres then being stretched along with the other elements of the nerve trunk. Additionally, as the funiculi are being stretched their cross-sectional area is being reduced. This introduces an intrafunicular compression factor which contributes to the continued deformation of nerve fibres. A point is ultimately reached when nerve fibres and vessels are ruptured inside the funiculi. However, the elasticity of the nerve survives until the perineurium ruptures which occurs later than the intrafunicular rupture of nerve fibres.

The epineurium is the loose areolar connective tissue which envelopes and separates the funiculi and forms an encircling sheath for the nerve trunk. It may, and often does, contain adipose tissue. Importantly it provides a packing for the funiculi which protects them from compression forces. In this respect the nerve is less vulnerable to compression where it is composed of many small funiculi separated by a large amount of epineurial tissue (Fig. 3). In such cases the deforming forces are dis-

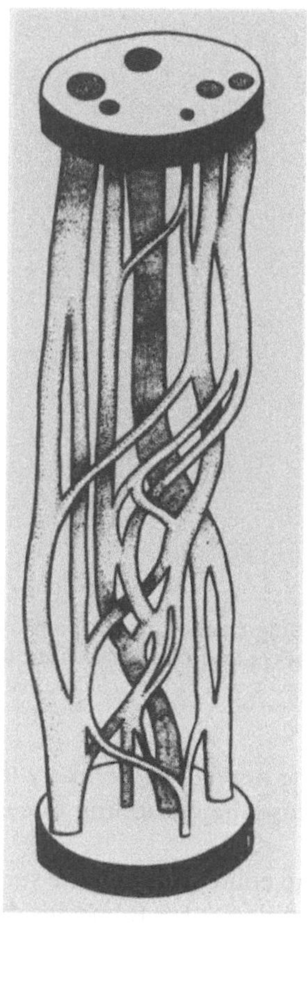

Fig. 1. Reconstruction of the funicular plexus of a 3 cm length of a peripheral nerve trunk

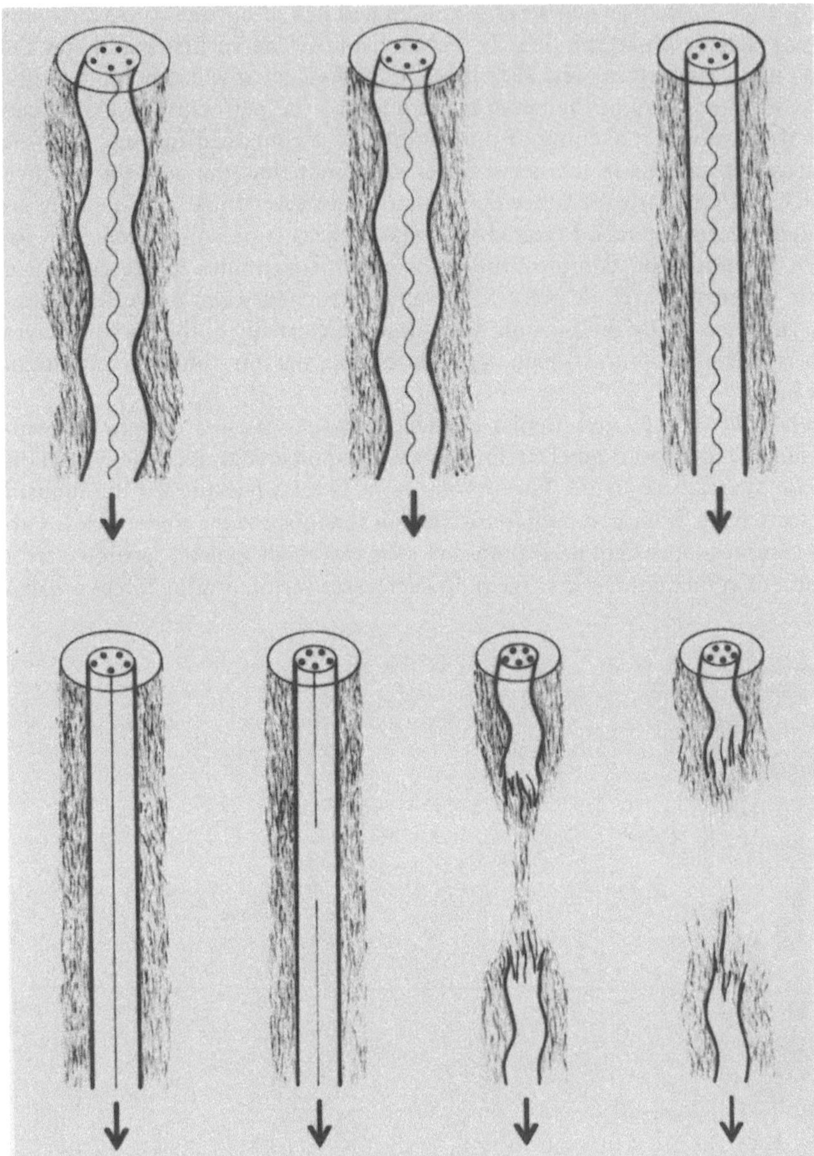

Fig. 2. Sequence of changes in a nerve trunk subjected to continuing traction to the point of mechanical failure. For simplification only one funiculus in the nerve and one nerve fibre in the funiculus are shown

sipated through the epineurial tissue. On the other hand the nerve is more likely to suffer when it is composed of a single funiculus in which case the deforming forces fall directly on the funiculus.

Blood vessels. The major nutrient vessels are found in the epineurium on the surface of the nerve or more deeply between funiculi. Only capillaries are found inside

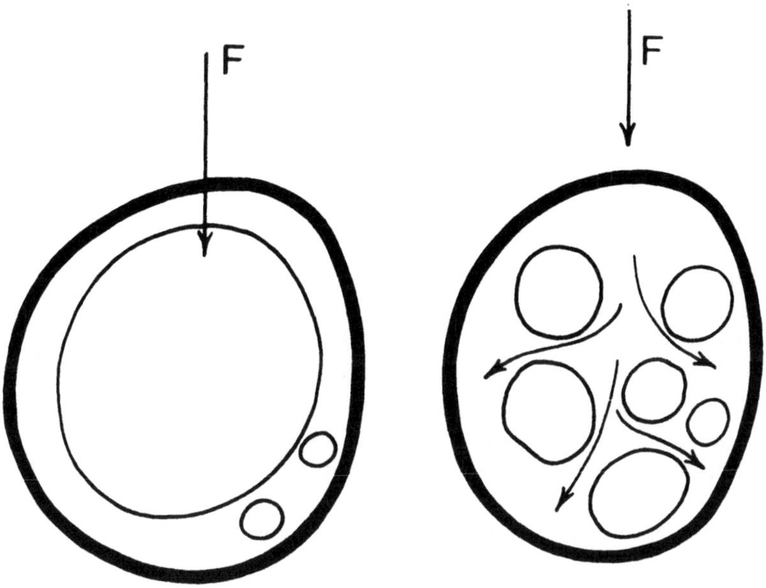

Fig. 3. The deforming effects of compression on nerve fibres are reduced when the funiculi are smaller and are separated by a large amount of epineurial tissue

funiculi except for the occasional arteriole found in an intrafunicular septum which indicates the impending division of a funiculus or the recent fusion of two funiculi.

The nerve fibres of the nerve trunk are well separated by perineurial and epineurial tissue from neighbouring vessels of any size that are in direct contact with the nerve.

Lymphatics. There are no lymphatics inside the funiculi, only endoneurial spaces which do not communicate with the lymphatics which are located in the epineurium. These lymphatics drain to regional lymph nodes.

The Intracranial Part of the Nerve

The intracranial part of the nerve differs in several important respects from the extracranial part.

1. Each nerve fibre is ensheathed in endoneurium, the collagen fibrils of which are finer than those found in the extracranial part of the nerve. All the nerve fibres are collected into a bundle in which they pursue a parallel course and are held together by endoneurial tissue. The nerve lacks a funicular structure.

2. The perineurium and the epineurium are absent. In the absence of these protective structural features, which offset the effects of stretch and compression, the nerve, though located intracranially, is now more vulnerable to damage from any deforming forces to which it may be subjected.

3. The undulations in the system which are such a feature of the extracranial part of the nerve are not as prominent a feature. This reduces the tolerance of the nerve fibres to stretch.

4. In the absence of funicular plexus formations, the nerve fibres maintain a localised position in the nerve.

5. Large vessels now obtain a direct relationship to nerve fibres in a manner not seen peripherally. Thus the superior cerebellar artery may indent or transfix the trigeminal nerve root (Sunderland, 1948).

6. The root entry zone, which involves the first few millimetres of the nerve root, presents special features which distinguish it from the remainder of the intracranial part of the nerve (Gamble, 1976; Carlstedt, 1977; Berthold and Carlstedt, 1977).

(i) A cone shaped core of the central nervous system extends outwards for a few millimetres into the centre of the nerve root. This gives two concentric zones to the transition region – an axial core with the structure of a central nervous system fibre tract with glial elements surrounded by a layer of peripheral nerve fibres separated by endoneurial spaces.

(ii) The cone of central nervous system tissue extends further outwards in sensory than in motor nerve roots.

(iii) In their passage from the peripheral to the central nervous system, myelinated nerve fibres do not temporarily lose their myelin sheaths, as was originally believed, though the myelin sheath does undergo a reduction in thickness.

(iv) The unmyelinated fibres come to be concentrated superficially and ventrolaterally.

(v) The blood vessels of the outer zone do not extend into the inner axial core, the latter having a poorer blood supply than the former.

(vi) The auditory nerve consists essentially of a fibre tract of the central nervous system in most of its length.

A. Classification of Nerve Injury

When the structural features of a cranial nerve that have just been outlined are examined in relation to the effects of injury to the nerve it will be seen that they provide a rational basis for a useful classification of nerve injury.

For the extracranial part of the nerve the classification identifies five degrees of injury of ascending order of severity (Fig. 4).

A *first degree injury* is one in which the architectural features of the nerve are preserved and there is no Wallerian degeneration. However, conduction is blocked at the site of damage, the nerve fibres conducting above and below the lesion but not across it. After a quiescent period conduction across the damaged segment returns and function is completely and rapidly restored. This is a physiological conduction block lesion.

A *second degree injury* is one which results in Wallerian degeneration of the nerve fibres distal to the site of the injury and for a variable but short distance proximal to it. However, the endoneurial sheath of each nerve fibre is preserved so that, following the removal of the axon and myelin debris of degeneration, the endoneu-

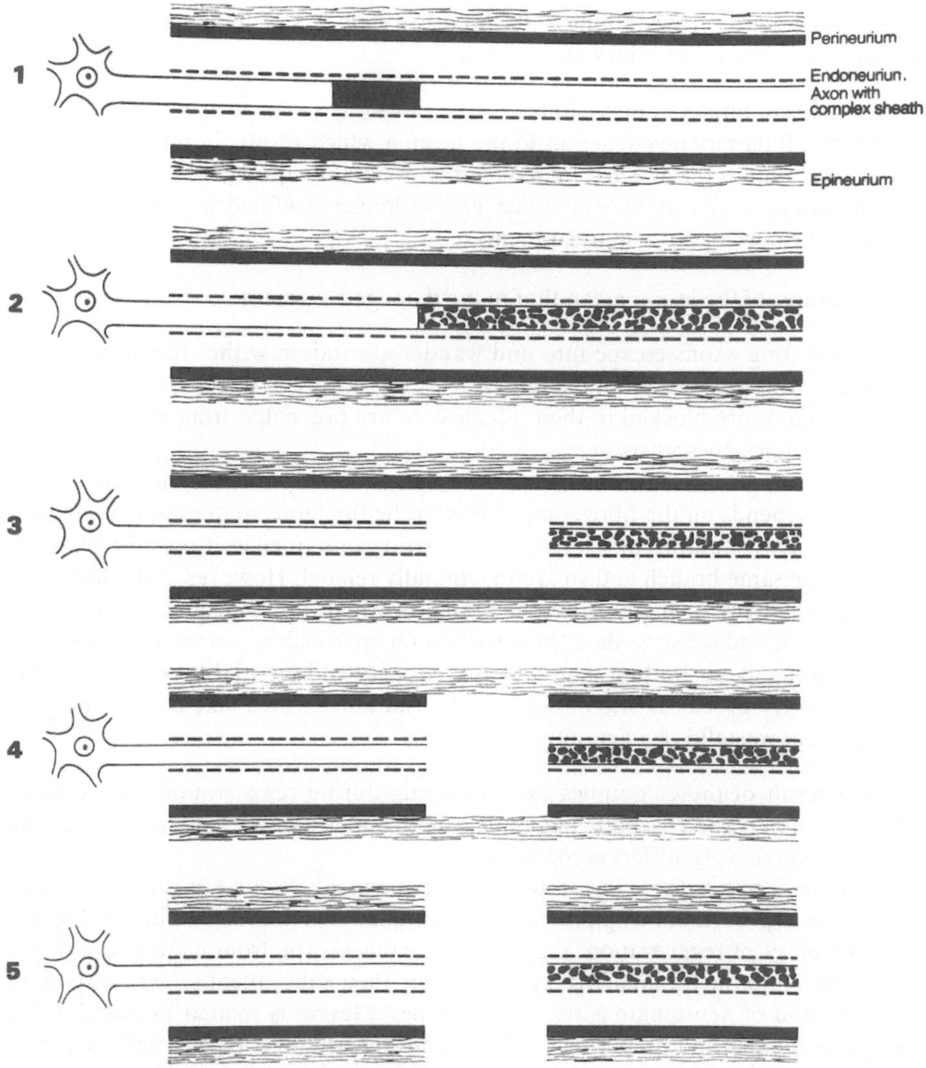

Fig. 4. A classification of nerve injury based on the progressive involvement of the axon, physiological conduction block followed by Wallerian degeneration, the endoneurial sheath, the funiculi and finally loss of continuity of the entire nerve trunk

rial tubes outlined by the endoneurial sheath of each nerve fibre are left occupied by Schwann cells.

After a latent period, the duration of which is influenced by the severity of the injury, the axons commence to regenerate and each, in its growth, is confined to the endoneurial tube which originally contained it. This ensures that regenerating axons are inevitably led back to the structures they originally innervated so that the restored pattern of innervation is precisely the same as the original. In this way function is fully restored.

The *third degree lesion* is an intrafunicular lesion in which the endoneurial sheath has been destroyed along with the other elements of the nerve fibre. Three consequences of such an injury are:

1. the loss of continuity of nerve fibres,
2. a general inflammatory reaction to the trauma which results in the formation of scar tissue within the affected funiculi at the site of the injury, and
3. regenerating axons, as they advance, are no longer confined to the endoneurial tubes which originally contained them.

These features of the lesion mean that in the damaged segment:

(i) regenerating axons escape into and wander at random within the disorganised tissue formed as a result of the injury;
(ii) some axons are blocked in their advance, or are prevented from entering endoneurial tubes, by scar tissue;
(iii) regenerating axons are free to enter foreign endoneurial tubes, the outcome of which depends on the fibre composition of the funiculus in question. Such erroneous cross-shunting of axons is of no great consequence if the fibres are all from the same branch and so are functionally related. However, if the fibres are representatives of many different branches which are functionally unrelated, e.g. motor and sensory, then the effects can be particularly damaging. Motor regenerating axons finding their way into sensory endoneurial tubes and cutaneous sensory processes into motor endoneurial tubes which take them to muscles represent wasteful regeneration.

As a result of these complications occurring during regeneration, the restored pattern of innervation is both incomplete and imperfect in comparison with the original, and recovery suffers accordingly.

A *fourth degree lesion* is one in which the funiculi are severed or ruptured, continuity of the nerve trunk being preserved by mangled funicular and epineurial tissue. With the onset of regeneration, regenerating axons escape from endoneurial tubes and funiculi into the traumatised segment where their subsequent growth is spent in the formation of neuromatous tissue. This type of lesion is treated by excising the disorganised tissue and preparing the nerve ends for whatever type of nerve repair is required.

A *fifth degree injury* is one which results in the loss of nerve trunk continuity.

Mixed lesions. In any nerve injury not all nerve fibres are necessarily affected to the same degree to give a lesion of uniform pathology. Some nerve fibres may suffer more than others so that the degree of involvement varies in different nerve fibres. This accounts for complex mixed lesions.

Partial lesions. In any nerve injury some nerve fibres and/or funiculi may escape damage to give a partial as opposed to a complete lesion.

Nerve Root Injury

In the case of the intracranial nerve roots, the absence of perineurial and epineurial tissue, and the simpler structure of the nerve, mean that the five degrees of injury characteristic of the extracranial part of the nerve are now reduced to three.

A first degree injury remains as a physiological conduction block lesion.

A second degree injury again leaves the endoneurial sheath intact but involves Wallerian degeneration followed by axon regeneration in which regenerating axons are confined to the endoneurial tubes which originally contained them.

A third degree injury involves rupture of the endoneurial sheaths of nerve fibres which means complete loss of continuity of the nerve root.

Mixed and partial lesions occur as in the case of the extracranial part of the nerve.

When the effects of trauma to the nerve root are studied it will be seen that:

1. more serious lesions are produced more readily;
2. intracranial lesions of any severity inevitably result in confused reinnervation with loss of discrete responses at the periphery. This complication of regeneration is aggravated by axon branching at the site of damage.

Acknowledgements: The illustrations used in this paper are from the author's book Nerves and Nerve Injuries, 2nd. ed., 1978 and are published with the permission of Churchill Livingstone, Edinburgh.

References

Berthold CH, Carlstedt T (1977) Observations on the Morphology at the Transition between the Peripheral and the Central Nervous System in the Cat. II. General organization of the transitional region in S_1 dorsal rootlets. Acta Physiol Scand Suppl 446:23–42

Berthold CH, Carlstedt T (1977) Observations on the Morphology at the Transition between the Peripheral and the Central Nervous System in the Cat. III. Myelinated fibres in S_1 dorsal rootlets. Acta Physiol Scand Suppl 446:43–60.

Berthold CH, Carlstedt T (1977) Observations on the Morphology at the Transition between the Peripheral and the Central Nervous System in the Cat. V. A light microscopical and histochemical study of S_1 dorsal rootlets in developing kittens. Acta Physiol Scand Suppl 446:73–85

Carlstedt T (1977) Observations on the Morphology at the Transition between the Peripheral and the Central Nervous System in the Cat. I. A preparative procedure useful for electron microscopy of the lumbosacral dorsal rootlets. Acta Physiol Scand Suppl 446:5–21

Carlstedt T (1977) Observations on the Morphology at the Transition between the Peripheral and the Central Nervous System in the Cat. IV. Unmyelinated fibres in S_1 dorsal rootlets. Acta Physiol Scand Suppl 446:61–71

Gamble HJ (1976) Spinal and Cranial Nerve Roots. In: Landon DN (ed) The Peripheral Nerve. Chapman and Hall, London, p 330–354

Sunderland S (1948) Neurovascular Relations and Anomalies at the Base of the Brain. J Neurol Neurosurg Psychiat 11:243–257

Experimental Studies on Neural Regeneration

W. KREUTZBERG, München/FRG

Interruption of the continuity of an axon leads to a number of morphological, metabolic and electrophysiological changes (reviewed by Lieberman 1971, Grafstein and McQuarrie 1978). These have been studied in our laboratory mainly in the facial nucleus, in the hypoglossal nucleus and in spinal motoneurons. Since the classical experiments by Franz Nissl in the last century the morphological changes occurring after axotomy are known under the term of chromatolysis or retrograde or axonal reaction. This describes a neuron with a dispersed Nissl substance with an excentric nucleus and with swelling of the cell body. The nature of the signal informing the nerve cell body on the traumatic event which occurred to its peripheral process is unknown. However, the signalling must occur rather briefly after the lesion since first changes can be seen within hours of injury. The signal seems to trigger what could be called the regeneration program of the nerve cell. Changes in messenger-RNA and in ribosomal-RNA have been seen very early in this process (reviewed by Austin and Langford 1980). Changes in RNA as measured by biochemical methods may be accompanied by the changes in the morphological organization of the granular endoplasmic reticulum. There is an enormous increase in free ribosomes as well as in ribosomes connected to cisternae of the r-ER. Frequently a pronounced accumulation of ribosomes is seen forming a nuclear cap. It seems reasonable to assume that this increase in the synthetic machinery of the neuron has to do with an increased production of neuroplasm which will be exported to the axon. Some of the enzymatic changes can also be seen in this context. For instance, there is a remarkable increase of the enzymes of the pentose phosphate pathway. This may contribute to the production of ribose needed in the synthesis of RNA (Kreutzberg 1963). Enzymes which are more involved in the synaptic function of the neuron may, however, decrease in the regenerating neurons. In the rat facial nucleus, for instance, as well as in the hypoglossal nucleus acetylcholinesterase almost disappears from regenerating motorneurons. In other species, for instance in the guinea pig, there is a decrease of AChE activity in the neuropil only (Kreutzberg et al. 1974; 1975). A very early response of a motor nucleus to nerve transection is also seen in its glucose consumption. If 2-deoxyglucose is used as an indicator for glucose utilization a striking increase is seen as early as 24 hours after the operation in both, the hypoglossal and the facial nucleus. This process continues for at least 4 weeks (Kreutzberg and Emmert 1980). The resolution of the autoradiography does not allow for a finer resolution, however, it seems that the complete motor nucleus and not only the chromatolytic neurons may be involved in this higher glucose utilization.

This finding already shows that changes during regeneration are not restricted to the motoneurons only. The microenvironment, i.e. neuropil, neuroglia and local capillaries are involved in the process too. There is, for instance, an increase in alcaline phosphatase activity in the local capillaries (Kreutzberg et al. 1974). There is a proliferation of microglial cells especially in the immediate environment of the motoneurons. The proliferation of these microglial cells leads to a remarkable change in the synaptic organization of the neuron since a displacement of synaptic terminals occurs on the soma and the stem dendrites of the neurons, and these places are taken by proliferated microglia cells. This leads to a loss of approximately 80 percent of the axosomatic synapsis (Blinzinger and Kreutzberg 1968). The proliferated microglial cells demonstrate a remarkably high activity of 5′-nucleotidase in their plasma membranes. This is a key enzyme for the production of adenosine, a substance with vasodilatory activity and probably trophic effects (Kreutzberg and Barron 1978).

It is generally accepted that the chromatolytic changes can be interpreted as a hypertrophy of the motoneuron aimed towards the production of material to substitute for the lost axon. The hypertrophy of the nerve cell center on the one hand and the demands of the growing axonal sprouts on the other impose a problem of logistics to the motor unit. Axonal transport is the vehicle to bring the newly synthesized material to its destination. As one would assume, there is an increase in transport of proteins in the axon during regeneration (Kreutzberg and Schubert 1971; Griffin et al. 1976). Constant supply of axoplasm to the proximal stump of the nerve results primarily in a considerable enlargement of the axon tip. This leads to the formation of typical growth cones from which axonal sprouting originates. We recently studied this sprouting process with scanning electron microscopy and could find that the growth cones have a rather unstable surface from which very delicate fine processes grow in great number (Kreutzberg 1979). Bundles of these axonal sprouts can be seen after a week growing into the peripheral tissue. The growth process in the regenerating nerve fibres may be in principle not very different from what can be seen also in tissue culture. To illustrate this, a film was shown during the conference on the regeneration of neurites growing out from neuroblastoma cells (N 18) after microsurgery with a microscalpel (Rieske and Kreutzberg 1978). In tissue culture the cinematography permits a direct observation of the events occurring after lesion of nerve fibers. The regeneration process seemed to start with the formation of ruffling membranes over the whole surface of the N 18 cells. This is followed by an elongation of small processes to longer neurites. The fibers have also been investigated by electron microscopy and a number of cytochemical methods (Isenberg et al. 1977 and 1978). From these investigations it seems clear that actin in the form of microfilaments plays a very important role in these processes. It is very likely that actin is also involved in the force generating mechanism driving axonal transport (Isenberg et al. 1980). Thus, this protein may be a very crucial substance for the regeneration of peripheral nerve fibers.

In summary, the neurobiology of the regenerating motor unit shows a very complex picture. It involves not only the injured nerve fiber but also the neuronal perikaryon, the satellite cells and the microvasculature in the nucleus of origin, as well as the Schwann cells and the sheath cells of the peripheral part of the nerve. A response of the neuron is important for the production of new axoplasm to substitute for the lost axon. Axonal transport is important to supply the growing fiber and the axonal sprouts with this newly formed material.

References

Austin L, Langford CJ (1980) Nerve regeneration: a biochemical view. Trends Neurosci 3:130–132

Blinzinger K, Kreutzberg GW (1968) Displacement of synaptic terminals from regenerating motoneurons by microglial cells. Z Zellforsch 85:145–157

Grafstein B, McQuarrie IG (1978) Role of the nerve cell body in axonal regeneration. In: Cotman CW (ed) Neuronal Plasticity. Raven Press, New York, p 155–195

Griffin JW, Drachman DB, Price DL (1976) Fast axonal transport in motor nerve regeneration. J Neurobiol 7:355–370

Isenberg G, Rieske E, Kreutzberg GW (1977) Distribution of actin and tubulin in neuroblastoma cells. Cytobiologie 15:382–389

Isenberg G, Small JV, Kreutzberg GW (1978) Correlation between actin polymerization and surface receptor segregation in neuroblastoma cells treated with concanavalin A. J Neurocytol 7:649–661

Isenberg G, Schubert P, Kreutzberg GW (1980) Experimental approach to test the role of actin in axonal transport. Brain Res 194: in press

Kreutzberg GW (1963) Changes of coenzyme (TPN) diaphorase and TPN-linked dehydrogenase during axonal reaction of the nerve cell. Nature 199:393–394

Kreutzberg, GW, Schubert P (1971) Changes in axonal flow during regeneration of mammalian motor nerves. Acta Neuropathol (Berl) Suppl 5:70–75

Kreutzberg GW, Tóth L, Weikert M, Schubert P (1974) Changes in perineuronal capillaries accompanying chromatolysis of motoneurons. In: Cérvos-Navarro J (ed) Pathology of Cerebral Microcirculation. Walter de Gruyter Verlag, Berlin

Kreutzberg GW, Tóth L, Kaiya H (1975) Acetylcholinesterase as a marker for dendritic transport and dendritic secretion. In: Kreutzberg GW (ed) Physiology and Pathology of Dendrites. Raven Press, New York, p 269–281

Kreutzberg GW, Barron KD (1978) 5′-Nucleotidase of microglial cells in the facial nucleus during axonal reaction. J Neurocytol 7:601–610

Kreutzberg GW (1979) Neurobiological factors influencing regeneration of facial motor neurons. Clin Plastic Surg 6:389–395

Kreutzberg GW, Emmert H (1980) Glucose utilization of motor nuclei during regeneration: a 14 C 2-deoxyglucose study. Exp Neurol, in press

Lieberman AR (1971) The axon reaction: a review of the principal features of perikaryal responses to axon injury. Int Rev Neurobiol 14:49–124

Rieske E, Kreutzberg GW (1977) Neurite regeneration after cell surgery with laser microbeam irradiation. Brain Res 148:478–483

Olfactory Nerve

(First Cranial Nerve)

Functional Testing and Disturbances of Olfactory Sense

C. HERBERHOLD, Hamburg/FRG

Clinical experience in problems of olfaction over the past 100 years or so has not gone beyond a stadium of qualitative description and phenomenological sampling of syndromes of olfactory disturbances. Certainly, one reason for this lack of clinical knowledge is that basic research has dealt with problems far away from physiological and especially from clinical questions. Instead of this, investigations emphasized structural properties of smelling substances to get contact with the nature of stimulation and were looking for signs of stimulus processing in a psychophysical or ecological manner.

The need, however, for clinically valuable possibilities for diagnosis and management of olfactory disorders has increased continuously. Then the conditions of life have improved the individual meaning of olfactory sensation, and the suffering from its disturbances enhanced, respectively. A sign of a personal or social feeling of inferiority of these patients is, for instance, the growing number of medical judgements dealing with the function of olfactory system.

In the current situation, the clinical olfactologist tries intensively:

1. to improve the olfactometrical testing procedures or to develop new ones
2. to gain further knowledge of the pathophysiology of the olfactory system.

I. Olfactometry

All the techniques of functional testing of sense of the smell are summarized in the term olfactometry. Problems of all proposed methods in olfactometry are based on the lack of knowledge of the specific stimulus energy as well as on the difficulty of reaching the hidden anatomical site of the peripheral olfactory cells in the upper nasal floor. Therefore all efforts for the development of suitable olfactometers aim at an exact determination of odors instead of the physical stimulating energy and at their transport to the olfactory epithelium without loss of molecules.

We prefer as first basic olfactometry for this and for practical reasons a modified *sniff bottle technique* in clinical every day life (Figs. 1 and 2). In the head space of suitable bottles above molar solutions of typical substances of the so-called seven basic odors, a stable gaseous odorous concentration develops, from which the patient nasally inspires through tubes (solution made of diethylester of phthalic acid). With this simple method we get surprisingly precise and reproductable informations on:

1. the olfactory thresholds, and
2. the qualitative and quantitative possibility of smell perception.

Table 1. Olfactometric thresholds; sniff bottle-technique

	Acetone	Eucalyptol	Phenyl-ethanol	α-Ionon	Isobutyric acid
Sniff bottle-technique	$x \cdot 10^{17}$	$x \cdot 10^{16}$	$x \cdot 10^{15}$	$x \cdot 10^{15}$	$x \cdot 10^{16}$
Literature	$x \cdot 10^{14}$	$x \cdot 10^{16}$	$x \cdot 10^{17}$	$x \cdot 10^{16}$	$x \cdot 10^{16}$

According to the literature our thresholds range between 10^{15}–10^{17} molecules per ml of the stimulating vapor (Table 1). The measurement is performed separately for each nostril and lasts about 10 minutes. The subjective answers of the patients are given with definite symbols in a formular, which allows quick visual orientation of the result (Fig. 3).

As a second method we utilize the *testing of gustatory smelling* which was inaugurated by Güttich in 1961. Here alcoholic aroma essences known in liquor production are orally offered for tasting. The complete flavour sensation occurs only if the senses of smell and taste are in normal function simultaneously. For securing the results, especially those of olfactory function, we ask the patient to taste twice, with closed nose and with the nose open. In patients with stopped nasal ventilation only taste sensations are described (Fig. 4). Using this hidden test of olfaction by oral application of testing solution this method is suitable for detection of aggravants and simulants.

Since registration of evoked potentials is matured as a practicable electrophysiological technique, objective measurements of sensory organs were developed based

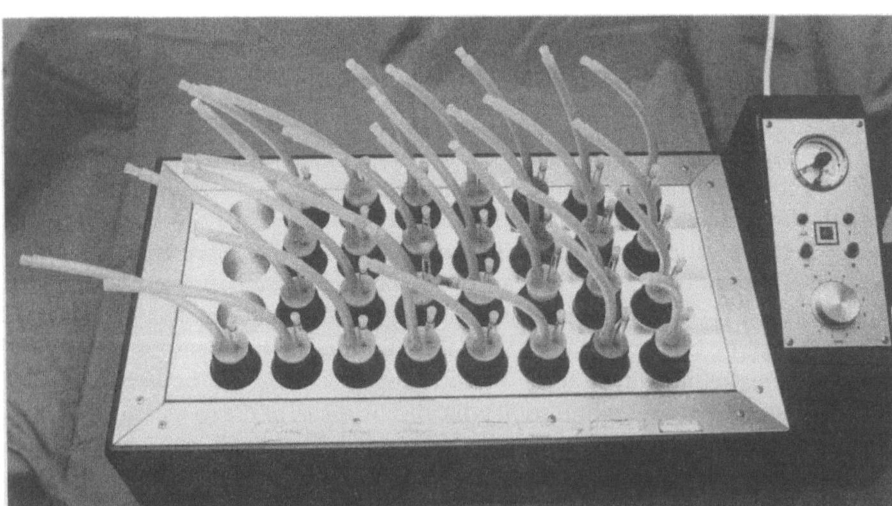

Fig. 1. Bottle collection in a thermostatic metal block. For each primary odor four molar concentrations were used

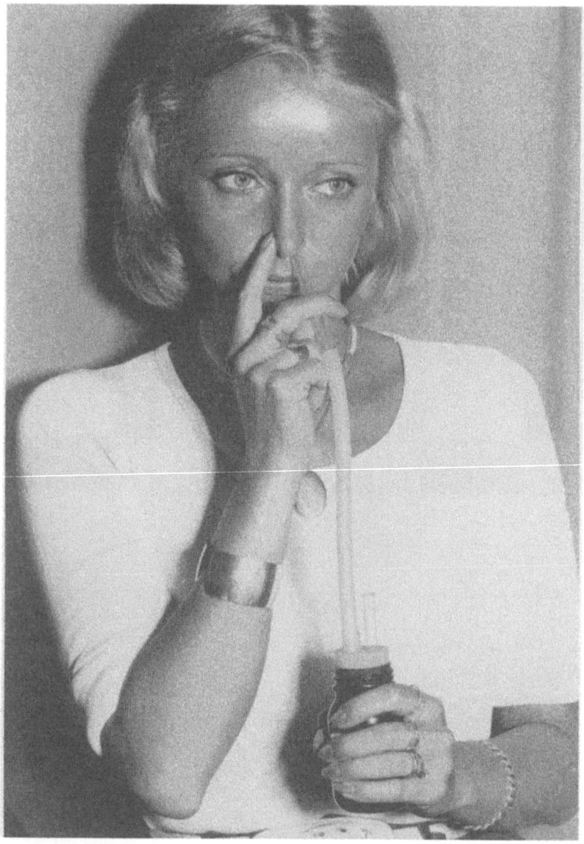

Fig. 2. Olfactometry with sniff bottle-technique (thermostated bottles). Inspiration from the head space through a silicon tube. In bottle openings a double perforated rubber

upon it. We were able to introduce a technique for registration of olfactory evoked potentials and to establish it in clinical work as *computer-olfactometry*. By an electronic control system the olfactory stimulus has a rectangular characteristic and is defined for timing and duration. The technique of registration is similar to electroencephalography. The electrodes are placed bitemporally and at the vertex (Figs. 5 and 6).

The odor is added to every fifth inspiration to avoid adaptation. The stimulus of 150 ms is repeated only 16 times and produces a well established evoked potential. Typically, a double peak develops, which we named the olfactory twin potential (Fig. 7).

The specifity of the evoked potential is demonstrated by the facts, that its amplitudes and latencies are dependent on stimulus intensity, that adaptation phenomena exist, and that after head injuries with interruption of olfactory pathway the potentials disappear. This is obviously correct for the chemosensible first potentials after 220 ms and the second chemosensory, the real olfactory peak, after 450 ms. Also,

Subjective olfactometry

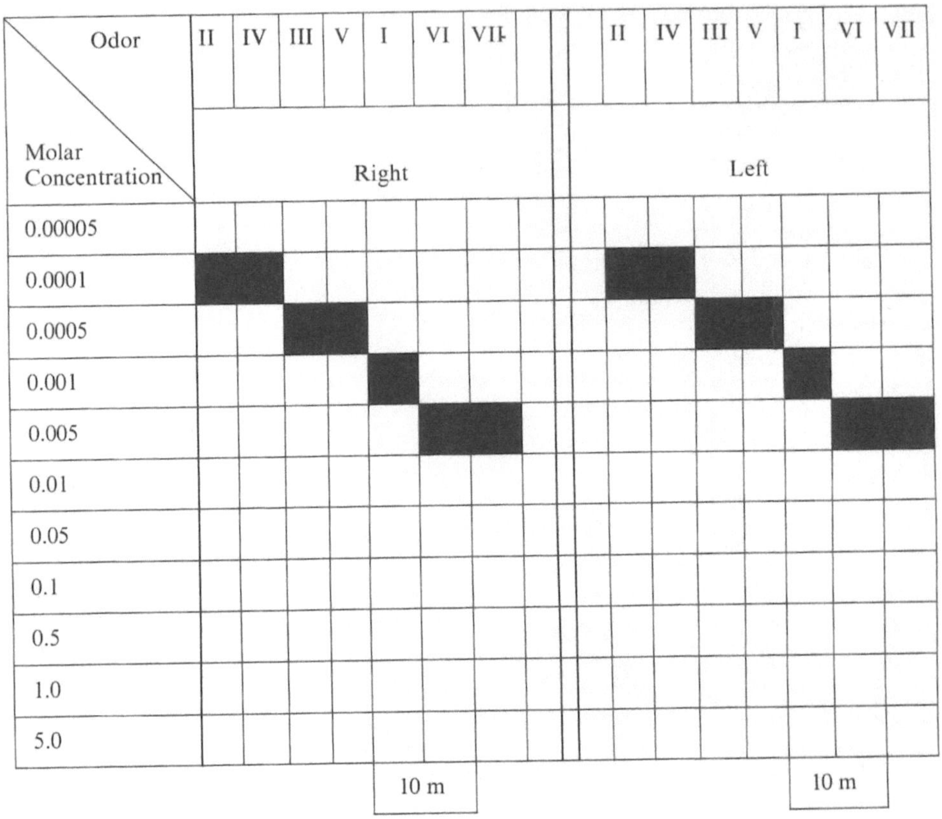

Fig. 3. Schedule. Symbols: I = Ethylbutyrat, II = Eucalyptol, III = Scatol, IV = Ionon, V = Menthol, VI = Acetic acid, VII = Thiophen, Φ: no perception,) (: olfactory threshold, +: recognition

Gustatory smelling

Name:		
	Nose closed	Nose open
Cherry with rum		
Cocoa with nut		
Apricot/brandy		
Half and half		

Fig. 4. Schedule.

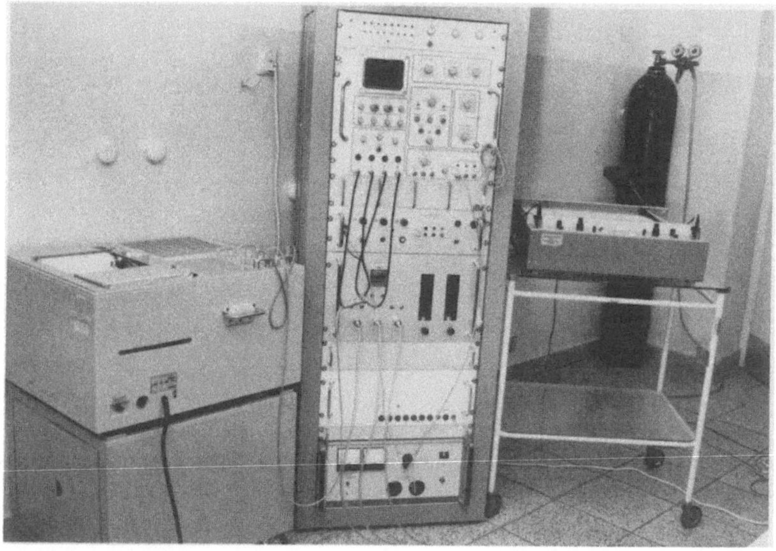

Fig. 5. Computer olfactometry, equipment. Stimulus generator (middle), EEG-amplifier (left), recorder (right)

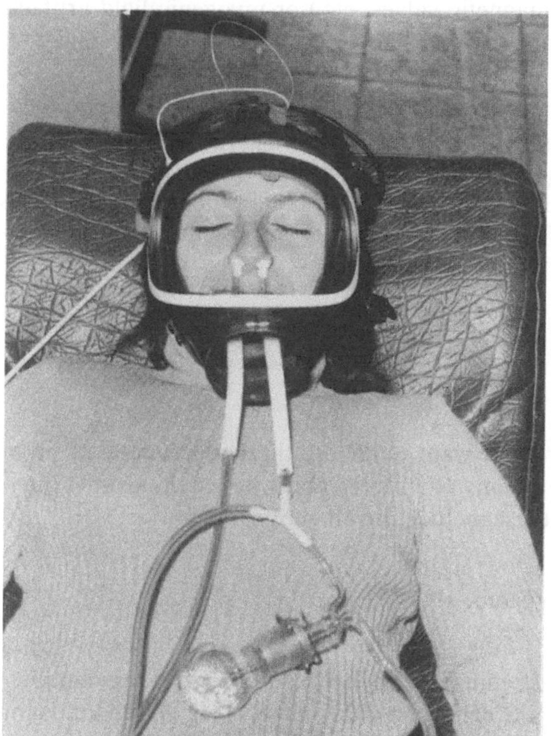

Fig. 6. Computer olfactometry. Stimulus application over panorama mask. Odor vapor in the bottle. Technique see Herberhold, 1973

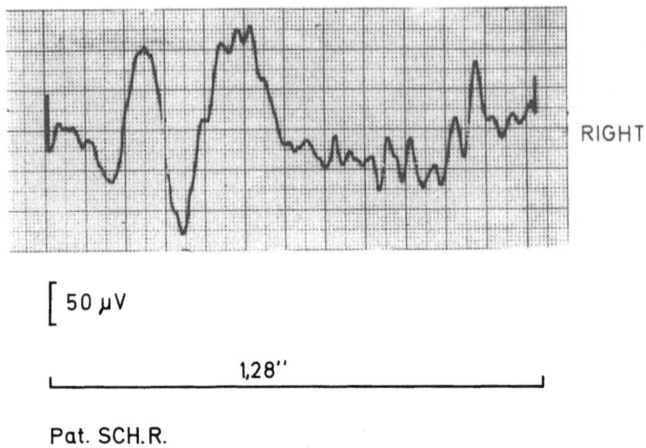

Fig. 7. Normal Computer olfactogram with typical twin-potential. First peak (from left) is equivalent of chemosensible, second peak of chemosensory i.e. olfactory activity

the potentials after head injuries show, that acoustic phenomena in connection with stimulation procedures (action of magnetic valves, etc.) or myogenic field artifacts by stimulus related eyelid contraction take no part in development of the olfactory evoked potentials.

With the computer olfactometry we have, for the first time, an objective measurement which allows registration of stimulus related electrical phenomena of the olfactory pathway itself, independent of patient's will. Thus we get clearer clinical results than with subjective measurements. Moreover, we obtain the first inside views in regular and disturbed functions of the sense of smell. To present, the method allows a semiquantitative interpretation.

II. Clinical

Out of the series of smelling disorders I want to choose three as example of problems with which the clinician is frequently confronted and which demonstrate interesting aspects of pathophysiology, these include the olfactory abilities in:

1. encephalitis disseminata,
2. after influenza or grippic infection, and
3. after head injuries.

In patients with encephalitis disseminata who are examined with the complete otoneurologic test-battery, utilizing the computer olfactometry (Fig. 8) the following properties became conspicuous again and again:

1. Potentials with broad basis,
2. split peaks,

3. one side changes, and
4. discrepancies between subjective and objective olfactometry.

Here, I especially want to keep our sights on the last point. In a careful interpretation of our results, which are similar with those of visual evoked potentials (personal communication by Müller-Jensen) it seems, that the central nervous system in these patients is able to integrate the afferent olfactory information to a normal or nearly normal perception, whereas the evoked cortical summing potential already demonstrates pathological changes. Phenomena following the electrical stimulation of the olfactory pathway obviously hurry on in advance of the clinical statement.

As a second example of the daily practice I want to cite smell disorders after influenza or grippic infections. These olfactory disturbances are much more frequent than generally assumed. There are reports declaring that 75 percent of the patients suffering from viral influenza develop disturbances of smell, 50 percent as hyposmia and the other 25 percent as anosmia and parosmia, respectively. The site of viral damage is still unclear. Our computer-olfactograms show, in cases of anosmia, the absence of the complete twin potential or of its sensory part. We want to conclude that the viral tropism to sensory epithelium and its neurites or to free nerve endings imply a peripheral damage. Naturally, here each therapy will remain full of problems. In some cases the administration of Zinc leads to a little improvement.

Lastly, we will consider head injuries. In this connection the first cranial nerve is the most frequently damaged among the twelve. That is certainly to be explained by the correlation of its anatomical course and the distribution of the traumatic mechanisms.

After head injuries the computer olfactograms show three types of slopes:

1. Summing potentials without any peak (Fig. 9)
2. Summing potentials with isolated loss of the sensory peak (Fig. 10) and
3. Summing potentials with isolated loss of the sensible peak (Fig. 11)

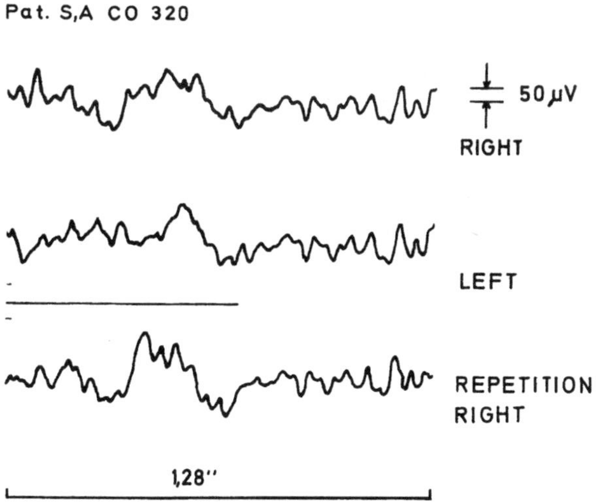

Fig. 8. Computer olfactogram in encephalitis disseminata (multiple sclerosis). See text

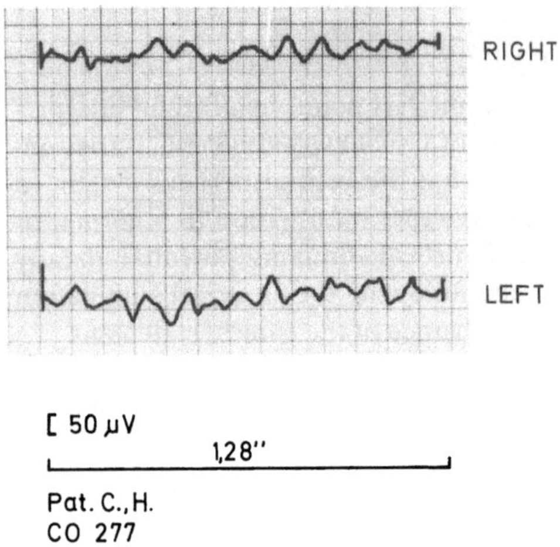

Fig. 9. Computer olfactogram after head injury. Total loss of any olfactory perception. Disappearance of the twin potential

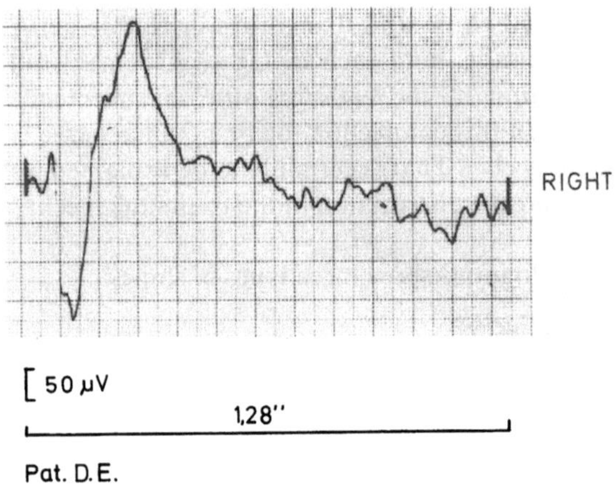

Fig. 10. Computer olfactogram after head injury. Loss of the chemosensory (olfactory) peak. Subjective: anosmia

Whereas the first type of registration is accompanied by total anosmia, the others can be combined with residual olfactory function. The non-appearance of the olfactory peak should be ascribed to peripheral damage in the area of lamina cribrosa or of the olfactory bulb and/or tract; the non-appearance of the sensible peak, to central damage.

Summarizing our own cases, Koch (1980) found, in agreement with the traumatic data, that about 75 percent of disorders of olfaction judged by us are basing on sagittal traumas, 42.5 percent after frontal and 32 percent after occipital traumas (Table 2). Surprisingly occipital traumas nearly completely lead to anosmia, whereas hyposmia after frontal trauma, too, appeared in 20 percent. Accompanying neurological symptoms were more often obvious after frontal than occipital traumas. Altogether the disorders of smell after head injuries prove to be

58% hyposmias,
40% on both sides and
only 2% unilateral anosmias (Table 3).

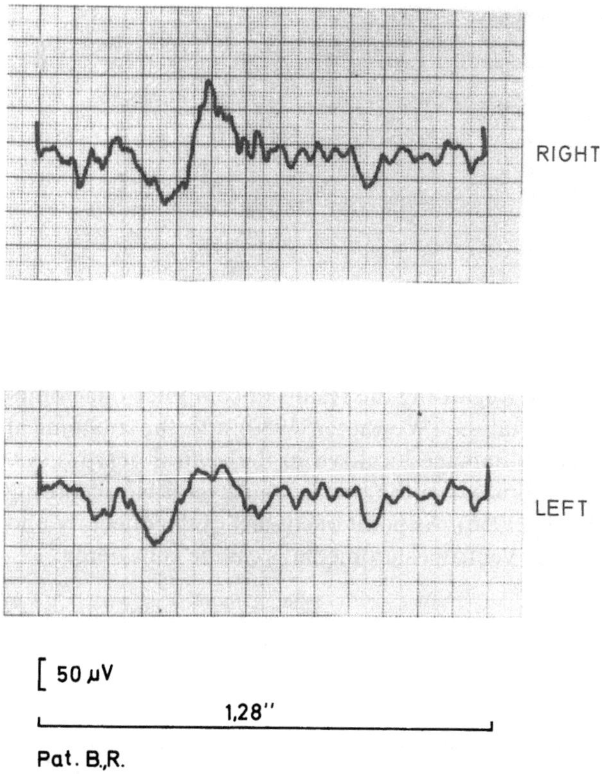

Fig. 11. Computer olfactogram after head injury. Loss of the chemosensible (trigeminal) peak. Subjective: Highgrade hyposmia

Table 2. Disorders of olfaction after head injury ($n = 47$)

After frontal trauma	42.5%
After occipital trauma	32.0%
After sagittal trauma	74.5%
After lateral trauma	8.5%
After bilateral trauma	4.3%
Others	12.7%

Table 3. Smell disorders of olfaction after head injury ($n = 47$); diagnosis by clinical evaluation

Hyposmia	58%
Anosmia, bilateral	40%
Anosmia, one side	2%

Table 4. Combined disorders of chemical senses after head injury ($n = 24/47 \triangleq 51\%$)

Distribution			
Hyposmia	–	Hypogeusia	46%
Hyposmia	–	Ageusia	25%
Anosmia	–	Hypogeusia	21%
Anosmia	–	Ageusia	8%

Remarkably often, we found by a precise examination, combined damages of both of the chemical senses (Table 4). Regarding the results of computer-olfactometry, experimental respiratory noise analysis (Westhofen 1980) and the anatomical facts, we must assume in such cases a damage localized in the central nervous system, and especially in the root of brainstem in the area of third ventricle according to Faber and Jung (1947), and Faust (1956). As point of contact of the olfactory and gustatory senses, the thalamic nucleus ventroposteromedialis can be considered.

III. Conclusion

By improvement of simple and further developments of more extensive testing procedures based upon electrophysiological phenomena we are now more and more able to elaborate precise information about olfactory disorders. Recording olfactory evoked potentials and simultaneous recording of stimulus following reactions on other neural pathways utilizing polgraphic studies promise deeper views in the pathophysiology of disorders of olfaction and evidence for localization of damage in the neural course of smell.

References

Faber W, Jung R (1947) Über Geschmacksstörungen bei Hirnverletzten und das Syndrom Anosmie-Ageusie. Nervenarzt 18:530–544

Faust C (1956) Das klinische Bild der Dauerfolgen nach Hirnverletzung. Thieme, Stuttgart

Güttich H (1956) Gustatorische Riechprüfung mit Riechstoffen und Mischreizschmeckstoffen. Arch Ohr, Nas- u. Kehlk-Heilk 178:408–414

Herberhold C (1973) Nachweis u. Reizbedingungen olfaktorisch u. rhinosensibel evozierter Hirnrinden-Summen-Potentiale sowie Konzept einer klinischen Computer-Olfaktometrie. Opladen

Herberhold C (1972) Computer-Olfactometric mit getrenntem Nachweis von Trigeminus- u. Olfaktoriusreaktionen. Arch klin exp Ohr-, Nas- u. Kehlk-Heilk 202:394–397

Herberhold, C (1976) Typical Results of Computer-Olfactometry. Rhinology 14:109–116

Koch G (1980) Olfaktologische Analyse von stumpfen Schädel-Hirn-Traumen. Auswertung von Computer-Olfaktometrien im Hinblick auf die Unfallmechanik. Inaug. Diss. Bonn

Westhofen M (1980) Lösen olfaktorische Reize atemreflektorische Reaktionen aus? Experimentaluntersuchung zur Frage eines sog. unwillkürlichen Riechtests. Inaug. Diss. Bonn

Clinical Aspects of Gustatory Sense

H. Schaupp, Frankfurt/FRG

There is a remarkable gap between the importance of taste for man and its clinical consideration which is evident not only in the limited diagnostic potential and the unsatisfactory differential diagnostic analysis of taste disorders but also in the inferior rank given to taste in the medical opinion and the carelessness of some surgeons with the chorda tympani in middle ear operations. Fortunately, taste as a phylogenetically seen old sense is little affectable against lesions of different kinds.

1. Congenital and hereditary conditions
2. Endocrine diseases
3. Atrophy of oral (lingual) mucosa
4. Infections
   a) Virus
   b) Bacteria
5. Exogen – toxic influences
   a) occupational (chemical)
   b) dental cleaning substances
   c) oral disinfectants
6. Irradiation
7. Pharmacons (drugs)
8. Lesions of peripheral (sensory) nerves
   a) Chorda tympani
   b) N. glossopharyngicus
9. Lesions in C.N.S.

Fig. 1. Etiology of the disorders of taste

Inborn and Inherited Impairments of Taste

Familial Dysautonomia

In familial dysautonomia, an inborn malformation of the nervous system, of the skin and mucous membrane with relative insensitivity against temperature and pain stimuli and no secretion of tears, there is also a dysplasia of the taste papillae with aplasia of taste buds. Pearson et al. (1970) found no taste buds at all in the circumvallate papillae of a child. Corresponding to aplasia of taste the thresholds for the four qualities are raised, sometimes to a degree, that even saturated solutions of salt (NaCl), sugar or urea cannot be distinguished from tap water. Since it is a malformation of the nerves it could be possible in some cases to initiate the secretion of tears and lower the taste thresholds by metacholine, a substance similar to acetylcholine.

Taste Blindness

The so called blindness of taste of a certain percentage of the population against phenyl-thio-carbamide (PTC) is a peculiar phenomenon, since these people have extremely high thresholds against all substances with the >C=S-group and many derivatives. The deficiency is transmitted recessively in a homozygote manner. The specifity of the impairment is emphasized by the fact that the thresholds of the other qualities and even the sensitivity against other bitter substances, for instance qui-

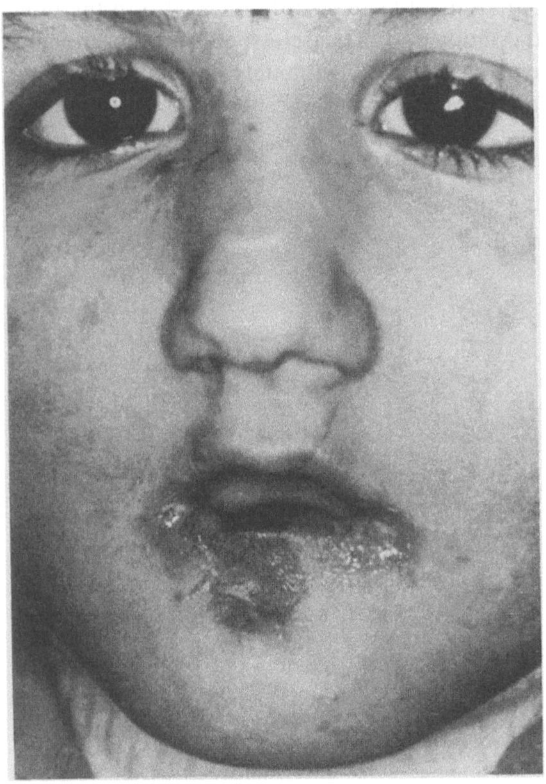

Fig. 2. A five year old girl whose parents were consanguineous (the grandfathers were brothers) with insensitivity to pain and temperature, lack of tears and reduced taste for all qualities. Note the multiple lesions of bites on the lips

nine, are normal. The percentage of "tasters" within a population depends on ethnic factors and is between 60 and 70%. There are interesting though not fully clarified connections between taste blindness and some severe diseases: for instance congenital athyreotic cretinism, nodular goiter, Downs's syndrome and ulcers of the duodenum. Kalmus (1971) supposes, that the difference between tasters and nontasters depends on the presence of a special protein or other molecules on the receptor membrane.

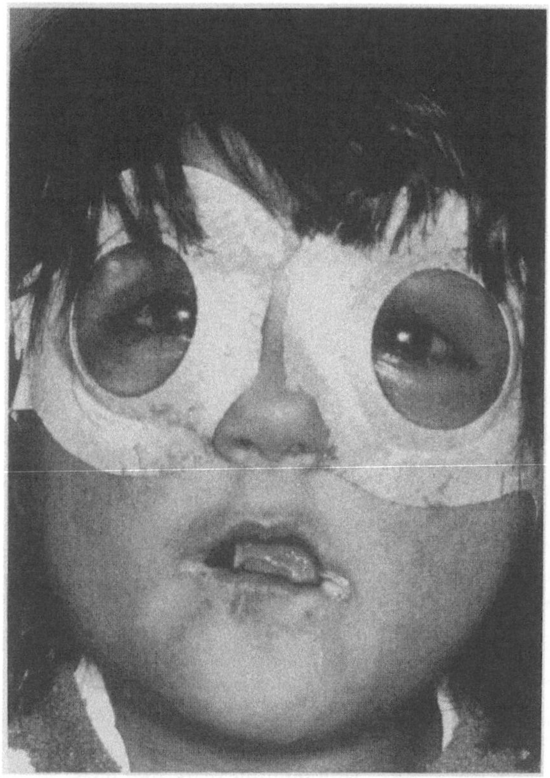

Fig. 3. The three and a half year old sister of the girl in Fig. 2 with similar symptoms of familial dysautonomia. Bite effects on the lips and keratitis

Taste Impairments in Endocrine Diseases

First communications about impairment of taste in alimentary diabetes were made 120 years ago and in diabetes the connections are best investigated. Almost all authors have found a hypogeusia in the diabetic. Schaupp and Seilz (1969) compared the electric thresholds of 227 diabetics with the thresholds of healthy persons of the same decades and found the thresholds to be significantly elevated at blood sugar levels over 180 mg percent. The significance of the deviation increases with rising blood sugar level.

We have also investigated taste in some other endocrine diseases of the thyroid gland and of the adrenocortical system, but significant rise of the electric thresholds could only be detected in a group of 22 patients with Sheehan's syndrome. The increase of the thresholds was highly significant in patients without hormone administration.

Further on we found slightly significant elevation of thresholds in patients with hypothyroidism. In general, alterations of taste under pathologic constellations have no importance, but in single cases severe hormonal impairments may at least be a co-factor of manifest taste disturbance.

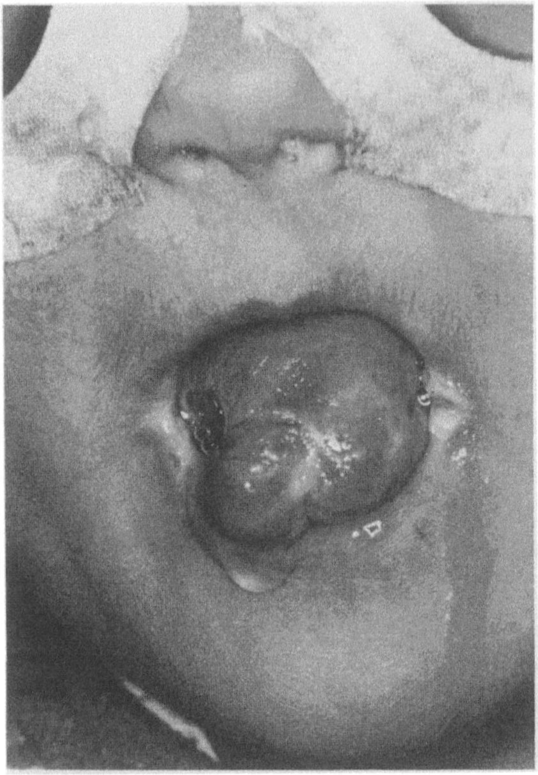

Fig. 4. Tongue of the girl (Fig. 3) with multiple scars after bites

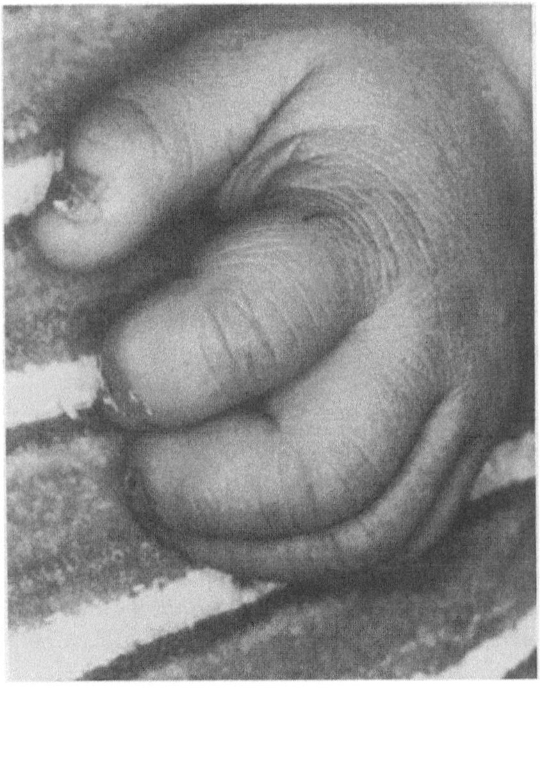

Fig. 5. Left hand of the girl (Fig. 3) with mutilation of the fingers as a consequence of uncontrolled bites

Disease	*Elgustometric threshold*
diabetes, alimentary	+
hypothyroidism	(+)
hyperthyridism	–
Sheehan's disease	+
Addison's disease	–
Cushing's disease	–
adrenogenital syndrome	–

+ = threshold increased, – = normal threshold
In 11 untreated pat. (=50%) with Sheehan's disease thresholds were highly significant elevated (P=0.0005).

Fig. 6. Electric taste thresholds in endocrine diseases

Acquired Disorders at the Periphere Taste Area

Taste Impairments After Atrophy of the Mucous Membrane

In atrophic processes of the mucous membrane of the tongue one can regularly find disturbances of taste. This becomes evident in cases of irregular atrophy where one can define the areas of hypogeusia precisely by electrogustometry. In patients with irregular atrophia as in red plane lichen of the tongue we observe equal quantitative decline of taste as well as dissociated impairment for the four qualities in the diseased areas.

With advancing age we also find a decrease of taste, a fact that had been correspondingly established by all investigators. The decline of sensitivity to sweet, salty, sour and bitter is essentially the same; all curves show a noticeable decline after the late fifties.

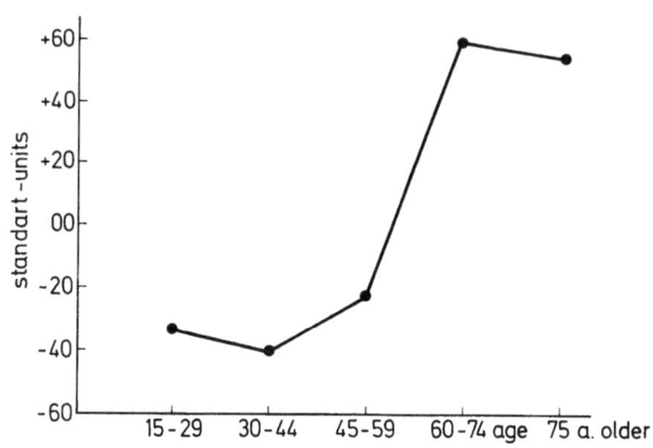

Fig. 7. Relationship between age and taste sensitivity (composite of four taste qualities) (after: Cooper et al. 1959)

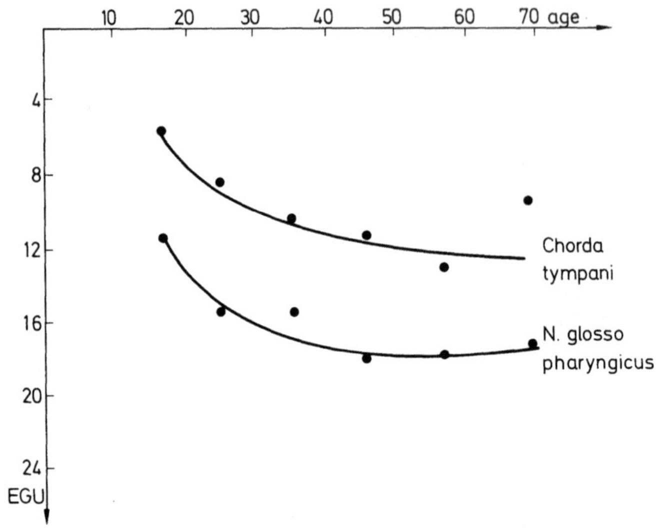

Fig. 8. Relationship between age and taste sensitivity; average of the electrogustometric thresholds of 109 test persons (from: Rossberg et al. 1966)

The decline of taste depends on atrophy and numerical reduction of taste receptors within the general atrophy of the mucous membranes. With advancing age one can find hydropic transformation of the sensory cells, subepithelial fibrosis and atrophia of the epithelium. The number of papillae decreases and in addition there is also a decrease in number of taste buds. In the circumvallate papillae they drop from 245 in infants to 88 in old men.

We do not notice this gradual decline of taste. But it is another situation in the rapidly progressing atrophia of the epithelium of the tongue as a symptom of gastric achylia under vitamin-A-deficiency. Several authors have found disturbances of taste up to severe hypogeusia and parageusia. In patients with Hunter's glossitis for instance a lowering of taste acuity for all four qualities could be proved and reproduced in animal experiments with vitamin-A-free food.

Impairment of Taste Caused by Infections

Bacterial and viral infections can leave longlasting impairments, partly as general hypogeusia, partly as dissociated alterations of the threshold of the single qualities.

Viral Infections

Disturbances of taste have been observed in 3 diseases:

influenza
epidemic parotitis
dengue.

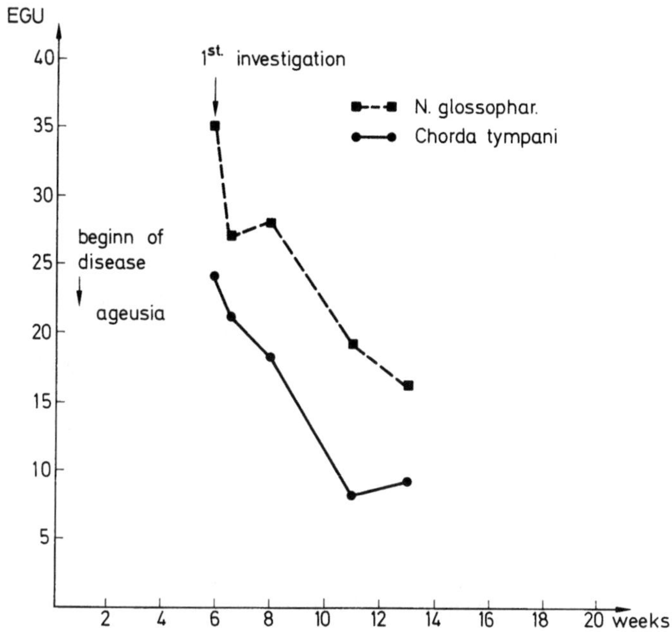

Fig. 9. Improvement of taste impairment after influenza in a 50 year old patient. Recovery after 11 weeks; thresholds in EGU

The alteration of taste as an almost characteristic and early manifestation of dengue is of diagnostic importance. More important is the impairment of taste by influenza, although, compared to the large number of influenza infections, isolated alterations of taste are a rare complication. Within eight years we could observe isolated hypogeusia in only four cases of influenza. Dysgeusia (and hypogeusia) begins in the early stage of the disease and lasts weeks to months with slow recovery. The impairment expresses itself in quantitative reduction of taste acuity up to ageusia or irregularity of taste pattern. It results in a flat, dull, alkaline sometime bitter taste. Far more often than an isolated impairment we find a combined disturbance of taste and smell in influenza. The site of the viral lesion is as yet unknown, but it can be assumed that it is not only an isolated neuritis of single nerves or superficial damage of the sensory end-organs. In some cases, where the impairment lasts for years as in one of our cases – ageusia and anosmia seven years after influenza – we may assume a central lesion especially when there are accompanying vegetative symptoms.

Taste Disturbances by Bacterial Infections

They are of less clinical importance than those after viral infections. Impairments after specific infections could as yet been observed after:

tuberculosis
endemic typhus
diphtheria,

in the latter perhaps as a consequence of diphtheric neuritis. Disturbance after unspecific bacterial infections are rare. Among the many patients with infections of the upper respiratory tract, there were only two with serious putrid sinusitis who had alterations of taste (parageusia as salty taste). After healing of the sinusitis, the dysgeusia also vanished. There is an interesting report by Rauh and Mros (1966) concerning six cases of dysgeusia (one with ageusia) in 24 patients with ozaena.

Exogen-Toxic Lesions of the Taste

After the clinical observation of a few cases of hypogeusia by toxic substances in industry Rossberg, Schaupp und Schmidt (1966) investigated 543 workers in the metal manufacturing industry and found that about 30 percent of the workmen had elec-

Substance	*Author*
tetrachlorethane	Moeschlin, 1956
tobacco smoke	Krut, Perrin and Pronte-Stewart, 1961 Kaplan and Glanville, 1964 Kaplan, Glanville and Fischer, 1965 Manzella and Ferrara, 1967
hydracine benzol benzine anilin and derivatives lacs and their solution mediums	Rossberg, Schaupp and Schmidt, 1966
rubber dust chromates Co	Schaupp, 1969

Fig. 10. Substances which cause threshold alteration or dysgeusia by chronic inhalation

tric taste thresholds above the normal statistic range. But a significant deviation could only be stated up to the decade of 30 to 40 years. In the higher decades the statistical diffusion in normal persons was so wide that significant deviations could not be found. Meanwhile we know several chemical substances with taste disturbing effects.

Only with some substances such as tetrachlorethan, hydracin, carbon monoxide, and benzol the alterations are clinically relevant in the sense of strong reduction of taste acuity, where in most other cases the alterations were not perceived as pathologic by the involved persons. Nevertheless we have to value disturbances of taste by chemical substances in industry as an analogue to noise deafness among those who work amid high noise levels.

Taste Disturbances by Tooth Pastes and Related Agents

In a broad series v. Heesen and Schaupp (1969) studied this special form of exogen taste impairment by testing nearly all commercial pastes, powders and liquids for tooth care. Wo got the following results:

1. All tooth pastes caused measurable electrogustometric decrease of taste acuity of different amount and duration.
2. The effects in the mean disappeared after 30 min., but there were pastes with measurable effects of about 70 min.
3. Within certain limits there is a direct connection between time of application and quantity of paste on one side and taste disorder on the other.
4. The modality bitter was impaired most seriously (up to 120 min. after routine application of the pastes), then sweet, salty and at least sour.
5. The disturbance was produced exclusively by one content of the pastes; the tensides. The most powerful toxic agent was sodium lauric sulfate. The lesions are probably produced by the interaction of the lipophilic groups of the tensides with the lipoids of the cell membrane.

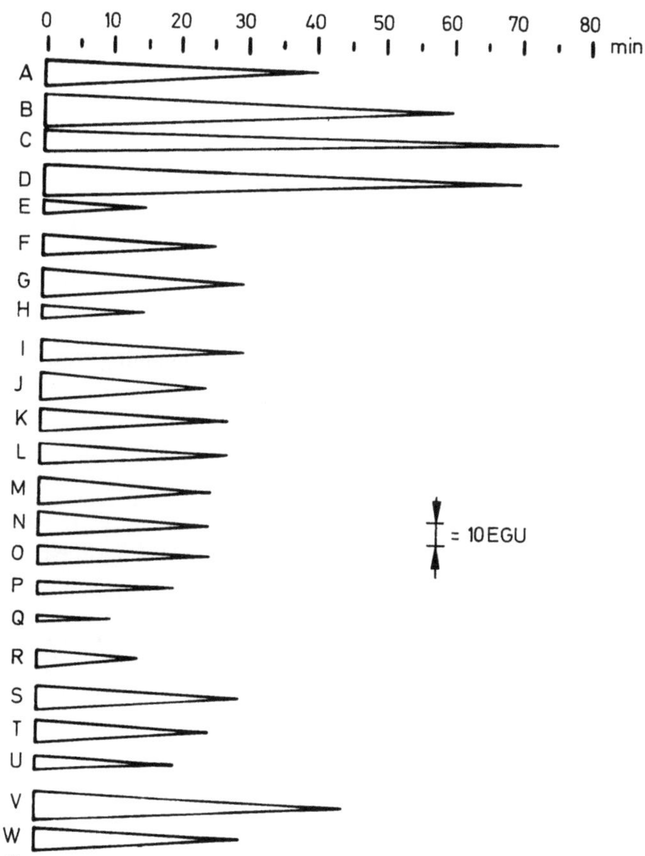

Fig. 11. Decrease of taste acuity of different amount and duration after routine application of commercial tooth pastes (A–X) in EGU (from: v. Heesen and Schaupp 1969)

Taste Disturbances by Mouth Disinfectants

Even substances used as medicaments in practice can display taste disturbing side effects, as preparations which contain

1. hexetidin and
2. chlorhexidin.

Hexetidin, a derivative of pyrimidine with good antibacterial and antimycotic qualities shows a structural analogy to thiamine and is competitive for the coenzyme

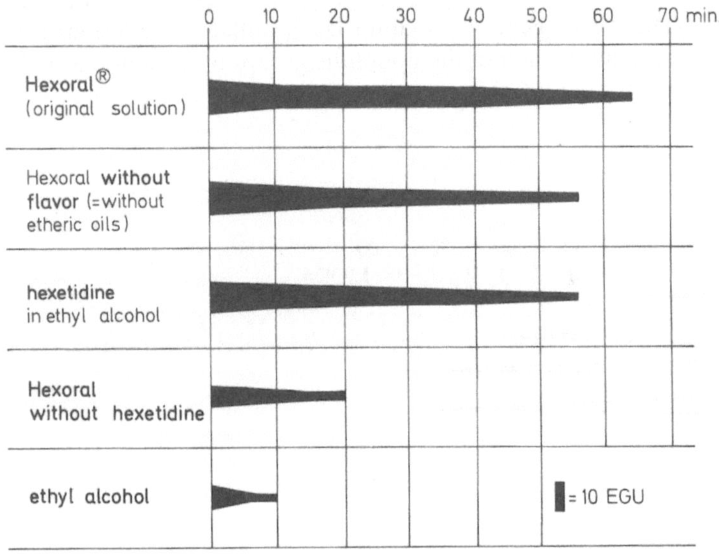

Fig. 12. Extent and duration of dysgeusia after rinsing with the hexetidin-containing Hexoral and its constituents (from: Schaupp and Wohnaut 1978)

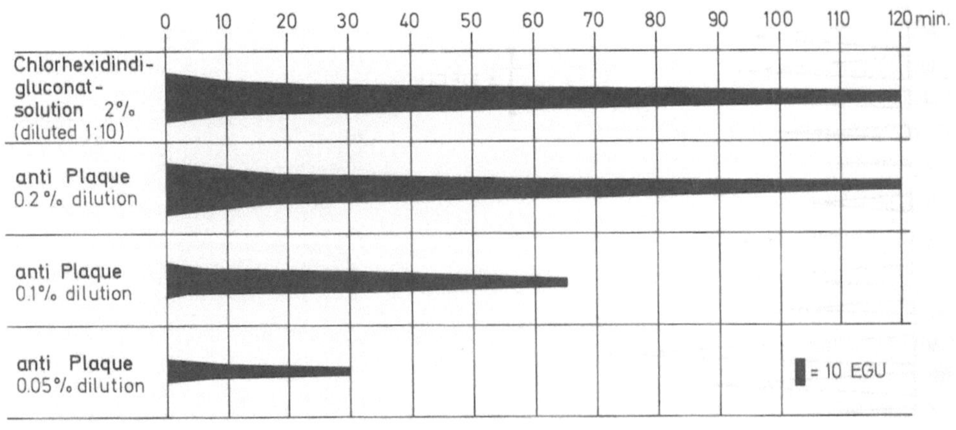

Fig. 13. Extent and duration of dysgeusia after rinsing with chlorhexidindigluconat-containing solutions (from: Schaupp and Wohnaut 1978)

thiamine pyrophosphate. It inhibits the pyruvate kinase reaction. So carboxylation is interrupted in bacteria and cells.

Chlorhexidin destroys the cytoplasmatic membrane and precipitates the cytoplasm.

All oral disinfectants after routine application had the effect of dropping taste acuity, which lasted up to 2 hours.

When the disinfectants were used several days in the normal concentration, disturbances of the taste could be measured even 24 hours after the last application. In equivalent concentrations chlorhexidin is more effective on taste than hexetidin. As the cause of dysgeusia or bitter dominance we found a dissociated lesion of the single taste qualities, in that sweet was most affected, bitter the less, whereas the other qualities were in between.

Radiogenic Impairments of Taste

Irradiation causes impairments of taste whenever applied therapeutically in tumor doses to the oral region. The impairments pass nearly as a natural law: they culminate during irradiation and recover extensively after the end of radiation. At this time the character of the dysgeusia changes permanently, as if the receptors of the single qualities were unequally sensible against radiation. In today's scheme of fractional irradiation the disturbances begin after approximately 2000 rad and reach the highest point at the end of the radiation period.

The four qualities react differently: sweet is most quickly affected, then salty, less and later bitter, and finally sour. At the peak level of damage, about the twentieth day, the impairment becomes so severe, that some patients are not able to distinguish even concentrated solutions of sugar, salt or quinine. When the sour quality seems to be more resistent, the sour "taste" could be also a sensible stimulus on the inflamed, irritable and aching epithelium and not a sensory sensation. Therefore in such patients the sour sensation is often connected with a burning sensation and the sour threshold difficult to determine. Altogether we can state, that taste recovers

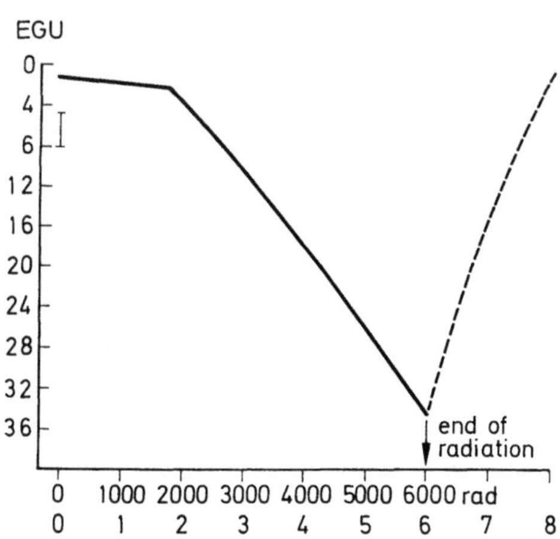

Fig. 14. Electrogustometric thresholds during and after gamma irradiation in the oral region of a 45 year old patient (from: Schaupp et al. 1972)

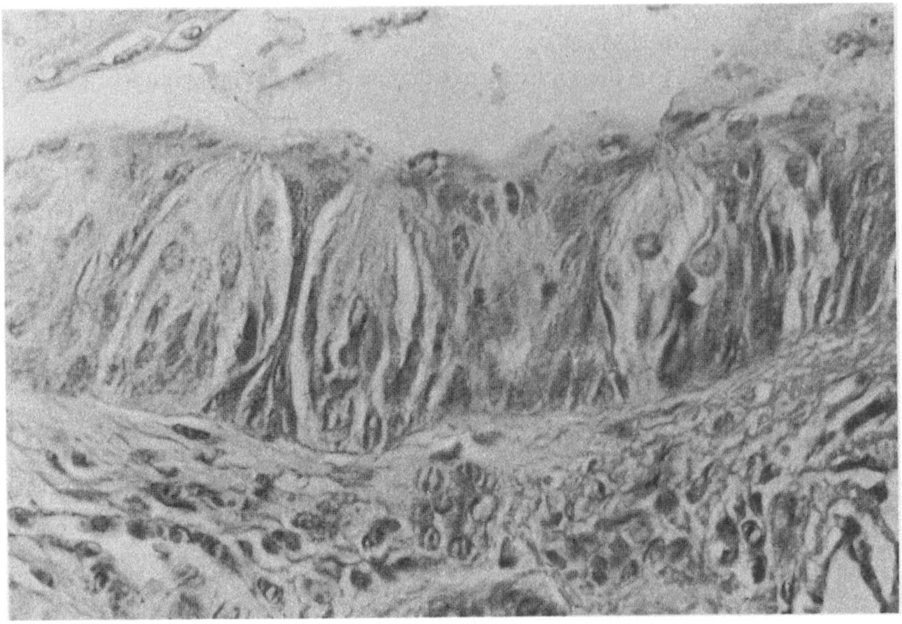

a

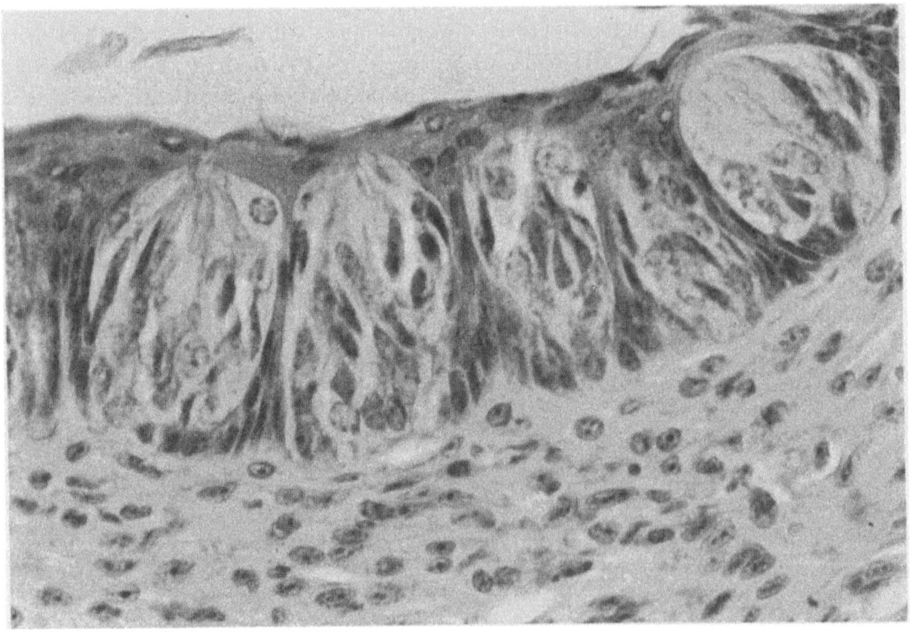

b

Fig. 15 a–c. Sections of the circumvallate papilla of mice. **a** without irradiation **b** after 6000 rad fractionated irradiation (200 rad/day) **c** 2 days after an acute irradiation with 4000 rad

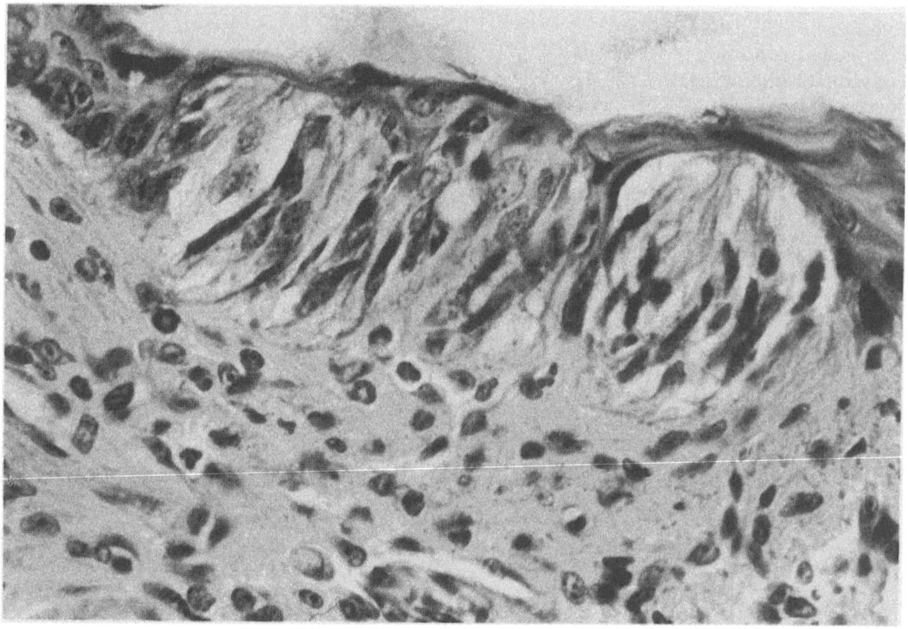

Fig. 15c

after the end of radiation within 100 days. But regeneration is not complete; it remains a slight permanent sensorial lesion which is measurable even after 13 years as a statistic quantity. And it is interesting that in case of a second radiation series the damage will come sooner and reach the utmost extent earlier, already occuring after four to eight days, apparently as a consequence of the previous damage. Radiogenic dysgeusia and ageusia depend on the fast change of the papillae, buds and taste cells, which have an average lifespan of only a few days (Beidler, 1963; Conger and Wells, 1969). Beidler noted that cells of different age will perceive different qualities. The ionizing rays stop the ingrowth of young cells and consequently comes a shift of the excitation pattern and diminution of one quality after another. In our experiments in mice (Schaupp, Bertram and Schulz-Freywald, 1972) we saw the earliest noticeable alterations of the taste buds after 3000 rad. After acute irradiation (with 4000 rad) which is about eight times (for buds) to 18 times (for cells per bud) as effective as fractionated, we found the signs of severe damage.

Radiogenic taste impairments are a severe charge for every patient because they occur just at the time of heavy local and general radiotherapy, and the appetite of the patient will be further reduced.

Taste Impairments Through Drugs

Protracted application of the following drugs may effect taste impairments (see Fig. 16 on page 53 above).

acetylsalicylic acid
oxifedrinehydrochloride
phenindion (2-phenylinandion-(1,3))
L-dopa
biguanides
antibiotics (lincomycin and ethambutol)
gold salts
cytostatics (azathioprin)
penicillamine (in 30% of cases; corrected by administration of copper)

Fig. 16. Drugs which can cause dysgeusia and hypogeusia after chronic medication

The clinical mechanisms of the impairment are as yet unknown. Only in the case of D-penicillinamine we know that the enzymes of the protein synthesis and other functional proteins are blocked. The effect of cytostatics (for instance Azathioprine) is probably similar to that of ionizing rays.

Taste Disturbance Through Lesions of Peripheral Nerves

Chorda Tympani

The sudden, abrupt dissection of an intact chorda is noticed by 80 percent of all patients. They state a numb, rough sensation on the paralysed side of the tongue and an altered taste to foods. Some complain of a metallic taste and – as a compensation – chew on the healthy side. The parageusia sometimes persists for years after cutting the chorda, in a case of Bull (1965) 21 years after mastoidectomy. In general about 32 percent of the patients with sudden dissection of the chorda will have permanent troubles. Slow destruction of the chorda in a chronic otitis for instance, will not be perceived. In many patients the chorda is, though preserved in continuity, so heavily injured in its function by the chronic infection that dissection has no consequences. In about 50 percent of patients with chronic epitympanal otitis we can find preoperative ipsilateral ageuisa. The sensorial redundance of the taste organ is obviously so wide, that vicarious taking over of the function by intact areas is easily possible. But it is a seeming balance; a restitution of taste in the denervated area will never take place and a medially well defined atrophy of the fungiform papillae will appear.

Bilateral division of the chorda produces permanent troubles in 80 percent of patients. They complain about dryness of the mouth and various, hetergeneous disturbances of taste: metallic taste, taste generally poorer; patients notice, that they do not have the awareness of tasting before the food reaches the back of the tongue and so appreciate the taste nearly too late.

This is important because of the big number of patients submitted to bilateral stapedectomy. Properly the preoperative electrogustometric investigation of all otosclerotic patients should be self-evident. Not only a dissection of the chorda, but also an overstretching can cause dysgeusia and is to be avoided. After overstretching we can observe permanent dysgeusia in seven percent of patients.

Conclusions

1. Sudden dissection of the chorda tympani nerve always leads to ageusia and in a high percentage of patients to transitory or even permanent troubles.
2. Overstretching of the chorda effects similar troubles, but the percentage is much less.
3. Whenever possible, the chorda has to be spared. Preventive or routine dissection of the nerve are on principle to be refused and declined.

Disturbance of Taste in Facial Paralysis

Loss of taste on the anterior two-thirds of the tongue is quite a common accompaniment of Bell's palsy; parageusia, however, is less frequent. Extent of lesion and prognosis are of course different in the facial nerve and chorda tympani and depend on the kind of lesion. The best prognosis for restitution of taste is in Bell's palsy. It is much poorer in herpes zoster of the ear and, of course, in traumatic palsies.

Krarup (1958 c) found dysgeusias in 84 percent of patients with acute Bell's palsy and among these ageusia in 35 percent.

In restitution, taste function returns earlier than motor function. In general the fibres of the chorda tympani regenerate earlier and more completely. Patients in which dysgeusia continues despite complete recovery of motor function are rare. The higher functional resistance of the chorda tympani can not only be seen in Bell's palsy but also in herpes zoster of the ear, even if the extent of lesions here is much higher. In most fresh cases there is a good coincidence between the first pathologic gustative and motor signs. Sometimes the dysgeusia (bitter taste) precedes the facial paralysis by up to 10 days.

Glossopharyngeal Nerve

A solitary peripheral paralysis of the glossopharyngeal nerve is, for topographic reasons, less frequent by far than paralysis of the chorda. A direct lesion of the nerve trunk is a rarity, though the nerve often lies very close to the tonsil, separated only by a thin muscular layer. A little more frequent are peripheral paralyses of the ninth nerve together with other nerve lesions as a complication of large abscesses or tumors of the base of the skull. We have seen six of these cases in which the taste deficiency had not been observed because of the more disturbing motor defects.

Of higher significance are disturbances of taste in the posterior third of the tongue as a consequence of cutting or streching the lingual rami of the glossopharyngeal nerve during tonsillectomy, or postoperative neuritis. As ageusia or parageusia the disturbances last up to 10 months and are described as dysgeusias and taste paresthesias with permanent bitter or sweet taste or simply as disgusting taste sensations for instance while taking in sweets. They are sometimes bilateral. Among 50 gustometrically investigated patients Tarab (1955) found ageusia in 8 percent, which lasted for more than three months in three patients. Most of the authors who have reported about the disorders suppose a raised sensibility of the taste fibres. The others comprehend the dissociated disturbances as a postoperative neuritis. Over a seven years' period we could observe only three patients with these lesions which lasted for up to seven months.

Central Lesions and Taste

Poisoning with Carbon Monoxide

The longest observation of taste disorders from CO intoxication were performed by Kittel (1966). He stresses, that in a certain percentage of acutely poisoned patients hypogeusia remains as a permanent defect. We can recall only one case in which taste disturbances restituted completely while the damage of the inner ears was irreparable.

The Syndrome of Anosmia – Ageusia

Faber and Jung (1947) first reported about this syndrome in soldiers with trauma of the brain. They stated a contusion of the brain near the wall of the III. ventricle where the sensory fibres of the mouth and nose region travelling together with the smell and taste neurons on a very close pathway is causative. According to the localization of the lesion the syndrome of loss of sensibility in the nose-mouth-region and anosmia – ageusia is very often accompanied by vegetative troubles as diabetes insipid, disturbed sleep, pathologic sweats, circulatory disturbance and disturbance of sexual potency, sometimes xerostomia. Of course the syndrome is not always strongly marked, and sometimes only an incomplete pattern appears. But it is more frequent than generally assumed. We can observe it with a frequency of about two to three patients a year. Especially with regard to forensic involvement it is important for the patients concerned that the physician knows the syndrome and does not regard patients who complain about this complex of lesions as simulators.

Disturbances due to Cerebral Focus

Lesions of the cortical representation of taste in the postcentral gyrus can evoke dissociated disturbances and agonizing taste paresthesias. In most of the reported cases they found hypogeusia for the hallucinated quality. Adler (1935) stated that nearly all cortical disturbances of taste are partial and affect only one to two qualities. As causes he discussed: local encephalitis, multiple sclerosis, cephalo malacic fibroses and meningiomas.

Summary

Many pathologic conditions are accompanied by disturbances of taste. There are patients in whom the cause is evident as in trauma and irradiation and others where we have only a slight suspicion of causality as in drug-borne impairments. The chapter gives a relatively short survey of the most important clinical causes of taste disorders and their degree, beginning with inherited disturbances and taste disorders in endocrine diseases, continued by disorders in the peripheral taste area after atrophy of the mucous membrane, infections, inhalative noxa, drugs and irradiation and finally traumatic lesions of the peripheral and central pathways. Physiologic, diagnostic and therapeutic aspects are not included.

References

Adler A (1935) Zur Topik der cortischen Geschmackssphäre. Z Neurol 152:25

Beidler LM (1963) Dynamics of Taste Cells. Wenner-Gren-Center Int. Sympos. Series Pergamon Press, Oxford London New York Paris 1:133–148

Bull FR (1965) Taste and the Chorda Tympani. J Laryngol Otol 79:479–493

Conger AD, Wells MA (1969) Radiation and Aging Effect on Taste Structure and Function. Radiat Res 37:31–49

Cooper RM, Bilash J, Zubek JP (1959) The Effect of Age on Taste Sensitivity. J Gerontol 14:56–58

Faber W, Jung R (1947) Über Geschmacksstörungen bei Hirnverletzten und das Syndrom Anosmie – Ageusie. Nervenarzt 18:530–544

v. Heesen W, Schaupp H (1969) Geschmackstörungen durch Mundpflegemittel. Arch klin exp Ohrenheilk 195:179–191

Kalmus H (1971) Genetics of Taste. In: Beidler LM Handbook of Sensory Physiology. Chemical Senses 2 Taste. Springer, Berlin Heidelberg New York, p 165–179

Kaplan AR, Glanville EV (1964) Taste Threshold for Bitterness and Cigarette Smoking. Nature 202:1366

Kaplan AR, Glanville EV, Fischer R (1965) Cumulative Effect of Age and Smoking on Taste Sensitivity in Males and Females J Gerontol 20:334–337

Kittel G (1966) Diskussionsbemerkung auf dem Jahreskongreß d. Südwestd. HNO-Ärzte in Karlsruhe 1965. Z Laryng Rhinol Otol 45:589–590

Krarup B (1958) Taste Reactions of Patients with Bell's Palsy. Acta Otolaryngol (Stockh) 49:389–399

Krut LH et al. (1961) Taste Perception in Smokers and Non-Smokers. Br Med J 11:384–387

Manzella G, Ferrara P (1967) Sull' importanza des pH della saliva mista umana nella stimolazione dei chimoricettori gustativi. Boll Mal Orecch 85:87–92

Moeschlin S (1965) Klinik und Therapie der Vergiftungen. Thieme, Stuttgart

Pearson J, Finegold MJ, Budzilovich G (1970) The tongue and taste in familial dysantonosmia. Pediatrics 45:739–749

Rauh Ch, Mros B (1966) Geruchsstörungen bei Ozaena. HNO 14:179–180

Rossberg G, Schaupp H, Schmidt W (1966) Geruchs- und Geschmacksvermögen bei Arbeitern der chemischen und metallverarbeitenden Industrie. Z Laryng Rhinol Otol 45:571–589

Schaupp H, Seilz J (1969) Geruch und Geschmack bei endokrinen Erkrankungen. Arch Klin Exp Ohr Nas Kehlk Heilk 195:179–191

Schaupp H (1969) Unpublished investigation

Schaupp H, Bertram KJ, Schulz-Freywald G (1972) Radiogene Geschmacksschäden. Z Laryng Rhinol Otol 51:336–343

Schaupp H, Wohnaut K (1978) Geschmacksstörungen durch Munddesinfizientien. Ein Beitrag zur Erkennung von Nebenwirkungen hexetidin- und chlorhexidinhaltiger Präparate. HNO 26:235–241

Tarab S (1955) Troubles de la gustation après tonsillectomie. Pract Oto Rhino Laryng 17:260–262

Some Remarks About the Olfactory Nerve from the Surgical Point of View

H. DIETZ, Hannover/FRG

The olfactory nerve, together with the smell-brain, is an important factor in the history of the development of the vertebrale animals. The human brain has evolved at the expense of the smell-brain, which for the human being is of almost no importance. Also, in neurosurgery the olfactory nerve is of no vital importance. It gains significance only because it is the first of the cranial nerves, and also quite vulnerable. But apart from those cases where one has to operate because of the olfactory nerve (meningioma of the olfactory region or rhinoliquorrhea through the lamina cribriformis) it rather hinders the surgeon who operates transfrontally. This is the reason why many surgeons think that if the local situation during surgery makes it necessary, the first cranial nerve may be easily sectioned. In fact, nowadays a perfect sense of smell is not as important for the human being as it had been for his vertebrates, where it was vital. In many cases of one-sided anosmia the patients had not even been aware of it and in those cases where it was known, it was not perceived as a major disadvantage. Reduced ability of the sense of smell usually is not experienced as a serious handicap. Accordingly, section of the olfactory nerve in the course of operation is even justified if it is done only to gain a better survey of the operating field or access to it.

Publications of neurosurgical procedures say nothing about the olfactory nerve. Wherever something is said about surgery in the anterior fossa or the frontobasis as a transpassing region towards the structures dorsal of the sphenoid wings, it is only mentioned that one should 'protect' the olfactory nerve as far as possible, but that one may, if necessary, section it, for example:

if it "hinders" the surgeon in the view,
if it disturbes the continuation of the operation,
if it threatens to rupture in cases of excessive tension,
if the olfactory bulb threatens to burst out of its bed.

The region of the lamina cribriformis presents great anatomic variations and as diverse are the circumstances the surgeon may find at the olfactory tract and bulb:

the length and thickness of the olfactory nerve may differ notably,
the consistency and therefore the resistance against compression and tension may be very diverse,
the olfactory bulb may sometimes be strongly adherent to the olfactory fossa,
at other times it may detach from its bed at the slightest touch,
the olfactory tract may tear off just behind the bulb and the bulb remains, as chained on strong fila olfactoria, firmly in the fossa,
several blood vessels may accompany the nerve and may be wounded or twisted and ruptured at the slightest touch,

Table 1. Olfactory nerve lesions

I. After operations in or through the anterior cranial fossa (102 patients)

Unilateral operation (83)			*Bifrontal* operations (19)	
Total anosmia	5×	(6%)	8×	(42%)
One-sided anosmia	14×	(17%)	4×	(21%)
Disturbances of smell				
one-sided	21×	(25%)	–	–
bilateral	10×	(12%)	–	–
Slight hyposmia only	8×	(10%)	7×	(37%)
Normal sense of smell	25×	(30%)	–	–
	83	(100%)	19	(100%)

II. After frontobasal head injury with anterior fossa fractures

Findings	Preoperative (128)		Postoperative (102)	
Examined cases	*61*	*(48%)*	*102*	*(100%)*
Total anosmia	13	(21% v. 61)	14	
One-sided anosmia	15	(24.6%)	56	
Disturbance of smell				
one-sided	5	(8%)	8	
bilateral	1	(1.6%)		
Normal sense of smell	14	(23%)		
Findings not usable	13	(21%)		
	61	(100%)	102	
No examination	67	(52% v. 128)		

in some cases the olfactory tract is of such a tough consistency, as if it were a true nerve,
it may bleed quite strongly from the vascular connections to the ethmoidal arteries when detaching the bulb from the fossa,
sometimes the fossa, after detaching the bulb, remains completely dry.

Because of these many variations it is not always possible to protect the olfactory nerve when using a transfrontal or frontolateral-subfrontal procedure. Especially in cases of a fronto-lateral access (for example, towards the hypophysis, or on aneurysma of the anterior communicating artery) it is recommended not to prepare the nerve in its full length but to visualize it only in its middle and posterior parts and to lift it slightly. An anatomic preparation is not possible. Quite often anosmia is seen in the postoperative period, although the surgeon thought that he had protected the nerve. It is often believed that due to a loosening of the fila olfactoria blood enters into the lamina cribriformis, thus causing loss of function by secondary tissue alteration. Such a finding which normally is final and not reversible can only be observed in the postoperative period but cannot be changed. It is almost impossible to find in the literature results of postoperative check-ups about the ability to smell after having undergone a transfrontal operation.

We have gathered material about the postoperative status of the sense of smell from two groups, each consisting of 102 patients, who in the last 8 years underwent:

I. a one-sided or bilateral transfrontal operation (hypophyseal adenomas, aneurysms, lateral sphenoid wing meningiomas, frontal lobe tumors, etc.),
II. operation after a frontobasal head injury because of rhinoliquorrhea.

In the first group, the non-traumatic cases, in 83 patients with a one-sided transfrontal operation we found a disturbance in the sense of smell in 70 percent: that is; a complete anosmia in five patients, a one-sided anosmia in 14, and 39 suffered a disturbance of sense of smell. Twenty five patients (30 percent) remained without any handicap. In 19 patients after a bifrontal operation, a complete anosmia was noticed in eight, one-sided anosmia in four, and no or only a slight hyposmia in seven. Eight patients were not aware of suffering a disturbance, 21 were not bothered by it.

In the second group, the frontobasal injuries, 61 patients underwent an examination of sense of smell before the operation. Out of these 34 (56 percent) suffered a disturbance (six hyposmia, 28 anosmia, from these 13 complete and 15 one-sided). Of the non-examined cases, in two thirds olfaction was not tested, in one third it was not possible to examine because of the mental state or because of the injuries. In these patients it was noticed during the operation that the olfactory tract or bulb was injured fortythree times on one side and eight times on both sides. In 19 patients the nerve was cut by the surgeon in order to cover the defect with a galeaperiost plastic (13 times one-sided, 6 times on both sides). Thus, in 70 patients we found anosmia during the postoperative check-up (14 times complete, 56 times one-sided). This means that within the traumatic cases over five times more anosmias were found (69 percent) than in patients with tumors or aneurysms.

In the literature much can be read about posttraumatic disturbances of olfactory sensation. The percentage in frontobasal injuries is quoted between three and eighty percent, if one considers that the traumatic consequences also can be related to the central smell system or that local changes in the mucous membranes of the nose during the acute phase make evaluation difficult. Meanwhile, when damage exists in connection with an injury, it depends vitally on the skill and care of the surgeon to avoid damage to the olfactory nerve during operation. We found 23 percent non-traumatic postoperative anosmias.

Preservation of the Olfactory Tract Following Operation on Anterior Communicating Artery Aneurysm Using Bifrontal Craniotomy, and Its Functional Prognosis

J. SUZUKI, T. YOSHIMOTO, and K. MIZOI, Sendai/Japan

Introduction

Various methods for approaching anterior communicating artery (AComA) aneurysms have been reported [1, 2, 3, 4, 6, 8]. Since the bilateral feeding and draining arteries can be identified and preserved, the entire area around the aneurysm exposed, and damage to normal brain tissue avoided, we have come to use bifrontal craniotomy by means of which the aneurysm can be approached between the cerebral hemispheres with maximum safety and certainty [3, 6]. The one shortcoming of this method, however, has been that damage to the olfactory tracts has been inevitable.

Between 1961 and 1979, 1500 patients with directly operated cerebral aneurysms were treated at the Department of Neurosurgery, Institute of Brain Diseases, Tohoku University. Five hundred and nine of those cases were aneurysms of the AComA (Table 1). From this experience, we have realized that preservation of the olfactory tract is possible in such cases, even when bifrontal craniotomy is used [5]. In the current paper we report the methods used for preservation of the olfactory tract and discuss the functional prognosis for olfaction, based upon our experience since 1976.

Table 1. Total aneurysm patients treated by direct intracranial operation from 1961 to 1979.

Site of AN	No. of cases	Deaths in hospital (%)
AcomA	509	32 (6.3%)
IC	345	20 (5.8%)
MC	265	10 (3.8%)
AC	79	3 (3.8%)
VB	44	2 (4.5%)
Mult.	258	22 (8.5%)
Total	1500	89 (5.9%)

AcomA = anterior communicating artery. IC = internal carotid artery; MC = middle cerebral artery; AC = anterior cerebral artery; VB = vertebrobasilar system; Mult = multiple aneurysms

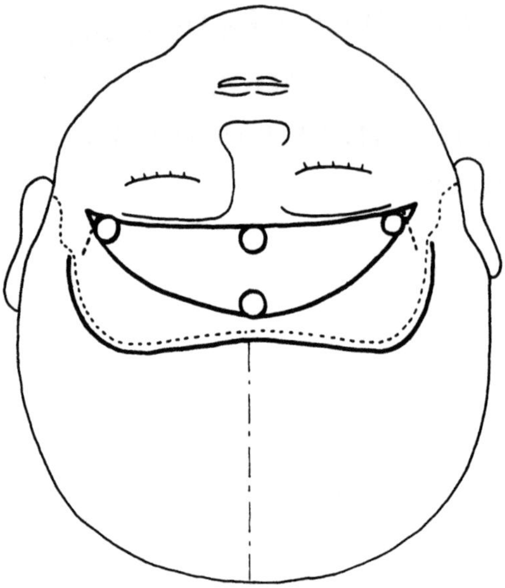

Fig. 1. Skin incision and craniotomy

I. Operative Technique

The surgical technique used in preservation of the olfactory tract when treating AComA aneurysms using bifrontal craniotomy is as follows: The skin is incised slightly posterior to the frontal hair line. Four burr holes are made as shown in Fig. 1, and the anterior edge of the bone flap is cut down frontally as close to the orbital edge as possible. Infrequently, the frontal sinus is opened, but there is little danger of infection if sufficient care is taken. After cutting the dura mater and falx, treatment of the olfactory tract begins.

A unilateral frontal pole is gently retracted away from the anterior fossa and the arachnoid membrane and small blood vessels in contact with the dura mater are carefully cauterized. In doing so, the portion of the olfactory bulb adhering to the cribiform plate of the olfactory tract can be seen. The contralateral olfactory tract is then approached in the same manner. The tracts are then bluntly separated from the frontal lobe, a process which is easily accomplished as far as two cm from the olfactory bulb. However, since there is danger that one of the olfactory tracts can easily be separated too extensively, if both tracts are not treated together, the left and right olfactory tracts are separated alternatively little by little (Fig. 2). At the portion of the basal frontal lobe to which the olfactory tract adheres, the tract is separated from the brain with a thin spatula. If even a small amount of arachnoid membrane, fibrous tissue or blood vessels remains adherent to the olfactory tract, it can be pulled and damaged during the operation due to an only slight movement of the frontal lobe. The key to successful separation of the tract from the brain is never to apply pressure in a downward direction posteriorly from the olfactory bulb, but to continually apply upward pressure (toward the olfactory bulb) on the frontal lobe to which the tract is adherent. The proximal portion of the olfactory

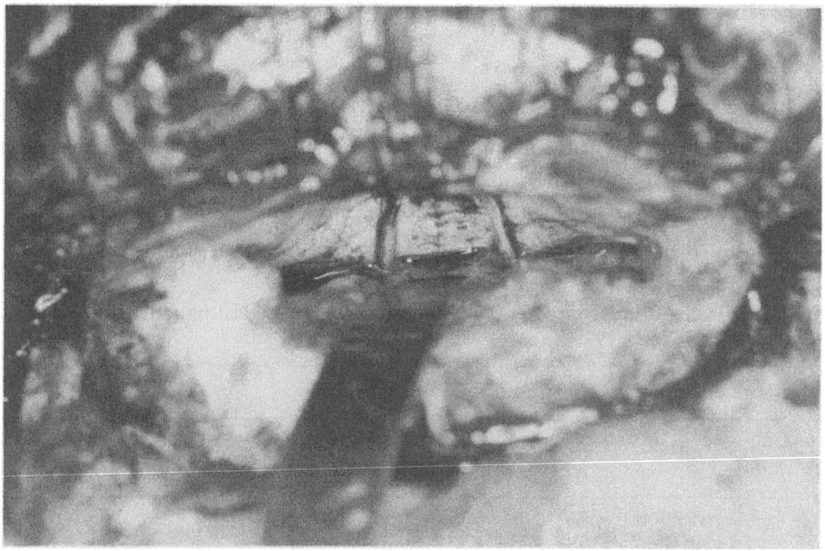

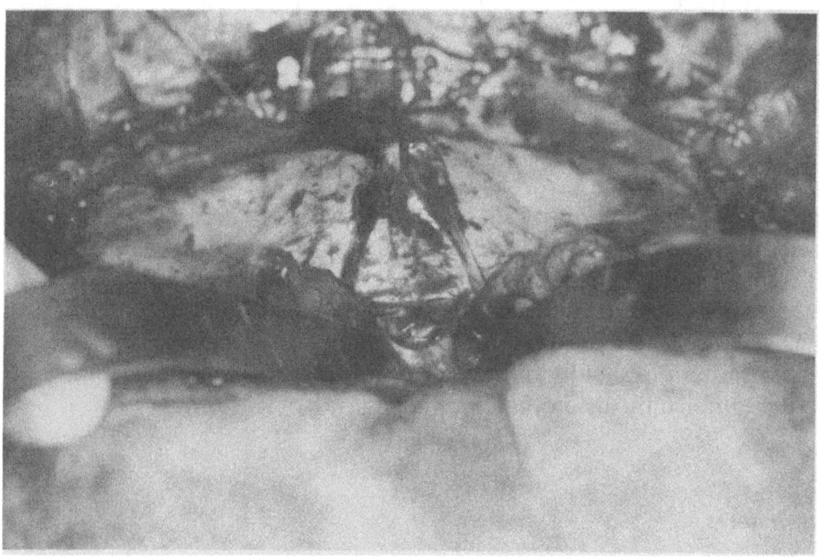

Figs. 2 and 3. Preservation of the bilateral olfactory tracts

tract is found at the termination of the internal carotid artery, but it is not necessary to separate the tract from the brain that far. Rather, separation as far as about 1.5 cm anterior to the termination is sufficient (Fig. 3).

Upon completion of this process, the bilateral A_1 portions of the anterior cerebral arteries are identified and the aneurysm is treated using the interhemispheric approach. The olfactory tract will not in any way be an obstruction during treatment of the aneurysm.

II. Cases of Olfactory Tract Preservation and Its Functional Prognosis

1. Subjects and Methods

Subjects were the 110 patients with AComA aneurysm treated between 1976 and 1979. Radical treatment of the aneurysm was performed in all cases using bifrontal craniotomy by one of the authors (J. Suzuki). The operative results and follow-up results after four to 48 months are shown in Table 2.

Table. 2. Operative results on discharge and at follow-up review in 110 patients with AcomA aneurysms treated from 1976 to 1979.

Results on discharge		Results at follow-up review					
Result	No. of cases (%)	Excel-lent	Good	Fair	Poor	Dead	Lost to follow-up
Excellent	68 (61.8%)	66	0	1	0	0	1
Good	21 (19.1%)	14	3	0	1	3	0
Fair	10 (9.1%)	4	2	2	0	1	1
Poor	9 (8.2%)	0	0	2	1	3	3
Dead	2 (1.8%)						
Total	110	84 (77.8%)	5 (4.6%)	5 (4.6%)	2 (1.9%)	7 (6.5%)	5 (4.6%)

By examination of the records of all 110 patients, preservation of the olfactory tract was determined. Next, the presence of olfaction was investigated by postal questionnaire in all cases except two hospital deaths. Finally, objective study of olfaction in 55 patients, chosen at random, was made by an otorhinolaryngologist. The following tests were administered using a T and T olfactometer [7]: detection thresholds, recognition thresholds, and the alinamin test. The overall capability for olfaction was determined by the otorhinolaryngologist.

2. Results

a) Operative findings

Both olfactory tracts were preserved in 38 of the 110 patients (35 percent), one tract preserved in 35 patients (32 percent), both were damaged in 29 patients (26 percent), and the condition unclear due to incomplete records in eight patients (7 percent). In relation to the year of surgery, it was found that 53 percent of the patients with bilateral damage were operated upon in 1976, 15 percent in 1977, 15 percent in 1978, and 16 percent in 1979 (Table 3).

b) Subjective olfaction

Forty two of the 108 patients questioned replied that olfaction was normal (39 percent), 52 responded negatively (48 percent), and in 14 patients (13 percent)

Table 3. Preservation of the olfactory tract as determined by operative findings in the 110 patients with AcomA aneurysm treated from 1976 to 1979.

	1976	1977	1978	1979	Total (%)
Bilateral preservation	5	12	13	8	38 (35%)
Unilateral preservation	7	17	4	7	35 (32%)
Bilateral damage	17	6	3	3	29 (26%)
Unclear	3	5	0	0	8 (7%)
Total	32	40	20	18	110

determination was impossible due to late death, consciousness disturbance or failure to respond to the questionnaire. It was found that 47 percent of the patients with bilateral olfactory tract preservation reported normal olfaction, whereas 34 percent with unilateral preservation and 33 percent with bilateral damage reported normal olfaction (Table 4).

c) Results of objective testing of olfaction

Investigation was made of 48 patients, excepting only seven in whom nasal disorders causing disturbances of olfaction were found (four reporting olfaction, three reporting no olfaction). It was seen that 21 of the 25 patients (84 percent) reporting normal olfaction were found objectively to be normal and four (16 percent) were anosmic. All of the patients reporting no olfaction were found objectively to be anosmic. In relation to the operative findings, it was seen that of the 23 patients with bilateral preservation, 15 reported normal olfaction, 14 of whom were found objectively to be normal and one of whom was anosmic. All eight patients reporting anosmia were found objectively to be anosmic. Among the 13 patients with unilateral olfactory tract damage, four reported normal olfaction, three of whom were found objectively to be normal and one anosmic. All nine who reported no olfaction were found to be anosmic. Among the eight patients with bilateral olfactory tract damage, three reported normal olfaction, two of whom were found objectively to be normal and one of whom was anosmic. All five who reported no olfaction were found objectively to be anosmic.

Table. 4. Relationship between the presence of subjective olfaction and the operative findings of the olfactory tracts.

		Operative findings of the olfactory tracts				Total
		Bilateral preservation	Unilateral preservation	Bilateral damage	Unclear	
Subjective olfaction	Present	18	12	9	3	42 (39%)
	Absent	16	21	12	3	52 (48%)
		4	2	6	2	14 (13%)
	Total	38	35	27	8	108 cases

Table. 5. Results of objective testing of olfaction.

Operative findings (cases)	Subjective olfaction (cases)		Objective study of olfaction (cases)			
Bilateral preservation (23)	present	(15)	normal	(14)	anosmia	(1)
	absent	(8)	normal	(0)	anosmia	(8)
Unilateral preservation (13)	present	(4)	normal	(3)	anosmia	(1)
	absent	(9)	normal	(0)	anosmia	(9)
Bilateral damage (8)	present	(3)	normal	(2)	anosmia	(1)
	absent	(5)	normal	(0)	anosmia	(5)
Unclear (14)	present	(3)	normal	(2)	anosmia	(1)
	absent	(1)	normal	(0)	anosmia	(1)
Total (48)	present	(25)	normal	(21)	anosmia	(4)
	absent	(23)	normal	(0)	anosmia	(23)

III. Discussion

Until recently, it has been thought inevitable that olfactory tract damage occurs during bifrontal craniotomy and no systematic investigations of the methods for preservation have been reported. Only the brief statement concerning the olfactory tract by Pool, who has reported treatment of a large number of AComA aneurysms using bifrontal craniotomy, can be found: 'One frontal pole is retracted very gently and gradually until the olfactory tract can be seen and divided by cautery'. From our experiences using bifrontal craniotomy, we have found bilateral olfactory nerve damage in 26 percent of our patients, but the frequency of such damage has gradually decreased. In 1970, 17 of 32 cases of 53 percent had olfactory tract damage, but in 1977 and 1978, only 15 percent and, in 1979, 16 percent had bilateral damage. It is concluded, therefore, that by using this method the olfactory tract can be preserved in a large percentage of such patients. In other words, the greatest drawback of bifrontal craniotomy can be overcome, allowing for this operative approach to be used not only for AComA aneurysms, but also for brain tumors, etc.

We have also investigated the quality of olfaction in our patients with unilaterally or bilaterally preserved olfactory tracts. Eighteen of the 38 patients with bilaterally preserved tracts (47 percent) and 12 of the 35 patients with unilaterally preserved tracts (34 percent) reported normal olfaction. Such results are somewhat contrary to expectations, especially the fact that some 42 percent of the patients with bilateral preservation reported anosmia. This is probably due to damage to the olfactory bulb itself, despite the fact that the olfactory tract appeared to have been preserved intact. Such findings indicate that still further care must be taken at operation.

Among the findings concerning subjective sense of olfaction, it is especially interesting that one third of the patients who had their bilateral olfactory tracts damaged or severed during operation reported normal olfaction and that two of the three who were tested objectively were found to be normal. There are currently various internationally accepted examination methods with regard to vision and hearing, but similar methods for olfaction have not been devised. This is thought to be due to the fact that certain aspects of olfaction remain ambiguous and perhaps not subject to objective measure. The T and T olfactometer [7] used in the current study was constructed with the cooperation of departments of otorhinolaryngology, physiology, and psychology from 14 universities with the support of the Ministries of Education and Public Welfare. It is thought to be a reliable instrument for measuring olfactory function. Regardless, there are still many uncertainties concerning olfaction in general. In order to discuss olfactory disturbances with any degree of certainty, it will therefore be necessary to consider operative findings, subjective symptoms, the results of objective tests of olfaction, etc. and still collect larger numbers of patients.

Summary

Based upon 110 patients with AComA aneurysm approached via bifrontal craniotomy, we discuss preservation of the olfactory tracts and the functional prognosis for olfaction.

1. It is possible to preserve the olfactory tracts bilaterally or unilaterally in over 80 percent of such patients.

2. With regard to the correlation between surgical findings and subjective sense of olfaction, it was found that 51 percent of the patients with bilateral preservation, 37 percent with unilateral preservation and 33 percent of those with bilateral olfactory tract damage reported normal olfaction.

3. Objective examination of olfaction by an otolaryngologist showed that 84 percent of the patients reporting normal olfaction had normal olfaction indeed, whereas all of those reporting no olfaction were anosmic.

References

1. French LA, Chou SN, et al. (1966) Aneurysm of the anterior communicating artery. J Neurosurg 24: 1058–1062
2. Kempe LG, Vander Ark GD (1971) Anterior communicating artery aneurysms. Gyrus rectus approach. Neurochirurgia (Stuttg) 14:63–70
3. Kodama N, Ebina T, et al. (1978) Surgery of anterior communicating artery aneurysm – from the experiences of 346 cases –. Brain Nerve (Tokyo) 30:895–909 (English abstract)
4. Pool JL (1972) Bifrontal craniotomy for anterior communicating artery aneurysms. J Neurosurg 36:212–220
5. Suzuki J, Hori S (1973) A new surgical method for anterior communicating artery aneurysms – without doing damage to the brain and olfactory nerve. Operation (Tokyo) 27:1079–1084 (Jpn)
6. Suzuki J, Kodama N, et al. (1979) Surgical treatment of Anterior Communicating Artery Aneurysms: From the experiences of 346 cases. In: Suzuki J (ed.) Cerebral Aneurysms – experiences with 1000 directly operated cases. NEURON, Tokyo p 238–243
7. Takagi S (1979) Olfaction. Otolaryngology (Tokyo) 25:634–644 (Jpn)
8. Tindall GT, Kapp J, et al. (1970) A combined technique for treating certain aneurysms of of the anterior communicating artery. J Neurosurg 33:41–47

The Nervus terminalis

A. PERNECZKY, Vienna/Austria

Three so-called nerves enter the telencephalon from the region of the nose. They constitute the fila olfactoria, the nervus vomeronasalis and the nervus terminalis. The nervus vomeranasalis connects the vomeronasal organ with the olfactory bulb, which area is connected with the amygdaloid complex. These connections and the similarity in structure of the accessory bulb and the main olfactory bulb suggest that the vomeronasal nerve is a special differentiation of the olfactory system. The third nerve of this region, the nervus terminalis, was mentioned first by Fritsch (1878) in vertebrates, who noted the position of such root fibers on the dorsal surface of the telencephalon. To Pinkus (1895) belongs the honor of tracing it from the nasal sac to the preoptic recess in protopterus. This first reasonably definite account of the nerve led to its being termed the nerve of Pinkus.

Material and Method

We investigated morphologically the olfactory region in three representatives of the selachian (shark) and in human embryos. First we dissected under the operating microscope and then we made histological slides using special stains.

Results

In the shark the nervus terminalis is macroscopically also a thick, independent nerve lying ventromedially from the olfactory tract and olfactory bulb (Fig. 1). The nerve has a larger ganglion in his intracranial course.

In human embryo of 95 mm length we found the nervus terminalis entering the ventromedial portion of the telencephalon, in the region of the lamina terminalis by small roots. Traced peripheralward, the small nerves run along and medially the olfactory tract and olfactory bulb. They pass through the lamina cribrosa, reach the nasal septum. These are numerous small ganglia scattered along the intracranial course of the nerve (Fig. 2).

The histological investigations showed that the caliber of the fibers constituting the nervus terminalis is like that of preganglionic and postganglionic fibers of the sympathetic system. The cells in the ganglia of the nervus terminalis are multipolar, bipolar and pseudounipolar.

Discussion

The nervus terminalis is found in all representatives of the vertebrates except the birds. The nerve is described in man by Johnston (1913), Brookover (1914),

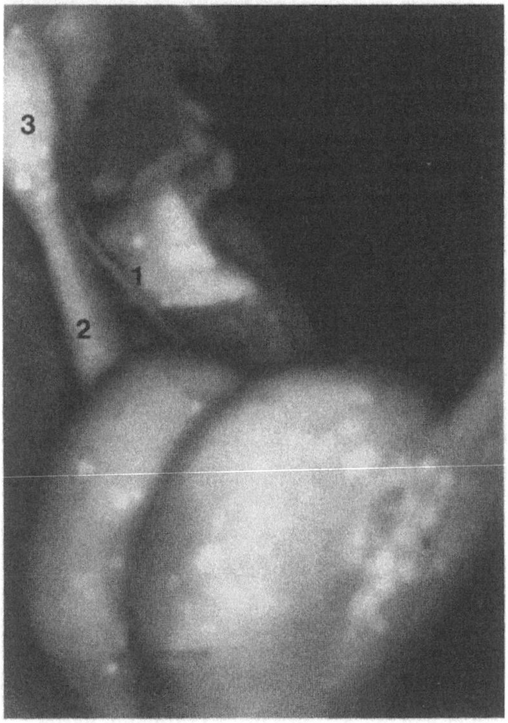

Fig. 1. The nervus terminalis in shark. *1* N. terminalis, *2* olfactory tract, *3* olfactory bulb

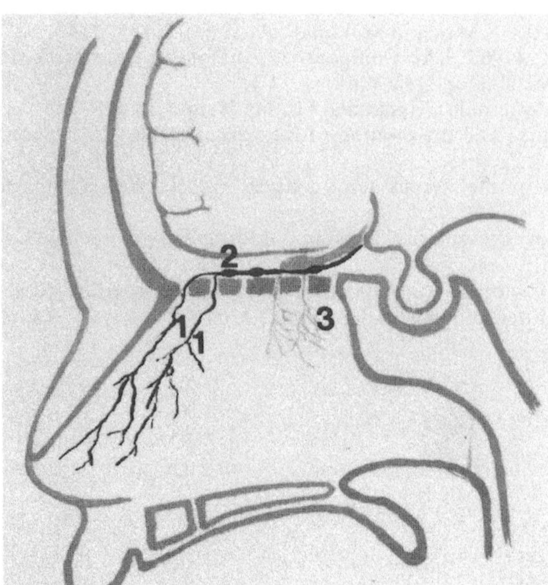

Fig. 2. The nervus terminalis in man (parasagittal section). *1* N. terminalis, *2* Ganglion of n. terminalis, *3* N. olfactorius

McCotter (1915), Larsell (1918), Pearson (1941), Clara (1959) Kappers et al. (1967). Brookover (1914) found, that sympathetic chain connections with the sphenopalatine nerve and ganglia are present. Larsell (1918) considered the nervus terminalis as vasomotor, an interpretation in agreement with the earlier suggestion of Huber and Guild (1913). Johnston (1913) stated, that 'in all vertebrates there is a receptive component in the nervus terminalis supplying ectodermal territory'. The different types of cells in the ganglia of the nervus terminalis (Pearson 1941, DeVanna 1951) show the mixed character of the nerve.

Conclusion

The nervus terminalis includes sensory fibers and vegetative efferent components and enters the telencephalon in the region of the supraoptic recess, so anterior to (and essentially dorsal to) the sulcus limitans diencephali. Therefore the nerve is homologous, in a broad way, to the dorsal spinal and lateral cranial nerves.

References

Brookover CH (1914) The Nervus terminalis in adult man. J Comp Neurol 24:131–136

Clara M (1959) Das Nervensystem des Menschen. Thieme, Leipzig

DeVanna F (1951) Distribuzione periferica del Nervo terminale e sue cellule nei mammiferi. Arch Ital Anat Embriol 56:1–18

Fritsch G (1878) Untersuchungen über den feinen Bau des Fischgehirnes. Gutmann, Berlin

Huber GC, Guild SR (1913) Observations on the peripheral distribution of the nervous terminalis in Mammalia. Anat Rec 7:253–271

Johnston JB (1913) The Nervous terminalis in Reptiles and Mammals. J. Comp Neurol 23:97–122

Johnston JB (1914) The Nervous terminalis in Man and Mammals. Anat Rec 8:185–214

Kappers CUA, Huber GC, Crosby EC (1967) The Comparative Anatomy of the Nervous System of Vertebrates, Including Man. Hafner, New York

Larsell O (1918) Studies on the nervous terminalis: Mammals. J Comp Neurol 30:198–215

McCotter RE (1915) A note on the course and distribution of the nervus terminalis in man. Anat Rec 9:43–58

Pearson AA (1941) The development of the nervus terminalis in man. J Comp Neurol 75:39–55

Pinkus F (1895) Die Hirnnerven des Protopterus annectus. Morphol Arb (Schwalbe) 4:275–304

Pinkus F (1905) Über den zwischen Olfactorius- und Opticusursprung das Vorderhirn (Zwischenhirn) verlassenden Hirnnerven der Dipnoer und Selachia. Arch Anat Physiol Suppl Bd. 447–492

Olfactory Nerve

M. Samii, Hannover/FRG

At the suggestion of Professor Suzuki we have been working this year on the technique of preserving the olfactory nerve in all our operative procedures in the anterior cranial fossa. Our experiences confirm the results of Professor Suzuki. As an example I would like to demonstrate the following patients, in whom the preoperatively intact sense of smell remained preserved postoperatively.

The first case is a spontaneous frontobasal cerebrospinal fluid fistula with slight hyposmia. After performing four drill holes a bifrontal osteoplastic craniotomy and ligation of the superior sagittal sinus was accomplished. Both olfactory nerves were then dissected free up to the chiasm angle. Afterwards a typical pedceld galea-periostal plastic up to the sphenoid plane was accomplished. Fixation sutures were applicated between both olfactory nerves and also one suture lateral to each (Fig. 1).

In the next patients we face a bilobed aneurysm of the anterior cerebral artery with severe intracerebral bleeding. Both olfactory nerves are prepared free above the sphenoid plane and over the optic nerves. The anterior cerebral arteries are also exposed. One can see the exact topographic relation between the olfactory nerve and optic nerve and both anterior cerebral arteries (Fig. 2a). Exposure of the

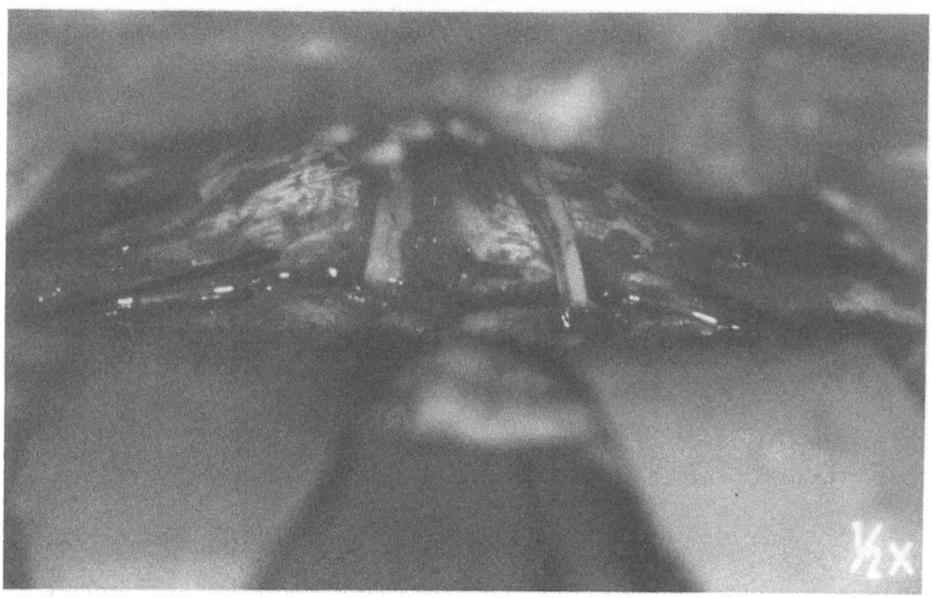

Fig. 1. Bifrontal approach to the anterior cerebral fossa with preservation of the olfactory nerves in a patient with frontobasal cerebrospinal fluid fistula. One can see the fixation sutures between both olfactory nerves and also one suture lateral to each

aneurysm of the anterior communicating artery (Fig. 2b). Clipping of the aneurysm with preservation of the anterior communication artery. Both olfactory nerves are kept in continuity. In this case also the preoperatively intact sense of smell was preserved postoperatively.

Obviously, for most people the sense of smell means a vital function of life, whereas its absence, for example in some professions, might be felt almost as an invalidity. I am of the opinion that we have to attempt this procedure based on the pioneer work of Professor Suzuki and our results.

In addition I would like to comment on tumors of the olfactory nerves, which should be mentioned in this connection. Unfortunately, the olfactory nerves in case of these tumors are either completely destroyed in their function before surgery, or the radical nature of tumor removal requires the sacrifice of the olfactory nerves.

The olfactory or esthesio-neuromas are very rare tumors. In the world literature, according to Blockmanis, until 1972 only 40 cases are mentioned. Skolnik and co-workers reported on a five year survival rate of 52 percent. The frequency of local recurrence, according to these authors, is about 50 percent, and the formation of metastases into the regional lymphatic nodes and the lungs is about 20 percent. Therefore, these tumors are clinically malignant, although micromorphological malignant signs are rarely present. The opinions as to therapy differ enormously. Tringwald (1966) as well as Caballes (1965) have pointed out that olfactory neuromas are radiosensitive. However, they cannot be cured by radiotherapy alone.

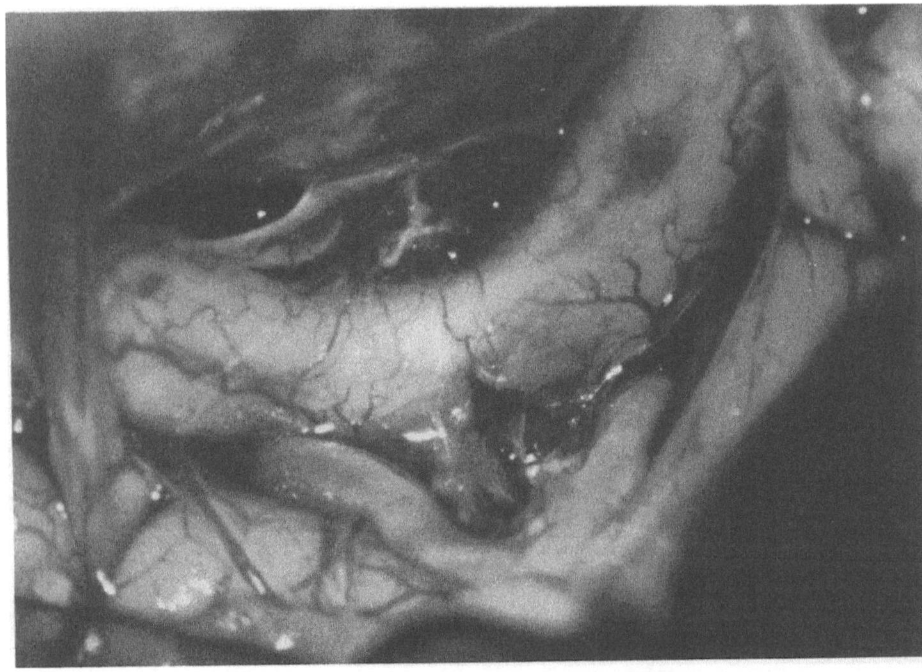

Fig. 2a. Both olfactory nerves are dissected free above the sphenoid plane and over the optic nerves in a patient with an anterior communicating artery aneurysm. The anterior cerebral arteries are also exposed. One can see the exact topographic relation between the olfactory and optic nerve as well as the anterior cerebral arteries

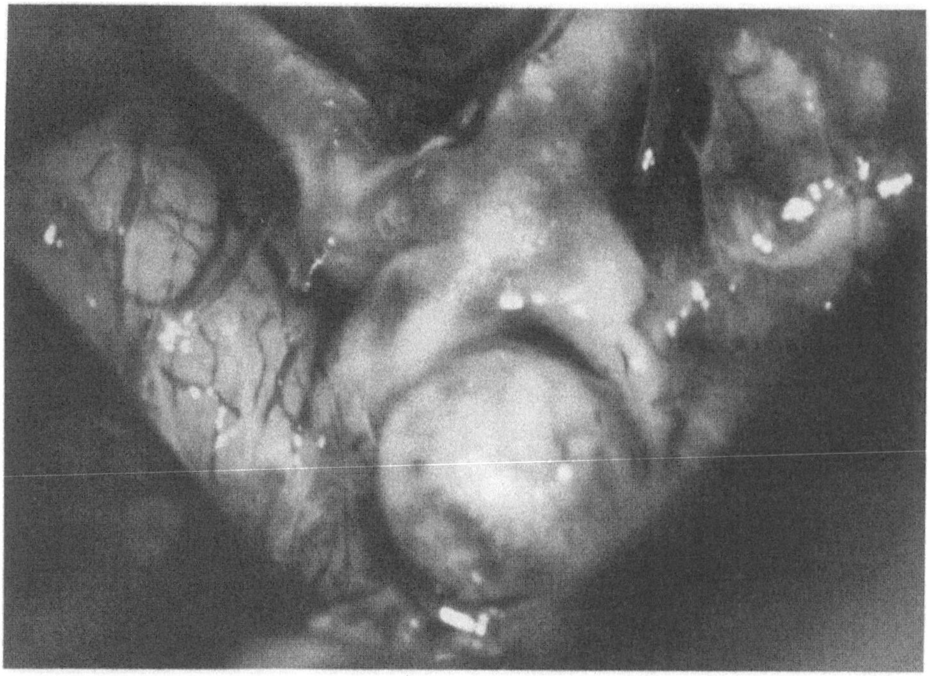

Fig. 2b. The same patient as Fig. 2a. Exposure of the bilobed aneurysm of the anterior communicating artery

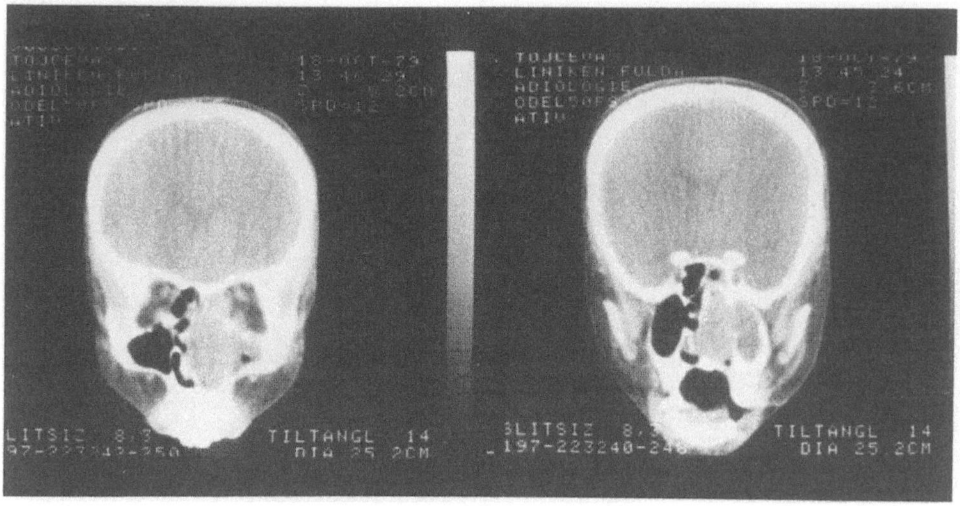

Fig. 3a. CT scan of a 29 year old patient with a large tumor of the left nasal cavity with partial involvement of the adjacent paranasal sinuses. Histological examination resulted in a so-called olfactory neurocytoma

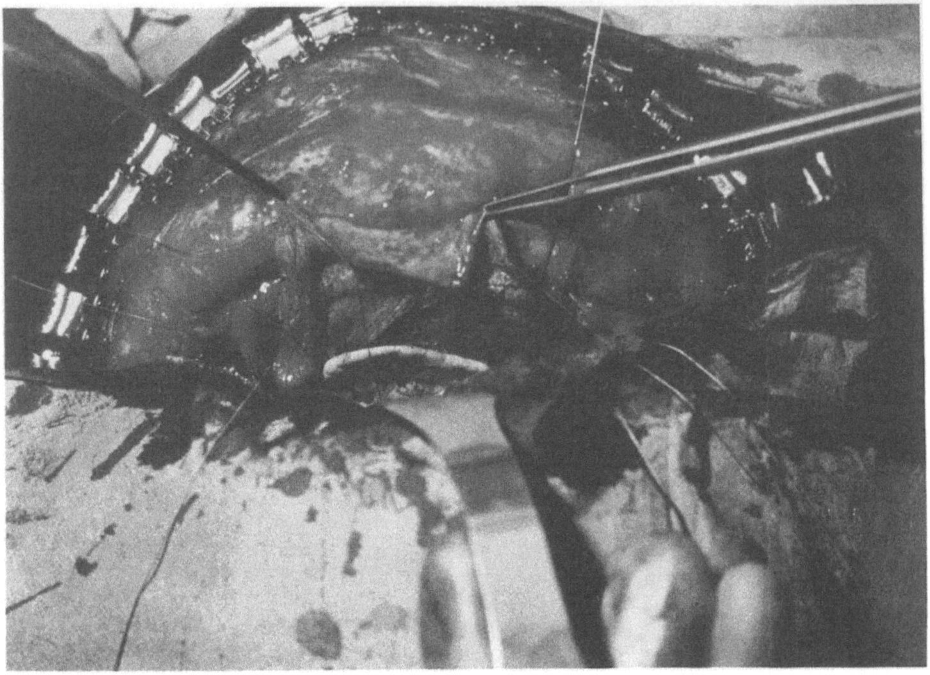

Fig. 3b. The same patient as Fig. 3a. After resection of the dura protecting the lamina cribosa, the ethmoid roof and the anterior part of the sphenoid plane, the crista galli was removed. One can see the reconstruction of the skull base in three layers by dura flaps, Palacos R as well as pediceld galeaperiostal flap

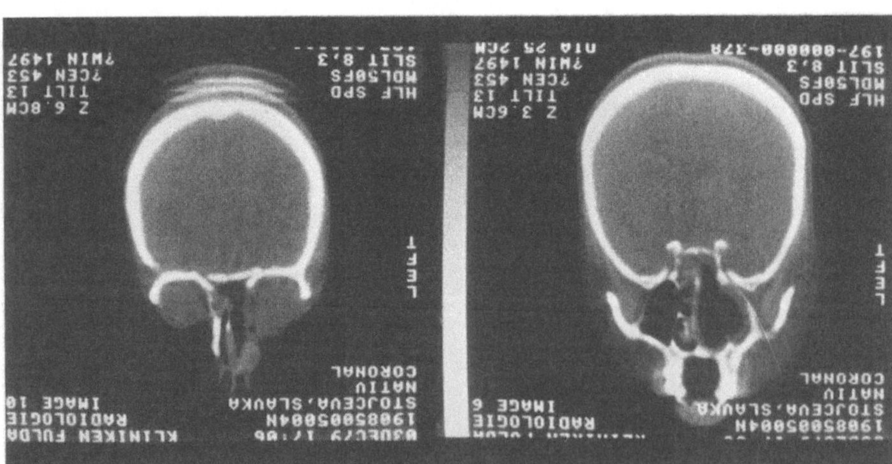

Fig. 3c. The same patient as Fig. 3a and b. Postoperative CT scan. The tumor is totally removed and the skull base defect is bridged by means of Palacos

Because of the malignant biological behaviour of the tumor, radical operation with removal of the tumor matrix is necessary (Huet et al. 1953).

A 29 year old Yugoslavian patient contacted Professor Draf and myself because of disturbance of nasal breathing. The histological examination of the grey-reddish, slightly bleeding tumor, which had grown into the vestibule of the nose on the left side, resulted in a so-called olfactory neurocytoma. CT scan demonstrated a large tumor of the left nasal cavity with partial involvement of the adjacent paranasal sinuses. Skull base destruction was not confirmed (Fig. 3a). After bifrontal craniotomy, both olfactory nerves were dissected up to the optic nerve and transected there. Subsequently the olfactory tract was lifted up to the front, and the olfactory fibres were transected. After resection of the dura protecting the lamina cribrosa, the ethmoid roof, and the anterior part of the sphenoid plane, the crista galli was removed and the osseous skull base shifted caudally. We then performed reconstruction of the skull base in three layers by dural flaps, Palacos R as well as a pediceld galeaperiostal flap (Fig. 3b). In the next step the rhinosurgical exposure and removal of the tumor block including the mucous membrane and the adjacent bone was performed by W. Draf. Fig. 3c demonstrates the postoperative CT scan: The tumor was totally removed and the skull base defect bridged by means of Palacos.

References

Blockmanis A (1972) Esthesioneuroepithelioma: A report of two cases and discussions of the management. Can J Otolaryng 1:43

Caballes RL (1965) Psammona bodies in olfactory neuroblastoma. Laryngoscope 75:1749

Huet PC et al. (1953) Un cas d'andiohistiocytome des fosses nasales. Ann Otolaryngol (Paris) 70:785–789

Skolnik EM et al. (1966) Olfactory neuroepithelioma. Arch Otolaryngol 61–67

Tringwald FR (1966) Olfactory placode tumors. Laryngoscope 76:267

Optic Nerve

(Second Cranial Nerve)

Optic Nerve, Topographic Anatomy *

J. Lang, Würzburg/FRG

Optic Canal

The optic canal represents from the point of view of practical medicine an important, and biologically interesting portal between the insides of cranium and eye cavity: through the short canal a nerve together with its layers and the ophthalmic artery reach the orbita. A corresponding large vein does not exist. In newborns it is like a canal outlet to the intracranial side which in the mid-canal region and in the orbital exit looks like a rounded and on-point standing triangle or ellipse. The average length of the upper wall of the canal is 5.13 mm and of the lower wall 4.0 mm. Especially during the first two years of life the penetrating cylinder grows to a one-sided and, on the cerebral opening, flattened cylinder.

The orbital cross-section of the canal has an oval shape. Surprisingly, however, the caudal wall of the canal expands postnatally only about 20 percent. The cranial wall, on the other hand, expands about 91 percent of its length, i.e., from 5.13 mm to 9.80 mm. The main growth (30 percent) takes place between birth and second year, and between the eight and ninth year (21 percent) and up to eleventh year of age 93 percent of the adult values are reached. The shortest diameter of the canal cross-section (optic-taille) is located in about the middle of the canal. In newborns it is 3.56 and in adults, on the average, 4.63 mm in size. During the first year of life, the canal expands about 26.4 percent and postnatally totally about 30 percent. The limit values for the upper wall of the canal in our investigations vary between 7.3 and 12 mm. Maniscalco and Habal (1978) give the average length of the upper wall of the canal as 9.22 (5.5–11.5) mm. On the basis of their findings, the average width of the intracranial aperture is 7.18 (5.0–9.5) mm and of the orbital aperture 4.87 (4.0–6.0) mm. This value, as well, is in agreement with our findings, since the optical-taille in adults have an average value of 4.63 (4.0–5.1) mm. The canal width expands on average from 3.56 in newborns during the first trimenon, to 4.23 mm, i.e. about 19 percent. The average height of the canal, measured in the region of optic-taille parallel to the orbit level, is in newborns 4.0 mm whereas the major growth (23 to 96.5 percent of the adult value) occurs up to second year. The average height of canal in adults is 5.1 (4.1–6.2) mm.

The roof of the optic canal in adults according to Maniscalco and Habal (1978), is on the average 2.09 (1.0–3.0) mm thick. We emphasize that two mm rostral to the intracranial aperture postnatally the roof parts of the optic canal are significantly attenuated (see Fig. 1). This part in adults and aged people is covered by a dura lamelle so as to form a regular dural optic canal. Occasionally, from the medial or lateral sides of the upper wall of the canal, tongue-like processes are

* Supported by Deutsche Forschungsgemeinschaft

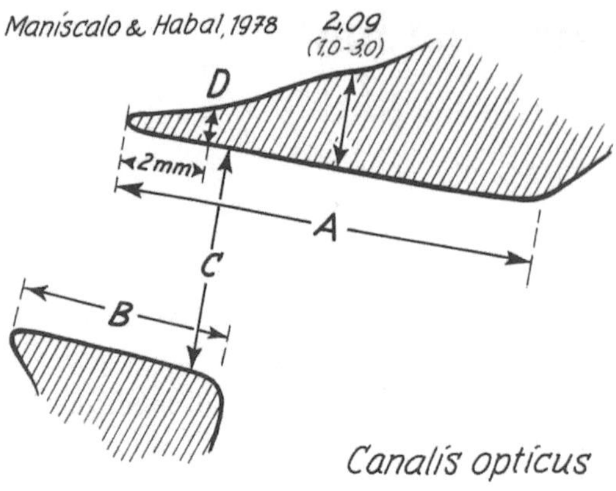

	A	B	C	D
neon.	5,13 (4,5-6,0)	4,0 (3,5-5,0)	4,0 (3,5-5,0)	2,24
2 y.	6,67 (6,0-8,0)	4,85 (4,5-5,5)	4,92 (3,4-6,0)	1,48
ad.	9,80 (7,3-12,0)	4,80 (3,0-9,3)	5,10 (4,1-6,2)	0,75

Fig. 1

projected into the dura lamelle. It is to be emphasized that in one to two percent of adults there are canals of 1 to 2 mm in length and in width, which penetrate the lower radix of the small wedge-bone lining. On the basis of the findings of Adachi, 1927, and angiographic analysis, it is maintained that, with the same percentage, ophthalmic arteries traverse through these canals.

Optic Canal and Pneumatisation of its Wall

Van Alyea, 1941, found that in about 40 percent of the cases the sphenoid sinus reaches the optic canal and thus can surround its upper and lower wall. Less often (in the case of incomplete development of sphenoid concha) the posterior superior ethmoid cells grow towards dorsal and border directly on the optic canal which is 0.5 mm or less and which sometimes shows dehiscences. According to Maniscalco and Habal, 1978, the wall of the optic canal, especially on the orbital aperture, is quite strong having an average thickness of 0.57 (0.4–0.74) mm (origin of muscles) and hence in case of decompressions must be removed by the transethmoid route. In their investigations, the optic canal in 25 percent of the cases was surrounded completely by ethmoid cells. The average length to be removed in cases of transethmoid decompressions, as measured by Maniscalco and Habal, should be 7.3 mm (see Fig. 2).

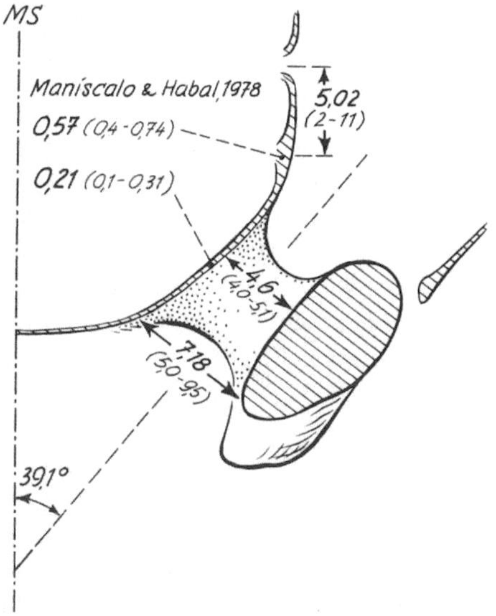

Fig. 2. Canalis opticus

Optic Nerve, Layers, and Vascularisation

The intracranial part of the optic nerve is surrounded by a relatively thick pia mater which sends numerous septs into the nerve. Its blood supply takes place via internal carotid, anterior cerebral, and ophthalmic arteries. In the region of membraneous optic canal there are up to 70 μm wide anastomoses between the dura and nerve vessels. It is to be emphasized that in the subdural slit of this region, especially in the medial and lateral aspects (and also on the tuberculum

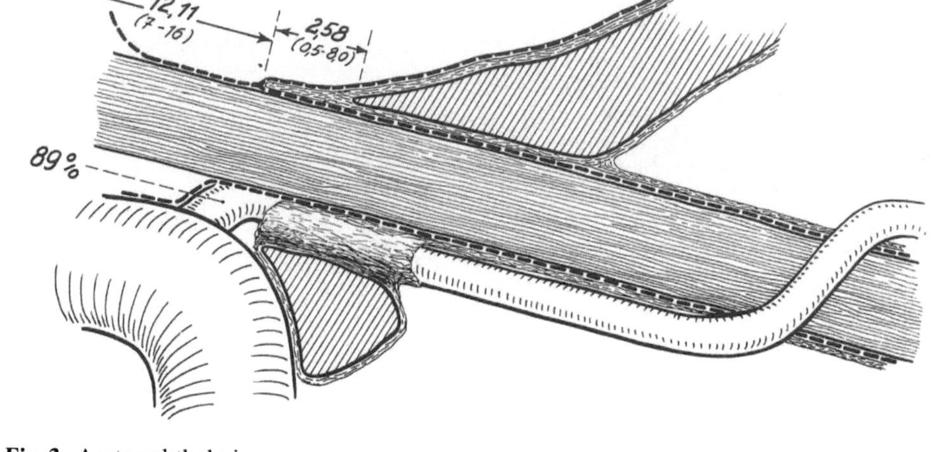

Fig. 3. Aorta ophthalmica

sellae), 100–500 μm long, finger-shaped or complicated form of villi project into the subdural gap. They contain particularly wide capillaries (25 μm). It is assumed that they are involved in the production, and possibly in the resorption, of a subdural fluid, the presence of which was suggested by Penfield, 1924.

Within the optic canal the nerve is followed by its pia layer. The dura mater continues through the canal as a dura-periost layer up to the periorbit. There, the dura-periosteal layers dissolve into a dura layer which make up the dura of optic nerve and a periost layer which becomes periorbit. Also the arachnoid husk can be identified through the whole canal as well as in that part of the nerve lying in the eye cavity. In the optic canal, numerous cords of connective tissue run between the dura-periosteal layer, arachnoid and pia mater of the nerve (Fig. 3).

Ophthalmic Artery

The usually 1.25 mm wide ophthalmic artery stems mostly from above the dural perforation of the internal carotid artery (see Fig. 3). Then it proceeds forward and lateral (normally overcast by optic nerve) and enters in 40 percent medial to the optic nerve, in 35 percent in the middle below it, and in 25 percent laterally below the optic nerve into optic canal and then in the dura-periost layer. In 78 percent of the cases, it reaches the orbita lateral and below the nerve (Fig. 4). Zuckerkandl, 1884, has once observed a case where the ophthalmic artery crossed over the upper side of the nerve in the canal. Such a crossing over on the upper side of the nerve is seen intraorbitally in 85 percent of Europeans, in 93.5 percent of Japanese

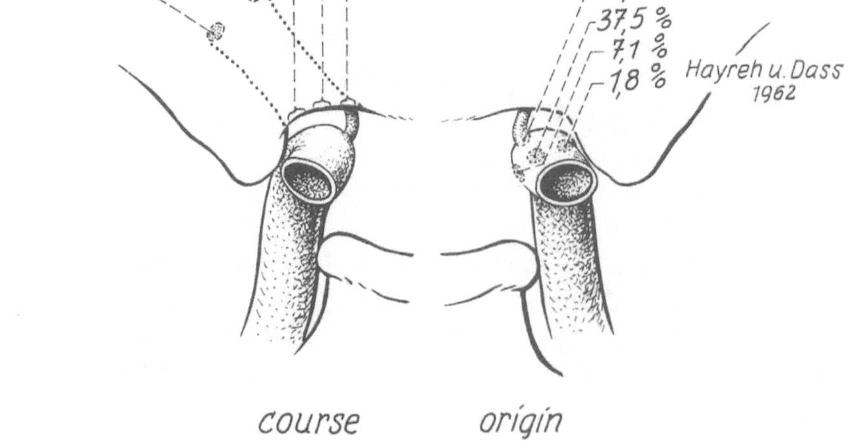

Fig. 4. Aorta ophthalmica

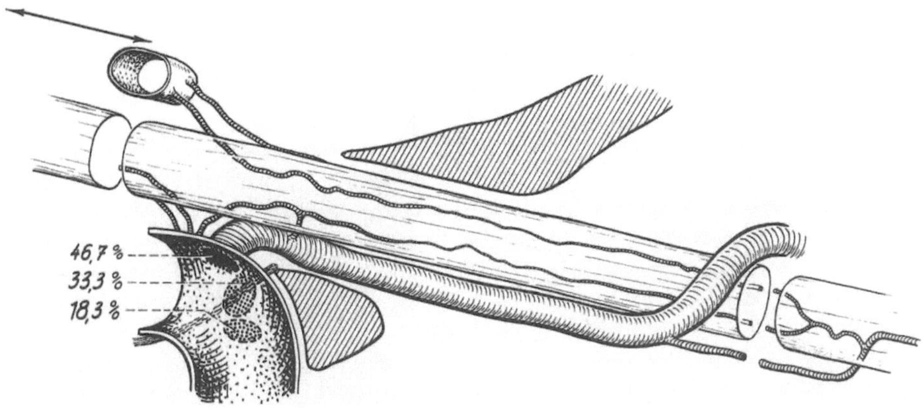

Fig. 5. Nervus opticus, vascularisation

(Fig. 5). A crossing of the artery below the nerve inside the orbita has been observed in Europeans 15 percent, in Japanese 6.5 percent. According to Singh and Dass, 1960, in two percent of the cases the entire opthalmic artery arose from the middle meningeal artery and entered either through the superior orbital fissure, lateral end; or through a so-called meningo-orbital foramen into the orbit. An anastomosis between the anterior branch of middle meningeal artery and the ophthalmic artery occurs regularly. It is to be noted that the optic nerve is about five mm longer than the distance between the posterior aspect of the ocular bulb and apertura orbitalis canalis optici, something that was already known to the post anatomists: Reserve length in eye ball movements.

Intraorbital Aperture of the Optic Canal and Common Tendonous Annulus

In the region of optic apex the origins of eye muscles form a double pierced tendonous funnel. An upper, medial oval opening with vertical long axis surrounds the optic nerve and the ophthalmic artery; and a lower lateral perforation which encloses the oculomotoric, abducent and nasociliar nerves. It is stressed that the oculomotor nerve divides itself, often behind its entering portal, into ramus superior and ramus inferior. Between the opening known by Meckel as Foramen n. oculomotorii or as pars nervosa inferior and the one for optic nerve and ophthalmic artery known as pars optica, there is normally a tendonous angle which connects the beginning parts of the muscle rectus medialis with those of the rectus superior muscle. Above, directly next to and together with the muscle rectus superior stems the muscle levator palpebrae superioris from a tendonous ring. Somewhat further away from it emerge the muscle obliquus superior. The muscles rectus lateralis (partly) and rectus inferior stem from the lateral aspect of the pars nervosa, and laterally above also the muscle rectus superior. The trochlear, frontal and lacrimal nerves as well as the ramus anastomoticus of the lacrimal artery and the superior

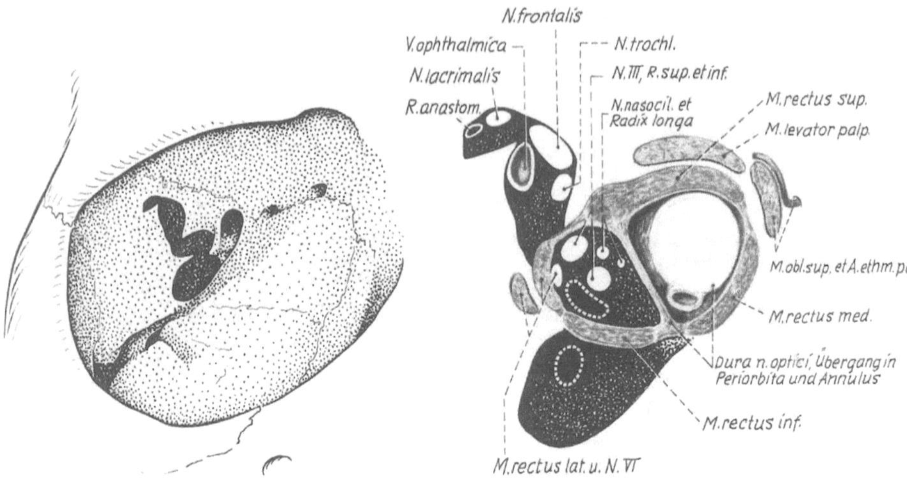

Fig. 6. Annulus tendineus communis (Topography – Axis optic canal)

ophthalmic vein transverse the region of superior orbital fissure laterally and above the tendonous annulus. In cases of transcranial decompression of the optic nerve (Fig. 6), it is of significance that in the very posterior region of the orbital roof the trochlear nerve crosses over to the medial side directly below the periorbit and the anterior clinoid process, which is often grooved by the nerve (see Fig. 7). Finally, I would like to point out that not only the orbital muscle with its fibers reaches the region of cavernous sinus, but also the fatty tissues of the orbita, of the medial angle of the superior orbital fissure, and of the pterygopalatine fossa lead to the cavernous sinus. Figure 5 shows the intracranial and intraorbital vascularisation of the optic nerve through the central retinal artery and an accessory artery of the optic nerve. It is to be emphasized that the vagina externa n. optici (= dura mater) and the arachnoid layer of the internal vagina which contains also arachnoid villi that can project into the subdural gap, are normally widened directly behind the bulbus oculi ampullär. In case of sudden intracranial pressure-rise, the average diameter of this retrobulbular expansion should be about 1.1 mm larger than in the control groups (Muller and Deck, 1974). The intraorbital length of the optic nerve is in newborns about 24.5 mm, in adults between 29.3 and 31.6 mm (Ares). According to Schaeffer, 1924, the total eye-to-chiasma length of the optic nerve is, on the average, 44.4 mm right and 41.9 mm left.

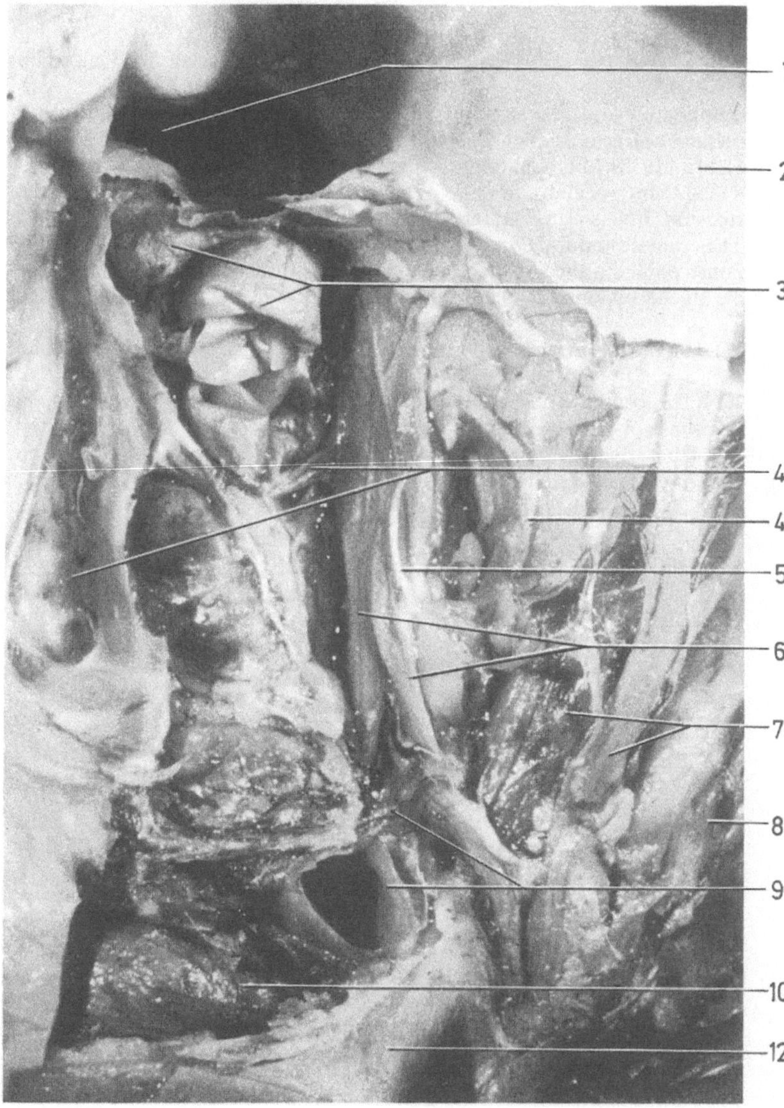

Fig. 7. Orbit. roof removed. *1* = nasofrontal duct; *2* = frontal sinus, large; *3* = anterior superior ethmoid cells; *4* = N. et A. ethmoidalis ant. and olfactory fossa; *5* = opthalmic artery; *6* = medial twig of frontal nerve; *7* = M. obliquus sup. and N. IV; *8* = frontal nerve and M. levator; *9* = lacrimal artery; *10* = posterior ethmoid cell (in contact with optic canal); *11* = sphenoid sinus (mucosa); *12* = optic canal (dura periosteal)

Summary

The optic canal, its postnatal growth and relations to paranasal sinuses are described. The origin and course of the ophthalmic artery and the optic nerve are demonstrated.

References

Adachi B (1928) Das Arteriensystem der Japaner. Bd. I u. II. Kyoto: Verlag der Kaiserlich-Japanischen Universität

Alyea OE van (1941) Sphenoid sinus. Anatomic study, with consideration of the clinical significance of the structural characteristics of the sphenoid sinus. Arch Otolaryngol 34:225–253

Maniscalco JE, Habal MB (1978) Microanatomy of the optic canal. J Neurosurg 48:402–406

Muller PJ, Deck JHN (1974) Intraocular and optic nerve sheath hemorrhag in cases of sudden intracranial hypertension. J Neurosurg 41:160–166

Penfield WG (1924) The cranial subdural space (A method of study). Anat Rec 28/4:173–175

Schaeffer JP (1924) Some points in the regional anatomy of the optic pathway, with especial reference to tumors of the hypophysis cerebralis and resulting ocular changes. Anat Rec 28:243–279

Singh S, Dass R (1960) The central artery of the retina. I. Origin and course. Br J Opthalmol 44:193–212

Singh S, Dass R (1960) The central artery of the retina. II. A study of its distribution and anastomoses. Br J Opthalmol 44:280–299

Zuckerkandl E (1884) Über den Circulations-Apparat in der Nasenschleimhaut. Wien: Kaiserl.-Königl. Hof- und Staatsdruckerei

Optic Nerve. Clinical Examinations and Findings

K. HOFFMANN, Hannover/FRG

Introduction

When discussing clinical pathology of the optic nerve, it must always be kept in mind that the second cranial nerve is not a 'nerve' in the sense of peripheral neurology. It is ontogenetically, morphologically and functionally a tract of the Central Nervous System equal to the spinal cord. That means regarding its clinical pathology that the optic nerve cannot only be affected by diseases of the eye itself, either circulatory, inflammatory, degenerative or neoplastic in origin. As part of the CNS it is prone also to cerebral conditions. It follows that pathological findings and their early diagnosis have a great value not only for the eye, but even more for the general health or even the life of the patient.

Methods of Clinical Examination

The clinical examination of a patient with suspected disease of the visual system, especially the optic nerve, has to start with a medical history taken as carefully as possible. For the experienced physician this alone may be the final clue for making his diagnosis. It has to be taken into account, however, that patients with optical disease frequently have other disorders of the CNS, and conversation or cooperation may be difficult. Relatives or friends should be consulted. Headache, nausea and vomiting, disseminated symptoms as well as a vascular history or a history of metabolic disorders give significant hints. Any kind of visual impairment, unilateral or bilateral, the onset, duration or periodicity can be of immense diagnostical value.

The ophthalmological examination of a patient with a suspected disease of the visual pathways must be divided into two different parts:

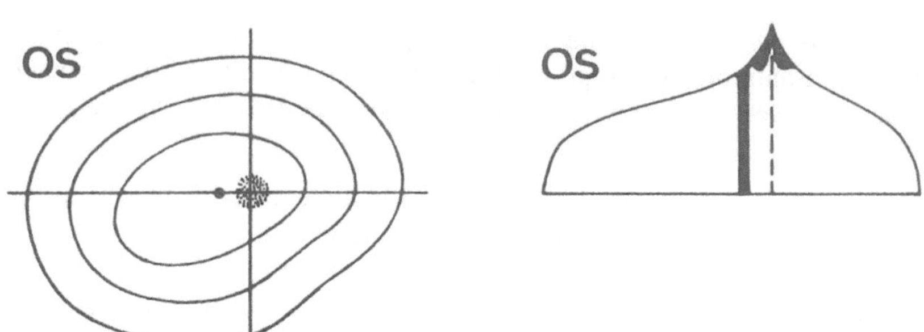

Fig. 1. Impairment of central visual acuity = relative central scotoma (right: static, left kinetic perimetry)

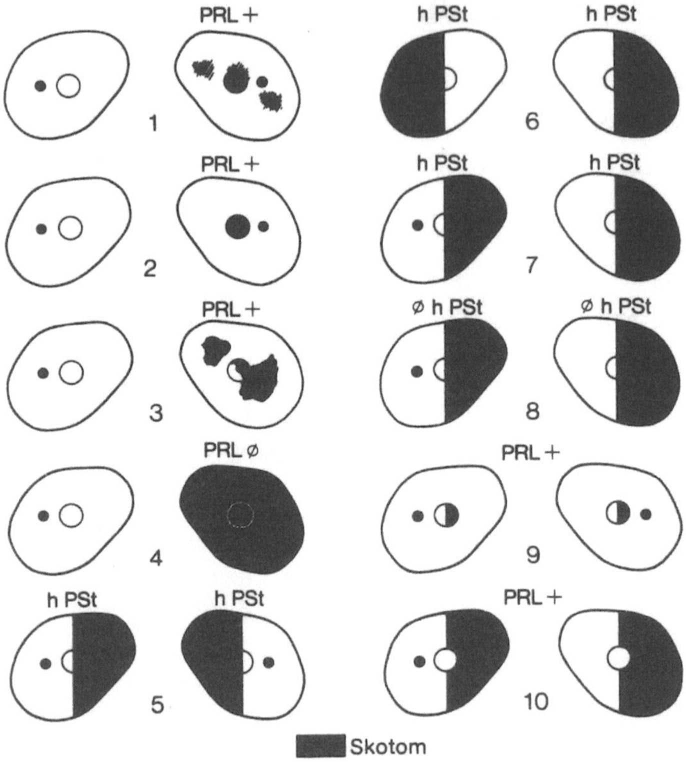

Figs. 2 and 3. Synopsis of visual field defects: (*1–7*) retina to corpus geniculatum laterale, (*8*) radiatio optica, (*9*) visual cortex, (*10*) other parts of the fissura calcarina, (*P*) papilla nervi optici, (*PRL*) pupillary reflex to light, (*hPSt*) hemianopic loss of pupillary reflex

1. the *subjective examination,* which is the test of visual acuity as well as visual field. The results are of great, but by no means equal value: since an impairment of visual acuity may be a more alarming symptom for the patient, visual field defects can give very detailed diagnostic help. The importance of the examination of the visual field, especially also for follow-up studies, cannot be overemphasized.
2. the *objective examination,* including the position and motility of the eyeball, further neuro-ophthalmological signs such as ptosis and pupillary reaction. Of utmost value, however, is fundoscopy with inspection of the optic nerve-head, the optic disc.

ad 1. a) The investigation of visual acuity should include distant vision with the appropriate spectacle correction. The acuity of near vision may give some information as to the possibility of accommodation and on the fixation area.

ad 1. b) If impairment of visual acuity was complained of or is detected or suspected, the examination of the visual fields should start with the testing of the central field area in order to determine the presence and localisation of central or paracentral scotomas (Fig. 1). The examination of the peripheral visual field is an

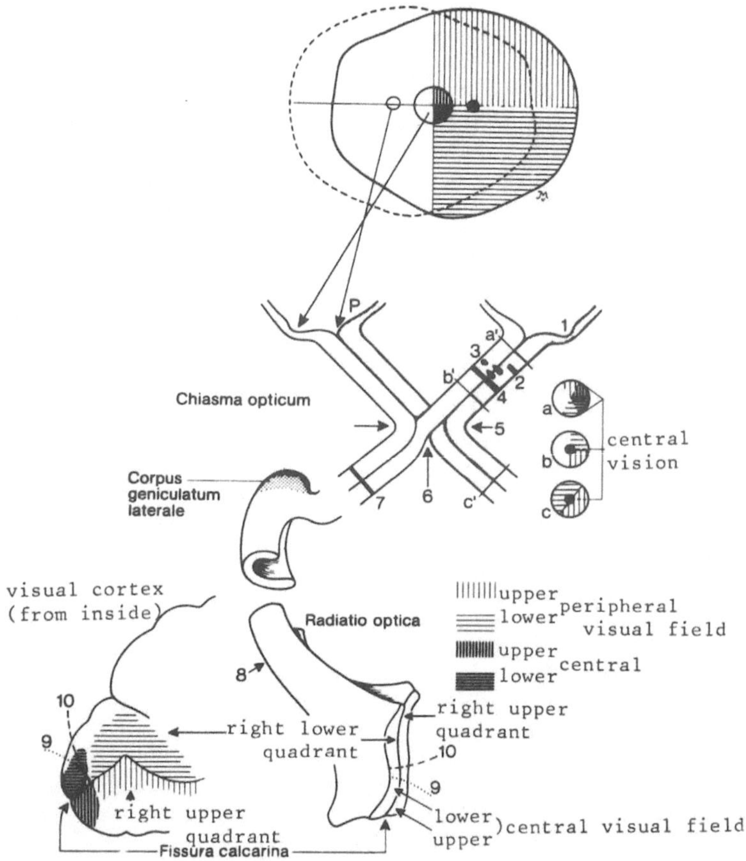

Fig. 3

absolute demand in any neuro-ophthalmological investigation. After gross information by the confrontation-test, perimetry has to be performed as carefully as possible. A synopsis of different types of visual field defects and their topic value is given in Figs. 2 and 3. The importance of the visual fields, especially also in the follow-up of undiagnosed or even known lesions, may be demonstrated by three case-reports:

1. This 46 year old patient was admitted to the eye-clinic because of blurring of vision on right eye. Visual acuity R 0.2, central scotoma of 5° diameter. Pallor of the optic disc. Because of lack of any other ophthalmological and neurological symptoms (spinal fluid normal) the diagnosis was optic neuritis. Follow-up was recommended. One year later a sudden attack of severe headache: severe subarachnoid hemorrhage from a right-sided walnut-sized infraclinoidal aneurysm. Now a quadrant-shaped visual-field defect of the right eye (Figs. 4 and 5) was found.
2. This 58 year old colleague noticed, when playing tennis, a scotoma in the temporal part of his right visual field. Left eye with slight reduction of visual acuity and minimal central scotoma. No further ophthalmological abnormalities, no neurological defects, spinal fluid normal. Follow-up of visual fields showed

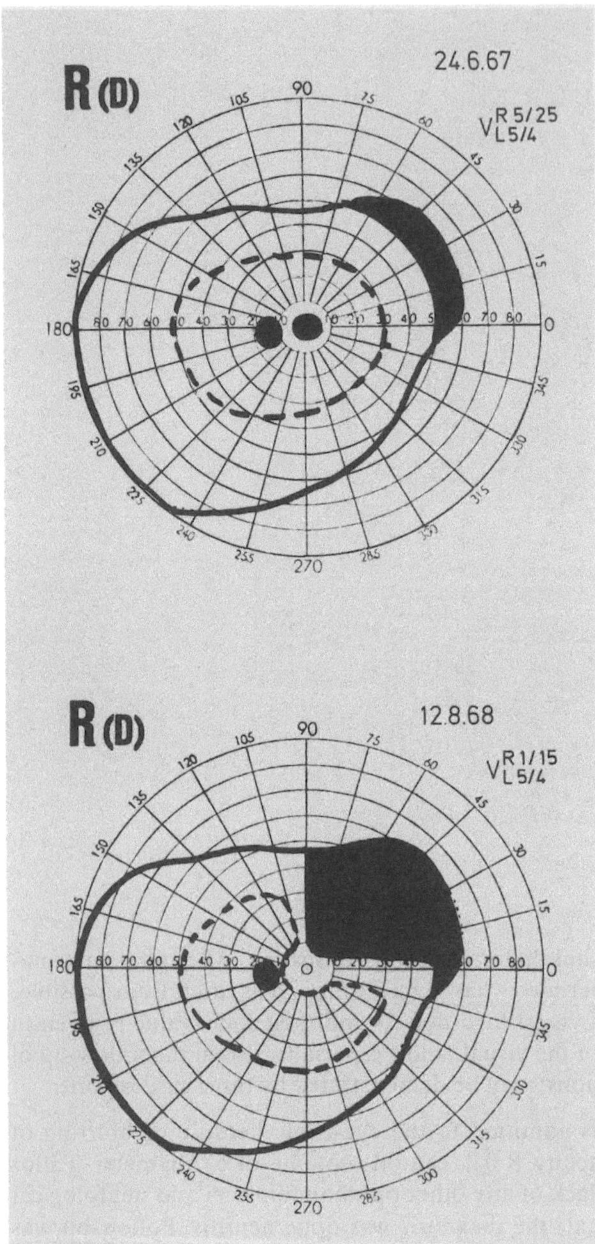

Fig. 4. Visual fields with central scotoma (24. 6. 67) and quadrant-shaped visual field defect (12. 8. 68)

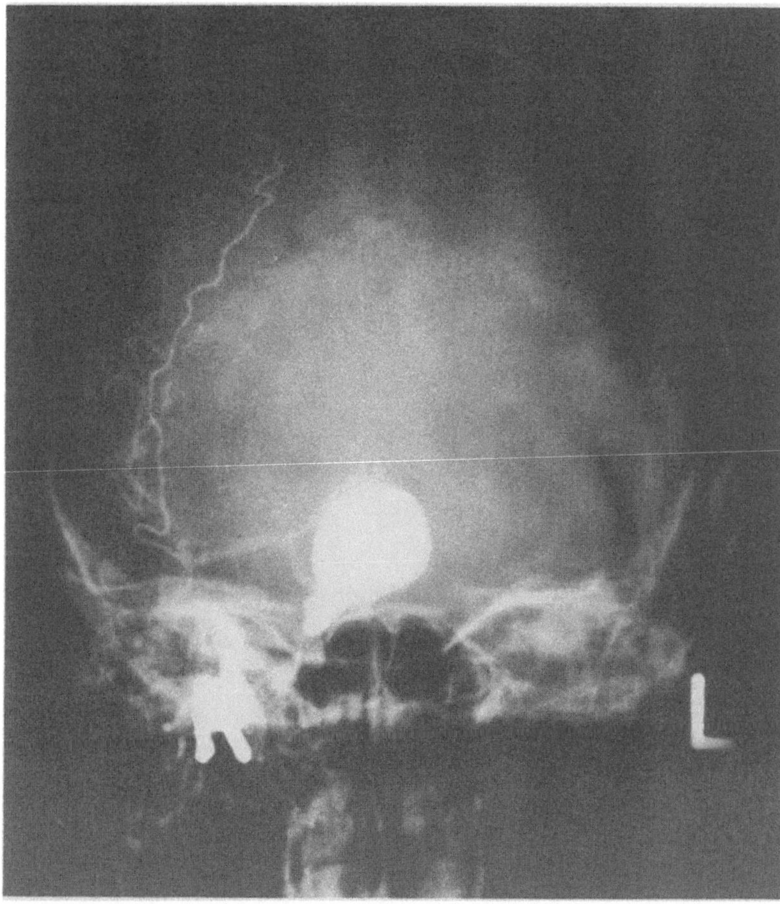

Fig. 5. Angiogram of right carotid artery showing large infraclinoidal aneurysm

decrease, at last increase of scotomas. When peripheral defects on the left eye appeared, angiography of carotid artery was performed and showed a chiasma-tumor (histologically craniopharyngioma) (Figs. 6 and 7).

3. This 55 year old patient had undergone several craniotomies because of meningioma of the sphenoid region. During the last five years of follow-up studies of visual fields and visual acuity no further impairment could be noted. CT-examinations showed no further progress (Figs. 8 and 9).

ad 2. Out of the objective tests of examination fundoscopy has by far the greatest importance. Without invasive procedures we can easily see and judge the head of the optic nerve. The evidence of edema, hemorrhage, new vessels, pallor, especially of its temporal part, where lies the macula-papillary bundle, can be detected. The diagnosis of papillitis, papilledema or optic atrophy has to be established. In case of prominence of the disc the visual function as a rule allows

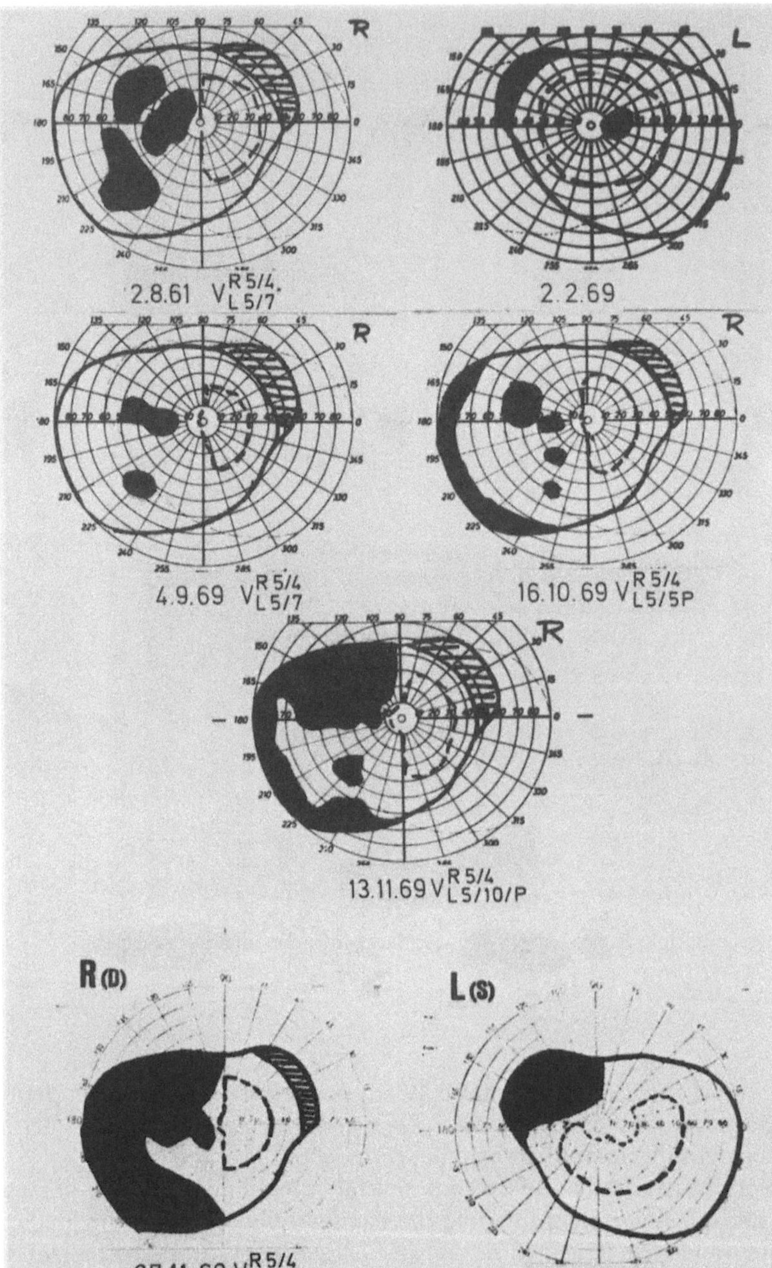

Fig. 6. Follow-up of visual field defects with progress and amelioration of paracentral scotomas

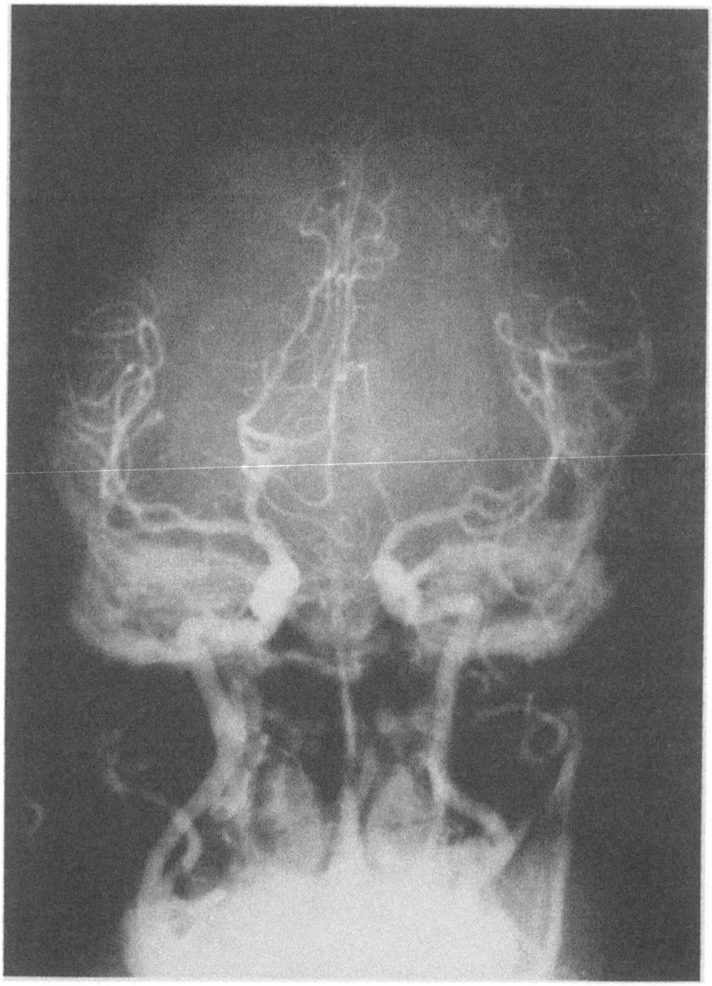

Fig. 7. Simultaneous angiogram of both internal carotid arteries demonstrating chiasmal tumor (craniopharyngioma)

one to differentiate papillitis and papilledema: blurring of vision up to severe impairment on one side, no defects on the other. The full clinical picture of papilledema is well-known (Figs. 10, 11):

1. increased redness of the disc
2. slight haziness and blurring of the margin
3. physiological cup in the center of the disc is filled, grey streaks appear along the central vessels
4. slight turgescence of the veins, which are enlarged; artery – vein ratio 1:3 or even 1:4
5. absence of venous pulse of the disc

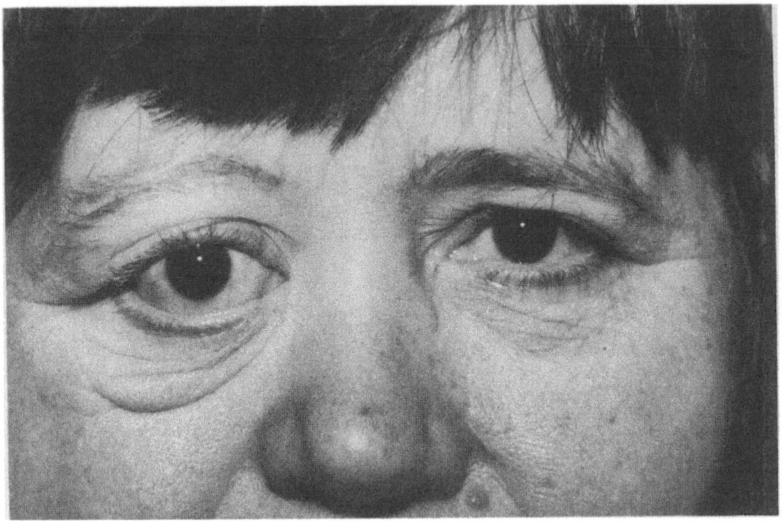

Fig. 8. Pat. with exophthalmos of right eye due to meningioma of the sphenoid

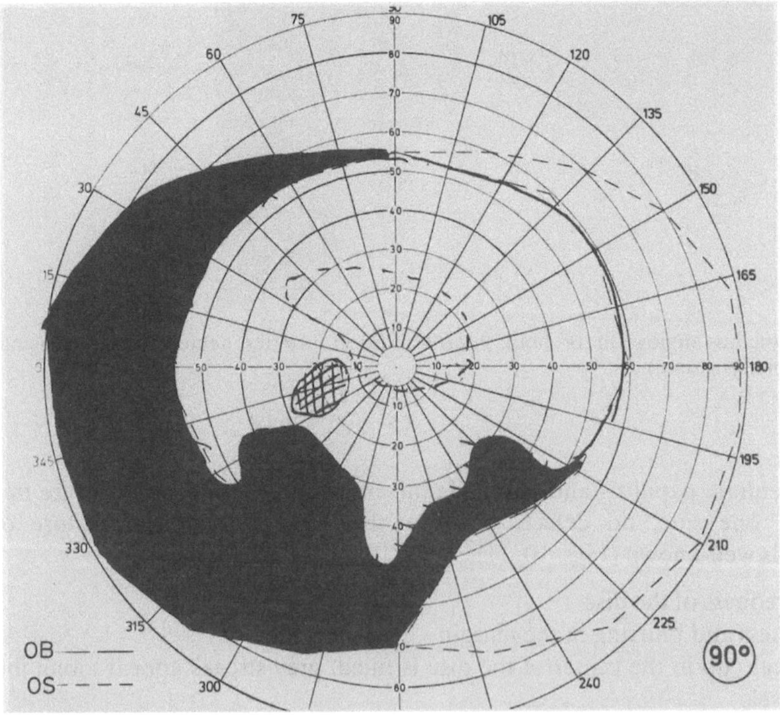

Fig. 9. Same pat., five year follow-up of visual field defect without progress

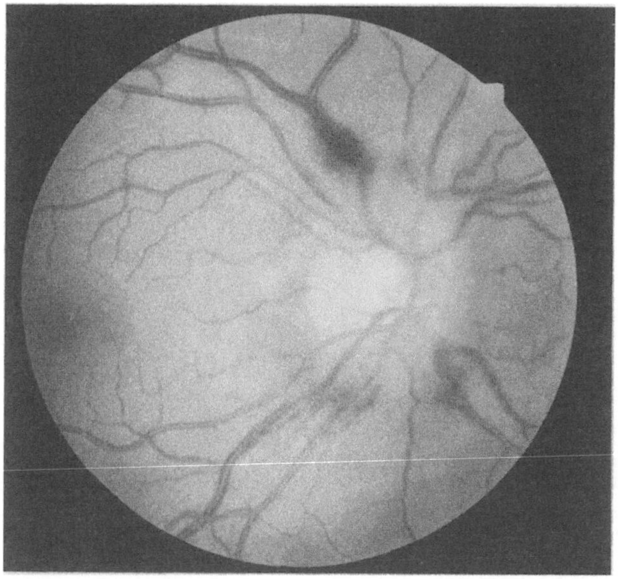

Fig. 10. Papilledema due to increased intracranial pressure in a case of brain tumor

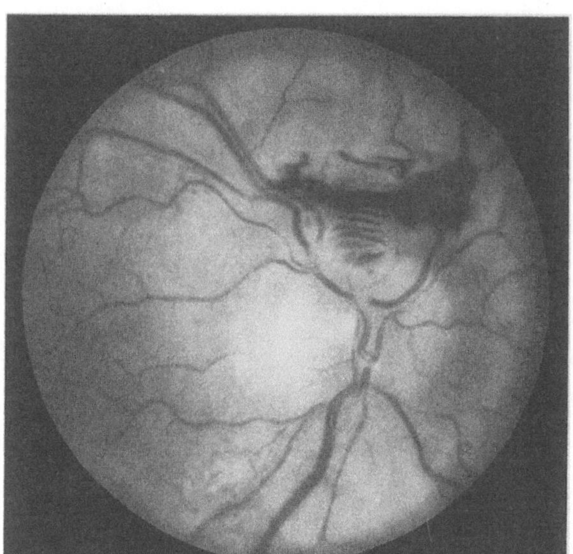

Fig. 11. Papilledema with extensive peripapillary hemorrhage typical for acute onset of increased intracranial pressure (subarachnoid hemorrhage)

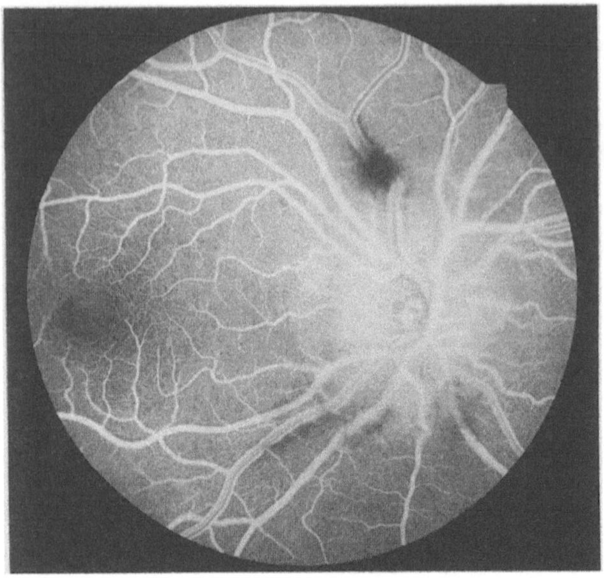

Fig. 12. Fluorescein-angiogram of papilledema (Fig. 10) showing congestion of capillaries in the region of the optic disc. Diffuse extravasation of fluorescein

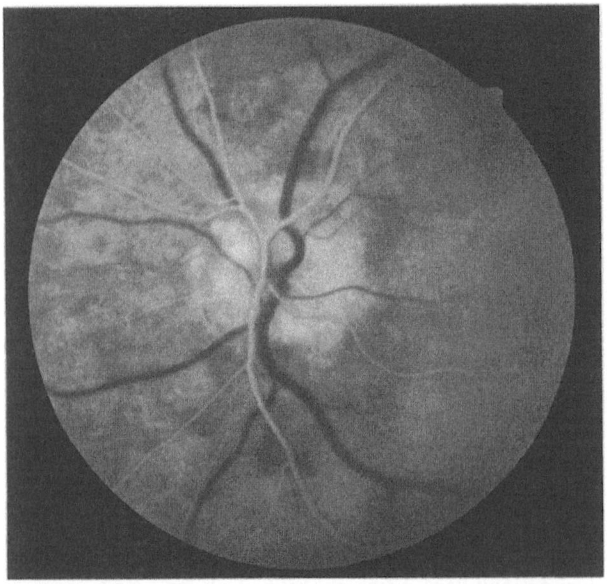

Fig. 13. Optic nerve head with partially buried "drusen"

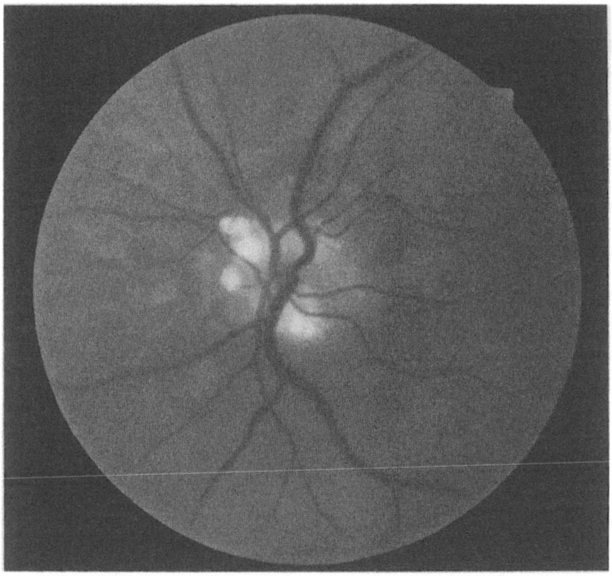

Fig. 14. Fluorescence of "drusen" of Fig. 13 can be demonstrated in a fluorescein-angiogram

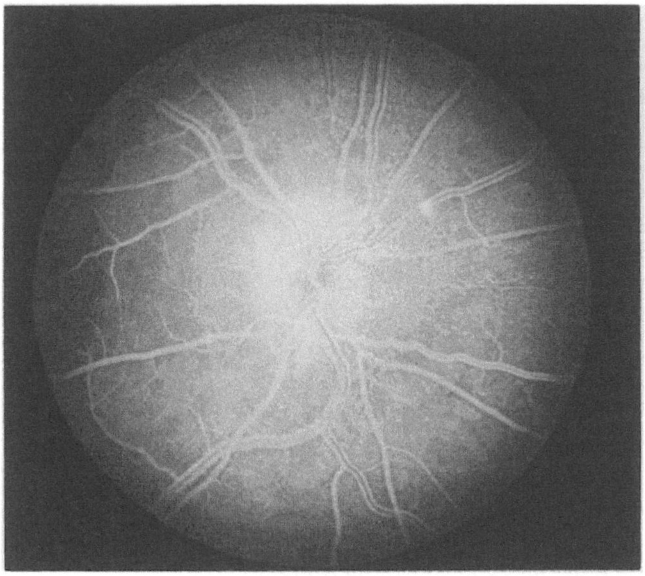

Fig. 15. Fluorescein-angiogram of papillitis: Compared with the findings in papilledema (Fig. 12). Congestion of capillaries is less, extravasation of fluorescein more extensive

6. forward protrusion of the disc-up to 8 dptr., mushroom-like shape of the disc, vessels bending over the margin
7. occurence of flame shaped hemorrhages in the nerve-fiber layers

In order to rule out abnormalities of the disc, fluorescein-angiographic studies can be very helpful (Fig. 12). Buried 'drusen' can be ruled out (Figs. 13 and 14), edema can be proved (Fig. 15). The incidence of papilledema in cases of brain-tumor is shown in Table 1. On the other hand we see the incidence of brain-tumors in cases of papilledema given by a neurosurgeon (Table 2). It is interesting to

Table 1. Incidence of papilledema. In cases of Brain-Tumor (Tönnis 1953)

3033 tumors
1827 papilledema
→ = 60%

Table 2. Incidence of brain-tumors. In cases of papilledema (Bregeat 1956)

734 papilledemas
653 tumors
→ = 89%

Table 3. Causes of papilledema (Marchesani, 1936)

Tumor	186 = 61.2%	←
Abscess	6	
Tuberculoma	2	→
Aneurysm	1	= 64.1% spacetaking lesions
Blood- and vascular dyscrasias	44 = 14.5%	
Diffuse inflammations	16 = 5.2%	
unknown etiology	19 = 6.3%	

Table 4. Papilledema in brain tumor related to age (Brégeat, 1956)

1 to 5 years	81%
5 to 10 years	77%
10 to 20 years	66%
20 to 30 years	69%
30 to 40 years	62%
40 to 50 years	61%
50 to 60 years	48%
60 to 70 years	43%

compare the statistics of an ophthalmologist concerning the different causes of papilledema (Table 3). Another interesting fact is the incidence of papilledema in brain-tumor related to age (Table 4). Discussion is going on as to whether vascular factors are of importance, or whether the different distribution of brain-tumors in children, located more frequently in the posterior fossa, is the explanation.

When discussing pathological findings of the optic disc, it has to be remembered that in cases of hyperopia hypotension of the eyeball and 'drusen', buried or not, forward protrusion of the optic nerve head can be present.

At the end of most diseases of the optic nerve, as a consequence of lesions within the third neuron, that means between the ganglion cells of the retina and the geniculate body, optic atrophy develops. As we know, the degeneration does not only proceed in a central direction, as it is the rule since the fibres have their origin in the ganglion cells of the retina, but it also proceeds periphererically, so that even the ganglion cells themselves degenerate. When the optic nerve is cut, optic atrophy can appear within two weeks up to three months after injury.

The ophthalmoscopic diagnosis of optic atrophy seems to be easy. But it has to be underlined, that the diagnosis can never be made only because of the morphological picture! Since we know that the optic nerve gets its blood supply not from the central retinal artery, but from the circle of Zinn and Haller out of the posterior ciliary artery system, we have to keep in mind that even a white optic disc does not mean visual defect. If there is no visual defect, either acuity or field loss, the diagnosis of optic atrophy is not established.

As numerous as the diseases of the optic nerve can be, so, consequently, is the etiology of optic atrophy:

1. congenital atrophy
2. consecutive atrophy – secondary to retinal disease and destruction of the ganglion cells
3. circulatory atrophy
4. pressure and traction atrophy
5. post-inflammatory atrophy – local inflammation from optic neuritis or perineuritis
6. as a part of the central nervous disease (e.g. multiple sclerosis, tabes, neuromyelitis optica)
7. metabolic disorders – e.g. diabetes
8. toxic atrophy – tobacco, alcohol, arsenic, lead etc.
9. traumatic atrophy
10. atrophy of unknown origin, e.g. Leber's o.a., hereditary etc.

Conclusions

The ophthalmological examination, especially visual field examination and fundoscopy, is part of the basic clinical examination of patients with suspected disease of the visual pathways. The results of visual field examination can be of extreme value in the diagnosis of the presence and site of such lesions. Fundoscopy allows by noninvasive technique the direct inspection of the anterior part of the optic nerve.

References

1. Brégeat P (1956) L'oedème papillaire. Masson & Cie., Paris
2. Janzen R (1975) Neurologische Diagnostik, Therapie, Prognostik. Enke, Stuttgart
3. Karbowski M, Bischoff A (1978) Die Häufigkeit der Stauungspapille bei Hirntumoren. Acta Neuropathol (Berl) 5:203–209
4. Marchesani O (1936) Symptomatologie des Nervus opticus (einschließlich Stauungspapille). In: Bumke v O, Foerster O (eds) Hirnnerven/Pupille, vol 4. Springer, Berlin, p 38
5. Tönnis W, Borek WF (1953) Großhirntumoren des Kindesalters. Zbl Neurochir 13: 203–209

Diagnosis of Optic Nerve Lesions with Newer Techniques of Computerized Tomography

G. A. Meyer, J. P. Davis, D. L. Daniels, W. E. Gager, and V. M. Haughton, Milwaukee/USA

Indroduction

Conventional radiography, polytomography, angiography, orbital venography, and pneumoencephalography as well as orbital ultrasound studies have all played a valuable role in the diagnosis of lesions of the optic nerves and chiasm. However, some cases of progressive visual loss still defy definitive diagnosis prior to exploration. In an effort to enhance diagnostic precision, the authors have utilized a prototype CT/T 8800 scanner with conventional and metrizamide enhanced computerized tomography in the diagnosis of optic nerve and chiasm lesions at the Medical College of Wisconsin since 1977.

The safety and efficacy of metrizamide enhancement of the subarachnoid space of the optic nerves was studied experimentally and clinically (Davis, 1979). Prior data has indicated continuity of the subarachnoid space of the optic nerve and the intracranial cerebrospinal fluid spaces (Shimojyo, Gargano, et al., 1966; Levine, Bronstein, 1955; Field, Brierley, 1949; Tsukahara, Yamashita, 1975). Two of these reports suggested the possibility of damage to the optic nerve by instillation of foreign material into the adjacent space (Tabaddor, 1973; Manelfe, Pasquini, et al., 1978). Accordingly, radiographic and histologic study was performed of cat and monkey optic nerves and leptomeninges after injection of metrizamide into the theca and optic nerve sheaths (Haughton, Davies, et al., 1978; Haughton, Davis, et al., 1980). Another study determined the normal contours and dimensions of the optic chiasm both by detailed study of a cadaver specimen and by measurement of the chiasm in 41 CT scans performed for reasons other than visual system impairment (Daniels, Haughton, et al., 1980). Details of the methods used in both studies have been published in the references noted above.

I. Imaging of the Intraorbital Portion of the Optic Nerve with Metrizamide Enhancement of the Subarachnoid Spaces

Subtle lesions of the optic nerves continue to pose diagnostic difficulties and therefore we evaluated opacification of the subarachnoid space of the intraorbital optic nerve as a diagnostic technique. We felt the technique might be valuable in determining, for example, whether an optic nerve enlargement represented intramedullary tumor such as a localized optic nerve glioma or an extramedullary tumor such as an optic sheath meningioma. Furthermore, there is a suggestion in the literature that the operability of the latter lesions might be correlated with patency at the subarachnoid space through the area of the meningioma (Fox, Debrun, et al., 1979). Another possible application of the technique might be the

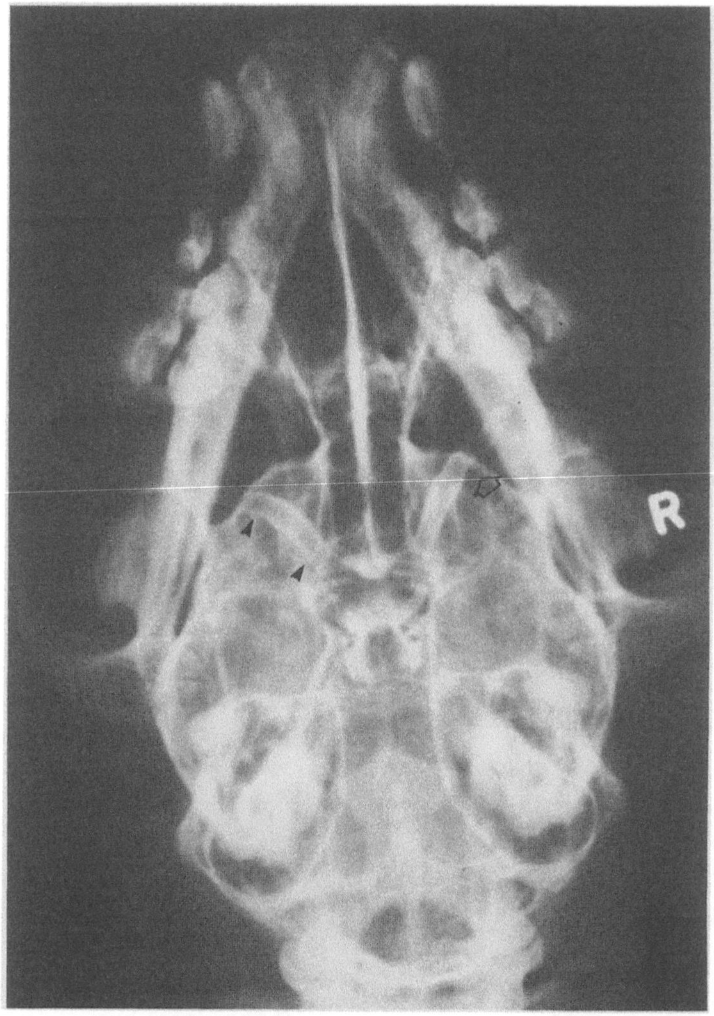

Fig. 1. Radiographic visualization of the metrizamide filled, normal, left, cat optic nerve (*arrow points*). The right optic nerve (*open arrow*) is displaced anteromedially by a plastic sphere

evaluation of retinal neoplasms extending caudally along the optic nerve possibly indicating the need for more radical resection such as orbital exenteration rather than simple enucleation.

The initial study involved normal and experimentally disordered optic nerves in 15 cats. Satisfactory conventional radiographs demonstrating opacified nerve sheaths were obtained with a high success rate (54 out of 55 studies) (Fig. 1). Immediate morbidity related to the contrast was low. Two animals had myoclonic jerks and another two had seizures. After this early experience all animals were premedicated with Diazepam 0.15 mg/kg. No further seizures were experienced.

The optic nerve sheaths and the leptomeninges of the optic nerve were studied histologically in 10 animals. Detailed histologic evaluation with myelin and connective tissue stains showed no significant pathologic change in animals having a single study with a concentration of metrizamide not exceeding 450 mgs/cc.

A subsequent study involved two macaque monkeys. There were nine successful studies using conventional radiography in twelve attempts in these animals. In three cases the basal cisterns failed to fill and there was extension of the contrast medium over the cerebral convexities because of improper positioning. Seizures occured in two cases.

A study of the human cases was less successful. We obtained good CT imaging in only one of nine cases despite sufficient metrizamide to opacify the chiasmatic cistern at fluoroscopy in all cases (Fig. 2). This case was a teenage female who was suffering from von Recklinghausen's disease complicated by bilateral optic pallor. The study was done primarily to rule out a cervical spinal cord tumor. Six ml of metrizamide with concentration of 170 mgs per ml were instilled in the lateral decubitus position via lumbar puncture. In all of the eight additional cases, insufficient contrast was found in the optic nerve sheath to allow visualization on the CT scans despite instillation of up to six ml of 300 mgs/ml metrizamide via Cl-2 puncture in the ventral decubitus position. After instillation, the metrizamide was slowly run up the ventral aspect of the C.S.F. axis and placed in the chiasmatic cistern under fluoroscopic control. The optic nerve sheath was then placed dependent to the chiasmatic cistern for two to 10 minutes to allow mixing of the

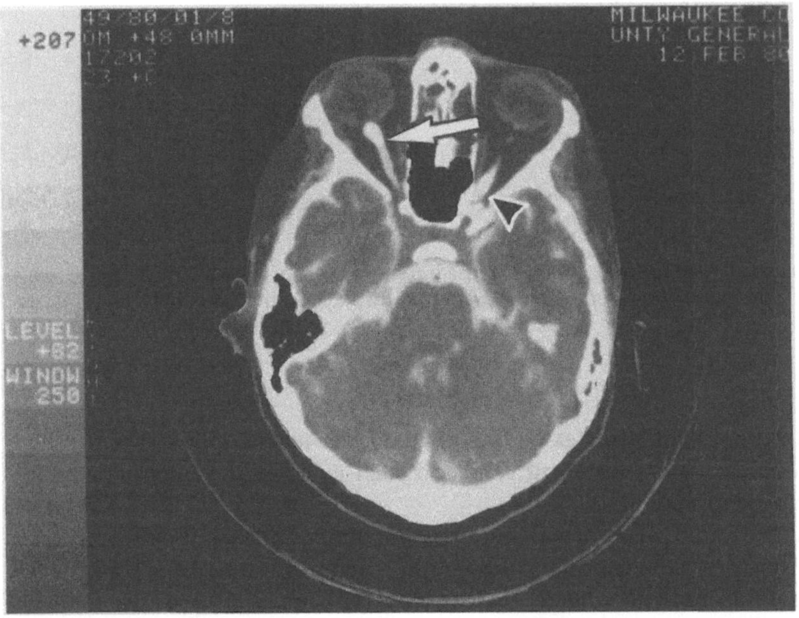

Fig. 2. CT visualization of optic nerves in a 13 year old girl. The right optic nerve sheath is seen anteriorly (*white arrow*) and the left posteriorly (*arrow point*). In adjacent slices both nerves were well seen throughout their intraorbital portions

contrast material with the intraorbital subarachnoid fluid. There were no serious difficulties in any of the nine cases. The morbidity was two cases of headache and one of vomiting. All cases were premedicated with Valium and all were placed in the 30 degree head-up position for at least eight hours following the study.

Small changes in the attenuation numbers of the optic nerve sheath following metrizamide instillation are not excluded by our study. However, due to the small volume of the optic nerve, visualization is essential for the procedure to have an important clinical role. One possible means of obtaining better visualization is the use of osmotherapy immediately prior to study to shrink the size of the optic nerve and perhaps increase the patency of the intraorbital subarachnoid space. However, until a more reliable technique is developed intraorbital optic nerve imaging cannot be considered a standard neuroradiologic procedure.

II. Imaging of the Optic Nerve from the Optic foramen to the Chiasm

The intracranial portion of the optic nerve was seen in each of the 41 'normal' cases evaluated primarily for chiasmal size and configuration. The nerves were best seen when the plane of the axial study was at or just negative to Reid's baseline or perpendicular to it.

The diagnostic efficacy of routine and contrast enhanced CT was evaluated in 34 cases of compression of the intracranial portion of the optic nerve by suprasellar

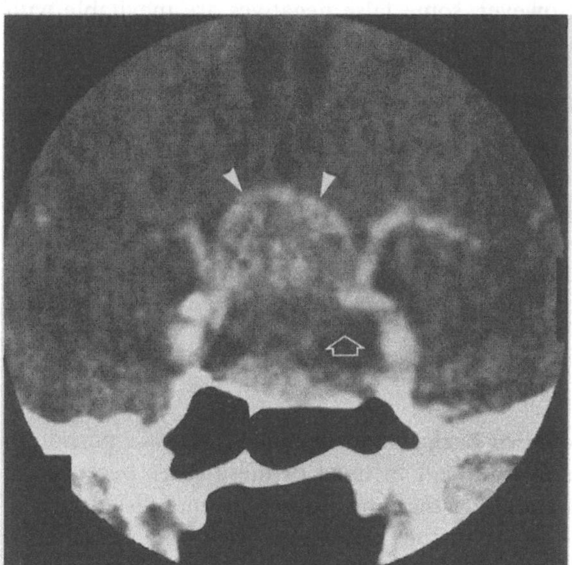

Fig. 3. Coronal CT demonstration of a pituitary adenoma in a 30 year old woman. The contrast enhancing suprasellar dome (*white arrow points*) is encroaching on the third ventricle. The less dense areas (*open arrow*) within the enlarged sella were proven to be cystic at surgery

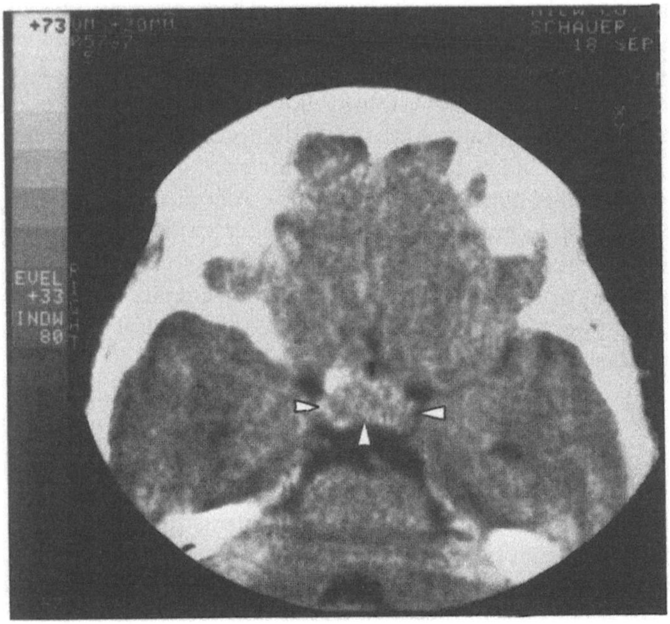

Fig. 4. Hyperdense chiasmal glioma (*arrows*) with focal calcification shown in this unenhanced axial CT scan

lesions causing visual deficit. Thus far, there have been no false negatives and only one false positive (See below). However, some false negatives are inevitable with very small lesions.

1. Pituitary Adenomas with Suprasellar Extensions – 20 Cases

Only one of these 20 lesions had significant calcification and this was in the capsule of the tumor only. The degree of intravenous contrast enhancement was highly variable as one might expect due to the high incidence of cyst formation and degeneration in these tumors. In none of the tumors was the contrast enhancement greater than the normal cavernous sinus or pituitary gland. In the usual case the diagnosis was suggested by the contiguous extension of a lesion occupying an enlarged sella turcica (Fig. 3).

2. Optic Gliomas – 7 Cases

Five of seven of these lesions extended back to and included at least a portion of the optic chiasm. Diagnosis was not difficult in most of these cases because the dimensions of the optic chiasm were larger than the range of normal listed later in the paper. In four cases, the tumor tissue was hyperdense before contrast enhancement (Fig. 4) and three were not (Fig. 5). There were irregular intraparenchymal calcifications in two. None of the optic gliomas showed significant intravenous contrast enhancement even though this has been reported by other investigators. Two of the six cases have been confirmed at operation. Two suffer from von Recklinghausen's disease and one has subsequently received radiation therapy. All four unoperated cases are being followed with serial scans.

Three of the seven cases had polytomographic pneumoencephalography in addition and two had instillation of subarachnoid metrizamide. Neither of these latter studies contributed to the diagnosis in a material way. There was one false positive diagnosis of optic glioma. The chiasm was markedly asymmetric, but, at surgery the smaller side was found to be atrophic. There was one false tissue diagnosis, an atypical teratoma which was initially thought to be optic glioma. The lesion enhanced dramatically suggesting a more aggressive tumor. The correct diagnosis was established by surgical biopsy.

3. Craniopharyngiomas – Five Cases

The diagnosis of these five cases was suggested by focal calcification largely in the capsule but occasionally in the intraparenchymal portion of the tumor. One of the lesions was apparently confined to the sella turcica and four of the five had at least a portion of the tumor within the sella turcica. One of these was a giant tumor extending into the cerebellopontine angle and another was atypical in that it was a relatively small and surgically removable lesion in a 70 year old female (Fig. 6). None of the five lesions enhanced dramatically with intravenous contrast. Most had subtle enhancement in small portions of the capsule.

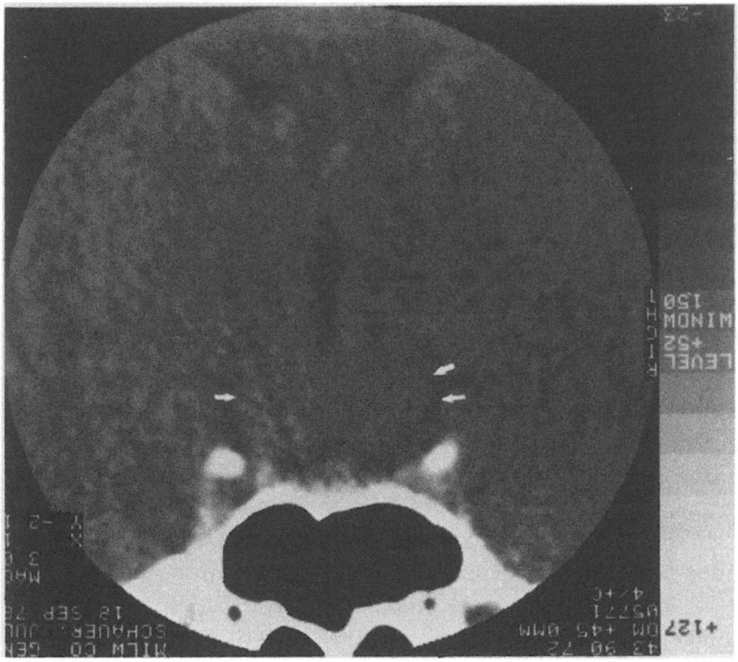

Fig. 5. Isodense chiasmal glioma with left (*single arrow*) and right (*double arrow*) margins outlined in the basal cisterns in this unenhanced coronal CT scan

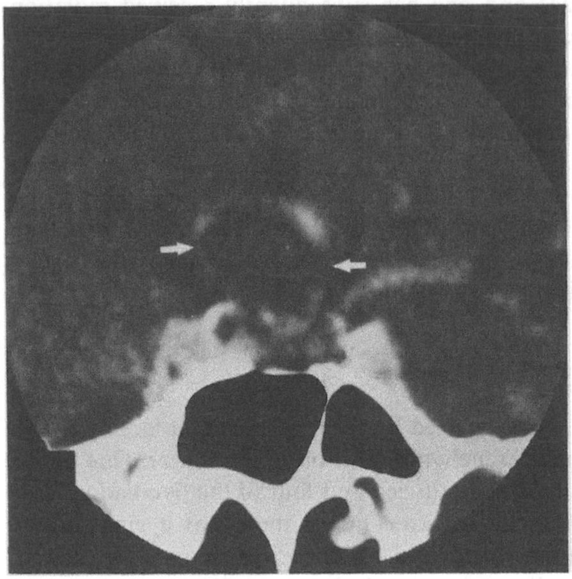

Fig. 6. Coronal CT image of a craniopharyngioma in a 70 year old woman (*arrows*). The capsular density is in part due to calcification and in part enhancement

4. Meningiomas – Two Cases

One of these two lesions was calcified and both had very dense and uniform intravenous contrast enhancement. One additional case was thought to be a meningioma but was proven to be a giant aneurysm following angiographic study. This case was atypical in that there was extensive bony erosion in the parasellar area and no calcification in the wall of the aneurysm.

III. The Shape and Dimensions of the Normal Optic Chiasm as Determined by CT/T 8800 Study

An initial survey study was done of a cadaver head with 0.15, 0.5 and 1.0 cm slice thicknesses performed at seven angles in the axial plane from –25 to +30 degrees to Reid's baseline. Coronal scans were also obtained in a plane perpendicular to the diaphragma sellae at 0.15 and 0.5 cm slice thicknesses. The shape and dimensions of the chiasm in the AP and lateral planes were determined on the axial projections and in the vertical dimension on the coronal projection.

Following this, 41 'normal' cases were studied in those patients having CT scans for reasons other than involvement of the anterior visual system. Most of these cases had 0.5 cm thick slices performed at a +10 degree angle from Reid's baseline. Sixteen of the 41 cases had coronal slices performed at either 0.15 or 0.5 cm slice thicknesses in a plane perpendicular to the diaphragma sellae.

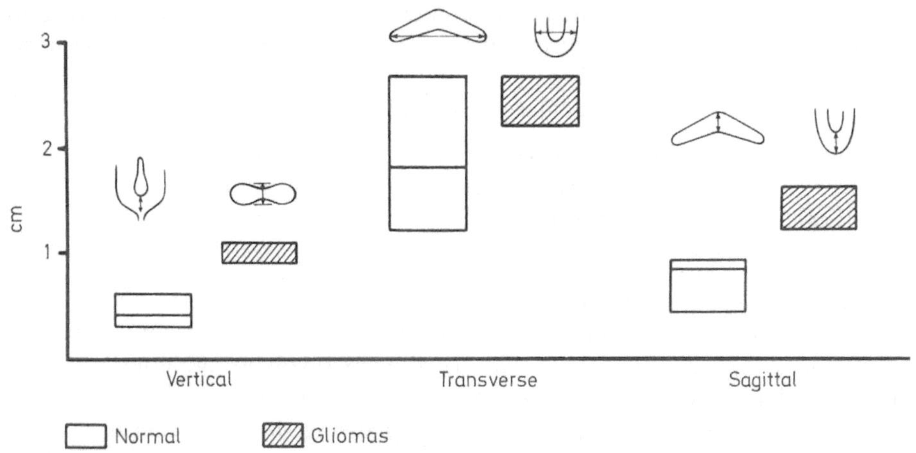

Fig. 7. Table and cross-sections of normal chiasmal configuration. Also, normal and abnormal measurements

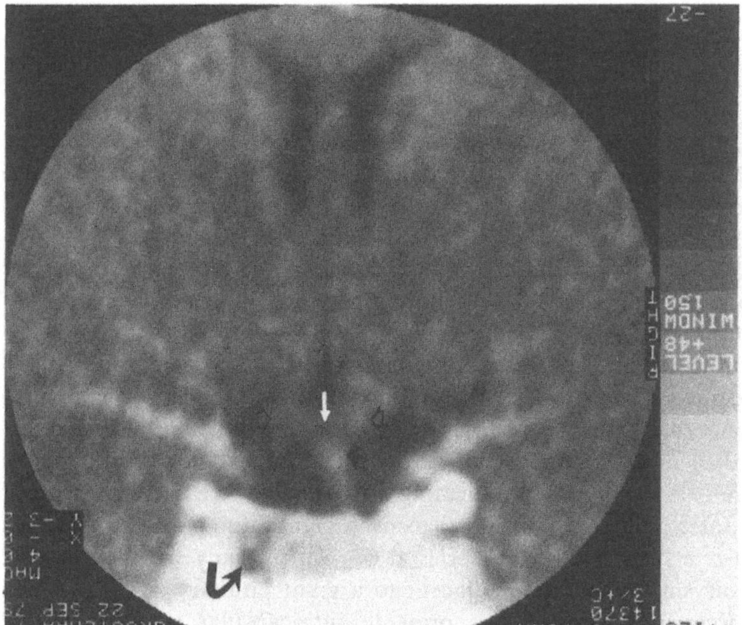

Fig. 8. Chiasm of normal size and shape (between *open* and *white arrows*). The white arrow is within the optic recess of the third ventricle. The infundibulum (*black arrow*) is deviated to the right by a microadenoma (*curved arrow*)

In axial projections the optic nerves and chiasm were either 'U' or boomerang-shaped with some transitional forms seen. In the coronal dimension the chiasm was either 'U' or dumbbel-shaped (Fig. 7).

The dimensions of the optic chiasm in the three planes were as follows:

Transverse	– 1.5 cm (normal range 0.9 to 1.8 cm – coronal)
	1.8 cm (normal range 1.2 to 2.7 cm – axial)
Vertical	– 0.4 cm (normal range 0.3 to 0.6 cm – coronal)
AP	– 0.8 cm (normal range 0.4 to 0.9 cm – axial)

In general, the normal optic chiasm was quite easily distinguished because of its smooth contour and isodense homogeneous appearance without significant intravenous enhancement (Fig. 8). The six gliomas involving the optic chiasm all produced enlargement above the normal ranges listed above.

In summary, the optimal technique for visualizing the optic chiasm is a slice thickness of 0.15 or 0.5 cm at an axial angle of either zero or + 10 degrees to Reid's baseline. Coronal scans are best performed in a plane perpendicular to the diaphragma sellae (or Reid's baseline) at 0.15 cm slice thickness. When it is desired to visualize the intracranial portion of the optic nerve, the best axial angle is –10 degrees, and when the optic tract is being evaluated the optimal angle is +20 degrees (both with reference to Reid's baseline). The single most useful portion of the CT scan study has been the coronal scan at 0.15 cm slice thickness with and without intravenous contrast enhancement.

Conclusions

High resolution CT scanning is by far the most efficient diagnostic study for the evaluation of lesions affecting the optic nerves and chiasm. We had few false positives or negatives, thus far, in 34 cases of tumors compressing the optic nerves and/or chiasm. The error rate in tissue diagnosis is 10 percent.

Orbital ultrasound studies continue to be used as valuable screening studies for orbital mass lesions. Rarely is orbital venography used to aid in the evaluation of vascular lesions of the orbit.

We have continued to utilize cerebral angiography in most of our tumor cases. The information gained is often crucial to the successful management of meningiomas and is indispensable with aneurysms. Determining the position of major vascular structures adjacent to the tumor can be of crucial importance to the operating surgeon. There is a recent report indicating a markedly increased incidence of aneurysms of the anterior circle of Willis adjacent to giant pituitary adenomas. We have encountered one such case in our series, a 67-year-old lady with an internal carotid artery aneurysm immediately adjacent to a giant pituitary adenoma. The aneurysm was successfully clipped just prior to intracapsular removal of the adenoma.

Polytomography with or without pneumoencephalography has not often been useful in our recent series of cases. We do not feel that the information gained justifies routine use.

In two cases we have had some difficulty determining the precise position of the optic chiasm when the patient has manifested a large suprasellar extension of a pituitary adenoma without bitemporal visual field defects. In both of these cases the optic chiasm remained positioned anterior to the tumor mass near the anterior communicating artery but theoretically an extremely post fixed chiasm might allow such a tumor to separate the anterior communicating artery from the optic chiasm. It would be of value to the surgeon to know of this situation but current technology does not allow precise visualization of the chiasm in many cases with large suprasellar extensions.

It is apparent to us that the precise determination of the anatomical relationships altered by suprasellar tumors is increasingly more crucial to successful treatment. Ther are at least four commonly used surgical approaches, namely, transsphenoidal, subfrontal, dorsal interhemispheric, and sphenoid ridge. Additionally, there are alternative methods of administering radiation therapy, which may be used as the primary treatment mode. The authors are confident that the application of these neuroradiologic methods will facilitate more effective treatment.

References

Daniels DL, Haughton VM, Williams AL, Gager WE, Berns TF (1980) Computerized tomography of the optic chiasm. Radiology, in Press

Davis JP, Haughton VM, Harris GJ, Eldevik OP, Gager WE (1979) Cat optic nerve imaging with metrizamide. Invest Ophthalmol Visual Sci 18:272–277

Field EJ, Brierley JB (1949) The retro-orbital tissues as a site of outflow of cerebrospinal fluid. Proc R Soc Med 42:447

Fox AJ, Debrun G, Vinuela F, Assis L, Coates R (1979) Intrathecal metrizamide enhancement of the optic nerve sheath. J Comput Assist Tomogr 3(5):653–656

Haughton VM, Davis Jp, Eldevik OP, Gager WE (1978) Optic nerve sheath imaging with metrizamide. Invest Radiol 13:544

Haughton VM, Davis JP, Harris GJ, Ho K (1980) Metrizamide optic nerve sheath opacification. Invest Radiol (In Press)

Levine S, Bronstein M (1955) The optic nerve sheath pathway. Arch Ophthalmol 54:544

Manelfe C, Pasquini U, Bank WO (1978) Metrizamide demonstration of the subarachnoid space surrounding the optic nerves. J Comput Assist Tomogr 2:545–547

Shimojyo S, Gargano F, Ellerman N, David N (1966) Contrast radiography of the optic nerve sheath. Neurology (Minneap) 16:1621

Tabaddor K (1973) Unusual complications of iophendylate injection myelography. Arch Neurol 29:453

Tsukahara I, Yamashita H (1975) An electron microscopic study of the blood-optic nerve and the fluid-optic nerve barrier. Albrecht von Graefes Arch Klin Ophthalmol 196:239

Misinterpretation of Progressive Visual Disturbances

H.-P. JENSEN, H. KLINGE, and U. MUHTAROGLU, Kiel/FRG

Introduction

Signs of altered visual perception are often misinterpreted in patients with intracranial tumors, particularly if compression of the optic nerve or the chiasm causes unilateral visual deterioration or if visual field defects are uncharacteristic, if mental disorder hinder the patients' perception and criticism or if other organic disturbances are predominant.

Material

During the last four and a half years we have treated 21 patients in whom, to some extent over a period of months and years, amblyopia was etiologically misinterpreted. Computed tomography was carried out relatively late and, in most cases, not expecting an intracranial tumor.

In table 1 we have listed the histological findings of 21 surgically treated patients and the initial diagnosis. Of the 12 meningiomas four were classified as tuberculum sellae meningiomas, four of the sphenoid ridge, three of the olfactory groove, and a very small meningioma was found in the optic foramen. Furthermore we found three pituitary adenomas, two craniopharyngiomas, two central gliomas, and two aneurysms.

Table 1. Clinical misinterpretations of visual disturbances

Histologic findings		Visual disturbances clinically misinterpreted as:					
		vascular optic atrophy	retrobulbar neuritis	optico-chiasmatic arachnoiditis	toxinic amblyopia	vegetative disorder	strabismus
Meningioma	12	4	2	2	1	1	2
Pituitary adenoma	3	2				1	
Craniopharyngioma	2	1				1	
Oligodendroglioma	1					1	
Malign. glioma	1				1		
Aneurysm	2	2					
Number of cases	21	9	2	2	2	4	2

In table 2 the reasons for misinterpretation of impaired vision are assembled.

1. In 4 cases unilateral impairment of vision was tolerated or not realised by the patient

A 57 year old female with a large aneurysm of the internal carotid artery tolerated visual loss of the left eye for years. She did not enter hospital until deterioration of vision of the right eye occurred.

A 43 year old teacher suffered from an increased need for sleep, hypotonia, steady increase in weight and impaired potency. Progressive unilateral deterioration

Table 2. Reason for misinterpretation of amblyopia

	no. of cases: 21
1. unilateral impairment of vision	4
2. uncharacteristic visual field defect	4
3. frontal lobe-syndrome	4
4. pituitary-diencephalic disorder	3
5. chronic alcoholism	2
6. from infancy	2
7. high grade myopia	1
8. mental deficiency	1

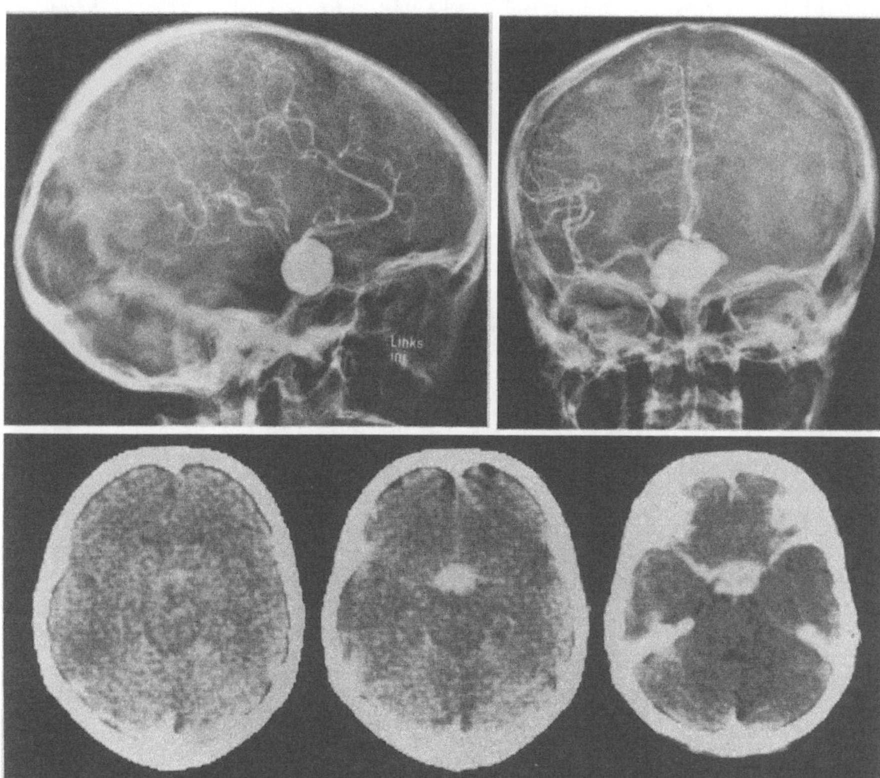

Fig. 1. Aneurysm of the internal carotid artery.

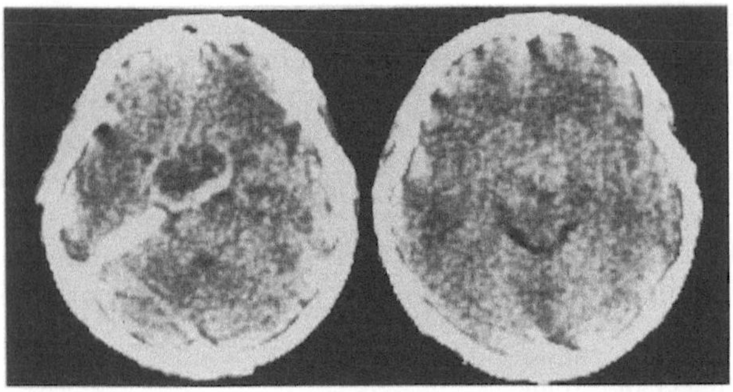

Fig. 2. Cystic pituitary adenoma.

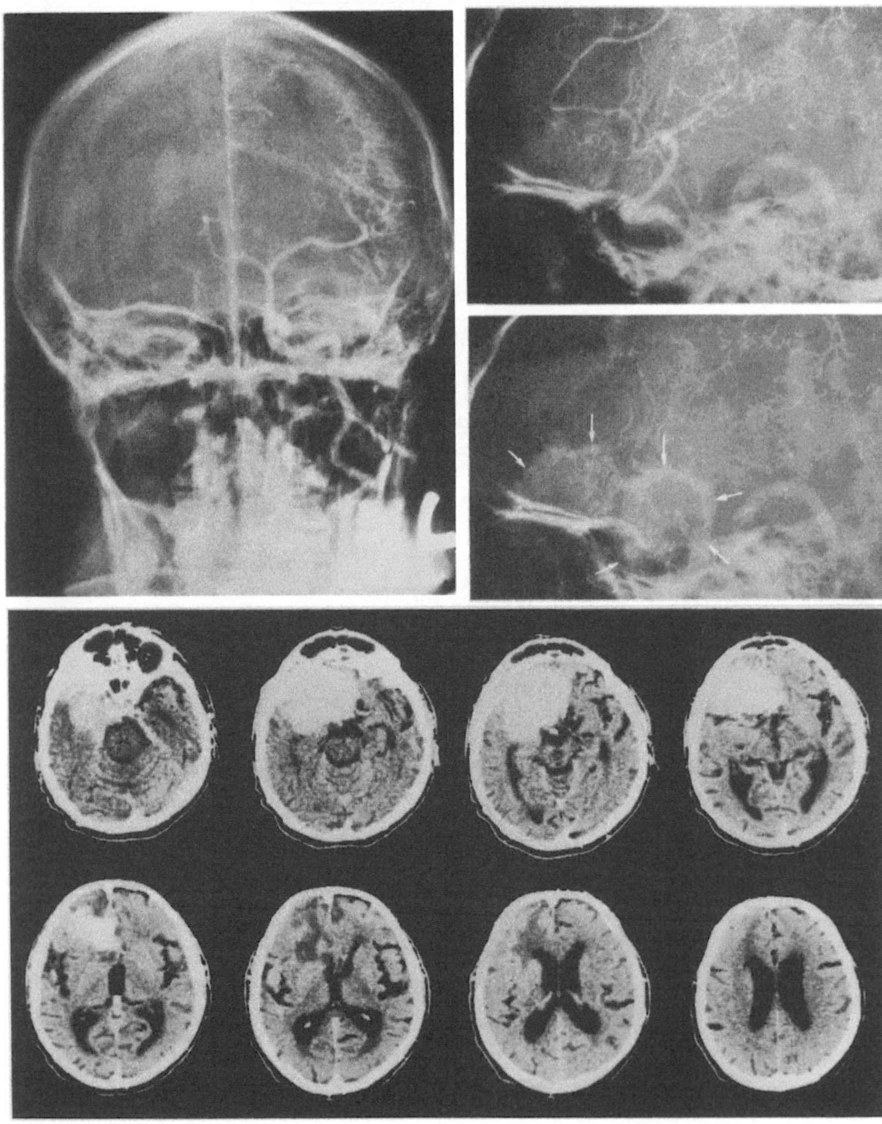

Fig. 3. Meningioma of the sphenoid ridge.

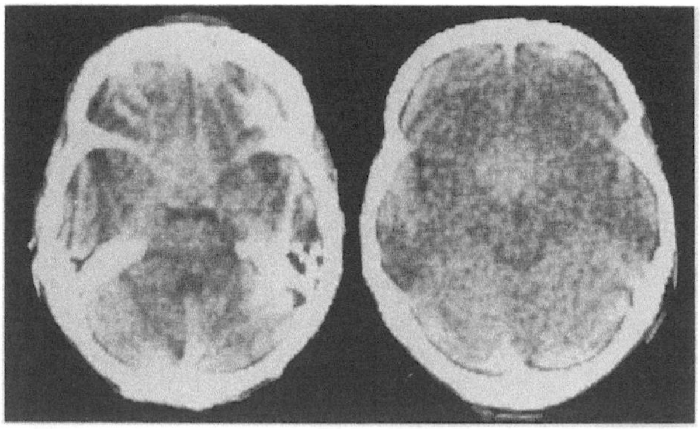

Fig. 4. Meningioma of the tuberculum sellae.

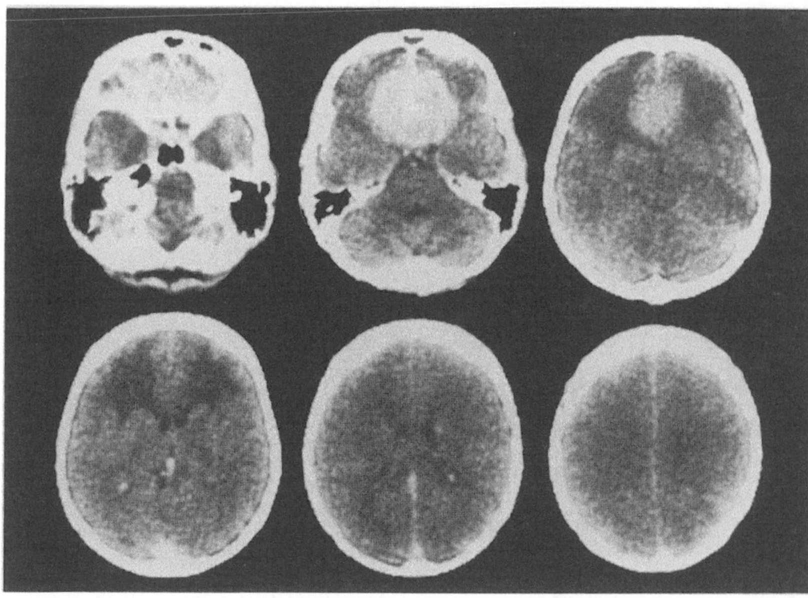

Fig. 5. Meningioma of the olfactory groove.

of vision did not disturb him for years. After he had broken his glasses an ophthalmologic examination followed revealing atrophy of the left optic nerve and left-sided concentric visual field defect. Further examination confirmed a left-sided cystic pituitary adenomy.

A 73 year old dentist had tolerated impaired vision of the left eye for 30 years. The first ophthalmologic examination two years ago revealed atrophy of the left optic nerve. At that time he could not decide on the recommended neurological examination, but underwent diagnostic procedure and surgical removal of the sphenoid ridge meningioma when vision of the right eye worsened.

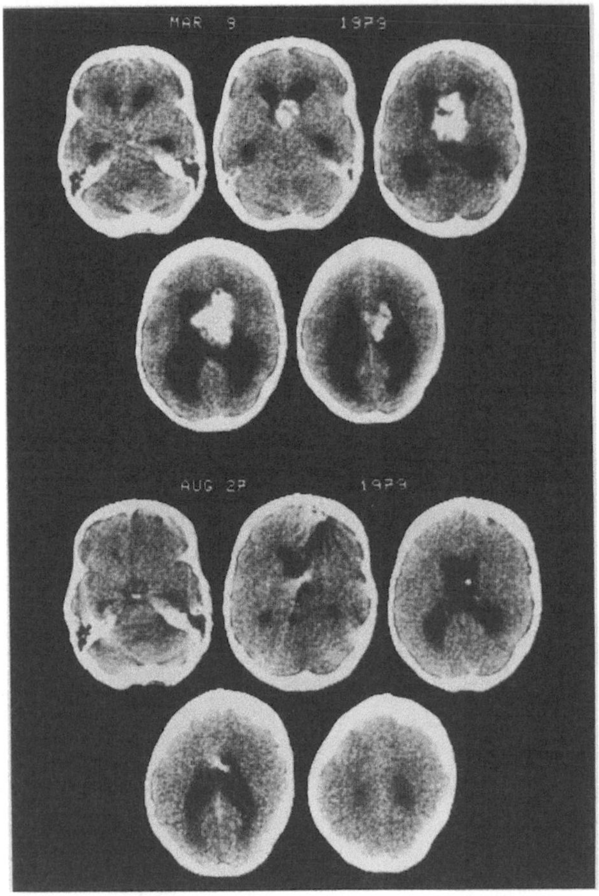

Fig. 6. Oligodendroglioma pre- and postoperatively.

2. Uncharacteristic visual field defects were found with three meningiomas of the tuberculum sellae and one pituitary adenoma.

A 54 year old female had suffered from loss of visual perception for two days after a narcosis 22 years ago. Twelve years ago atrophy of the left optic nerve was diagnosed. 11 and eight years ago neurological examinations performed in university hospitals, including angiography and pneumencephalography, showed no abnormality. Two years ago, after an abdominal operation, loss of vision on both sides appeared temporarily after which a right temporal visual field defect remained. Arachnopathia optico chiasmatica was suspected but finally computed tomography showed a meningioma of the tuberculum sellae. After surgical removal of the tumor slight improvement of vision was evident.

3. Three patients with frontal meningiomas and one with a craniopharyngioma showed marked frontal lobe syndromes, therefore impairment of vision was confirmed very late.

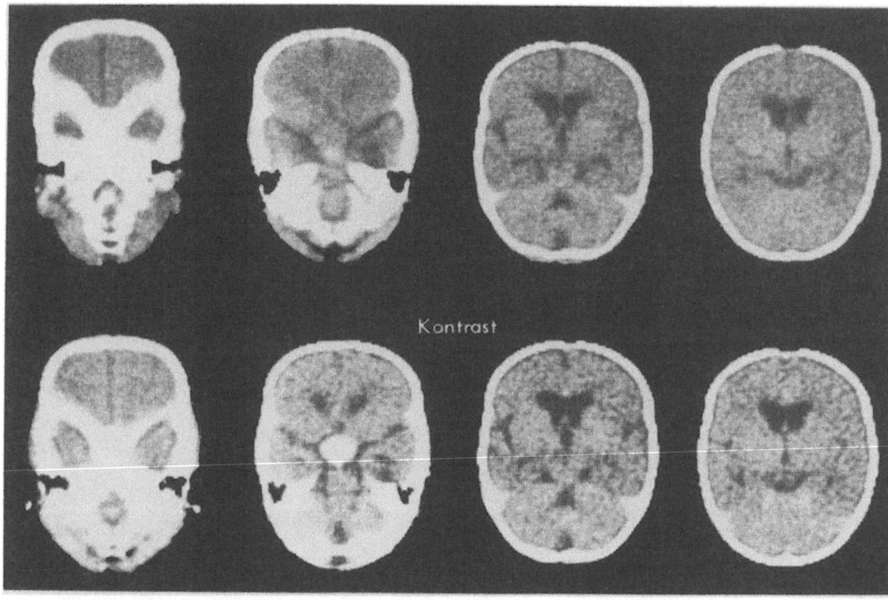

Fig. 7. Sella meningioma in a six months old child.

To illustrate this group we show a 58 year old patient with a meningioma of the olfactory groove which was not diagnosed until loss of vision of the right eye and only light-perception in the left eye was evident.

4. Marked diencephalic dysfunction was found in patients with a craniopharyngioma, a meningioma of the sphenoid ridge and a central oligodendroglioma.

The latter case was a 26 year old student, who was being treated for more than one year due to vascular headache, vertigo and attacks of hypotonia. Blurred vision when reading and watching television was interpreted as circulatory disorder. After loss of vision of the right eye and rapid deterioration of vision of the left, high-grade choked discs on both sides were discovered. After surgery circulatory function was no longer impaired, however vision improved on the left side only.

5. Two patients were being treated by psychiatrists due to chronic alcoholism, showing dyschromatopsia, and deterioration of vision. A meningioma of the tuberculum sellae and a central glioma were diagnosed very late.

6. Impairment of visual perception in children is frequently discovered at a very late stage.

A six months old child had primarily normal growth and development. After 3 months with the aid of CT scanning a suprasellar meningioma was verified compressing the chiasm.

A five year old girl showed left proptosis and slight ptosis as well as an asymmetry of the cranium from birth.

Computed tomography was carried out after the child became tearful, showed signs of defiance and became more and more clumsy. A giant meningioma of the left hemisphere was revealed. Deterioration of vision was not established until

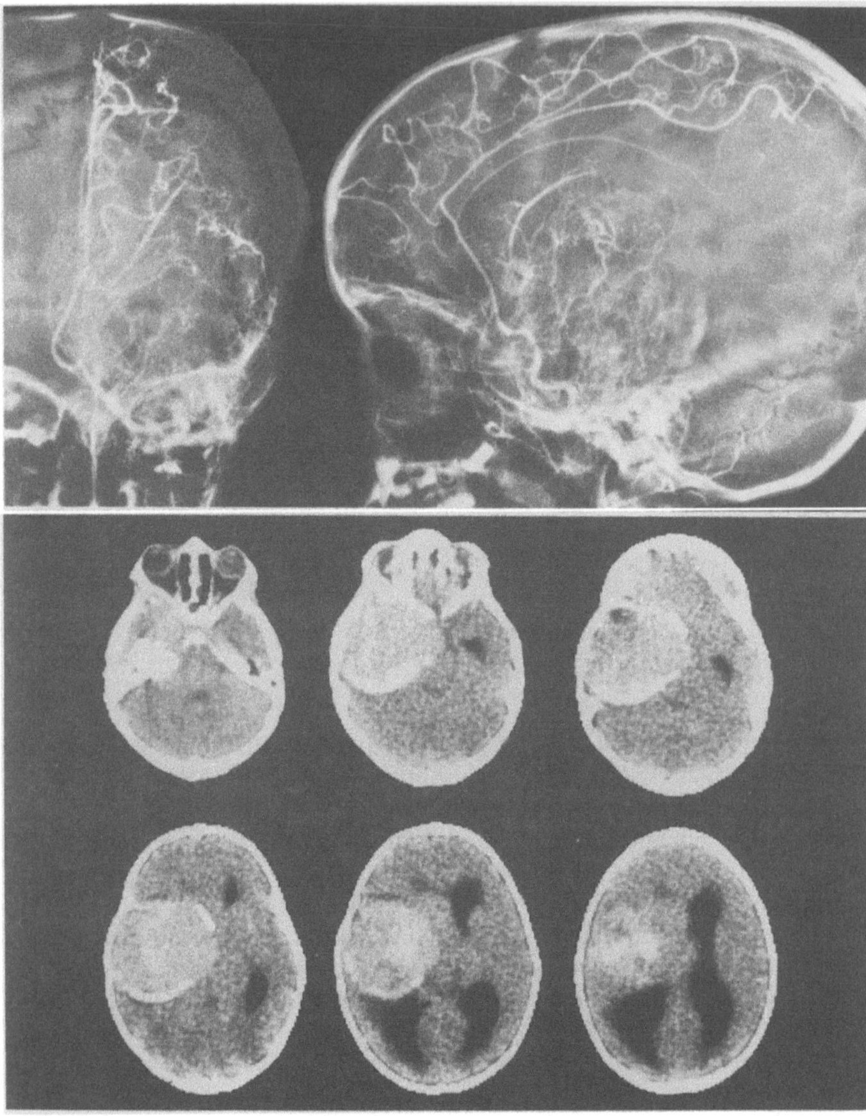

Fig. 8. Meningioma of the sphenoid ridge in a five year old child.

ophthalmologic examination showed choked discs on both sides. Vision improved rapidly after removal of the tumor.

7. Transiant bitemporal constriction of the visual field had been present in a 53 year old intensely myopic patient for many years. After a sudden onset of visual impairment CT scan revealed a very small hyperdense lesion within the sella. At operation a hematoma in the size of a peanut was found in old scar tissue and a small thrombosed aneurysm of the anterior communicating artery, not detected angiographically, was clipped.

8. The last case concerned a pituitary adenoma in a senile patient.

Conclusion

With the aid of CT scanning we easily diagnosed tumors in the region of the optic nerves in 21 patients, whose impairment of vision over a period of months and years was misinterpreted. The presentation of the reasons for the misinterpretation should encourage neurologists and ophthalmologists to carry out CT scanning at an early stage.

Transcranial Decompression of Optic Nerve After Trauma

J. Brihaye, Brussels/Belgium

The decision to operate, the operative technique and the appraisal of results in surgery of traumatic amaurosis are in relation with the clinical data, themselves dependent upon the pathology of the lesion. Therefore, before dealing with the surgical treatment, we will examine the clinical course and, afterwards, we will discuss the pathological factors which can be considered as responsible for the loss of vision.

As was previously demonstrated by the author [1], we have to consider two main clinical situations according to whether the visual loss is contemporaneous with the trauma or as it occurs some time after the trauma.

Visual loss, contemporaneous with the trauma, can be complete (amaurosis) or partial.

Amaurosis is recognized by the association of mydriasis with the abolition of the pupillary reflex to light, and by the occurrence of optic atrophy which appears a variable time after the injury, dependent upon the more or less remote site of the lesion on the optic nerve. Usually the nerve is injured at the level of the optic canal and the optic atrophy is observed 4 or 6 weeks afterwards.

In most cases, immediate amaurosis is irreversible, although a partial or total spontaneous recovery may rarely occur within the hours or days following the trauma. Favory and Sedan [9] have observed immediate amaurosis of a few minutes duration in boxers. In our department we saw a patient, 42 years old, who fell from his motor bike; he did not lose consciousness but was immediately blind. Within minutes he recovered the vision of the right eye, but the left eye remained amaurotic with the development of an optic atrophy.

The frequency of traumatic amaurosis is difficult to determine. Many injured people are in a comatous or non-responsive state; therefore, in the absence of a careful examination of the eyes it is not possible to know if there was a total but transitory loss of vision. So it is with patients who complain of amaurosis at the time of their recovery from unconsciousness; we do not always know if the amaurosis developed early or later.

When the visual loss is immediate but partial, one notices a sudden fall of the visual acuity associated with perimetric alterations.

We have seen cases with an abrupt but stable decrease in visual acuity as well as progressive deterioration of the vision up to an amaurosis. Turner [21] observed in 10 patients a visual acuity less than 1/10 and between 1/10 and 10/10 in 23 other people.

The fundus oculi in general has a normal appearance. The perimetric alterations are unpredictable. We have observed concentric narrowing as well as quadrantal or horizontal hemianopia, inferior or superior. The outline of the deficit is usually irregular [1].

Spontaneous recovery is as rare as is in those patients with immediate and total loss of vision.

Delayed visual loss can occur a short time (a few hours up to a few days) after the trauma or several weeks or even months later. In cases of an early visual alteration, as reported by Pringle [15] and Calmettes et al. [5], the decrease of the visual acuity is progressively rapid and the clinical course is similar to retrobulbar neuritis, more especially as the visual loss is often associated with a central scotoma. In rare cases, the decrease in vision occurs much later after the trauma and is due to slow compression of the optic nerve. In one of our patients [2] the lesion was a traumatic aneurysm of the carotid artery just beneath the optic nerve. In other cases, the lesion was an osseous callus in the optic canal or a secondary adhesive arachnoiditis [12, 19].

These differences in the clinical course are the direct expression of the underlying traumatic pathology which depends partly on the anatomical characteristics of the optic canal and optic nerve. We must recall the existence of the falciform ligament at the superior border of the intracranial optic foramen, the irregular shape of the optic canal with its narrowest and thickest portion at the intraorbital optic foramen [13], the importance of the vascular network in the pia-

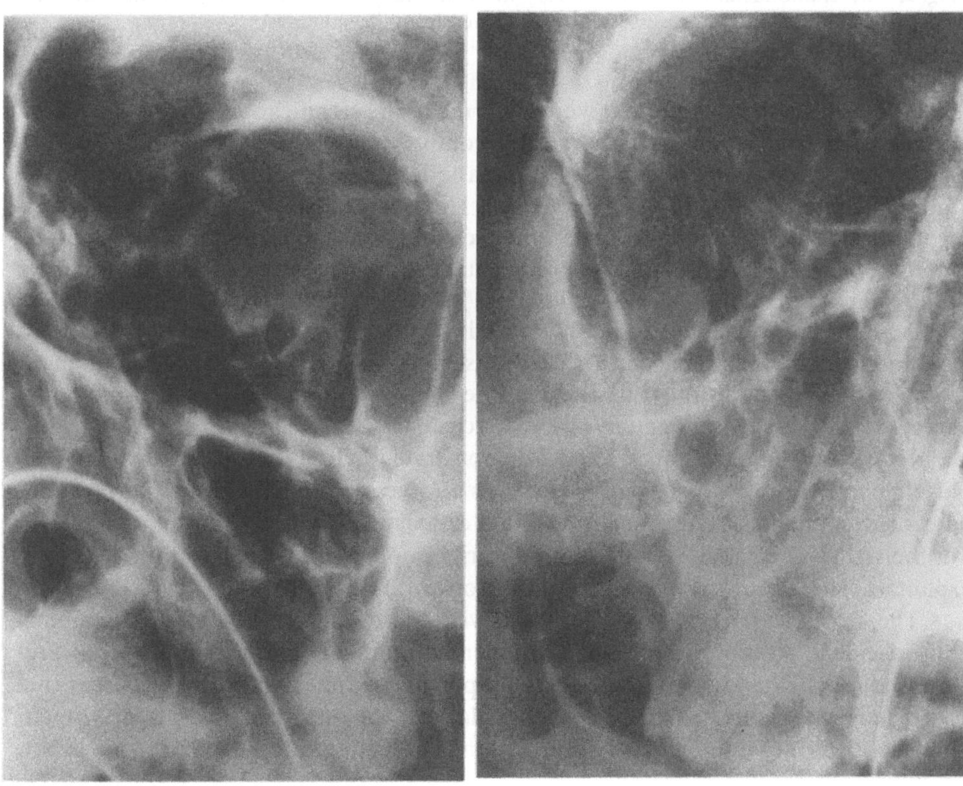

Fig. 1. The left optic foramen (left side of the figure) has a normal appearance. The right optic foramen is completely disrupted

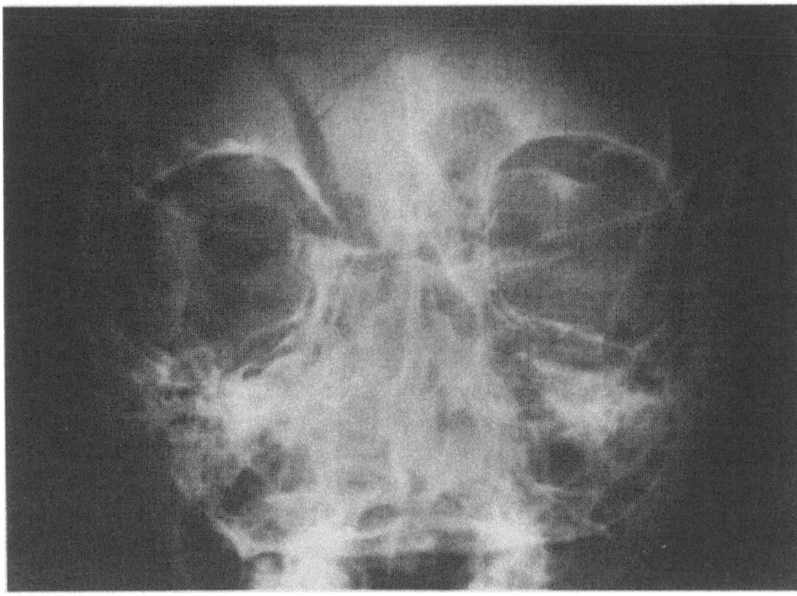

Fig. 2. The cranio-facial dislocation is very marked and particularly serious on the left side where the anterior clinoid process is partly detached from the sphenoid

mater of the nerve [3]. Later on, we will correlate the significance of these anatomical peculiarities in regard to the surgical decompression of the optic nerve.

We must consider two kinds of traumatic lesions of the optic nerve, some of mechanical and others of vascular nature. However, most of the time, no macroscopic lesion of the optic nerve is noted during surgical exploration or at postmortem examination. We must therefore understand that the pathogenic theories still remain partly hypothetical.

Among the mechanical causes, tear and torsion of the nerve due to traction at the moment of the impact are rarely observed. Experimental work on human cadavers have demonstrated that tear of the chiasm occurs before that of the optic nerves [7, 14]. Likewise, fracture of the optic canal is not frequently associated with a laceration of the nerve. Figs. 1 and 2 demonstrate fractures of the canal with lesion of the nerve. The first case (Fig. 1) concerns a 25 year old man who was involved in a car accident. He sustained a cranio-facial dislocation and a comminuting fracture of the right optic canal. At operation, the right optic nerve was lacerated by bone splinters. The amaurosis was contemporaneous with the injury and irreversible.

The second case (Fig. 2) concerns a 22 year old man who suffered a fatal motor bike accident. At admission he had an open cranio-facial fracture. Both eyes were a-reflectic to light. At operation, the right optic nerve appeared normal whereas the other nerve was contused and markedly enlarged; the optic canal was largely open but there was no improvement of the vision. The patient did not survive his brain injury.

Such a traumatic laceration of the optic nerve accounts for an immediate and probably irreversible amaurosis. Contusion can be responsible of a secondary

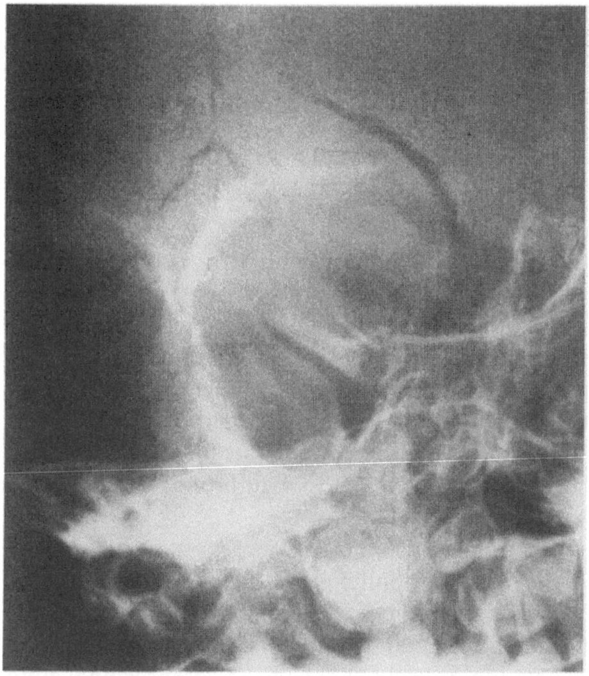

Fig. 3. A bone splinter encroaches upon the optic nerve in the optic canal

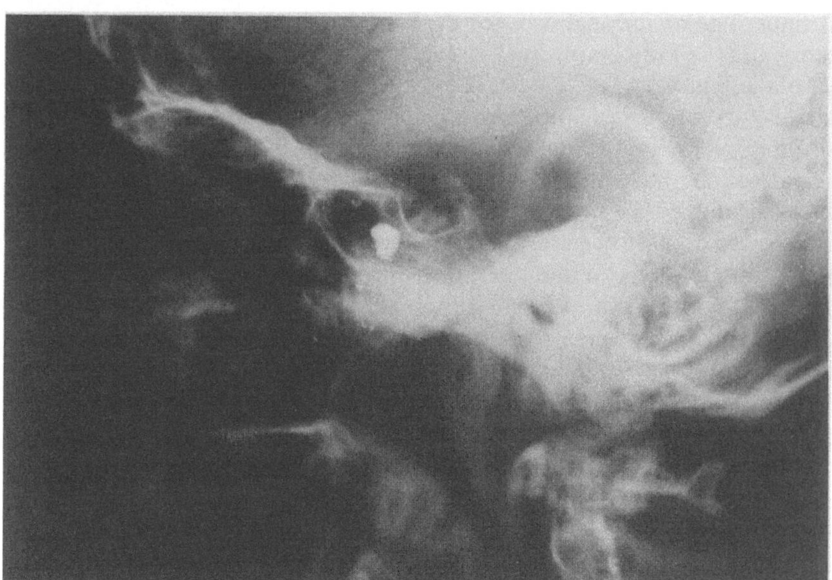

Fig. 4. Lateral view of the skull. Bullet in the sphenoidal sinus and fracture of the floor of the sella turcica

edematous reaction with enlargement of the nerve which results in compression inside the optic canal. This delayed compression of the optic fibers can explain an early delayed loss of vision.

We have seen linear bruising of the upper part of the optic nerve in relation with the meningeal falciform process as well as edematous reaction and enlargement of the nerve. Although this observation was made in only a few cases, it is evident that direct traumatic injury of the nerve can account for immediate or early delayed loss of vision. The patient in figure 3 concerns a child of one and a half year of age who fell from the first floor of his house. After two days of coma he rapidly regained consciousness. Four days after the fall, a right mydriasis was observed for the first time and the skull X-rays demonstrated a right frontal fracture and a bone splinter protruding into the right optic canal. The boy was transferred to our department 10 days after trauma. At operation, the optic foramen appeared normal and the nerve had a normal appearance at this level; on the other hand, there was a comminuting fracture of the roof of the optic canal. The optic nerve was liberated from bone fragments. No improvement of vision occurred after operation.

Figs. 4, 5 and 6 concern a 54 year old man who made an attempt at suicide with a revolver. He shot himself under the chin. The bullet was stopped at the skull base in the sphenoidal sinus. No neurological signs except for an immediate and irreversible left amaurosis were observed. Fundus oculi and perimetry of the right eye were normal. Left optic atrophy appear within 5 weeks. Leakage of cerebrospinal fluid through the sphenoidal sinus occurred soon after the trauma. X-rays of the skull show the bullet in the sphenoidal sinus, a fracture of the floor of the sella turcica and small metallic fragments around the optic canal. The patient was operated on through a transphenoidal route for extraction of the bullet and grafting of the sphenoidal sinus. The optic canal was not explored but it can be inferred from the clinical history and the radiographs that a severe contusion of the nerve occurred at the moment of the injury.

Vascular factors are often put forward in order to explain posttraumatic alteration of the optic nerve. Pringle [15] in 1922, raised the hypothesis of a compressive hematoma in the sheaths of the optic nerve. Out of 174 postmortem examinations, he noticed hemorrhage in the sheaths in 19 cases with or without fracture of the optic canal. But unfortunately there was no clinical correlation with these necropsic observations. While operating on three patients, 2, 3 and 4 weeks respectively after the trauma, Pringle observed distension of the sheaths by hemorrhage, but no improvement of the vision occurred after drainage of the blood.

With respect to this pathology one cannot forget that the optic subarachnoid space is in free communication with the cerebral subarachnoid space. Therefore blood in the sheaths of the nerve does not mean that it is responsible for the loss of vision. Moreover, the usual observation of a normal fundus oculi does not support the mechanism of a compressive hemorrhage. There is no doubt that such a hematoma could account for delayed and progressive loss of vision, but to present we do not know of any conclusive report with clinical correlation.

In reference to vascular lesions of the traumatized brain, it has been implied that lesions of the small parenchymatous vessels in the nerve may be responsible for immediate amaurosis. Mechanical strain on these small vessels would explain microscopic foci of thrombosis and hemorrhage into the nerve [8, 16, 18, 20, 21]. This hypothesis is attractive in that many perpendicular small arteries which derive from the vascular network in the pia mater enter the nerve; this anatomical distribution imperils the vascularization of the nerve if it is displaced, more especially as the sheaths of the nerve are firmly attached to the optic canal [13]. However, once again, we note the lack of postmortem verification in published reports.

A third vascular factor, arterial spasm, could play a role in some cases of early delayed loss of vision. We have discussed this pathology while reporting the clinical observation of a 34 year old man, injured in a car accident. He had a left non-reactive mydriasis at the first examination. There was a fracture of the left optic foramen. A left carotidography demonstrated segmental spasm of the ophthalmic artery at the level of the optic canal. Another angiogram, 7 days later, showed that the spasm of the ophthalmic artery had disappeared but small extravasation of the contrast media could be seen at the site of the optic canal and this extravasation

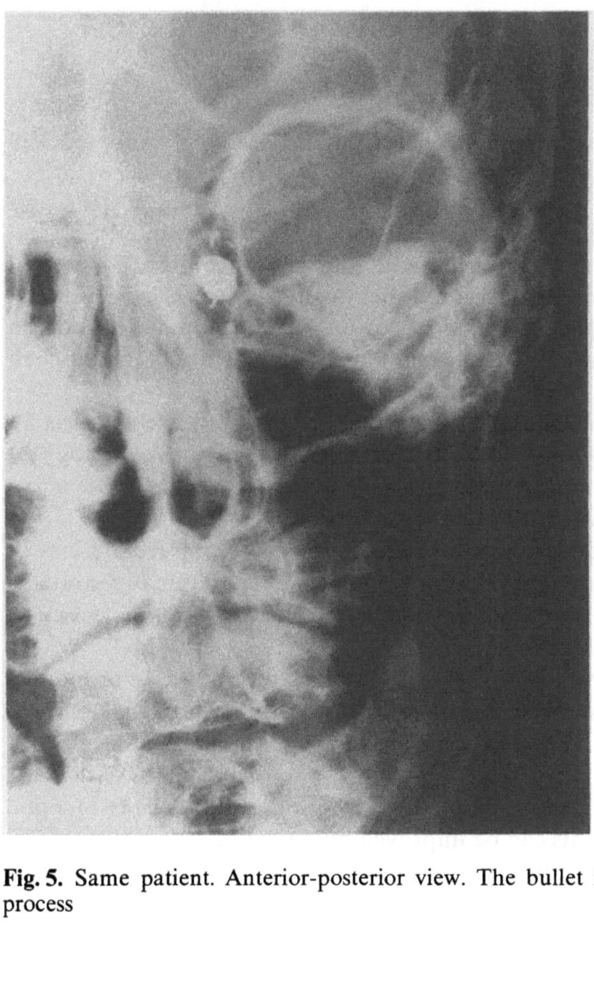

Fig. 5. Same patient. Anterior-posterior view. The bullet is seen under the anterior clinoid process

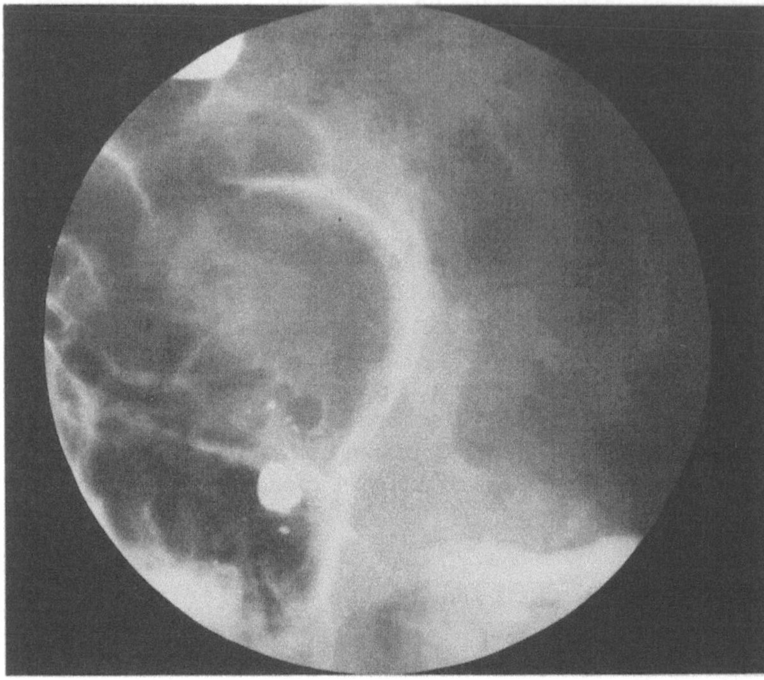

Fig. 6. Same patient. Oblique view. Metallic fragments around the optic canal are well demonstrated

was felt possibly to indicate injury of the arterial wall by a bone splinter. Surgical exploration took place 4 weeks after the trauma: the optic nerve had a normal appearance and size; no compression could be demonstrated. There was no improvement of the amaurosis [4]. Of course we can only outline a parallel between the loss of vision and the spasm of the ophthalmic artery without making an inference.

Nevertheless, for a long time, spasm of the retinal arteries was theorized as an explanation for the very transitory amaurosis or blindness in the pathology of boxing [9, 17]. We are inclined to think that spasm of the arteries of the optic nerve could play a role in some cases of posttraumatic amaurosis.

This transitory vasomotor disturbance could account for an immediate loss of vision with subsequent and progressive improvement. When traumatic strain is more severe, the functional disturbance could be replaced by organic vascular lesions, responsible for irreversible amaurosis.

Exceptionally, the progressive loss of vision takes place several weeks or months after the injury, and is known to be due to a callus of the optic canal or to a traumatic arterial ectasia [2, 12]. Secondary glial hyperplasia has also been described [19].

Considering the above discussion about the pathogenic mechanisms in optic trauma, it appears that few patients can be improved by operation.

Release of the optic nerve from a compressive or irritative factor remains a reasonable indication for operation. X-rays of the optic canal will demonstrate compound fractures, disruption of the canal and bone splinters, lesions which warrant surgical exploration.

Edema of the nerve may also warrant a surgical decompression. C.T. scan allows a fairly good appreciation of the diameter of the nerve though this demonstration is not so easy for the intracanalicular portion.

Clinically, when there is either a delayed visual disturbance, or a secondary aggravation, or an immediate but partial loss of vision, operation appears indicated. Otherwise, operation may be required because of other associated lesions (leakage of cerebrospinal fluid, etc.) and the surgeon will take this opportunity to explore the opto-chiasmatic region. In other cases, operation must be postponed because of a severe and life-threatening condition of the patient.

With respect to operative techniques, the interval between the trauma and the moment of the operation, and the extent of the decompression have to be considered. It is well known that nerve fibers are susceptible to compression which provokes extensive demyelination within the first week [6].

Therefore, to wait 3 or more days before performing a decompression can be too long a delay, and the quality of results may be improved if the decompression is carried out as soon as possible after the trauma.

To decompress the optic canal properly means more than incision of the falciform process and opening of the optic foramen. Because of the anatomical characteristics of the canal and in order to make certain that the whole length of the nerve is decompressed, it is mandatory to open the canal completely. In addition to the decompression of the bone we incised the sheaths of the nerve in two cases of edematous enlargement but that did not improve the results.

In fact, one cannot find in the literature an adequate series of cases operated by the transfrontal route with a well defined technique. The only thing about which everybody does agree is that surgical results are rather poor.

Our personal experience is also disappointing: out of 56 patients operated on for unilateral loss of vision, only 3 with edema of the nerve and 4 with laceration improved after operation. The only patient who responded to decompression of the nerve was the one with a traumatic pseudo-aneurysm of the carotid artery. In all other cases, the optic nerve had a normal appearance and size. But it should be stated that all operations were not performed by the same neurosurgeon and that the delay as well as the extent of decompression were quite different from one patient to another.

In conclusion, with regard to decision for or against operation, doubt still persists in relation to the correct attitude.

In spite of the poor results, we are of the opinion that operation is indicated providing that:

1. further studies would be better controled;
2. the shortest delay would be made in operating the patients;
3. decompression of the optic nerve would be systematically extended to the whole length of the optic canal.

In fact, we must learn why the quality of results is better when the decompression is performed by the transethmoidal route [10, 11]. The extent of the decompression, probably larger in every case with the transethmoidal approach, seems to be the most important factor in success or failure if the nerve has not been destroyed by the original injury.

References

1. Brihaye J (1954) – Lésions des nerfs optiques dans les traumatismes fermés du crâne. Acta Chir Belg 9:891–912
2. Brihaye J, Mage J, Verriest G (1954) Anévrysme traumatique de la carotide interne dans sa portion supraclinoïdienne. Acta Neurol Belg 54:411–438
3. Brihaye-Van Geertruyden M, Brihaye J (1956) Etude de la vascularisation du nerf optique. Archives de Biologie 67:569–581
4. Brihaye J, Brihaye-Van Geertruyden M, Jeanmart L (1976) Spasm of the ophthalmic artery in a case of posttraumatic amaurosis. Acta Neurochir (Wien) 33:319–324
5. Calmettes, Deodati, Anduze, Delfour (1953) Deux cas de traumatisme du nerf optique. Rev Otoneuroophthalmol 25:393–395
6. Clifford-Jones RE, Landon DN, Mc Donald WI (1980) Remyelination during optic nerve compression. J Neurol Sci 46:239–243
7. Coppez H (1929) Le mécanisme des lésions du chiasma dans les fractures du crâne. Arch Ophthalmol 46:705–716
8. Daum S, Guillaumat L, Ferrey B (1950) L'atteinte du nerf optique constatée précocement après un traumatisme cranien fermé constitue-t-elle une indication opératoire. Rev Otoneuroophthalmol 22:485–487
9. Favory A, Sedan J (1951) Traumatologie oculaire du boxeur. Arch Ophthalmol 11: 428–456
10. Fukado Y (1975) Results in 400 cases of surgical decompression of the optic nerve. In modern problems in ophthalmology. S Karger 14:474–481
11. Kennerdell JS, Amsbaugh GA, Myers EN (1976) Transantralethmoidal decompression of the optic canal fracture. Arch Ophthalm 94:1040–1043
12. Lillie WI, Adson AW (1934) Unilateral central and annular scotoma produced by callus from fracture extending into optic canal. Arch Ophthalmol 12:500–508
13. Maniscalco JE, Habal MB (1978) Microanatomy of the optic canal. J Neurosurg 48: 402–406
14. Osterberg G (1938) Traumatic bitemporal hemianopia (sagittal tearing of the optic chiasm). Acta Ophthalmol 16:466–474
15. Pringle JH (1922) Atrophy of the optic nerve following diffused violence to the skull. Br Med J 2:115–157
16. Rodger FC (1943) Unilateral involvement of the optic nerve in head injuries. Brit J Ophthalmol 27:23–33
17. Sedan J, Allies P (1951) Contrôle de la P.A.R. au cours même d'un knock-out. Rev Otoneuroophthalmol 23:374–377
18. Symonds CP (1945) Discussion on the ocular sequelae of head injuries. Trans Ophthalmol Soc UK 65:3–19
19. Tavernier Guillaumat Rosier (1950) Arachnoïdite optochiasmatique traumatique avec atrophie optique et cécité d'un oeil, puis deux ans plus tard baisse de l'acuité visuelle de l'autre oeil. Amélioration bilatérale de la vision à la suite d'une encéphalographie et d'une trépanation. Rev Otoneuroophthalmol 22:487–490
20. Traquair HM, Dott NM, Russell WR (1935) Traumatic lésions of the optic chiasm. Brain 58:398–411
21. Turner JWA (1943) Indirect injuries of the optic nerve. Brain 66:140–151

Microsurgical Transethmoidal Optic Nerve Decompression: Experience in 700 Cases

Y. FUKADO, Tokyo/Japan

Injury of the optic nerve is a complication most frequently seen in blunt head trauma, especially that caused by traffic accidents. In the past 18 years, an optic nerve injury was diagnosed in 750 cases with impaired vision after blunt head trauma. To improve the visual function in these patients, surgical decompression of the optic nerve may be indicated. In previous papers the results in 600 cases of such surgery done by the transethmoidal route were reported (Fukado, 1975, 1978). Since then, an improved surgical technique has been used under an operating microscope and the number of cases operated upon has reached 700, so that a more complete survey of the results and the method of surgery can be made. This paper will deal with the details of this surgical technique and the postoperative results of these 700 cases.

An optic nerve injury after blunt head trauma can be diagnosed from the characteristic clinical signs. The characteristic clinical signs are loss, or sluggishness of the direct light reaction of the pupil on the affected side (100 percent), a wound in the lateral part of the eyebrow (92 percent) and bleeding from the nose (76 percent). X-Roentgenograms do not show a fracture around the optic canal in every case.

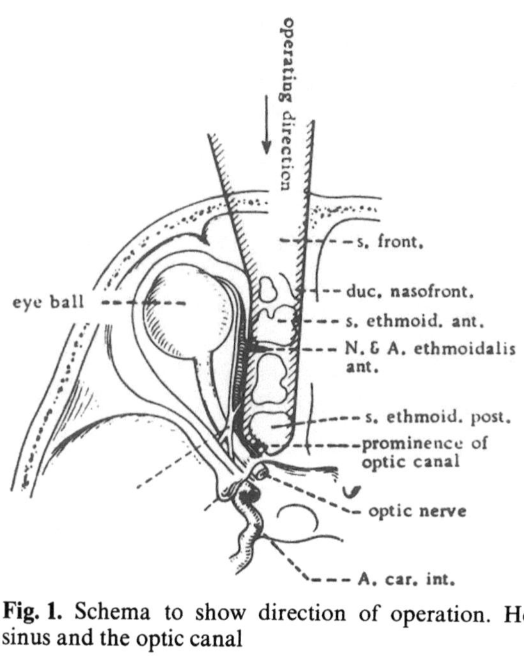

Fig. 1. Schema to show direction of operation. Horizontal section through the ethmoidal sinus and the optic canal

This is not only because of individual variation in the anatomy of the skull but also because the optic nerve injury may occur by the distortion of the canal at the moment of injury without a fracture.

The principle of this operation is illustrated in figures 1 and 2. The anterior wall of the ethmoidal sinus is removed and the optic canal is reached through the sinus. The inner wall of the optic canal is removed, taking care that the periosteum and the dural sheath of the optic nerve are spared.

The operation is done under local anesthesia, except in children, with one ml of two percent procaine hydrochloride. A straight skin incision, 40 mm long, is made along the inner wall of the orbit from the medial part of the eyebrow down to the lacrimal sac. The underlying periosteum is elevated from the bone as widely as possible. An oval piece of bone (15×10 mm^2) is removed from the junctional area of the processus frontalis of the maxillary bone, the ethmoidal and the frontal bones. The ethmoidal sinus can clearly be seen. The mucous membrane of the ethmoidal sinus is anesthetized with a gauze tampon immersed in four percent xylocaine solution and bleeding is stopped with adrenaline. The mucous membrane and the septa of the sinus are carefully removed to reach the depths of the sinus. Great care must be taken not to perforate the thin medial wall of the orbit and not to tear the optic nerve. At the very deepest end of the ethmoidal sinus, which in 40–45 mm deep, one can find the prominence of the optic canal.

At the deepest part of the ethmoidal sinus, the thin inner wall of the orbit is perforated with a spatula and a small piece of bone (about 10 mm in diameter) is removed. From this hole the inner wall of the optic canal, which is seen as a prominence, is removed as much as possible. Since the inner wall of the optic canal

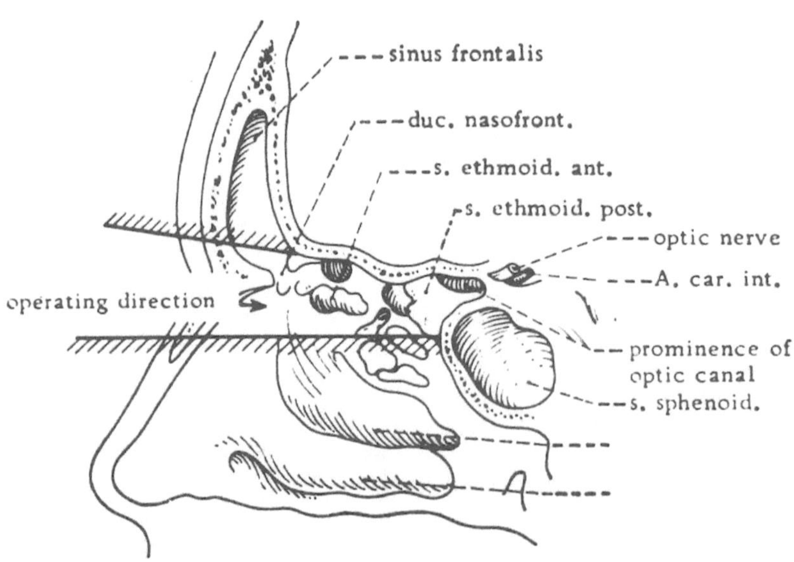

Fig. 2. Schema to show direction of operation. Sagittal section through the ethmoidal sinus and the optic canal

is thickest at its orbital end, further removal of the inner wall of the optic canal can be done with ease. During these procedures the direct light reaction of the pupil is examined and the patient is asked whether or not any visual improvement is recognized. In some cases an immediate improvement is reported.

Sometimes anatomical variations are encountered, such as where the optic canal runs in the deepest and upper end of the ethmoidal sinus and no bony prominence representing the optic canal can be recognized. In this case, after the inner wall of the orbit is perforated, the upper wall of the ethmoidal sinus is removed, then one can usually see the white optic nerve covered with its dural sheath.

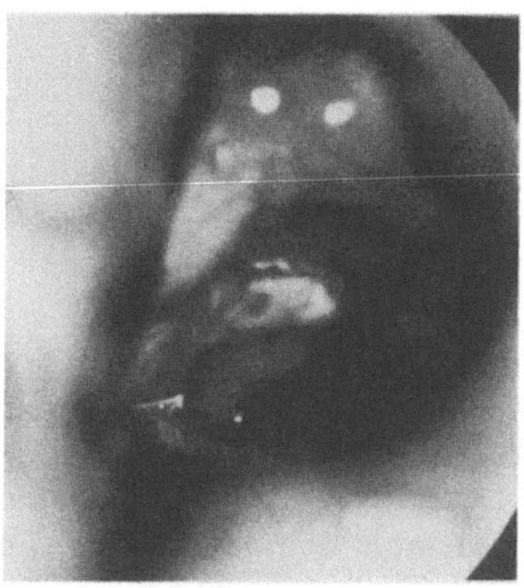

Fig. 3. The exposed optic nerve with its dural sheath

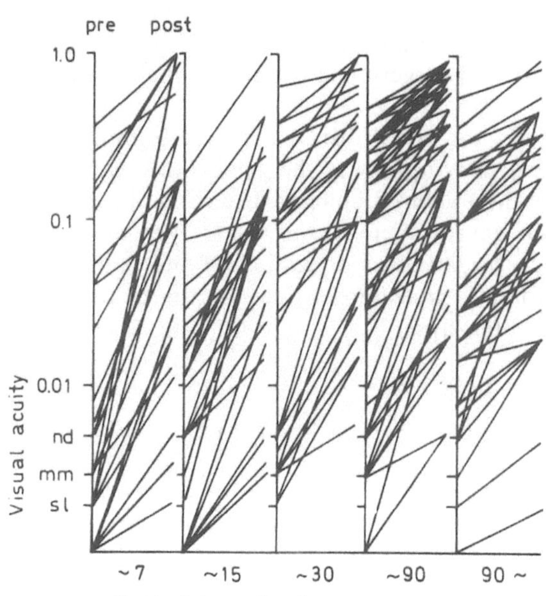

Fig. 4. Results of surgery. Postoperative visual acuity was determined after 6 months. The patients were divided according to the interval between the injury and surgery

Hemorrhage from the surrounding bone and mucous membrane is arrested with gauze tampon immersed in adrenaline. No gauze tampon should be used postoperatively. When the area around the optic nerve is clean and the hemorrhage has stopped, the periosteum of the maxillary and frontal bones are sutured together with catgut. The skin wound is sutured with nylon. The exposed optic nerve covered with its dural sheath is demonstrated in figure 3. Postoperative care is simple and the patient may remain an ambulatory case.

The postoperative improvement in the visual acuity is illustrated in figure 4 and table 1, where the patients are divided according to various intervals between the

Table 1. Results of surgery in recent 300 cases

within	7 days	23/54	43%
within	15 days	26/60	43%
within	30 days	31/73	42%
within	90 days	27/77	35%
over	90 days	14/36	39%

surgery and the injury. The postoperative visual acuity was determined at six month intervals. In cases where the operation was performed within seven days after the injury, remarkable improvement was obtained. With a longer interval after the injury the improvement is less, but a considerable number of cases can still obtain better postoperative visual function even after as long as 90 days. These cases were followed up to one year and none showed any deterioration of visual function. Improvement of the visual acuity, of course, depends on the severity of the damage of the optic nerve. From these results, however, one can say that the shorter the interval between the injury and surgery, the better postoperative visual improvement can be expected.

As evidenced by the present results, the visual disturbance due to optic nerve injury is a result of the physiological interruption of the optic nerve caused by hemorrhage, edema, compression by the fractured bone or distortion of the canal. It is, therefore, possible to obtain an improvement in the vision even more than three months after the injury. Since surgical decompression of the optic nerve described in this paper is a safe and easy procedure, it may be the treatment of choice even after a long posttraumatic time lapse.

References

Fukado Y (1975) Results in 400 Cases of Surgical Decompression of the Optic Nerve. Bleeker GM Orbital Disorders. S. Karger, Basel p 474–481

Fukado Y (1978) Results in 600 cases of surgical decompression of the optic nerve. Shimizu K XXIII Concilium Ophthalmologicum, Kyoto, Excerpta Medica, Amsterdam-Oxford p 1136–1137

Childhood Optic Gliomas. Microsurgical Treatment

W. Koos, A. Perneczky, and H. Schuster, Vienna/Austria

Over the decades there have been many excellent reviews of the literature (Byers, 1901; Hudson, 1912; Lundberg, 1935; Davis, 1940; Eggers et al., 1976; Oxenhandler and Sayers, 1978), but no present uniform therapeutic management of childhood optic gliomas exists. These gliomas remain a rare and controversial entity in the spectrum of intracranial tumors in children. Based on the cases treated at the Neurosurgical Department of the University of Vienna, a total of 36 patients ranging from one to 15 years of age, we would like to point out the surgical possibilities that have been opened up after the introduction of microsurgical techniques 10 years ago.

Material

The average age of the 36 children at the time of the operation (Table 1) was six and a half years, the youngest patient being 10 months and the eldest one 15 years. Both sexes were equally affected. In 14 patients (Table 2) the tumor was located in

Table 1. Age at diagnosis of optic gliomas ($n = 36$)

Age (yrs.)	no. of patients
– 1	1
1 – 5	14
6 – 10	15
11 – 15	6
	36

the area of the optic nerve. One child with a purely intraorbital glioma had a second tumor growing in the contralateral intracranial section of the optic nerve, which affected also parts of the chiasm. This patient was included among the seven cases of the group comprising children with gliomas of the optic chiasm. In 15 other cases, the tumor already affected the hypothalamus.

Surgery and Results

In the description of the surgical treatment and the postoperative results, we would like to distinguish between those cases where the tumors affected only the optic nerve and those where the tumor was localized in the chiasm and the hypothalamus.

Table 2. Gliomas of the optic pathways and hypothalamus (Dept. of Neurosurgery Vienna, 1964 – 1979)

Localization	of Patients	of Operations
Optic nerve		
Orbital section	6 (1)	
Orbital and intracranial section	6	14
Intracranial section	1	
Orbital and intracranial section and chiasm	1	
Optic chiasm		
Chiasm and intracranial section of optic nerve	5	8
Chiasm and intracranial section of optic nerve and hypothalamus	2	
Hypothalamus		
Optic chiasm and hypothalamus Hypothalamus and optic chiasm and thalamus	15	17
Total	36	39
Ventriculo-atrial shunts for hydrocephalus		11

1. The method of choice in treating gliomas of the optic nerve is the total extirpation of the nerve section containing the tumor (Table 3). Intraoperative histological control can offer a guarantee for the total removal of the tumor (Fig. 1). Usually the roof of the orbit has to be removed and the optic canal opened, in order to clarify the extent of the tumor. In three patients, in whom it was possible to establish with certainty that the tumor has affected the bulb, the latter has been removed as well. All of our 13 patients whose tumor had affected only the optic nerve have remained free of any complaint over the entire 16 year period of observation.

2. Six of the children suffering from gliomas of the chiasm and the hypothalamus were operated on prior to the introduction of the operating microscope; in the 19 other operations the operating microscope was used (Table 4). The tumors which involved the chiasm and had not at all or only to a small extent grown into

Table 3. Gliomas of the optic nerve ($n = 13$)

Operations	14
Extirpation of the optic nerve	11
Enucleation of the bulbus (plus optic nerve)	3
Postoperative condition	
Good (quoad vitam)	12
Fair (cosmetically)	2
Postop. death	0

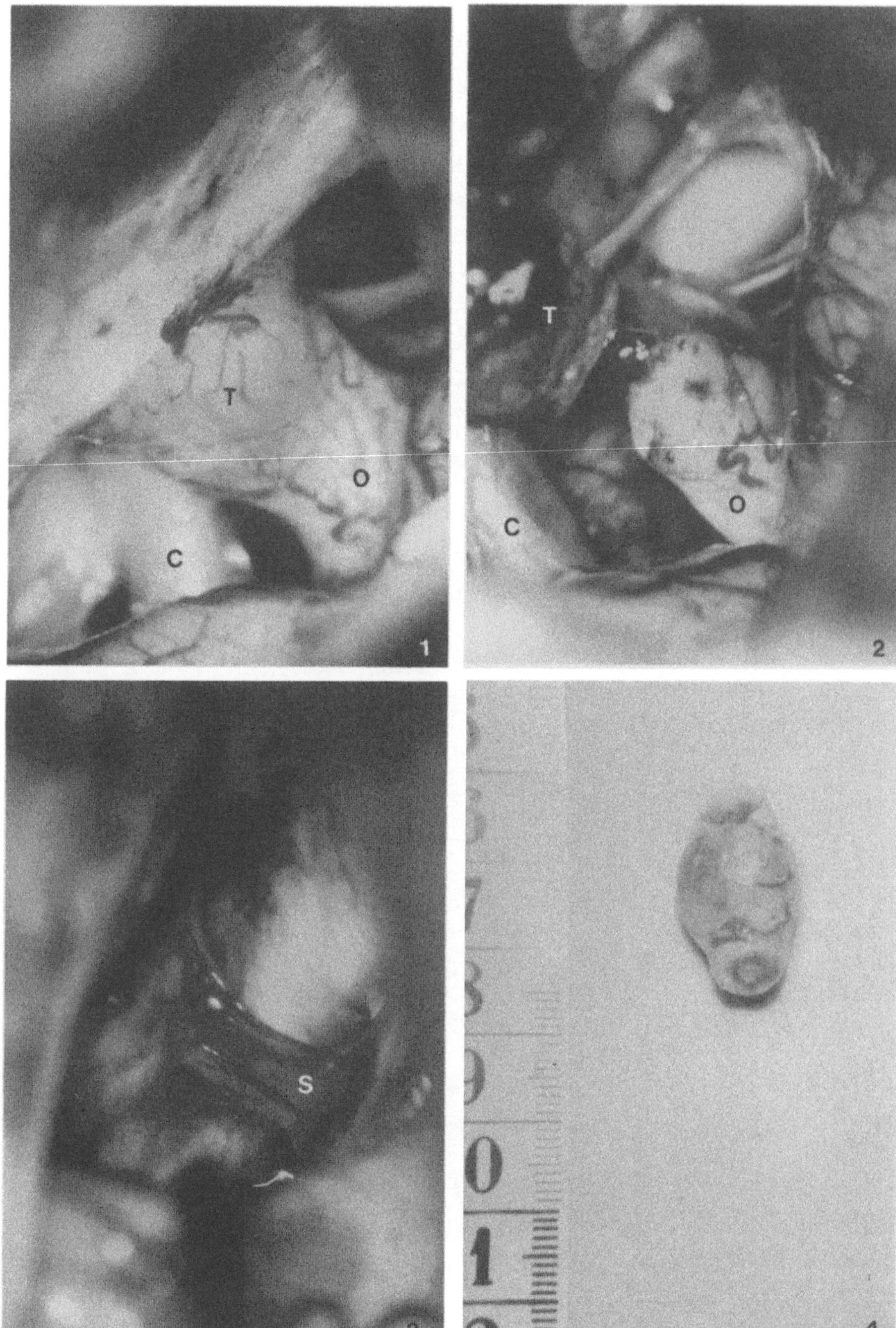

Fig. 1. Glioma of the left optic nerve with intracranial expansion of 3 mm. *1* The tumor in situ. *2* Transsection of the optic nerve centrally of the tumor. *3* The pituitary stalk after total removal of the glioma. *4* The resected tumor. *O* left optic nerve; *C* left internal carotid artery; *S* pituitary stalk; *T* tumor

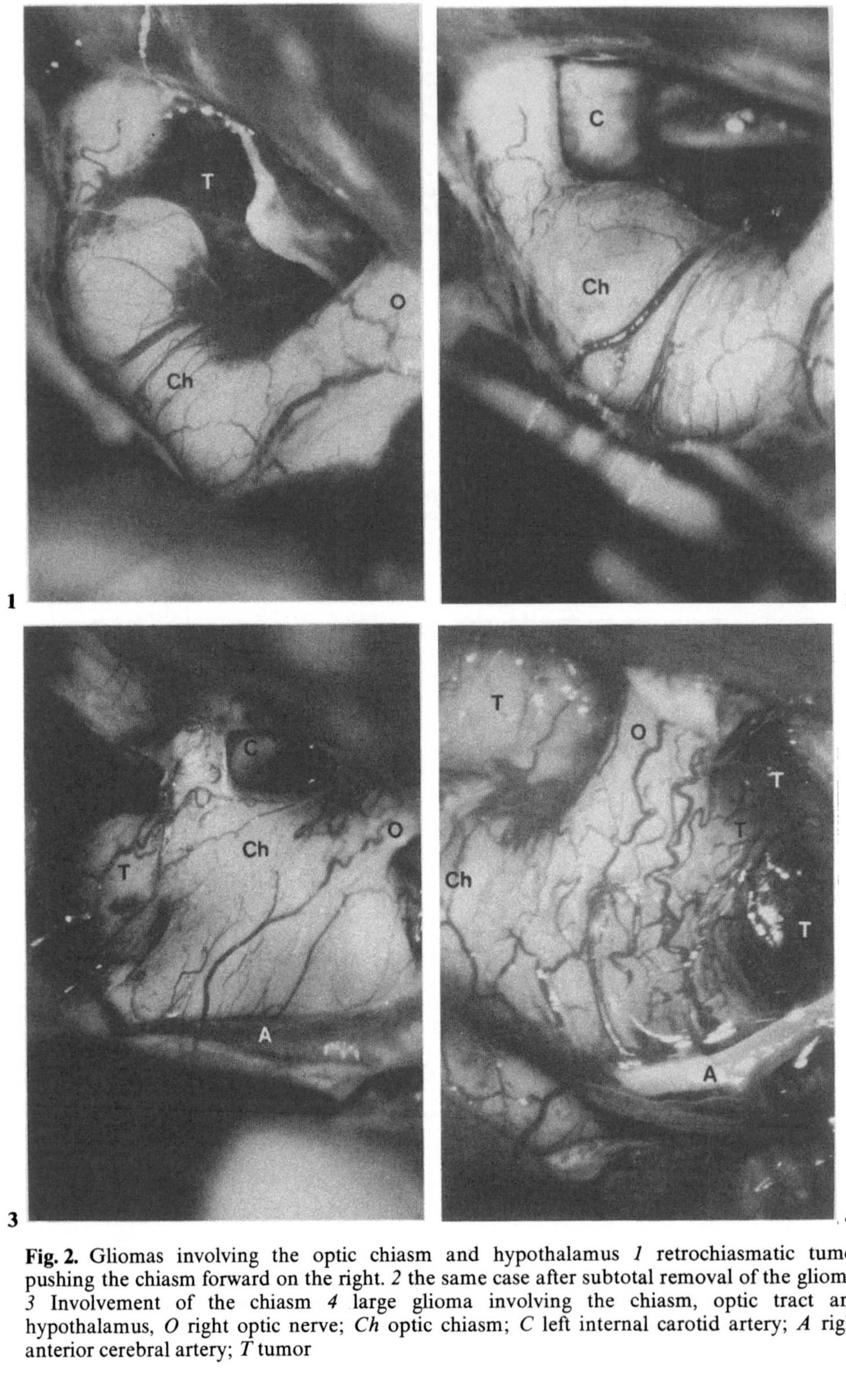

Fig. 2. Gliomas involving the optic chiasm and hypothalamus *1* retrochiasmatic tumor pushing the chiasm forward on the right. *2* the same case after subtotal removal of the glioma. *3* Involvement of the chiasm *4* large glioma involving the chiasm, optic tract and hypothalamus, *O* right optic nerve; *Ch* optic chiasm; *C* left internal carotid artery; *A* right anterior cerebral artery; *T* tumor

Table 4. Gliomas of the chiasm and hypothalamus

Operations	25
S̄ microscope	6
C̄ microscope	19
Subtotal extirpation	
ca. 80% of tumor	14 (13 C̄ microscope)
ca. 30 – 40% of tumor	10 (5 C̄ microscope)
Biopsy	1 (1 C̄ microscope)
Reoperation	2
VA-shunt (prior or after tumor operation)	11
Postop. radiotherapy	21 (+ 2 reop. pts)
Postoperative condition	
Good	11
Fair	5
Postop. death	7
(4 : 1 week after op. S̄ microsc.)	
(1 : 3 years after op. S̄ microsc.)	
(1 : 1 year after reop. C̄ microsc.)	
(1 : 4 days after op. C̄ microsc.)	

the hypothalamic structures (Fig. 2) could be removed in 80 percent (14 cases). In 10 patients where the tumor extended without any delimitation towards the floor of the third ventricle, the operation was performed to serve two purposes: (a) decompression of the optic nerves, the vessels and the hypothalamus; (b) protection of the still functioning fibres of the optic nerves and the chiasm. In 11 children, a ventriculo-atrial shunt was used because of hydrocephalus.

Two patients who had first been operated upon without the microscope had to undergo a second operation during which the operating microscope was used. These are the two patients who died, one four days and the other one year after the second operation. Five other children died, four of them immediately after the operation, one of them three years later. All of them were operated upon prior to the microsurgical area.

During the follow-up examinations of all 16 patients still alive, the condition of one patient, 15 years after the operation was poor; the child had become blind in both eyes, showed evidence of increased intracranial pressure and of hypothalamic deficiency. Carotid angiography, ventriculography and CT scan showed an inoperable tumor, so that only a ventriculo-atrial-shunt was carried out. All other patients are fully capable of going to school or work, only three of them suffer from scotomata or a reduction in visual acuity which is corrected, however, by means of glasses. Three children are still on hormonal substitution therapy. All three patients have insufficient production of the somatotropic hormone and ACTH. None of the patients suffer from a deficiency in gonadotropic hormones or in antidiuretic hormone.

Discussion and Conclusions

In this series, as in the literature, optic gliomas occurred in children predominantly in their first decade of life. Visual morbidity topped the list of presenting symptoms (Table 5). Recklinghausen's disease was a well known associated entity; in our series 33 percent (Table 6) (Davis, 1940; Marshall, 1954; Oxenhandler and Sayers, 1978).

The operative management of optic gliomas can pragmatically be divided into two anatomic categories: 1. the therapy of unilateral optic nerve gliomas and 2. the therapy of those with chiasmal or more extensive posterior involvement. In the treatment of unilateral optic nerve gliomas age is certainly a factor, as perimetry and reliable visual acuities are often impossible to perform in young children.

Table 5. Preoperative signs and symptoms in 36 patients with optic gliomas

Impaired vision	22
Optic atrophy	18
Papilledema	12
Exophthalmos	11
Visual field defects	8
Amaurosis	8
Impaired extraocular motions	5
Proptosis	3
Diencephalic syndrome	11
Increased intracran. pressure	9
Hydrocephalus	8
Impaired consciousness	4
Hemiparesis	4
Seizures	2
Extrapyramidal disturb.	2
V. Recklinghausen's disease (café-au-lait spots)	12

Table 6: Gliomas of the optic system and hypothalamus (case collection of literature: $n = 180$)

Localization	Literature	(Author's cases)
Extracranial	19%	(16%)
Extra- and intracranial	16%	(19%)
Intracranial	65%	(65%)
	100%	(100%)
V. Recklinghausen's signs		
Literature-series	30%	
Author's cases	33%	

Resection of the tumor first requires radiologic evidence of extent (Plain Roentgenograms, CT scan and fractional polytome pneumoencephalography. A transfrontal orbital approach can be used for the primary resection, sparing the globe for cosmetic purposes, according to Dandy (1922) and Housepian (1969). The approach to chiasmal and/or hypothalamic involvement is both diagnostic and therapeutic. However, in patients with hypothalamic tumor, exploration should be undertaken to rule out the possibility of a tumor other than an optic glioma and perhaps to carry out a decompression of the vascular and nervous structures of the suprasellar region.

The role of radiation therapy in chiasmal and hypothalamic gliomas remains uncertain. Taveras et al. (1956) and Bouchard (1966) showed that improvement of the clinical symptoms can also be achieved by radiotherapy without operation; life expectancy is relatively high. Based on our experience, however, microsurgical treatment combined with subsequent radiotherapy has certain definite advantages: (a) histological diagnosis of the tumor; (b) preservation of optic structures and vital areas of the CNS; (c) rapid restoration of largely normal function through decompression of still functioning nervous structures and therefore a significant decrease of morbidity; (d) radiation therapy because no radical surgery has been performed.

References

Bouchard J (1966) Radiation therapy of tumors and disease of the nervous system. Lea & Fabiger, Philadelphia

Byers WGM (1901) Primary intradural tumors of the optic nerve: fibromatosis nervi optici. Stud R Victoria Hosp (Montreal) 1:3–82

Dandy WE (1922) Prechiasmal intracranial tumors of the optic nerves. Am J Ophthalmol 5:169–188

Davis FA (1940) Primary tumors of the optic nerve. (A phenomenon of Recklinghausen's disease). Arch Ophthalmol 23:735–821

Eggers H, Jakobiec FA, Jones IS (1976) Tumors of the optic nerve. Doc Ophthalmol 41: 43–128

Housepian EM (1969) Surgical treatment of unilateral optic nerve gliomas. J Neurosurg 31:604–607

Hudson AC (1912) Primary tumours of the optic nerve. R Lond Ophthalmol Hosp Rep 18:317–439

Koos WT, Miller MH (1971) Intracranial tumors of infants and children. Thieme, Stuttgart

Koos WT, Böck F (1974) Microneurosurgery of the chiasm – sella turcica region; in Bushe, Spoerri and Shaw: Progress in pediatric neurosurgery. Hippokrates, Stuttgart pp 187–191

Koos WT, Böck F, Salah S, Pendl G (1976) Microsurgery of gliomas of the optic nerves, the optic chiasm, and the hypothalamus; in Koos, Böck and Spetzler: Clinical Microneurosurgery. Thieme, Stuttgart, pp 58–63

Lundberg A (1935) Über die primären Tumoren des Sehnerven und der Sehnervenkreuzung. Inaugural Dissertation, Karolinisches Institut. Nordiska Bokhaudeln, Stockholm

Marshall D (1954) Glioma of the optic nerve, as a manifestation of von Recklinghausen's disease. Am J Ophthalmol 37:15–33

Oxenhandler DC, Sayers MP (1978) The dilemma of childhood optic gliomas. J Neurosurg 48:34–41

Schuster H, Koos WT, Zaunbauer F (1977) Results of Microsurgical Treatment of Gliomas of the Optic System and the Hypothalamus in Children. Mod Probl Paediatr 18:211–215

Taveras JM, Mount LA, Wood EG (1956) The value of radiation therapy in the management of glioma of the optic nerves and chiasm. Radiology 66:518–528

Wagener HP (1959) Gliomas of the optic nerve. Am J Med Sci 237:238–261

Optic Nerve Glioma: General Considerations and a Case Report

P. J. NAESSENS, L. F. DE WAELE, and J. KLUYSKENS, Gent/Belgium

Introduction

Symptoms, diagnostic procedures and treatment of optic nerve glioma are discussed. A case report is presented at the end of the paper.

Optic nerve glioma is a rather unfrequent tumor. The incidence, of course, varies in different studies, but from most of them it appears to be confined to childhood and early adult life. The earliest symptoms of this pathology are mostly characterized by a slowly progressive unilateral exophthalmos, which is not accompanied by pain. However, poor vision may also be an early sign and it may even be present a long time before the appearance of an exophthalmos. Ocular pulsation is rare. In a small percentage of cases a relation is found with neurofibromatosis of von Recklinghausen. In those cases café-au-lait pigmentation of the skin is encountered. The disease is mostly unilateral, but can also be spread from one optic nerve to the other via the optic chiasm.

From the neuro-ophthalmological point of view the following signs may appear either alone or associated:

- proptosis
- optic atrophy
- papilledema: elevation of the optic disc may be present, giving the appearance of papilledema instead of optic atrophy.
- venous congestion of the fundus
- diplopia as a result of strabismus.

The *diagnosis* should be made first of all by the clinical picture and then confirmed by a complete radiological study of the orbital structures. *Roentgenography* of the orbits is the first valuable investigation to be carried out. Orbital asymmetry may be apparent. The next important feature is the size of the optic foramina, which can be visualized by special incidences. In many cases of optic nerve glioma an enlargement of the optic nerve foramen is encountered on the affected side. *Polytomography* of the orbit is, of course, very helpful. *Carotid angiography* rarely helps in diagnosis, unless the optic chiasm is also affected. *Venous angiography* of the orbits may be helpful, but are rarely performed. Last but not least, the *C.T.Scan* has, in recent years, completely changed the diagnostic possibilities of intracranial and intra-orbital lesions. Computerized tomography does provide information which cannot be obtained by any other means of investigation. This examination will demonstrate the exact size and localization, as well as the extension of the tumor.

Pathology

The optic nerve glioma contains either a fine or a coarse reticulate structure of fibrillary cells. They are quite similar to astrocytomas and are arranged in bundles, which are separated from each other by connective tissue septae. In some cases oligodendrocytes may be encountered. Cystic spaces are not unfrequently present in these tumors and they are filled with mucous-like liquid. The tumor remains in its most characteristic form confined to one optic nerve, but it may spread to the other optic nerve via the optic chiasm.

Other intrinsic optic nerve tumors include hemangiomas, benign congenital tumors and a special type of melanoma of the nerve head.

Treatment

In the literature the treatment appears to be still controversial although some guidelines are given as to the two different groups of optic nerve glioma.

The first group comprises only the tumors confined to the orbital cavity proper or with a short extension via the optic foramen into the intracranial cavity (dumb-bell shape). In these cases there is no chiasmal involvement and surgical removal must be considered as the treatment of choice. The operative approaches are either by the lateral orbital way (Krönlein approach) or by the transcranial subfrontal way, or by a combination of both.

To the second group belong the tumors which spread from the optic nerve to the optic chiasm or to the hypothalamic region. Here an orbital decompression with tumoral biopsy can be advocated. Radiotherapy is generally considered in cases with chiasmal and hypothalamic involvement, although the result of radiation therapy is doubtful.

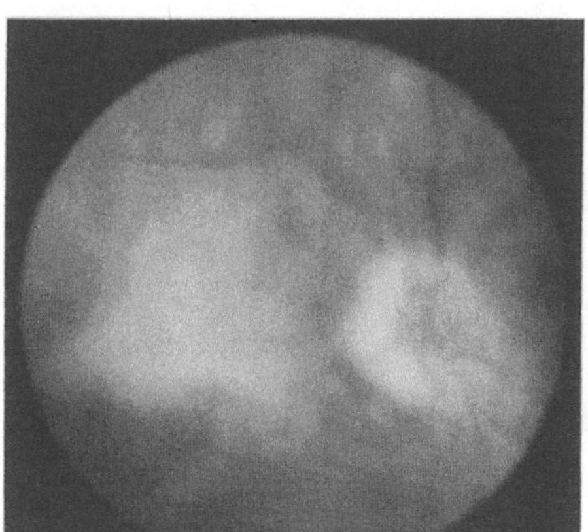

Fig. 1. Fundus: Macular edema with macular palor, narrow arteries and dilated veins

Case Report

A 4 year old boy presented with a convergent strabismus, proptosis, vision of 1/10 and optic atrophy of the right eye. The left eye was normal. On funduscopy macular edema was present with significant macular palor, very narrow arteries and dilated veins. Furthermore, there was generalized edema of the whole posterior pole of the right eye with optic nerve atrophy (Fig. 1).

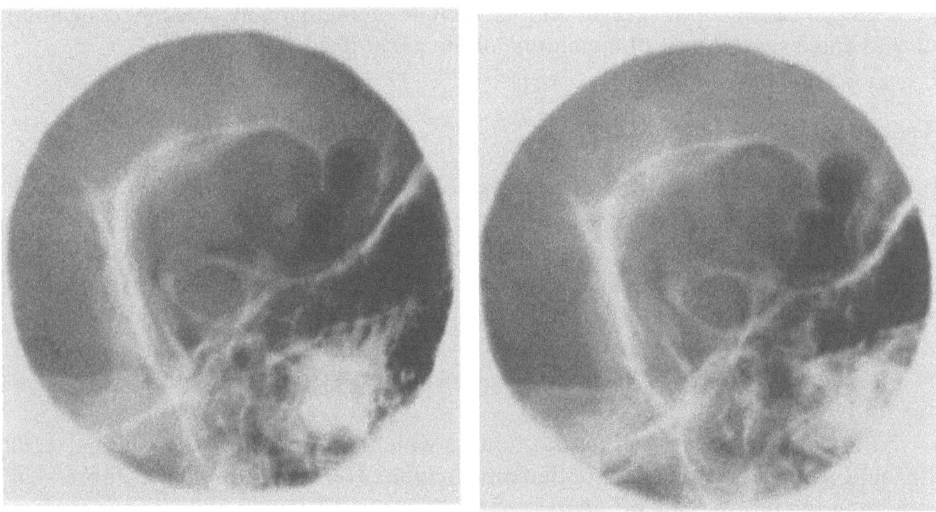

Fig. 2. Roentgenogram of the orbit: enlargement of the optic foramen

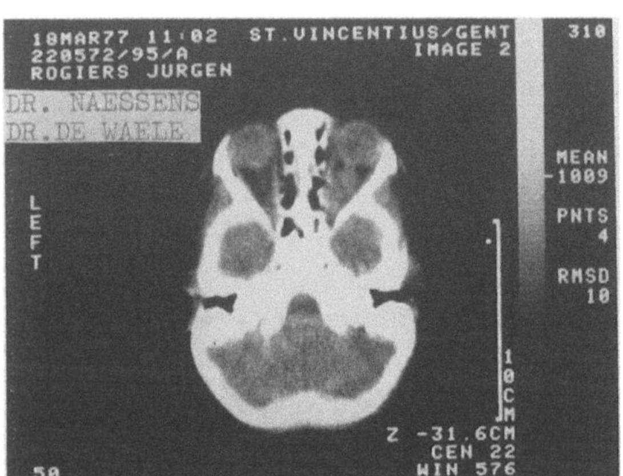

Fig. 3. C.T.Scan: Showing optic nerve glioma

On plain roentgenogram of both orbits the right optic foramen was grossly enlarged (Fig. 2).

Right carotid angiography was almost normal, except for a large venous branch near the base of the skull in the presellar region. C.T.Scan confirmed a mass lesion in the right orbit (Fig. 3).

Operation was performed through the subfrontal intracranial route. The optic nerve was first divided intradurally in front of the chiasm far away from any macroscopical tumor growth. Then orbitotomy was performed for surgical removal of the intra-orbital tumor portion. The pathologist reported a fibrillary astrocytoma of the optic nerve with mucous intratumoral cysts. Now, over three years later, the child is in perfect condition, C.T.Scan does not reveal any sign of recurrence.

References

Burger C et al. (1976) Surgical Pathology of the Nervous System and its Coverings. John Wiley and sons, New York, London, Sydney, Toronto, p 461–462

Clark RL et al. (1979) The Year Book of Cancer. Year Book Medical Publishers, Inc.

Delarue J, Laumonier R (1969) Anatomie Pathologique. Flammarion, Paris, p 2331–2332

Gawler J et al. (1974) British Journal of Ophthalmology, vol 58, No 6, p 571–587

Huber A (1976) Eye signs and symptoms in brain tumors. The C. U. Mosly Company, St. Louis, p 261–268

Karaguiosov L (1979) Surgical Treatment of Gliomas of the Optic Nerve and Chiasma. Acta Neurochir Suppl 28:411–412

Koos T, Miller MH (1971) Intracranial Tumors of Infants and Children. Georg Thieme Verlag, Stuttgart, p 172–175

Marajeva TG et al. (1979) Tumours of the Optic nerve and Chiasma in Children. Acta Neurochir, Suppl 28:409–410

Offret G et al. (1974) Anatomie Pathologique de l'oeil et de ses annexes. Masson & Cie, Ed, Paris, p 474–477

Russell S, Rubinstein LJ (1977) Pathology of Tumours of the Nervous System. Edward Arnold (Publishers) Ltd., London, p 308–311

Optic Nerve Compression by Pituitary Adenomas

R. FAHLBUSCH and F. MARGUTH, München/FRG

Visual field defects, impairment of visual acuity followed by optic nerve atrophy were first described by Harvey Cushing (1930) as chiasma syndrome. In 1928 this entity was pointed out to ophthalmologists in Scheveningen as being caused by operable suprasellar lesions. His definition, originally confined to primary optic atrophy and normal sella, now comprises all disturbances of the chiasma. Cushing's pioneer work in transsphenoidal (Cushing 1914) and transcranial pituitary surgery could be improved by microsurgical techniques (Guiot 1978, Hardy 1973) and endocrine diagnostic, developed in the last 10 years (Fahlbusch, Marguth 1978, 1979).

1. 'Chiasma-Syndrome'

Among 285 of our patients with suprasellar pituitary adenomas 13% had unilateral and 87% bilateral visual field defects (Fig. 1). In general the site of involvement of visual pathways can be localized by the pattern of the field defects. Bitemporal hemianopia localizes the tumor below the anterior part of the chiasm. This situation was found in more than half of the patients (151/285 = 53%), if all bitemporal defects are counted together. A left homonymous hemianopia with a defect to the right optic nerve localizes the tumor to the right tract, the right side of the optic chiasm and the right optic nerve. Also rarely observed was a lower temporal defect, which can be seen if the pars circularis of the anterior cerebral artery impinges on the upper part of the optic nerve. Central and paracentral scotomas with bitemporal hemianoptic pattern are considered to be early symptoms of chiasma disturbances, although they were observed in only 7% (19/285) of our patients. The frequency of visual defects in adenomas correspond well to the literature (Hollenhorst 1973, Stefanis et al. 1979, Huber 1977).

Whereas ten years ago 76% of our patients had visual field defects (Marguth, Fahlbusch 1969), only 33% presented a chiasma symptom in the last year (see Table 1). Today early diagnosis of pituitary adenomas has become possible by endocrine tests (Fahlbusch, Marguth 1978, 1979). The exact tumor localisation is given by computerized tomography of the skull (Fahlbusch et al. 1976).

Different factors can influence the chiasma syndrome (Fig. 2), which are related to the adenoma, the patient and the chiasma itself (Hollenhorst 1973, Stefanis et al. 1979). Thus the degree of visual impairment depends on the size of the adenoma, its symmetrical or asymmetrical extension into the suprasellar space, and the tumor consistency, which seem to lead in firm adenomas to higher loss of vision than in soft ones. Acute bleedings in adenomas can cause severe but still reversible symptoms. A tumor growing without capsule can reach a remarkable size without

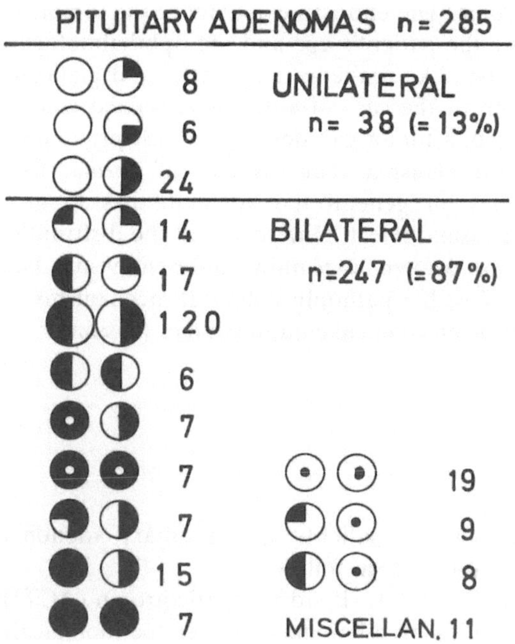

Fig 1. Visual field defects in 285 patients with suprasellar pituitary adenomas

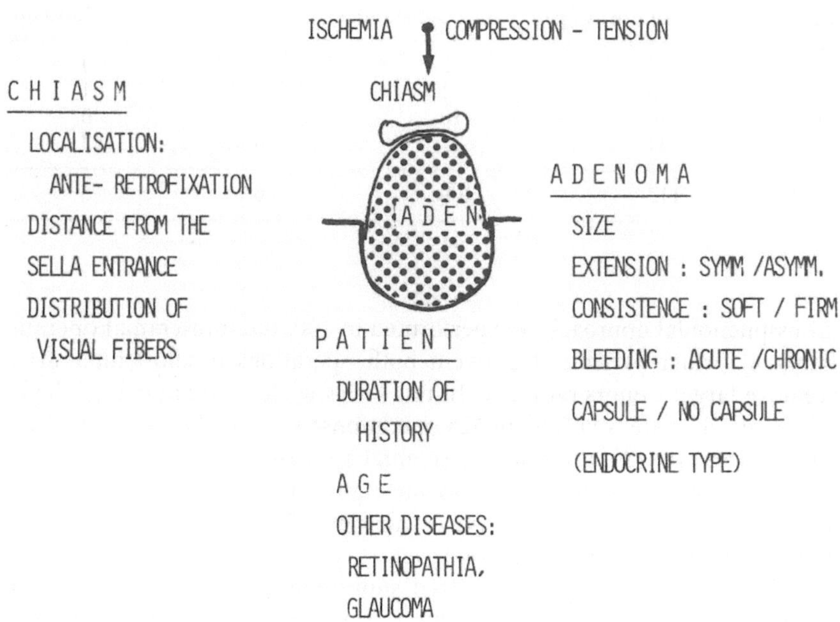

Fig. 2. Factors influencing the chiasma syndrome

causing any significant chiasma syndrome. The endocrine activity of the tumor has no remarkable influence. Furthermore the patient's age and the ophthalmological history are of importance. Other diseases like diabetic retinopathy and glaucoma may affect the optic nerve in addition. In the case of ante- or retrofixed chiasm, occuring in 5 and 10% of the population, a tumor can develop extensively into the suprasellar space without reaching the chiasma. The distance of normal fixed chiasm from the sella entrance varies, in general the adenoma has to grow 10–15 mm to suprasellar to cause a chiasma defect. Differences in the distribution of visual fibers within the chiasma are known, explaining different visual field defects with similar localized tumors. Possible pathophysiological mechanisms for visual field defects are ischemia as well as mechanical compression or tension.

2. Operative Management

In the last year, 1979, we operated on 112 patients with pituitary adenomas (Table 1). The endocrinological classification was as follows:

37 prolactin (PRL), 33 growth hormone (GH), 10 adrenocorticotropin (ACTH) producing adenomas. 32, i.e. one fourth of all adenomas were endocrinologically inactive.

Table 1. Endocrinological classification and surgical treatment in 112 patients (1979) with pituitary adenomas

Hormone excess	Number of pat.	T. sphenoid. op	Craniot.	Both op
PRL	37	32	2	3
GH	33	31	1	1
ACTH	10	10	0	0
'Inactive'	32	27	3	2
Total	112	100	6	6

The transsphenoidal approach was performed in 100, the transcranial operation in 6 patients. 6 further patients underwent both operations in short intervals, in order to remove larger tumors radically. In this series we lost no patient. In the last 10 years the mortality rate was 4.2% in 625 operations: 1.4% (7/496) after the transsphenoidal and 15% (19/129) after the transcranial approach.

Adenomas, extending symmetrically to the right and left optic nerve and the chiasm are no longer exposed by us via craniotomy. These adenomas would be removed today by the transsphenoidal approach.

Whereas large adenomas with lateralized suprasellar and parasellar extension are operated on microsurgically today by a small fronto-lateral approach in general.

3. Ophthalmological Results

Ophthalmological results up to now are not easy to document by any objective examination or calculation. Examinations of visual acuity and visual-fields were performed in the department of Ophthalmology of Munich university (Director: Prof. Dr. E. Lund). The percentage of visual impairment was calculated from both results – visual acuity and visual field examination, according to the technique recommended by the German Society of Ophthalmology (DOG) in September 78. For example normal vision is 0%, amaurosis 100%: bitemporal hemianopia is classified as 20% loss of vision, visual activity of 0.5 on both eyes also as 20%. In addition the loss of vision is 40%. This evaluation is based on the degrees of disablement used mainly for social insurances (Jefferson, 1978, presented a more detailed scoring system with special regard also to changes in patients with a higher degree of loss of vision). Roughly, the DOG system seems to be comparable to the techniques used firstly by Laws (1977), in order to interpretate visual results in patients before and after the transsphenoidal operation.

Out of our *transsphenoidal series* 76 patients were evaluated, operated on between 1975 and 79 (Fig. 3), when computerized tomography of the skull was introduced in our department and performed pre- and postoperatively. The symbols indicate the pathological condition and visual loss immediately before surgery. Ascending lines indicate postoperative improvement in vision. Position of symbols along abscissa indicates intervals between surgery and the earliest time –

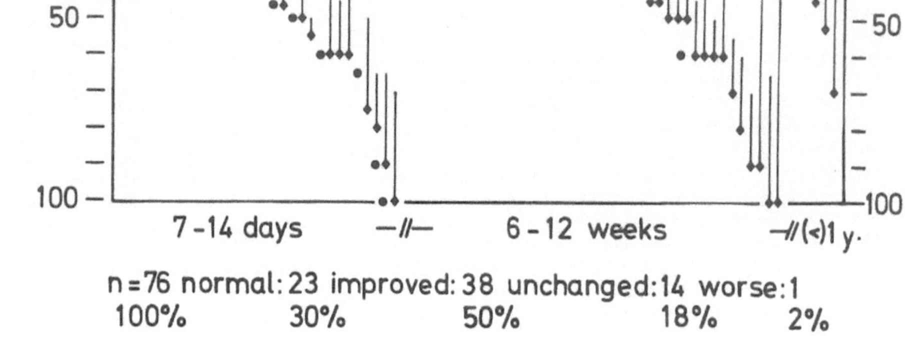

Fig. 3. Visual results in 76 patients with pituitary adenomas operated via the transsphenoidal approach. Symbols indicate the pathological condition and visual loss before surgery. Ascending lines indicate postoperative improvement in vision, descending lines deterioration. Closed circles indicate unchanged vision

7–14 days, 6–12 weeks and up to 1 year – in which the best ophthalmological results were achieved. 30% of the patients had normal vision, 50% improved, 18% remained unchanged, and only 1 patient worsened. – Nearly half of the patients had the best results just after the operation, more than half of the patients some weeks later and only a few patients (4/76) later up to 1 year. In general no normalisation could be obtained if the visual impairment was higher than 20–30% before the operation. Exceptions are patients with acute bleedings in the adenoma, who were operated upon very early. – Half of the 14 patients with unchanged vision had in the initial stage a higher degree of optic nerve atrophy. In 5 of these patients the tumor could not be removed totally. In 6 further patients subtotal removal led to improvements, but not to normalisation. Tumor residuals were assumed if the suprasellar capsule respectively the diaphragm did not herniate widely into the sella shown by postoperative CT-control.

The prognosis for visual recovery in patients over 65 years is considerably poorer than in younger ones: in our 18 patients no normalisation of vision was observed, and if vision had improved than hardly above the 20–30% limit (Fig. 4).

Among the patients with postoperative normal or improved vision, visual fields normalized in a higher degree and earlier, compared to visual acuity.

Impairment of vision in the first 3 days after the operation may indicate a second hemorrhage. Guiot (1978) described impairments as an effect caused by a pulling- or pushing-mechanism towards the chiasm which is located in a secondary empty-sella. A chiasma syndrome in the primary empty-sella syndrome is rarely

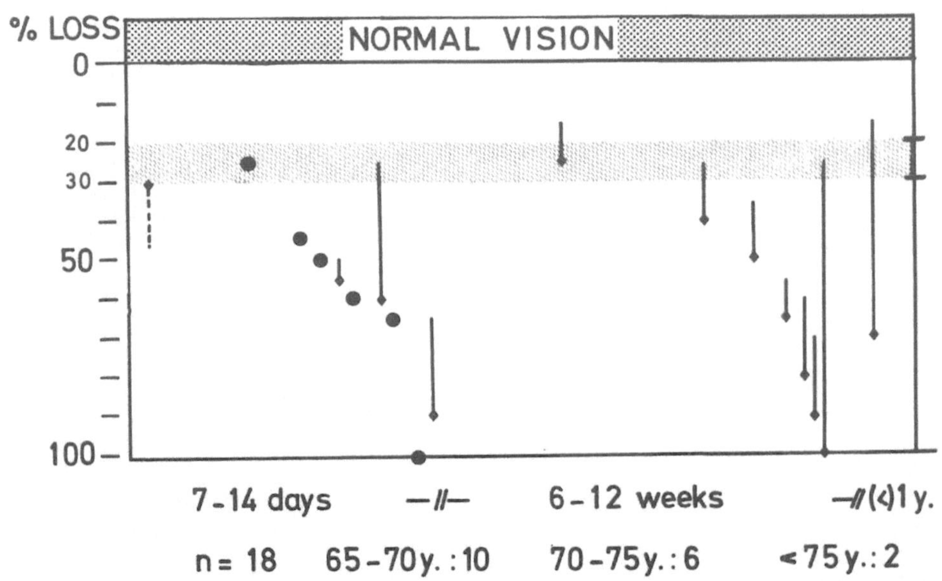

Fig. 4. Visual results in 18 patients, aged above 65 years, operated on via the transsphenoidal approach. (Symbols see Fig. 3.)

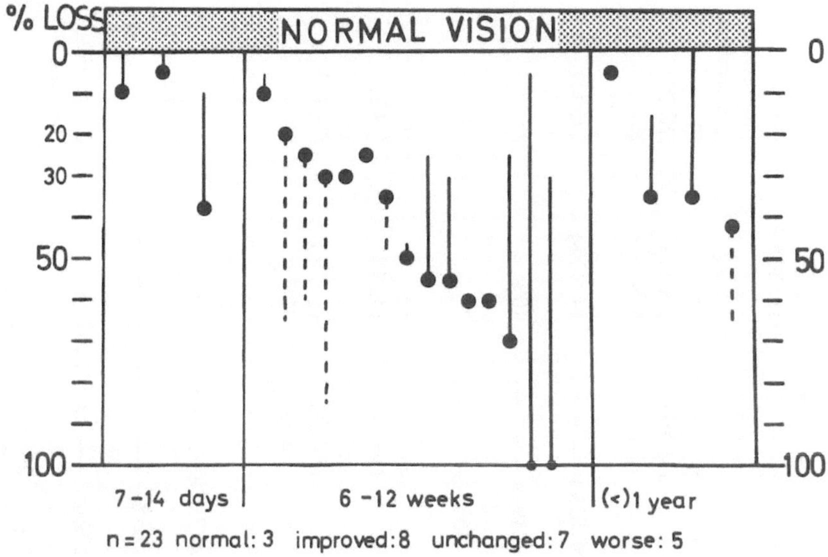

Fig. 5. Visual results in 23 patients with larger and 'giant' pituitary adenomas, operated on by craniotomy. (Symbols see Fig. 3)

seen (Cupps, Woolf, 1978). Besides 3 re-bleedings in 76 patients we could detect transitory impairments only in 4 patients. Thus we feel that filling the sella with muscle or cartilage is not necessary.

3 points shall be emphasized in explaining the result after *craniotomy* (Fig. 5): 1. these 23 patients had larger, asymmetrical tumors presenting a contraindication for the transsphenoidal operation. Additional 3 patients died postoperatively because of hypothalamic dysregulation. 2. Five out of 23 patients worsened – descending interrupted lines. 3. Only a few patients improved in the early phase. About 20% achieved their optimal results later, up to one year.

A summary about visual functions in 112 pituitary adenomas operated upon in the last 5 years (Table 2), via the transsphenoidal and transcranial approach, as well as both ways performed in short intervals shows: The chiasma syndrome in

Table 2. Visual function in 112 patients with suprasellar pituitary adenomas operated on between 1975 and 1979

Op	Sphenoidal	Craniotomy	Both ways	
normal	23 (30%)	3 (13%)	0	26 (23%)
improved	38 (50%)	8 (35%)	3 (23%)	49 (44%)
unchanged	14 (18%)	7 (30%)	5 (38.5%)	26 (23%)
worse	1 (2%)	5 (22%)	5 (38.5%)	11 (10%)
n=	76	23	13	112 (100%)

Table 3. Surgical decompression of the optic nerve and chiasm: Visual results for pituitary adenoma with transfrontal and transsphenoidal approach. (From: E. R. Laws et al. J. Neurosurg. 46 (1977) 717 – 722

Series	Dates (Total Cases)	Mortality Rate (%)	No. of Cases Analyzed	Normal	Improved	Unchanged	Worse
transfrontal (craniotomy) approach							
Cushing (Henderson, 1939)	1913 – 1932 (91)	4.5	88	← 62 (70.5%) →		18 (20.5%)	8 (9%) 'progressive deterioration'
Bakay, 1950; Olivecrona, 1967	1929 – 1947 (246)	11.4	202	19 (9.4%)	63 (31.3%)	67 (33.2%)	53 (26.2%)
Tönnis, et al., 1955	1933 – 1952 (264)	10.4	?	43%	19%	31%	7%
Heimbach, 1959; Krayenbuhl, 1958	1938 – 1956 (105)	9.4	95	← 79 (83%) →		11 (12%)	5 (5%)
Guillaume & Caron, 1958	1941 – 1957 (141)	12.0	~70	← 83% →		10%	7%
Fager, et al., 1973	1935 – 1972 (382)	13.0	197	← 45% →		?	9%
Olivecrona, 1967	1948 – 1959 (187)	14.0	136	17 (12.5%)	41 (30.1%)	59 (43.4%)	19 (14%)
Svien, et al., 1965	1950 – 1958 (?)	6.8	71	7 (9.9%)	38 (53.5%)	11 (15.5%)	15 (21.1%)
Ray & Patterson, 1971	1950 – 1969 (146)	1.2	106	~40%	~40%	18%	2%
transsphenoidal approach							
Cushing (Henderson, 1939)	1913 – 1932 (167)	5.3	159	← 114 (71.7%) →		39 (24.5%)	6 (3.8%)
Hamlin, 1962; Hirsch, 1957	1910 – 1962 (~425)*	~4.7	140	← 68% →			?
Demailly, et al., 1967; Guiot, 1967	1957 – 1972 (582)*	~1.24	63	26 (41.25%)	← 26 (41.25%) →		11 (17.5%) 'failures'
Laws & Kern, 1976	1972 – 1975 (139)	1.4	42	7 (16.7%)	29 (69%)	6 (14.3%)	0

112 patients became normal in 23%, improved in 44%, together 76%, remained unchanged in 23% and worsened in 10% (none of these patients became amaurotic after the operation!).

A comparison to earlier literature was given by Laws (1977) (Table 3) although no comparability seems to exist. However, the results in our transsphenoidal series seem to correlate in general with Laws (1977).

References

Cupps TR, Woolf PD (1978) Primary empty sella syndrome with panhypopituitarism, diabetes insipidus and visual field defects. Acta Endocrinol (Kbh) 89:445–460

Cushing H (1914) Surgical experiences with pituitary disorders (The Weir Mitchell Lecture). J Am Med Assoc LXIII, No. 18:1515–1525

Cushing H (1930) The chiasmal syndrome of primary optic atrophy and bitemporal field defects in adults with a normal sella turcica. Arch Ophthalmol 3:505

Fahlbusch R, Marguth F (1978) Developments in surgical treatment of pituitary adenomas. Neurosurg Rev 1/2:5–13

Fahlbusch R, Marguth F (1979) Concepts in neurosurgical treatment of pituitary adenomas. In: Marguth F, Brock M, Kazner E, Klinger M, Schmiedek P (eds) Neurovascular Surgery – Specialized neurosurgical techniques. Advances in Neurosurgery 7. Springer, Berlin Heidelberg New York

Fahlbusch R, Grumme Th Aulich A, Wende S, Steinhoff H, Lanksch W, Kazner E (1976) Suprasellar tumors in the CT-scan In: Lanksch W, Kazner E (eds) Cranial computerized tomography. Springer, Berlin Heidelberg New York

Guiot G (1978) Considerations on the surgical treatment of pituitary adenomas In: Fahlbusch R, v Werder K (eds) Treatment of pituitary adenomas. Thieme, Stuttgart

Hardy J (1973) Transsphenoidal surgery of hypersecreting pituitary tumors. In: Kohler PO, Ross GT (eds) Diagnosis and treatment of pituitary tumors. Exerpta medica – American Elsevier, Amsterdam New York

Hollenhorst RW, Younge BR (1973) Ocular manifestations produced by adenomas of the pituitary gland: analysis of 1000 cases. In: Kohler PO, Ross GT (eds) Diagnosis and treatment of pituitary tumors. Exerpta medica, American Elsevier, Amsterdam New York

Huj er A (1977) Chiasmasyndrome – Klinik Klin. Monatsbl Augenheilkd 170:266

Jefferson A (1978) The treatment of chromophobe pituitary adenomas by means of transfrontal surgery, radiation therapy and supportive hormone therapy. In: Fahlbusch R, v. Werder K (eds) Treatment of pituitary adenomas. Thieme, Stuttgart

Laws ER, Trautmann IC, Hollenhorst RW (1977) Transsphenoidal decompression of the optic nerve and chiasm. Visual results in 62 patients. J Neurosurg 46:717–722

Marguth F, Fahlbusch R (1969) Chirurgie der Hypophysentumoren. In: Kracht I (ed) Oestrogene-Hypophysentumoren. 15. Symp Dtsch Ges Endokrinol, Springer, Berlin Heidelberg New York

Stefanis G, Cavanaugh HD, Tindall GT (1979) Ophthalmological aspects of pituitary tumors. In: Tindall GT, Collins WF (eds) Clinical management of pituitary disorders. Raven Press, New York

Optic Nerve Compression by Meningiomas

K. Schürmann, Mainz/FRG

It is well known that the optic nerve can be compressed by meningiomas 1) in its whole course from the utmost periphery at the bulb, 2) in its retrobulbar portion, 3) within the dorsal cone of the orbit, 4) within the optic nerve channel and finally 5) intracranially between the chiasm and the optic nerve channel (see Table 1, Pt. 1–3).

In our series of 231 space occupying lesions of the orbit (Table 2), we observed 37 meningiomas which are to be distinguished from the special intracranial group of 44 meningiomas of the sphenoid ridge and suprasellar region with regard to their particular problems (Table 1, Pt. 4, see also second paper 'Tumor compression of oculomotor, trochlear and abducens nerve in cavernous sinus and orbit').

Among the 37 meningiomas which caused a compression of the optic nerve, we saw 24 meningiomas which were located in the anterior part of the orbit without any relation to the optic nerve sheath (Table 2 and 3). These meningiomas caused only a secondary compression of the optic nerve and mainly a dislocation of the

Table 1. Optic nerve compression by meningiomas

1 –	M. within the orbit	Retrobulbar without invasion of optic nerve sheath Retrobulbar optic nerve sheath m. (sheath of Schwalbe)
2 –	M. within the dorsal orbital tip	
3 –	M. within the optic nerve channel	
4 –	M. intracranial	– M. of the sphenoid ridge – inner third – M. of the sphenoid ridge – "en plaques" – M. of the sphenoidal plane – M. of the clinoid process – Suprasellar m.

Table 2. Space occupying lesions of the orbit

Meningiomas	– 37
Hemangiomas	– 37
Gliomas of the optic nerve	– 16
Lacrimal gland tumors (mixed t., cylindroma)	– 13
Mesenchymal tumors (fibroma, myxofibroma etc.)	– 24
(EPI) – dermoid tumors	– 15
So-called pseudotumor	– 34
Malignant neoplasms (sa, ca, meta, melanomas etc.)	– 26
Dubious classification	– 29
	231

bulb with diplopia. Their removal by orbitotomy is usually without problems. Therefore, they have the best prognosis with regard to full recovery of visual function and show no recurrence in follow up (Table 4 and Fig. 1 a and b).

In contrast, the eight meningiomas which originated from the optic nerve sheath as well as the menginiomas within the posterior muscle cone or within the optic nerve channel usually caused severe visual disturbances up to blindness. They were always followed by more or less severe visual dysfunction after microsurgical removal (Table 5). In two cases there was a recurrent tumor growth. In one case, the primary optic nerve sheath meningioma was located in the angle between the bulb and the optic nerve access.

Table 3. Intraorbital meningiomas

M. without relation to the optic nerve sheath (= M. within the anterior part of the orbit)	– 24
M. of the optic nerve sheath (of Schwalbe)	– 8
Hemangiopericytic meningioma (semimalignant)	– 2
Malignant meningioma	– 2
Micromeningioma of the optic nerve combined with a so-called pseudotumor	– 1
	37

Table 4. Intraorbital M. without relation to the optic nerve sheath – 24

= M. located within the anterior part of the orbit
= Caused mainly a dislocation of the bulb with diplopia
= Caused only a secondary compression of the optic nerve

Have therefore a very good prognosis in respect to visual function and diplopia recovery as well as to the cosmetic result after removal

no recurrence

Table 5. M. of the optic nerve sheath (of Schwalbe) – 8

Severe diminished visual function in every case until blindness

After removal:

Visual function ameliorated	– 0
Visual function unchanged (one case 0,9 and another 0,1)	– 2
Visual function worsened	– 3
Optic nerve resection necessary	– 3

Doubtful prognosis of visual function recovery in M. of the optic nerve sheath!

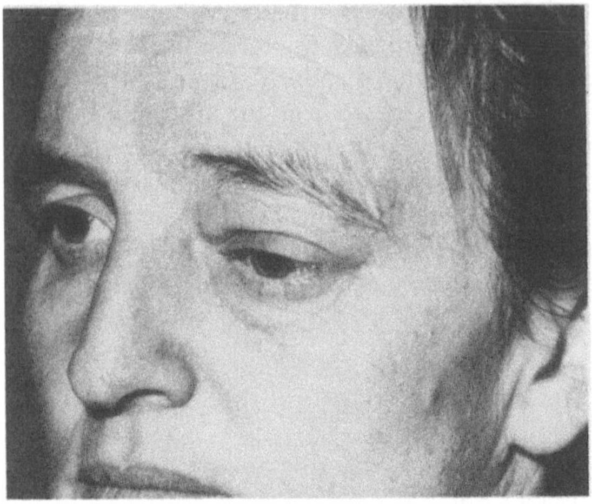

a

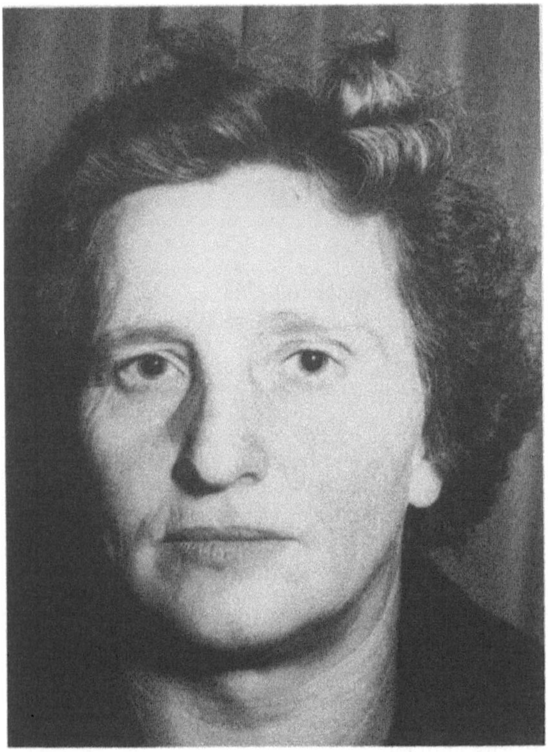

b

Fig. 1 a and b. a 35 year old woman with a meningioma within the anterior median part of the left orbit. Exophthalmos and dislocation of the bulb laterally and downward causing diplopia and a slight visual disturbance. **b** Full recovery after tumor removal by transcranial orbitotomy five years later. Optimal functional and cosmetic result

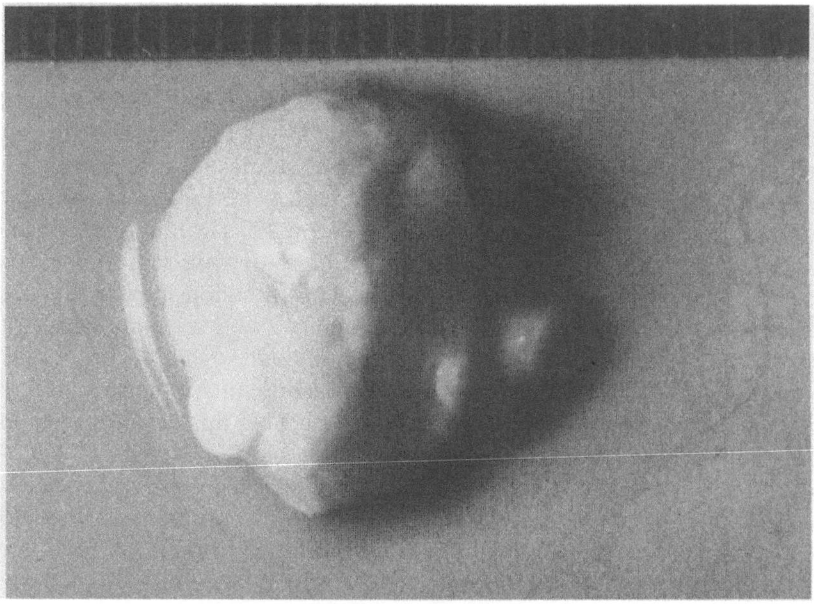

Fig. 2 a

Fig. 2 a. Tumor preparation of an optic nerve sheath meningioma of the posterior muscle cone and orbital part of the optic nerve channel. Tumor removal together with the total necrotic optic nerve

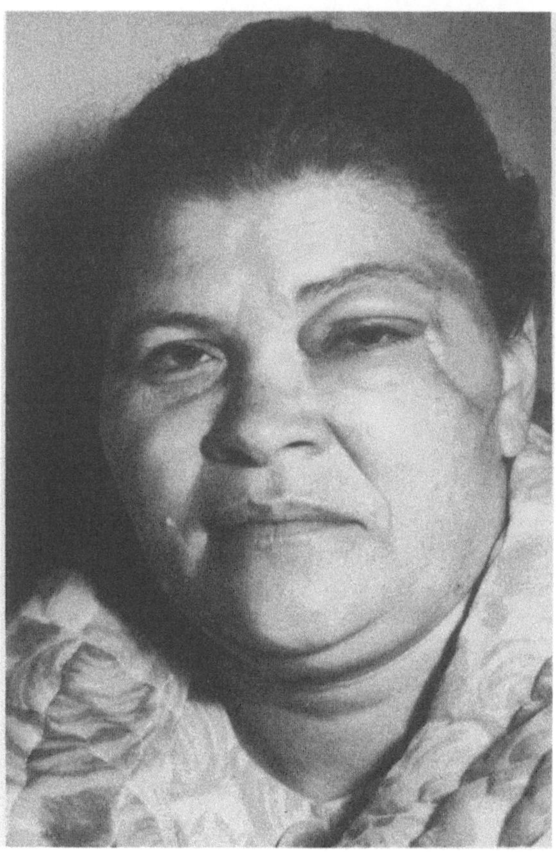

Fig. 2 b

Fig. 2 b and c. b 40 year old female patient of Fig. 2 a. Blindness in left eye. An opthalmosurgeon made an attempt to remove the posterior cone optic nerve sheath meningioma by an orbitotomia ossea lateralis (Krönlein's operation) without reaching the tumor. **c** The same patient as in 2 b one year after transcranial total removal of the tumor. Slight ptosis and abducens nerve paresis remained

It was a small tumor of 5 × 10 mm in size. The tumor was separated microsurgically from the optic nerve and the dorsal pole of the bulb to preserve the visual function. After its removal, the visual function had slightly deteriorated, but the tumor recurred after 11 years. The patient could be cured by a second, more radical operation. In the second case, the primary tumor was located in the dorsal muscle cone and visual function could be preserved by microsurgical removal. In this case, the recurrence of tumor growth followed after seven years and the tumor had invaded the surrounding bone and the ethmoidal cells. The tumor could be totally removed by recraniotomy and transfrontal orbitotomy with radical extirpation of the surrounding bone and sinuses. Histological examination showed that the recurrent tumor was a hemangio-pericytic meningioma with a semi-malignant character. I believe that optic nerve sheath meningiomas should be totally extirpated together with the optic nerve because of the difficulty of separating the encapsulated optic nerve from all tumor tissue. We performed this radical resection in three cases without recurrence over many years (see Fig. 2 a, b and c). Microsurgical isolation and removal of optic nerve sheath meningiomas and preservation of the optic nerve did not enable useful visual function to be maintained nor could a tumor recurrence be prevented. In my opinion, this must be borne in mind in the future.

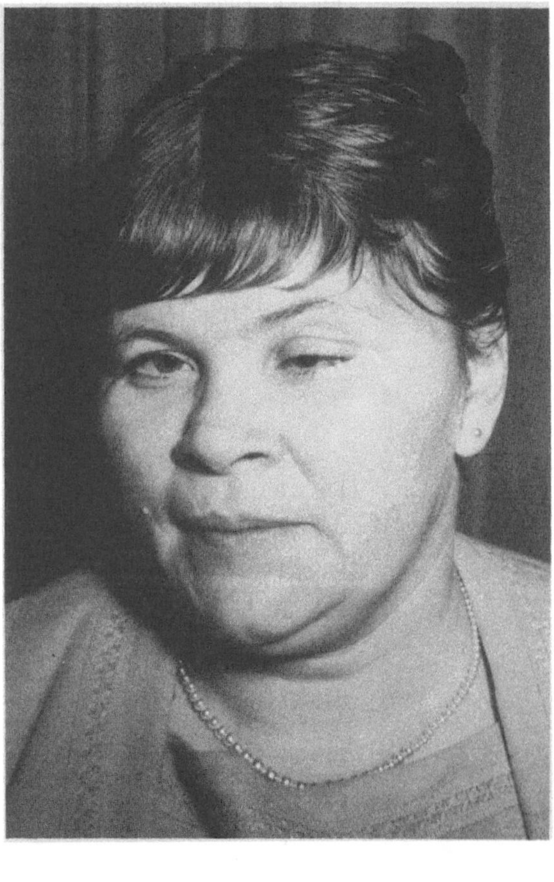

Fig. 2 c

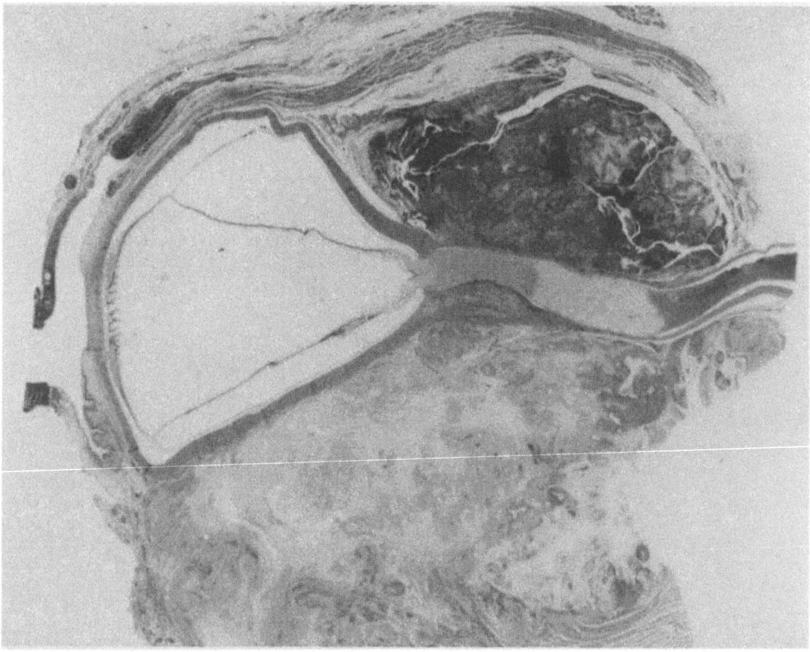

Fig. 3. Severe optic nerve atrophy by a rhabdomyosarcoma as an example of an optic nerve strangulation by encircling tumor masses

Which circumstances might be responsible for the observed postoperative worsening of visual function in meningiomas of the optic nerve sheath?

- an avoidable surgical lesion?
- particular variations of the vascularization of the optic nerve?
- reactive sheath fibrosis?
- poor regeneration capacity of central nerve?

We were unable to find any satisfactory answer to these questions. But we wish to stimulate basic researchers to tackle these problems.

One of my reflections is that the severe encircling strangulation of the optic nerve by tumor masses will cause a particularly serious vascular compression, followed by an extreme atrophy of the optic nerve with no real chance of recovery (Fig. 3). Further studies should be carried out in future.

Surgical Technique

It is not necessary to describe surgical techniques in detail. The common techniques such as orbitotomia simplex, orbitotomia ossea lateralis and orbitotomia transfrontalis by frontal osteoplastic craniotomy and their modifications are used depending on the individual situation. It is advisable in most cases to apply a limited lateral

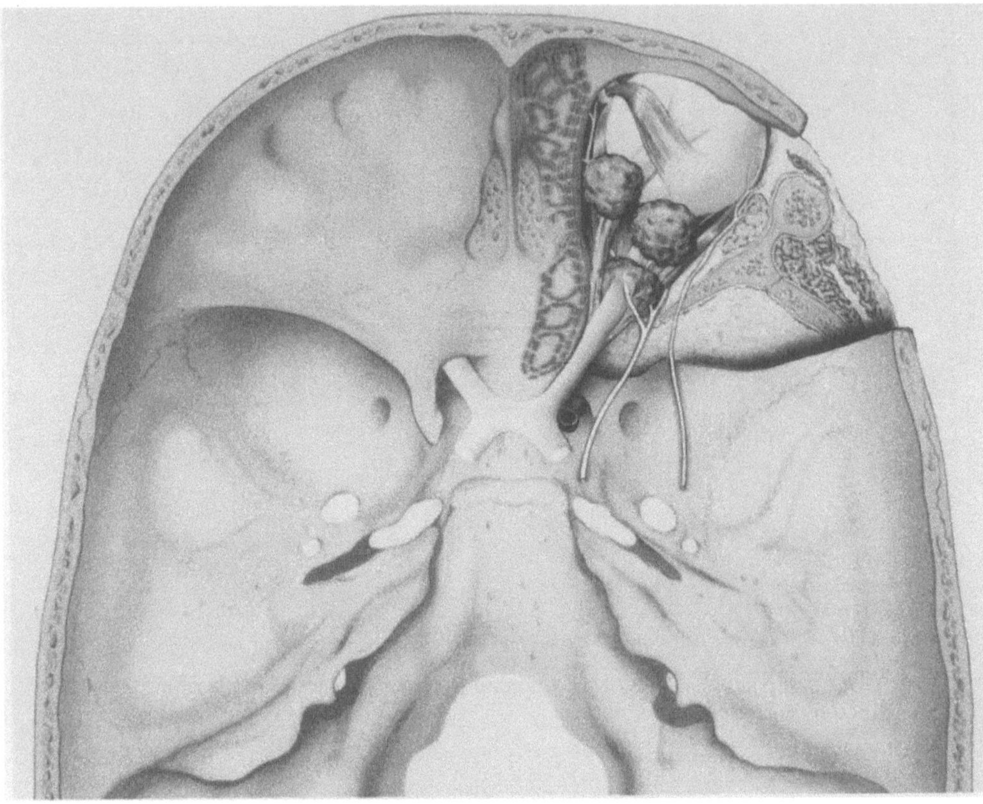

Fig. 4. Schematic picture of the extended bone resection not only of the orbital roof but also the lateral orbital wall and the sphenoid ridge up to the superior orbital fissure to obtain an optimal survey of the orbital content for better isolation of the important nerve elements within the posterior cone of the orbit

Table 6. Useful measures for reconstruction of anterior fossa dura with closure of opened sinuses and orbital walls reconstruction

Which material is available for plastic reconstruction?	
To replace dura mater	To replace bone
Autoplasty:	*Autoplasty:*
1 – Flap of the inner layer of galeaperiostium (with its blood supply)	1 – Orbital roof
2 – Flap of temporal fascia and/or temporal muscle (with its blood supply)	2 – Osteoplastic bone flap
3 – Free implant of muscle, fascia, fat of the leg	3 – Ribs
	4 – Pelvic crest
	5 – Tibial bone graft
Heteroplasty:	*Heteroplasty:*
– Lyophilizated dura	– Polymethylmethacrylate-plastic PALACOS

frontotemporal osteoplastic craniotomy for treating optic nerve sheath meningiomas. If the tumor is situated within the orbital cavity, the extradural approach is effective in most cases. However, in our experience a good survey of the orbital contents is necessary and only attainable with an extensive resection of not only the orbital roof but also the lateral orbital wall and sphenoid ridge up to the superior orbital fissure. In this way, the orbital contents can be largely exposed in a semicircle. Thus, there is enough room to isolate the functionally important nerve elements without danger of secondary iatrogenic nerve lesions. If necessary, the anterior clinoid process should also be resected with the possibility of opening the optic nerve channel (Fig. 4). Such an extended bone resection is mostly reconstructed by an appropriate Palacos Plasty (Table 6).

Summary

Meningiomas within the anterior part of the orbit and without connection to the optic nerve sheath have a very good postoperative prognosis with respect to all functions of ocular motility and vision as well as giving rise to excellent cosmetic result and absence of recurrence.

In contrast, meningiomas arising from the optic nerve sheath still represent a major problem which must be solved in future, particularly with respect to a desirable amelioration of visual function after removal as well as reduction of recurrent tumor growth.

However, this may remain wishful thinking.

Compression of the Optic Nerve by Cerebral Aneurysm – Based Upon the Experience in 1000 Operative Cases

J. SUZUKI, T. YOSHIMOTO, and Y. SAKURAI, Sendai/Japan

Introduction

Several reports dealing with compression of the optic nerve by cerebral aneurysms have previously been made, and it is generally held that such compression occurs in one to two percent of cerebral aneurysm patients [1, 8]. Most of these reports have been based upon autopsy materials rather than upon the operative findings and postoperative symptoms in directly operated patients.

Up to September of 1975, we had treated 1000 cases of directly operated cerebral aneurysms [11]. Here we report 13 patients presenting symptoms of compression of the optic nerve and discuss the effectiveness and necessity of the direct operation.

I. Subjects

Subjects included all patients showing preoperative visual field or visual acuity defects as symptoms of optic nerve compression, among the 1000 aneurysm cases which were radically treated (resection, aneurysm neck treatment, ligation and/or clipping) (Table 1). Thirteen such patients were found, including seven of the anterior communicating artery (AComA) and six of the internal carotid artery (ICA). Among the ICA patients, two were aneurysms at the ophthalmic artery

Table 1. Operative results in patients with saccular aneurysms at Tohoku University from June 1961 to September 1975.

Aneurysm Site	No. of Cases	Excellent	Good	Fair	Poor	Dead
ACoA	346	195	64	41	27	19 (5.5%)
ICA	246	143	44	20	22	17 (6.9%)
MCA	174	99	27	21	18	9 (5.2%)
ACA	49	31	5	6	5	2 (4.1%)
VBA	23	8	5	2	6	2 (8.7%)
Multiple	162	67	41	27	15	12 (7.4%)
Total no.	1000	543	186	117	93	61
%		54.3	18.6	11.7	9.3	6.1

AComA: anterior communicating artery, IC: internal carotid artery, MC: middle cerebral artery, AC: anterior cerebral artery, VB: vertebrobasilar system, Mult.: multiple aneurysm)

Table 2. Thirteen patients with saccular aneurysm showing preoperative visual acuity defects as symptoms of optic nerve compression.

Case	Sex	Age	Site of AN	Size (mm)	Operation	Results of surgery *
1	F	29	AcomA	20×20×20	Trapping	Excellent
2	M	16	AcomA	25×20×15	Resection	Excellent
3	M	47	AcomA	25×20×20	Resection	Good
4	M	29	AcomA	15×15×8	Resection	Excellent
5	M	38	AcomA	15×15×7	Resection	Good
6	M	23	AcomA	20×20×20	Resection	Excellent
7	M	43	AcomA	30×28×27	Resection	Died
8	M	40	ICA**	15×15×15	Clipping	Excellent
9	F	39	ICA**	30×25×20	Ligation	Died
10	F	58	ICA***	neck 4	Clipping	Excellent
11	F	66	ICA***	?	Clipping	Excellent
12	F	42	ICA***	neck 3.5	Clipping	Excellent
13	F	73	ICA***	15×13×12	Ligation	Excellent

F: Female M: Male, AcomA: Anterior Communicating Artery, An: Aneurysm, ICA: Internal Carotid Artery, *: 6M~9Year8M, **: Ophthalmic artery junction, ***: Posterior communicating artery junction, Excellent: capable of working, Good: Capable of working with minimum neurological symptoms

junction and four were aneurysms at the posterior communicating artery (PComA) junction. Investigation was made of the preoperative symptoms, surgical findings, particularly the relationship between the aneurysm and the optic nerves, and postoperative improvement of the symptoms. Ophthalmological examination of all 13 patients was performed by an ophthalmologist.

II. Results

1. AComA patients

All seven patients showed visual field and visual acuity defects as symptoms due to compression of the optic nerve by the aneurysm (Fig. 1). Visual acuity varied from null to 0.5, but five of the seven showed severe defects ranging from null to counting fingers at 2 m. Visual field defects included three patients with bitemporal hemianopsia, two with general contraction, one with nasal hemianopsia and one in whom the records were unclear. Operative findings indicated numerous large aneurysms: all were greater than 15 mm in diameter, and three were so-called giant aneurysms with diameters exceeding 25 mm. The aneurysms were located above the optic chiasma and laterally compressed both optic nerves. The sella turcica was found to be filled by the aneurysm in all cases (Fig. 2). Treatment consisted of trapping in one patient and resection of the aneurysm in six. Except for one patient who died due to postoperative hemorrhage during hospitalization and the patient treated by trapping in which no improvement of symptoms was observed,

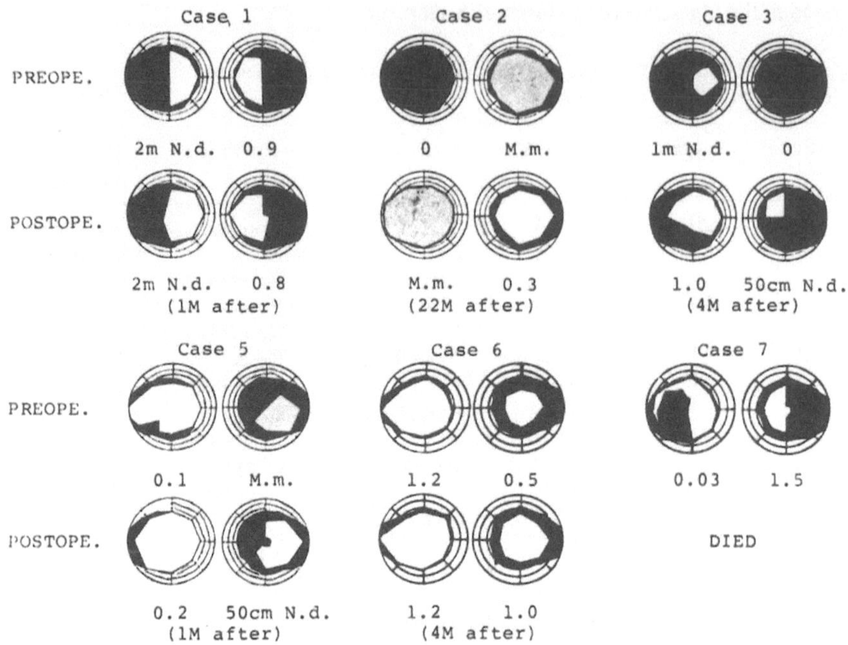

Case 1
Case 2
Case 3
PREOPE.
2m N.d. 0.9
0 M.m.
1m N.d. 0
POSTOPE.
2m N.d. 0.8
(1M after)
M.m. 0.3
(22M after)
1.0 50cm N.d.
(4M after)
Case 5
Case 6
Case 7
PREOPE.
0.1 M.m.
1.2 0.5
0.03 1.5
POSTOPE.
DIED
0.2 50cm N.d.
(1M after)
1.2 1.0
(4M after)

Fig. 1

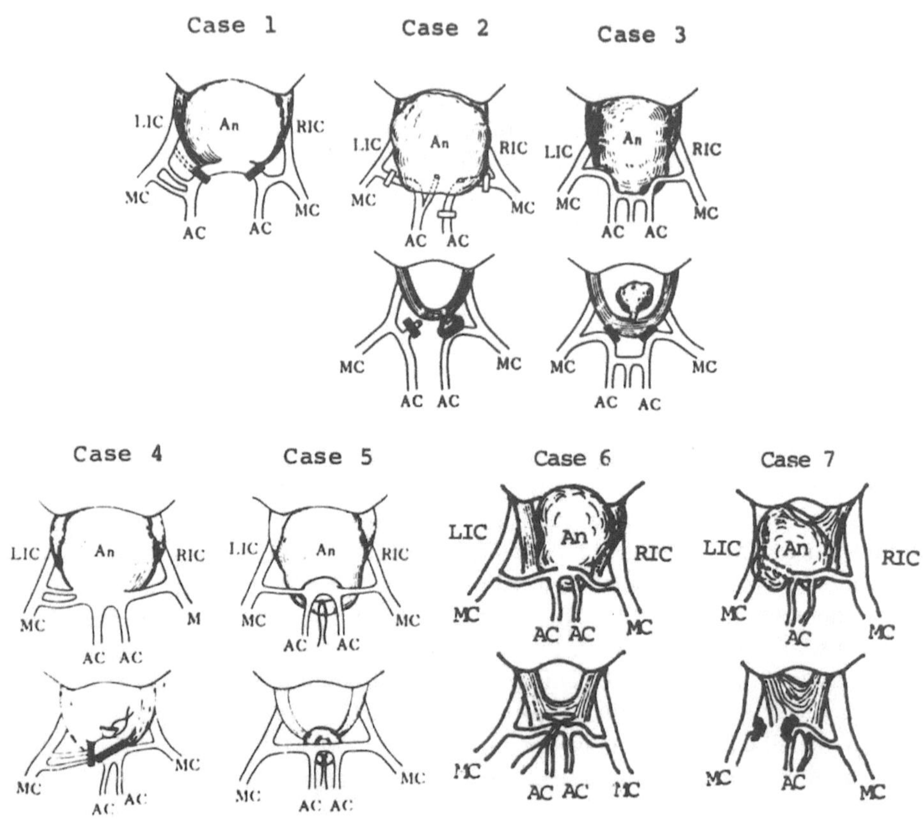

Case 1
Case 2
Case 3
LIC
An
RIC
MC
AC
Case 4
Case 5
Case 6
Case 7
M

Fig. 2

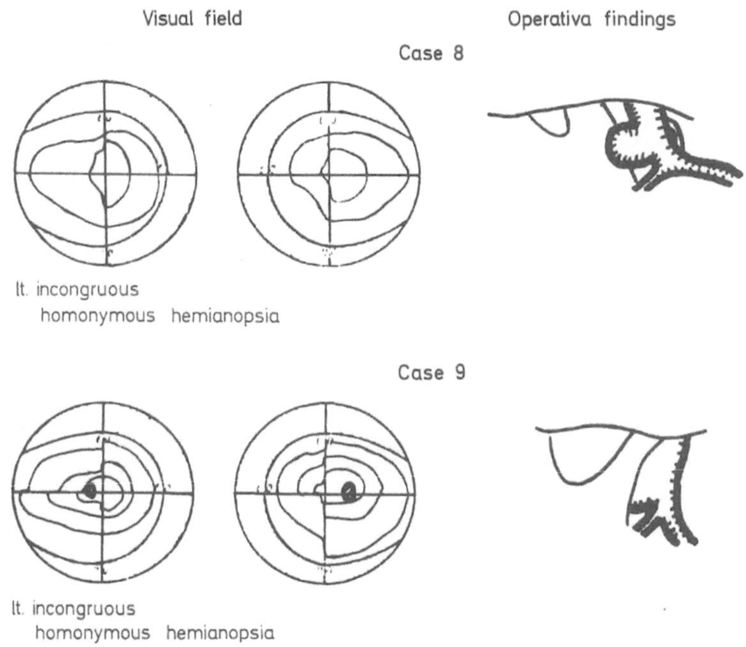

Fig. 3. Visual field defects and operative findings in two patients with aneurysm at the ophthalmic junction

all showed postoperative improvement, including two who showed nearly complete recovery (Fig. 1).

2. ICA patients

a) Two patients with aneurysm at the ophthalmic artery junction

Both patients presented with incongruous homonymous hemianopsia. Visual acuity was 0.4 and 0.8 on the affected side. No other ophthalmological abnormalities, such as symptoms of the oculomotor nerve, were seen (Fig. 3). The aneurysm in both patients was found at operation to have developed in a medial direction from the ICA and to compress the optic nerve and a portion of the optic chiasma in an upward direction. Clipping was successful in one case, but in the other a 30 mm giant aneurysm necessitated section of the optic nerve and ligation of the aneurysm neck. Kinking of the ICA occurred, and the patient died postoperatively while still hospitalized. The visual acuity of the surviving patient improved markedly from 0.4 to 1.2, but no improvement in the visual field was found.

Fig. 1. Changes of visual field defect and visual acuity after intracranial operation

Fig. 2. Operative findings and methods. *LIC:* Left internal carotid artery, *RIC:* Right internal carotid artery, *An:* Aneurysm, *MC:* Middle cerebral artery, *AC:* Anterior cerebral artery

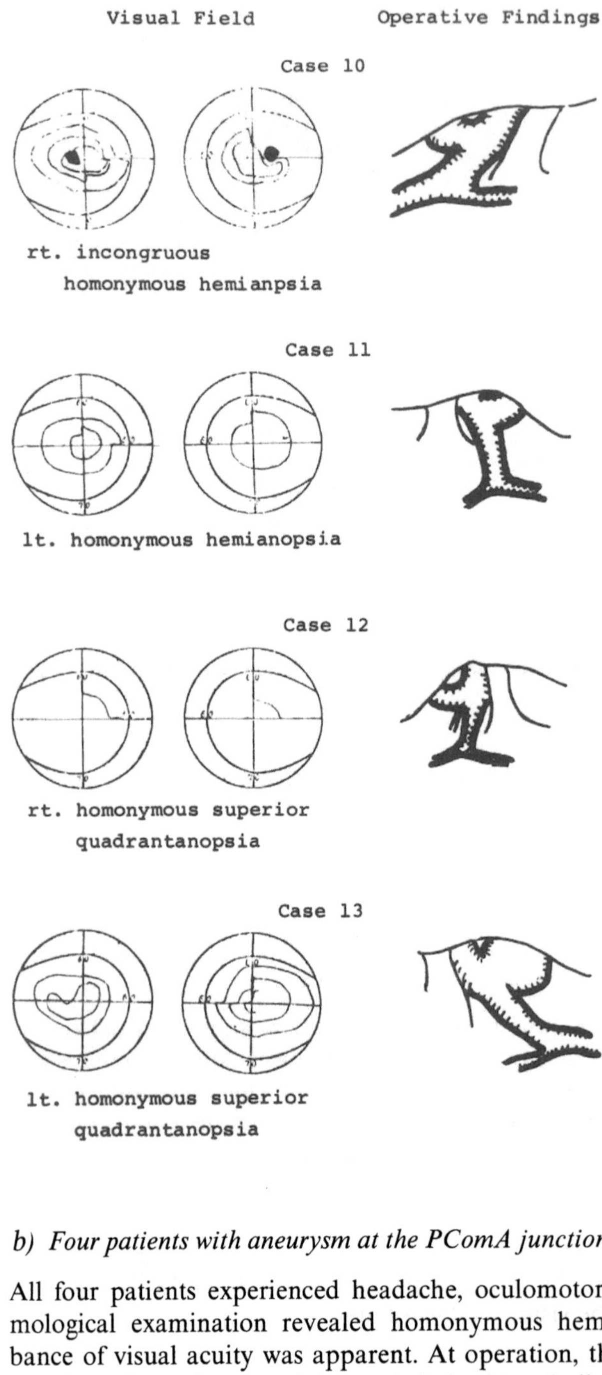

Fig. 4. Visual field defects and operative findings in four patients with aneurysm at the PComA junction

b) Four patients with aneurysm at the PComA junction

All four patients experienced headache, oculomotor defects and ptosis. Ophthalmological examination revealed homonymous hemianopsia (Fig. 4). No disturbance of visual acuity was apparent. At operation, the aneurysm in each case was found to have developed in an inferior-lateral direction from the ICA and to extend below the tentorium. There was consequently no direct contact between the aneurysm and the optic nerve, but the severe arteriosclerosis of the ICA seen in three of the four patients was found to result in compression by the ICA itself of the optic nerve from below. Clipping or ligation was performed in all patients. Postoperatively, no changes in visual field defects were found.

III. Discussion

The history of intra- and suprasellar cerebral aneurysms giving rise to bitemporal hemianopsia and other symptoms suggestive of brain tumor is long. Mitchell [3] reported an autopsy study in 1888, Horsley [3] reported a surgical case in 1885, and Cushing [7] indicated the existence of such lesions, although he himself had never experienced them. Nonetheless, the incidence of such lesions is known to be quite low – between one and two percent in the reports of neurologists and neurosurgeons [1, 8]. We experienced 13 such lesions among our series of 1000 aneurysm patients, but only nine patients (less than one percent of the total number of aneurysm patients) showed direct compression of the optic nerve.

Symptoms of optic nerve compression include visual field and visual acuity defects, the pattern of which differs according to the case. Among our AComA patients, such defects arose immediately following aneurysm rupture in two patients, and after one to 12 months in five. Atrophy of the optic nerve was apparent in two of the latter five patients.

With regard to the postoperative improvement in symptoms in these patients, it is known that treatment of only the neck of the aneurysm is insufficient; it is necessary to remove the body of the aneurysm itself to eliminate compression by the mass. The major problem, therefore, concerns the method of surgical treatment. In AComA cases, including giant aneurysms, the feeding and draining arteries of the aneurysm within the operative field must be completely opened and the neck of the aneurysm treated. First, adherence between the aneurysm and the optic nerve and surrounding blood vessels is ablated and the aneurysm neck treated. Finally, the aneurysm itself is ablated. For these purposes the best means for approaching the aneurysm is to use bifrontal craniotomy and an interhemispheric approach [6]. For treatment of the aneurysm itself, temporary occlusion of the feeding and draining arteries of the aneurysm is undertaken in order to achieve a dry field. Six of the seven AComA patients in this series were operated upon under moderate hypothermia (26 °C) to lengthen the permissible time of temporary vessel occlusion. Currently, however, prior to vessel occlusion, we administer 800 ml of 20 percent mannitol solution under normothermia and have obtained satisfactory results with temporary occlusion lasting up to 65 min [4, 5, 9, 10].

In our patients with aneurysms at the ophthalmic artery junction, clipping of the aneurysm neck was successful in one case, but extremely difficult in the other. Ultimately, ligation was performed, but the patient died. In such patients with giant aneurysms, methods such as carotid artery ligation in the cervical region should be considered following STA-MCA bypass surgery. Particularly from the viewpoint of postoperative improvement of symptoms, it is apparent that further study is necessary in these patients.

Finally, we have also studied the patients who presented visual field defects despite the fact that there was no direct compression of the optic nerve by the aneurysm. Judging from operative findings, it is thought that these patients had compression of the optic nerve by a severely sclerotic portion of the ICA. It is not certain whether the defects were due to the physical compression itself or due to defects in the vessels feeding the optic nerve. Since all of these patients were discovered by accident during examination for oculomotor nerve defects, it is thought that such findings are not particular to PComA aneurysms, but rather that there is a strong possibility that the sclerosis of the ICA itself is an important causal factor.

Summary

1. We have studied the 13 cases among our series of 1000 directly operated aneurysm cases who showed visual field and acuity defects due to compression of the optic nerve. Seven were AComA cases and six were ICA cases.

2. All of these patients had large aneurysms exceeding 15 mm in diameter. Four had giant aneurysms exceeding 25 mm in diameter.

3. For improvement of these symptoms, it is essential not only to treat the neck of the aneurysm, but also to ablate the aneurysm itself. For this purpose, great care must be taken in choosing the surgical method and the method for treatment of the aneurysm.

References

1. Jefferson G (1937) Compression of the chiasma, optic nerves and optic tract by intracranial aneurysms. Brain 60:447–497
2. Mitchell SW (1888) Aneurysm of an anomalous artery causing anterior posterior division of the chiasma of the optic nerves and producing bitemporal hemianopsia. Tr Am Neurol A 239–251
3. Pool JL, Potts DG (1965) Aneurysms and arteriovenous anomalies of brain. Hoeber Medical Division, Harper & Row, p 88
4. Suzuki J (1974) Method of prolongation of temporary stopping of the cerebral blood flow. Presidential address. 33rd Annual Meeting of the Japan Neurological Society. Sendai, Japan
5. Suzuki J, Yoshimoto T (1979) The effect of mannitol in prolongation of permissible occlusion time of cerebral artery – Clinical Data of Aneurysm Surgery. Neurosurg Rev 1:13–19
6. Suzuki J, Kodama N et al. (1979) Surgical treatment of anterior communicating artery aneurysms: From the experiences of 346 cases. In: Suzuki J (ed) Cerebral Aneurysms – experiences with 1000 directly operated cases. NEURON Tokyo p 238–243
7. Walsh FB (1964) Visual field defects due to aneurysms at the circle of Willis. Arch Ophthalmol 71:15–27
8. White JC (1964) Aneurysms mistaken for Hypophyseal Tumors. Clin Neurosurg 10: 224–250
9. Yoshimoto T, Suzuki J (1976) Intracranial defenitive aneurysm surgery under normothermia and normotension – utilizing temporary occlusion of major cerebral arteries and preoperative mannitol administration. Neurol Surg (Tokyo) 4:775–783 (Engl. abs)
10. Yoshimoto T, Sakamoto T, et al. (1978) Experimental Cerebral Infarction. Part 3. Protective effect of mannitol in thalamus infarction in dogs. Stroke 9:217–218
11. Yoshimoto T, Uchida K et al. (1979) An analysis of follow up results of 1000 intracranial saccular aneurysms with definitive surgical treatment. J Neurosurg 50:152–157

Optic Nerve Compression by Other Intracranial Etiology

M. SAMII, Hannover/FRG

After the previous discussions of compression of the optic nerve by pituitary adenomas, meningiomas and aneurysms, I should like to draw your attention to the relatively rare clinical pictures which through compression may also cause visual disturbances and scotoma.

Compression of the optic nerve chiasm by the floor of the III. ventricle may cause scotoma and decrease of visual function. Fig. 1 and Fig. 2 demonstrate computertomograms of two different patients with marked hydrocephalus. Whereas, in the case of the 26 year old patient (Fig. 1) we diagnosed a concentric scotoma with visual decrease of 10–20° preoperatively, we found complete normal ophthalmological findings in the 16 year old patient. The computertomograms (Fig. 2) definitely prove the enlargement of the third ventricle with extension into the sella turcica. In the ensuing discussion, Doctor Menzel will discuss in detail the follow up and results of visual disturbances caused by hydrocephalus.

According to our cisternotomographic investigations (M. Samii and J. Beck, 1970) the position and course of the optic nerve in the cranial caudal direction showed considerable variations. These variations were revealed by study of 50 normal pneumencephalotomograms. Fig. 3 shows an example of low location of

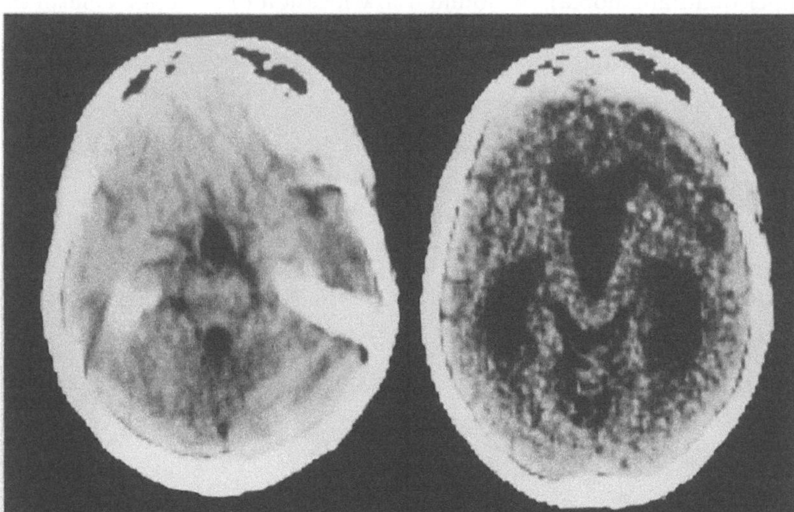

Fig. 1. CT scan of a 26 year old patient with concentric scotoma with visual decrease of 10–20°. Compression of the optic chiasm is caused by the floor of the third ventricle dilated by hydrocephalus

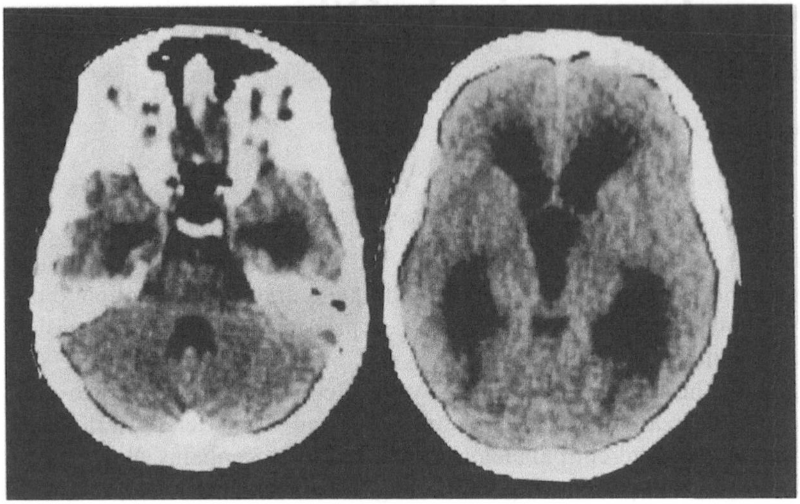

Fig. 2. Complete normal ophthalmological findings in a 16 year old patient despite hydrocephalus. The CT scan demonstrates enlargement of the third ventricle with extension into the sella turcica

the optic chiasm. It is located close to the diaphragma sellae. The largest distance of the optic chiasm from the diaphragma sellae was 10 mm (Fig. 4). Regarding the possible variations in the course of the optic nerves to the cranial caudal line, we have once again studied the pneumencephalographic films of 19 patients with visual disturbances in whom an intracranial space occupying process could be excluded with certainty. In three patients with visual field defect (temporal or bitemporal upper quadrantanopia), we found a low location of the optic chiasm in the cistern picture. A noticeable compression of the optic chiasm was caused by the

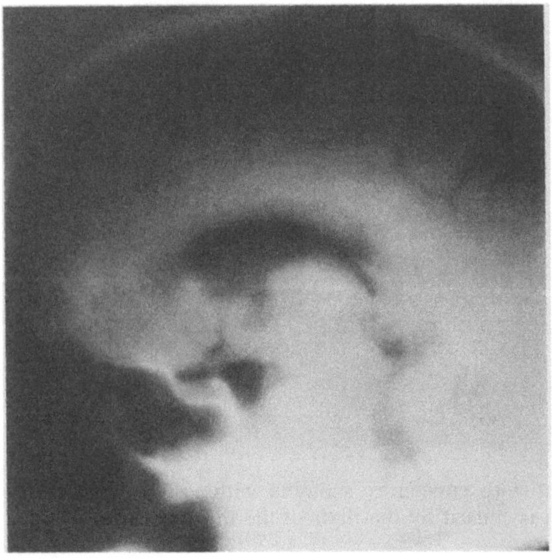

Fig. 3. An example of the low position of the optic chiasm in encephalo-cisternotomogram. The optic nerve is located close to the diaphragma sellae

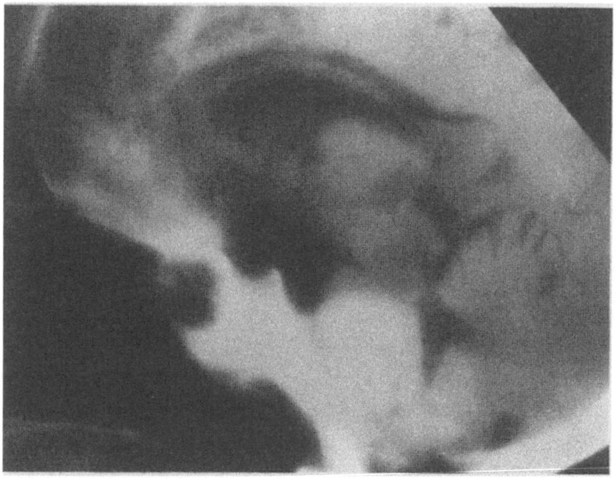

Fig. 4. Normal pneumencephalotomogram with the greatest distance of the optic chiasm from the diaphragma sellae

dorsum sellae (M. Samii, 1972). As an example I would like to discuss the following 40 year old woman: She was admitted to the hospital for clarification of a circulatory collapse. An insignificant impairment of the endocrinological findings and disturbances of the visual fields (bitemporal upper quadrantanopia) were found. Pituitary adenoma was therefore suspected and neuroradiological examinations suggested. An intracranial space occupying lesion could be excluded. The cisternotomogram, however, showed marked compression of the very low located optic chiasm caused by the dorsum sellae (Fig. 5). However, these examinations were retrospective studies and the patient therefore could not be called upon for operative treatment. In patients it is possible that these partial resection of the dorsum sellae could lead to functional improvement of the clinical syndrome.

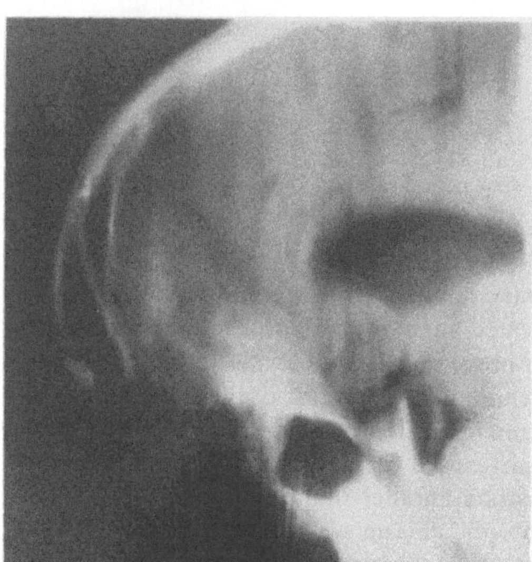

Fig. 5. Midline pneumencephalotomogram of a patient with bitemporal upper quadrantanopia. The soft tissue shadows of the optic chiasm are distinctly visible. The chiasm is located very low and is compressed by the dorsum sellae

a

b

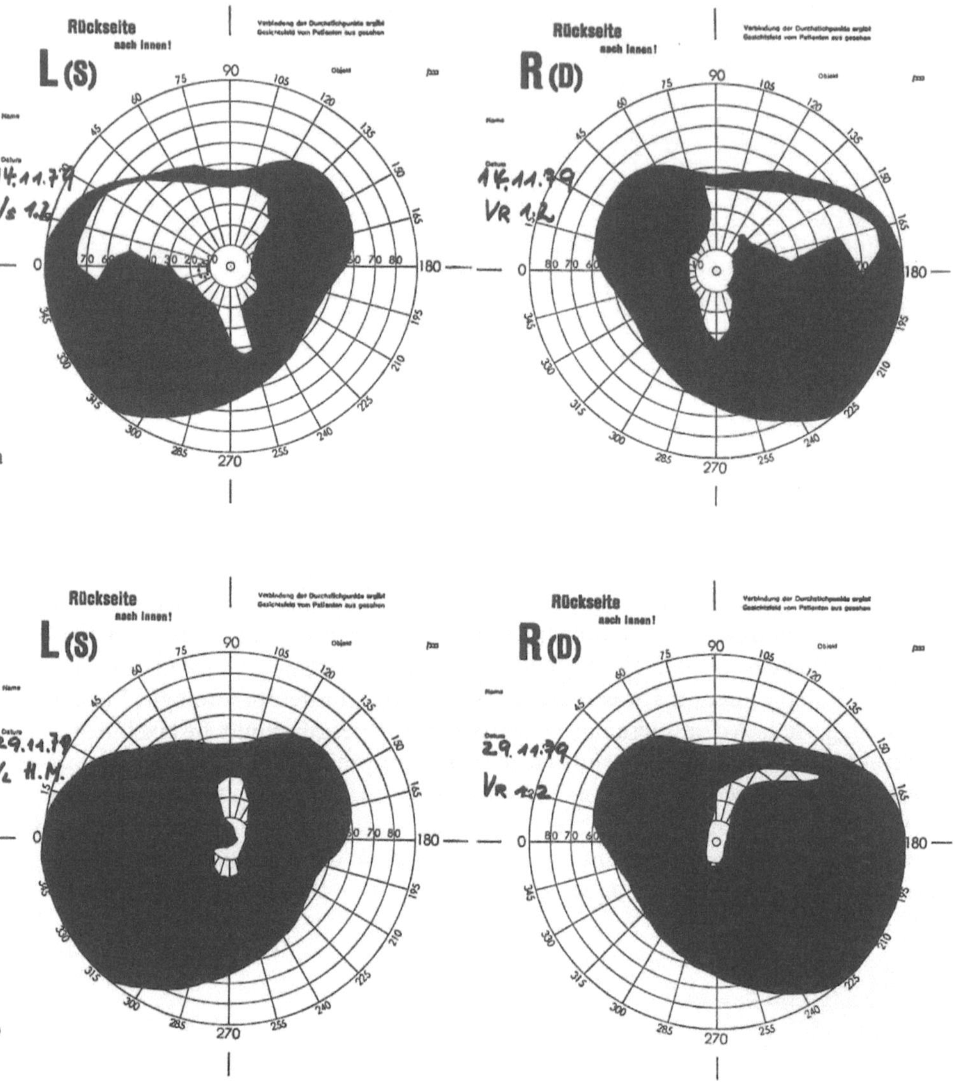

Fig. 6 a, b. Visual field deterioration over a two week period caused by vascular compression

Among 155 patients treated for pituitary tumors (M. Samii and K. Schürmann, 1978) we found in only five intrasellar located adenomas, a lower bitemporal visual field defect, which was not caused by compression of an adenoma. In these patients we discussed the possible etiology of arachnoiditis or neuritis of the optic nerve. In one patient, who showed the clinical picture of a bitemporal hemianopia, we found vascular compression to the optic chiasm caused by anomalies of both anterior cerebral arteries. I would like to demonstrate another interesting case of vascular compression of the optic nerves and the optic chiasm we operated upon in 1979. The 25 year old patient had been operated on, five years previously because of

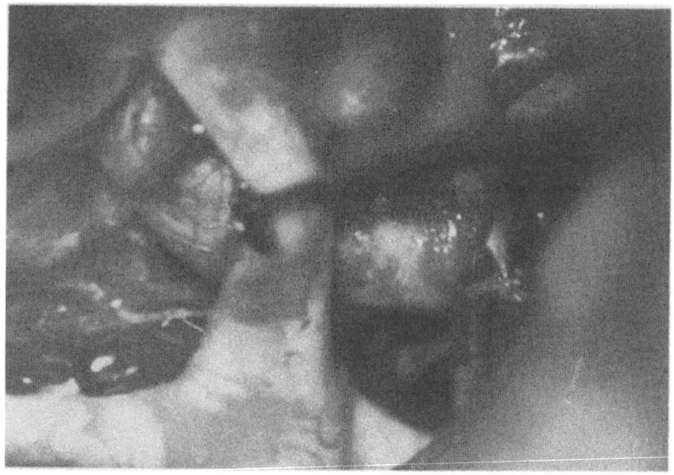

a

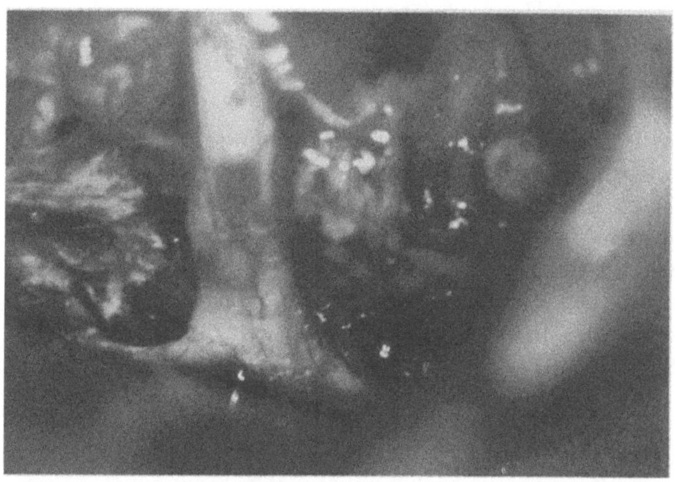

b

Fig. 7 a, b. The same patient as Fig. 6 a and b. Transfrontal optic nerve and optic chiasm exposure and decompression. The optic nerve is compressed by carotid and ophthalmic artery (**a**), after opening the optic canal a muscle piece is placed between the arteries and the optic nerve (**b**)

increasing scotoma and decrease of visual acuity with a diagnosis of arachnoiditis. The surgeon then found general alterations in the region of the arachnoidea and his attention was also drawn to the extremely large diameter of the internal carotid and ophthalmic arteries. Although a slight improvement of the ophthalmological findings could be ascertained after the intervention, the deficit persisted. Five years later the patient was admitted to the neurological clinic with increasing visual deficit on both sides (Fig. 6 a). Vision deteriorated over the next two weeks (Fig. 6 b). Carotid angiography demonstrated a medial location of both carotid arteries and deep location of the anterior cerebral artery. Based on acute amaurosis

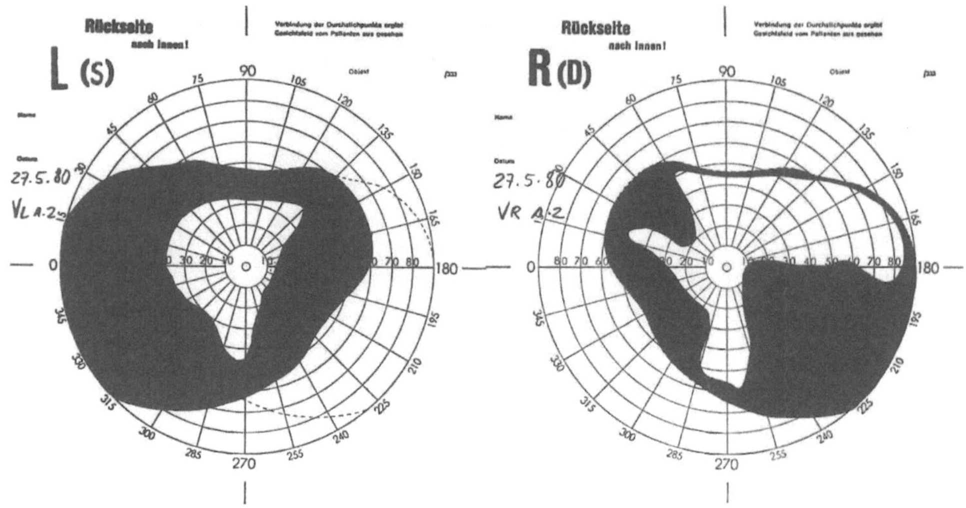

Fig. 8. The same patient as Fig. 6 and 7, six months after the operation. Impressive improvement in visual field defect

beginning 13 days later we performed an emergency operation despite exclusion of an intracranial space occupying process. Intraoperatively we could ascertain an extreme hypertrophy of both internal carotid arteries and the ophthalmic artery compressing both optic nerves (Fig. 7 a). Decompression was performed by means of muscle pieces after opening both optic canals (Fig. 7 b).

Postoperatively, we ascertained an impressive improvement in visual acuity and visual field defect. The last ophthalmological examination, six months later, demonstrated satisfactory visual fields (Fig. 8).

References

Samii M, Beck J (1970) Lage und Verlauf der Sehnerven im Cisternenbild. Radiologe 10: 456–459

Samii M (1972) Visual disturbances caused by a low located optic chiasm. Exerpta Medica, Intern Congress Series 306:48–55

Samii M, Schürmann K (1978) Operative treatment in relation to location and extension of pituitary adenomas. In: Fahlbusch R, v Werder K (eds) Treatment of pituitary adenomas. Georg Thieme, Stuttgart p 309–316

On the Pathogenesis and Prognosis of Lesions of the Optic Nerve in Hydrocephalic Patients

J. Menzel and Th. Rommel, Heidelberg/FRG

Hydrocephalus is associated with many neurological signs and symptoms. In reviewing the literature, we can point out that papilledema is a rare sign and occurs in about five to seven percent of all cases (Jensen, 1979). Optic atrophy with different degrees of reduction of visual acuity and/or visual field defects are observed with a nearly similar frequency. Concerning the pathomechanism, we know that the enlarged third ventricle compresses the optic nerves and/or the chiasm. In the same way, even compression of the pituitary stalk is possible (Hier, 1979). Neuroradiological evidence is given by ventriculography which demonstrates the enlarged third ventricle with emphasis of the optic recess (Fig. 1). CT scan shows dilatation of the third ventricle only (Fig. 2).

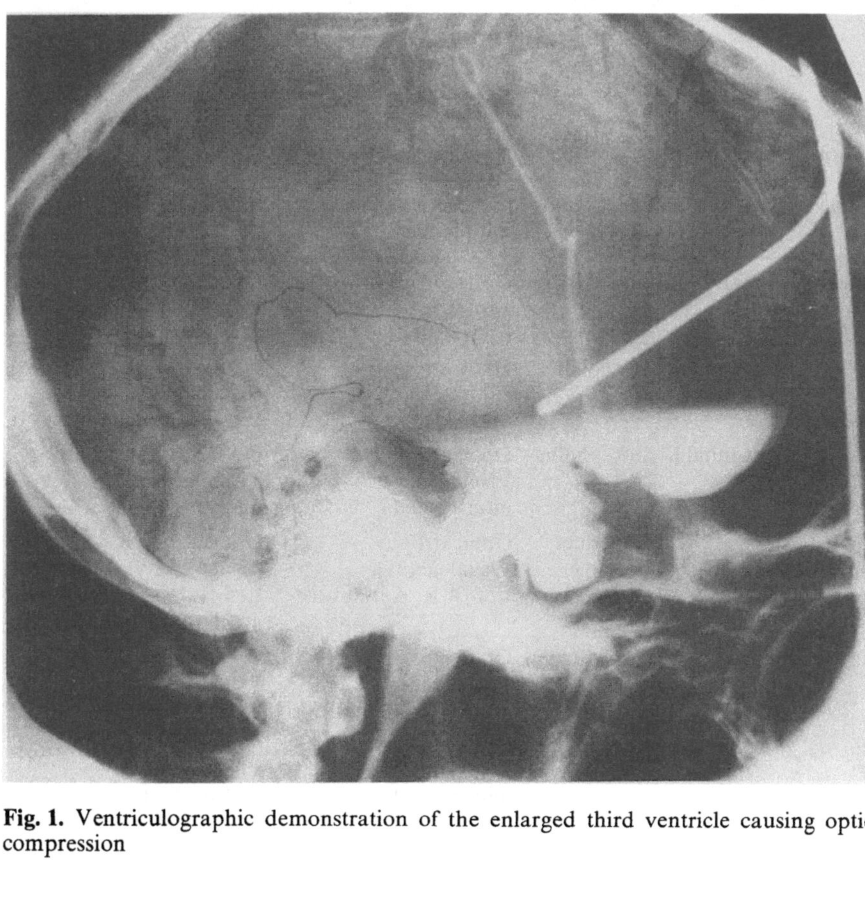

Fig. 1. Ventriculographic demonstration of the enlarged third ventricle causing optic nerve compression

Table 1. Follow-up in hydrocephalic patients with papilledema

Age	Sex	Cause of hydrocephalus	Papilledema	Follow-up
7 y	m	Meningitis	3 dptr.	disappeared normal visual acuity
14 y	m	Stenosis of the aqueduct	2 dptr.	disappeared normal visual acuity
13 y	f	Stenosis of the aqueduct	4 dptr.	disappeared normal visual acuity
61 y	m	GREITZ' syndrome	4 dptr.	disappeared normal visual acuity
31 y	m	Occlusion of the Foramen of MONROE	2 dptr.	disappeared normal visual acuity
48 y	m	Intraventricular cysticercosis	2 dptr.	disappeared normal visual acuity
15 y	m	Congenital hydrocephalus	2 dptr.	disappeared normal visual acuity
12 y	f	Congenital hydrocephalus	2 – 3 dptr.	disappeared normal visual acuity
22 y	m	Stenosis of the aqueduct	1 – 2 dptr.	disappeared normal visual acuity
8 y	f	Congenital hydrocephalus	1 dptr.	Optic atrophy

Table 2. Follow-up in hydrocephalic patients with optic atrophy

Age	Sex	Cause of Hydrocephalus	Ophthalmological symptoms	Follow-up
12 y	m	Stenosis of the aqueduct	Optic atrophy Visual acuity: L: 5/35 R: 1/35	Optic atrophy Visual acuity: L: 1/50 R: 1/50
8 y	f	Congenital hydrocephalus	Optic atrophy; Amaurosis	Optic atrophy Visual acuity: L: 5/20 R: Amaurosis
10 y	m	Congenital hydrocephalus	Optic atrophy; Visual acuity: undisturbed	Optic atrophy Visual acuity: undisturbed
15 y	m	Stenosis of the aqueduct	Optic atrophy; Visual acuity: L: 5/4 R: Amaurosis	Optic atrophy Visual acuity: L: 5/4 R: Hand movements
37 y	m	Stenosis of the aqueduct	Optic atrophy; Visual acuity: L: 1/12 R: Amaurosis	Optic atrophy Visual acuity L: 5/10 R: 5/20
12 y	f	Congenital hydrocephalus	Optic atrophy; Visual acuity: undisturbed	Optic atrophy Visual acuity: undisturbed

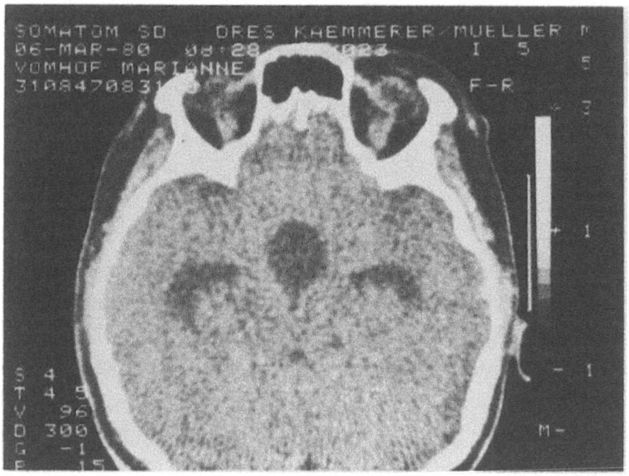

Fig. 2. CT scan of the same case

To judge the prognosis of optic system lesions in hydrocephalus we have analyzed 93 patients in a period from 1970 to 1979. Ophthalmological symptoms were observed in 37 cases, i.e. in 39.7 percent. The first table (Table 1) shows 10 patients with papilledema. Stenosis of the aqueduct was the most frequent basic disease. After CSF shunting papilledema disappeared in nine cases. Long-term examination showed normal visual acuity in these patients. Only in one case did optic atrophy follow papilledema. In this now 11-year-old girl visual acuity is considerably reduced. In a second group, six patients with optic atrophy are analyzed (Table 2). Underlying diseases included stenosis of the aqueduct and congenital hydrocephalus. All patients received CSF shunts and had longterm examinations. Preoperatively, two patients showed no deterioration of visual acuity. Follow-up investigations postoperatively demonstrate that optic atrophy is not reversible. In one patient visual acuity became significantly worse. In three cases slight recovery of vision was observed within two years.

In conclusion we can say:

1. Ophthalmological signs in hydrocephalic patients constitute 39.7 percent of our patients, which is a surprisingly high percentage.
2. Papilledema has a good prognosis after surgical therapy of hydrocephalus. Only in one case did optic atrophy develop.
3. Optic atrophy is not reversible and in two thirds of our cases was associated with diminished visual acuity. On the other hand slight improvements of important functional significance are observed within two years.

References

1. Hier DE, Wiehl AC (1979) Chronic hydrocephalus associated with short stature and growth hormone deficiency. Ann Neurol 2(3):246–248
2. Jensen F, Jensen FT (1979) Acquired hydrocephalus. A clinical analysis of 160 patients studied for hydrocephalus. Acta Neurochir (Wien) 46(3–4):243–256

Optic Nerve Compression by Processes of the Rhinobasis

W. Draf, Fulda/FRG

According to Wullstein (1972) the *rhinobasis* should be defined as that part of the skull base which is directly connected to the nasal cavity and the pneumatized system of the paranasal sinuses (Fig. 1). One should keep in mind that about two thirds of the osseus orbital walls are formed by the borders of the paranasal sinuses (Ganz 1977, Fig. 2).

Three groups of processes of the rhinobasis which may cause optic nerve compression must be considered (Table 1):

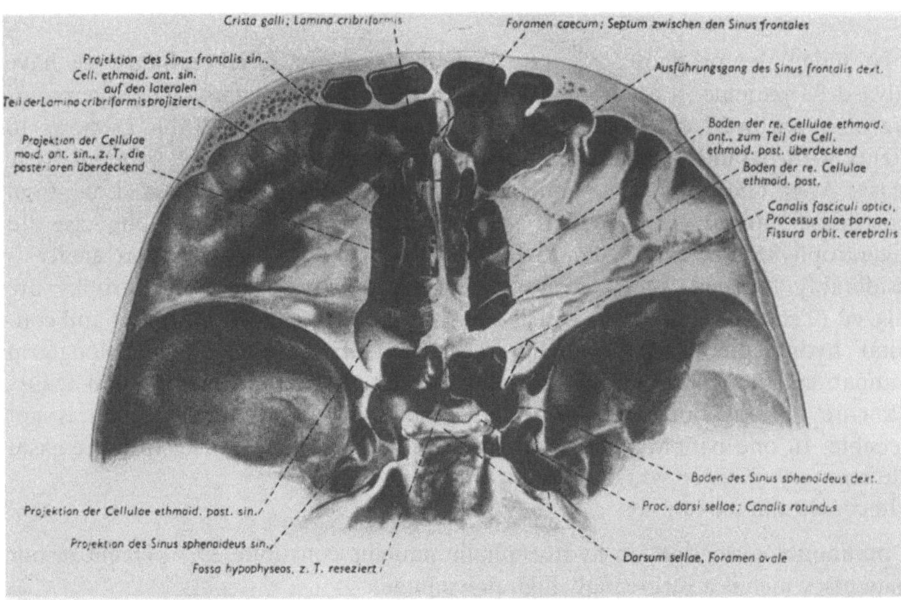

Fig. 1. Relationship between anterior skull base and the pneumatized nasal and paranasal sinuses system (Pernkopf 1957)

These three etiologic factors may cause more or less distinctive orbital apex-syndromes (Rochon-du Vignieaud 1893, Smith 1958, Table 2). Discussed as a pathogenesis are first the compression of cranial nerves II to VI, and second swelling of the tissue in the orbital apex. The symptoms are: Impaired vision or amaurosis, ptosis, diplopia, temporoparietal pain, and exophthalmus (Fig. 3).

Infections, especially acute and chronic sinusitis of the ethmoidal cells and the sphenoid sinus as well as *mucoceles* caused by infections or traumas can affect the optic nerve (Table 3).

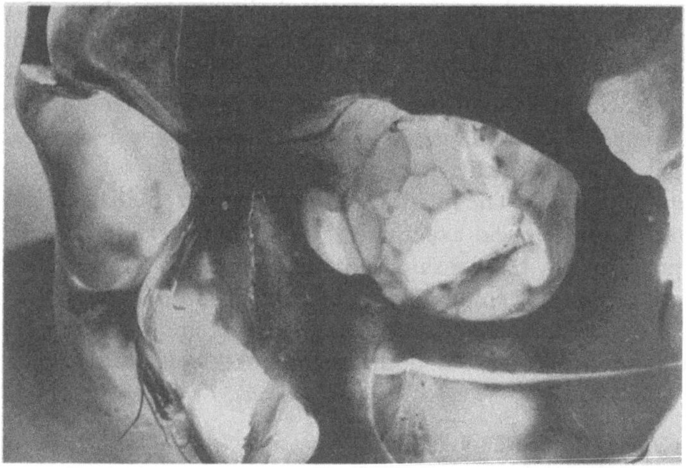

Fig. 2. Translumination of the facial skeleton. The maxillary and frontal sinus as well as the ethmoid cells forming a great part of the osseous orbit are visible

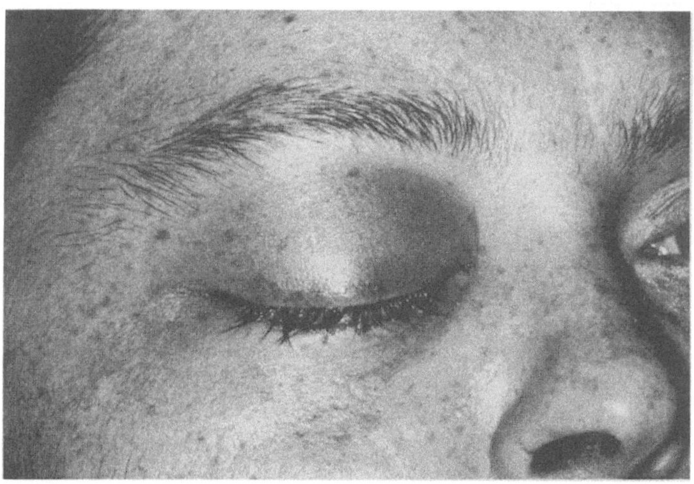

Fig. 3. Ptosis and Exophthalmus in orbital apex syndrome

Table 1. Optic nerve compression by processes of the rhinobasis

A. Infection
B. Trauma
C. Tumor

Generally, orbital complications due to infections including impaired vision or amaurosis are very rare. Marx (1913–1920) and Herrmann (1952–1957) found orbital complications in three to five per thousand patients. It is interesting that these data did not change with the use of the antibiotics (Table 4). Therefore one can say that isolated damage of the optic nerve caused by infection is a very rare event. Acute and chronic sinusitis (Table 5) can result either in an *orbital apex syndrome* or in a *retrobulbar neuritis*. The relationship between retrobulbar neuritis and sinusitis varies with various clinical experiences. Nevertheless, Hajek in 1915 stated that there is no proof for any relationship. Blindness caused by a mucocele of the sphenoid sinus has recently been described by Blum and Larson (1973), (Table 6). One should look for such a mucocele if there are symptoms as retrobulbar pain, orbital apex syndrome and/or destruction of the sella turcica.

Table 2. Orbital apex syndrome (Rochon-du Vigneaud 1833, Smith 1958)

Etiology:
Infection, trauma, tumor
Pathogenesis:
compression of cranial nerves II – VI
swelling of tissues in the orbital apex
Symptoms:
impaired vision or amaurosis
ptosis
diplopia
temporoparietal pain
exophthalmus

Table 3

A. infection	
1. acute	sinusitis
2. chronic	
3. mucoceles	

Table 4. Orbital complications

Marx (1913 – 1920)	3 – 5 percent
Herrmann (1952 – 1957)	

Table 5

Acute	Sinusitis	Orbital apex syndrome
Chronic		Retrobulbar neuritis

Trauma to the optic nerve (Table 7) can be caused by birth damage, accidents, operations, expecially transnasal and transmaxillary ethmoidectomy, local anaesthesia and the injection of contrast media. *Rupture of nutritive vessels* (Traquair et al. 1935) and *edema* of the optic nerve (Lazorthes and Anduze 1952) are the most important pathogenetic factors (Huber 1974). A postoperative orbital *haematoma* (Rawling 1904; Liebrecht 1912) can induce a lesion of the optic nerve.

Table 6. Mucocele of the sphenoid sinus

1. Retrobulbar pain
2. Orbital apex syndrome
3. Destruction of the sella turcica

Table 7. B. trauma to the optic nerve

Etiology:

birth damage, accident, operation

Pathogenesis:

rupture of nutritive vessels (Traquair et al. 1935)
edema of the optic nerve (Lazorthes and Anduze 1952)
orbital hematoma (Rawling 1904, Liebrecht 1912)
hematoma of the optic sheet (Hoelder 1879)
bone fragments (Berlin 1879)
rupture of the optic nerve (Liebrecht 1906)

Frequency:

0,5 – 5,2% in skull-brain injuries (Römer et al. 1973)
0,7% amaurosis in 4000 skull-brain injuries (Schmaltz and Schuermann 1971)
21% lesions of the optic nerve in 43 rhinobasal injuries which needed surgical treatment (Beuthner 1974)

A *direct lesion* of the optic nerve by bone fractures or its intracranial rupture is quite rare. Römer and coauthors (1973) reported a frequency of 0.5 to 5.2 percent injuries to the optic nerve in skull-brain-injuries based on the existing literature. Schmaltz and Schuermann (1971) found 0.7 percent amaurosis in 4000 skull-brain injuries. Beuthner described 21 percent lesions of the optic nerves in injuries of the rhinobasis in 43 patients, all of which needed rhinosurgical treatment (1974). Wuest (1949) saw a non-pulsating central retinal artery after rhinobasal trauma. After transmaxillary decompression of the orbit, the pulsation of this vessel returned. Damage of the optic nerve during endonasal and transmaxillary ethmoidectomy is a well known, but rare event according to the literature (Berendes 1962/63; Wirth 1963; Herrmann 1968; Oecken 1978; Langnickel 1978; Hansen 1967; Boette 1965; Schröder and Salzmann 1973). This complication is especially prone to occur if the frontal and sphenoidal sinuses are extensively pneumatized so that the optic nerve is surrounded only by mucous membrane (Fig. 4).

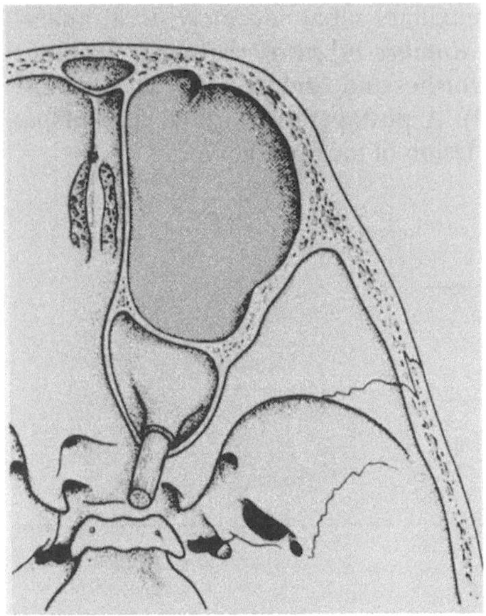

Fig. 4. Large frontal and sphenoidal sinuses. The optic foramen is surrounded by mucous membrane of the sphenoid sinus (Ganz 1977 according to Corning)

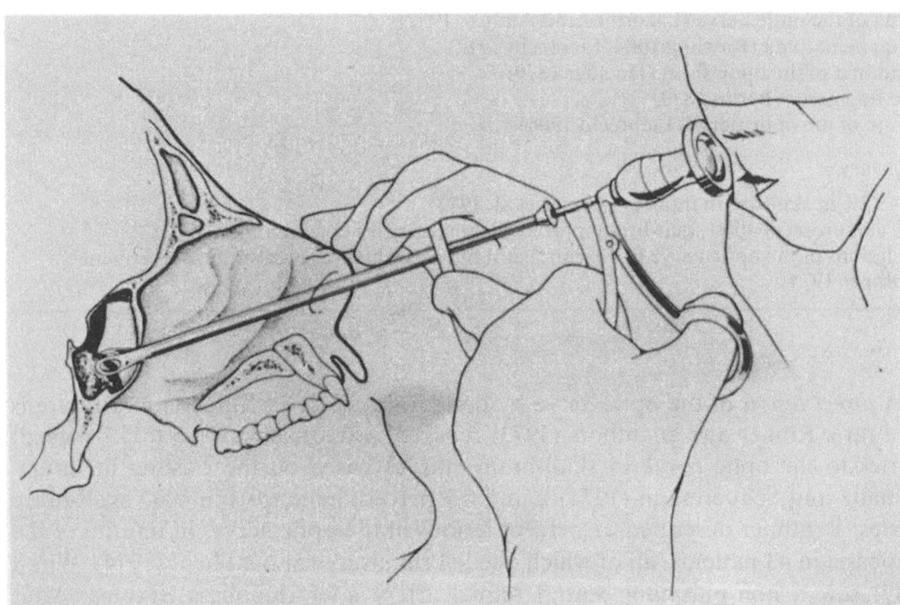

Fig. 5. Endoscopy of the sphenoid sinus with biopsy

In 1975 we published a case of irreversible amaurosis after endoscopy of the sphenoid sinus in a patient with carcinoma (Fig. 5). Postoperative haematoma was excluded by an immediate reexploration. Microscopical examination of the specimen showed absence of neural tissue. As pathogenetic factors of this lesion we discussed first an indirect overstretching and secondly a constriction of the nutritive vessels caused by irrigation of the sinus with a vasoconstricting solution (PRIVIN) used for haemostasis. Injury of the optic nerve is also possible after *local anaesthesia* (D. Hansen 1967; Schroeder and Salzmann 1973, Table 8). The optic nerve can be damaged by several mechanisms. Oecken (1978) published a case of transient amaurosis following *radiography of the maxillary sinus* with a *contrast medium* after a heavy fracture of the facial sceleton.

Table 8. Optic nerve lesion by local anaesthesia

1. Bleeding because of perforation of a vessel
2. Direct lesion by injection
3. Infiltration

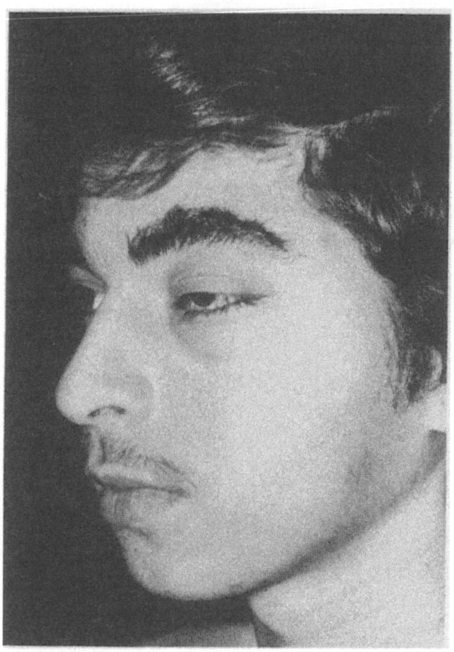

Fig. 6. Exophthalmus and ptosis caused by a large angiofibroma

If the optic nerve is involved by a *tumor* (Table 9) which is benign, the nerve can only be compressed by the tumor. Malignant tumors produce compression and often direct infiltration in addition. A 15 year old boy presented with a large but benign angiofibroma which had produced a typical orbital apex syndrome with exophthalmus, ptosis and almost a total amaurosis (Fig. 6). CT scan demonstrated

Table 9. C. Tumors

benign tumors	→	compression
malignant tumors	→	compression and infiltration

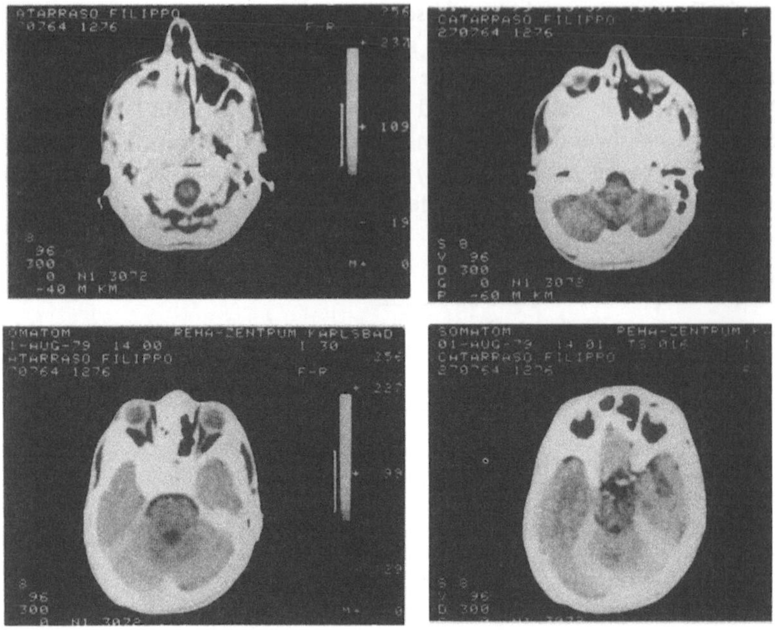

Fig. 7. CT scan of the tumor (Angiofibroma) noted in figures. (For this figure we thank Prof. Dr. J. P. Haas, Head of the Department for Radiology of Städtische Kliniken Fulda)

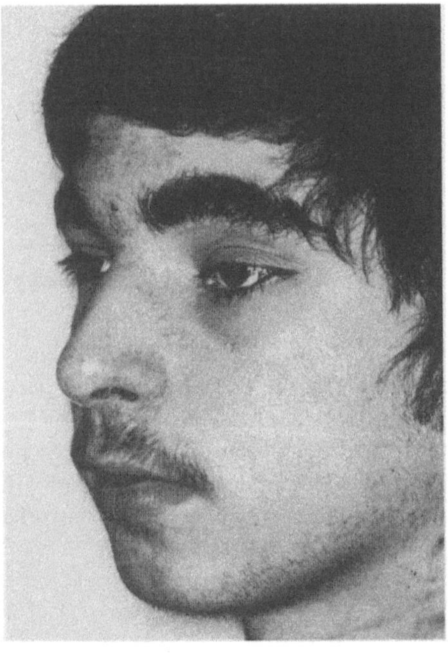

Fig. 8. The patient six months postoperatively

the extension of the process into the parasellar region on the left (Fig. 7). Via a lateral rhinotomy and using the microscope, it was possible to remove the tumor totally and to preserve the left optic nerve (Fig. 8). The vision improved greatly, but a small central scotoma remained.

In summary, infections, trauma and tumors of the rhinobasis may cause compression of the optic nerve. Early diagnosis and consequent surgical evaluation using the microscope can help to prevent permanent visual loss.

References

Berendes J (1962) Erblindung durch Komplikation bei Siebbeinoperation und Begutachtung zur Schuldfrage. HNO 10:182

Berendes J (1963) Grundsätzliches zur Begutachtung der iatrogenen Erblindung durch Siebbeinoperation. HNO 11:25

Berlin R (1879) Über Sehstörungen nach Verletzung des Schädels durch stumpfe Gewalt. Ber 12 Vers d Ophtal Ges Heidelberg 1879. Außerordentl Beilagen zu Klin Mbl Augenheilkd 17:9

Beuthner D (1974) Analyse zur Frage d N opticus-Dekompression – zugleich eine Übersicht über 10 Jahre präventivsanierende Versorgung von Rhinobasisfrakturen (1964–1973). Z Laryng Rhinol 53:830–835

Blum EMM, Larson A (1973) Mucocele of the sphenoid sinus with sudden blindness. Laryngoscope 83:2042

Boette G (1965) Verletzungen der Orbita aus der Sicht des Rhinologen. HNO 13:326

Draf W (1975) Die Endoskopie der Nasennebenhöhlen. Diagnostische und therapeutische Möglichkeiten. Z Laryng Rhinol 54:209

Ganz H (1977) Komplikationen der unspezifischen Nasen- und Nebenhöhlenentzündungen. In: Berendes J, Link R und Zöllner F (eds) Hals-Hasen-Ohren-Heilkunde in Praxis und Klinik. Band 1/I. Thieme, Stuttgart p 14.1–14.42

Hansen D (1967) Orbitale Komplikationen bei rhinologischen Eingriffen. HNO 15:300

Herrmann A (1968) Gefahren bei Operationen an Hals, Ohr und Gesicht und die Korrektur fehlerhafter Eingriffe. Springer Berlin Heidelberg New York

Hoelder R (1879) In: Berlin R (eds) Über Sehstörungen nach Verletzung des Schädels durch stumpfe Gewalt. Außerordentl Beilagen zu Klin Mbl Augenheilkd 17 p 9

Langnickel R (1978) Temporäre Erblindung nach endonasaler Siebbeinoperation. HNO 26:172–173

Lazorthes G, Anduze H (1952) L'ouverture du canal optique dans les lésions traumatiques récentes du nerf optique à propos de 10 cas opérés. Rev Neurol (Paris) 87:540

Liebrecht K (1906) Schädelbruch und Auge. Arch Augenheilk 55:36

Liebrecht K (1912) Schädelbruch und Auge. Albrecht von Graefes Arch Klin Ophthalmol 83:525

Oeken FW, Kessler L (1978) Fehler und Gefahren bei Routineeingriffen im HNO-Fachgebiet. Georg Thieme, Stuttgart

Pernkopf E (1957) Topographische Anatomie des Menschen. Bd 4, 1. Hälfte. Urban & Schwarzenberg, München Berlin Wien

Rochon-Du Vigneaud (1893) Quelques cas de paralysis de tons les nerfs orbitaires (ophthalmoplegie totale avec amourose et anesthesia dans le domaine de l'ophthalmique), d'origine syphilitique. Arch D'ophthalmologie, Tome treize

Römer F, Müller U, Bettag W (1973) Zur operativen Versorgung indirekter traumatischer Optikusläsionen. Klin Monatsbl Augenheilkd 163:327–331

Schmaltz B, Schuermann K (1971) Traumatische Opticusschäden. Probleme der Ätiologie und der operativen Behandlung. Klin Monatsbl Augenheilkd 159:33

Schroeder N, Salzmann H (1973) Sehnervenschädigungen nach Eingriffen im Nasennebenhöhlenbereich. Arch Klin Exp Ohr-, Nas- und Kehlk-Heilk 205:285

Smith AT (1958) Orbital apex syndrome. Ann Otol Rhinol Laryngol (St. Louis) 67:742
Traquair HM, Dott NM, Russel WR (1935) Traumatic lesions of the optic chiasma. Brain 58:398
Wirth G (1963) Entstehung einseitiger Amaurose bei Nasennebenhöhlenerkrankungen, insbesondere nach operativen Eingriffen. HNO 11:21
Wüst K (1949) Zur Behandlung d. drohenden Opticusatrophie infolge retrobulbärer Hämatome. Klin Monatsbl Augenheilkd 114:140
Wullstein HL (1972) Hat Terminologie zur Definition unseres Faches eine praktische Bedeutung? HNO 20:259–261

Follow up of Visual Defects After Optic Nerve Decompression

K. von WILD, M. SAMII, K. HOFFMANN, and L. OSTERWALD, Hannover/FRG

Repeated tests of the visual acuity and examination of the visual fields are still of utmost importance in the diagnosis and follow up of optic nerve lesions (Fig. 1) [1–5].

Since October 1977 we have operated upon 40 patients with visual field defects of one or both eyes due to various causes of optic nerve compression, as listed in Table 1. There were 19 pituitary adenomas, one craniopharyngioma, eight meningiomas, one glioma of the optic chiasm, one glioma of the frontal lobe, one spongioblastoma of the hypothalamic region, one mucocele of the ethmoidal cells, four aneurysms of the internal carotid and the anterior communicating cerebral artery, one compression of the internal carotid and anterior cerebral arteries, and three acute traumatic lesions. Using microscopical techniques we performed the decompression of the optic nerves by subfrontal approach in all but four tumors, which adenomas were operated by transsphenoidal route. Three traumatic lesions and one mucocele were treated via the transethmoidal approach.

Table 1. Etiology of optic nerve compression and restoration of function in the visual fields in 40 perisellar lesions (80 eyes)

Etiology of the disturbances	No. of cases	Function of visual fields			
		unchanged normal	improved	unchanged impaired	deteriorated
Pituitary adenoma	19	6	16	14	2
Craniopharyngioma	1		2		
Meningioma	8	6	2	5	3
Glioma of the optic chiasm	1			2	
Glioma of the frontal lobe	1			2	
Spongioblastoma	1		2		
Aneurysm	4	5	3		
Arterial compression	1		2		
Mucocele of the ethmoidal cells	1	1	1		
Head injury	3	3	3		
Total	40	21	31	23	5

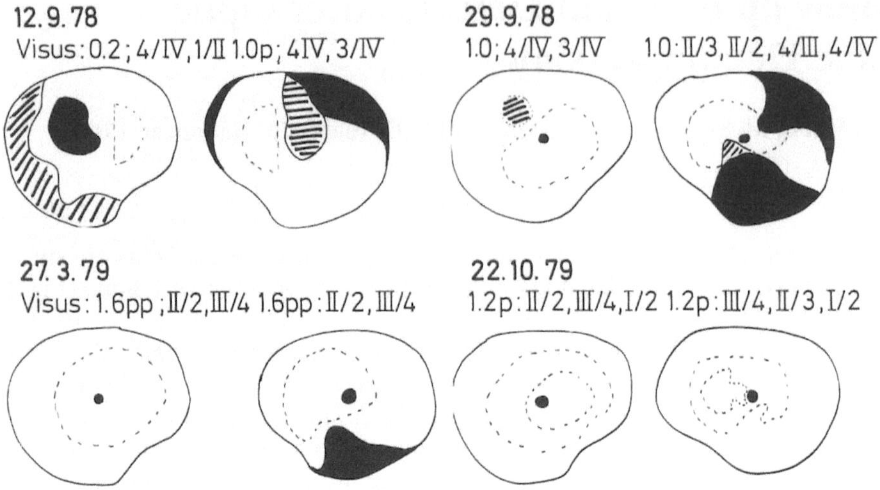

A

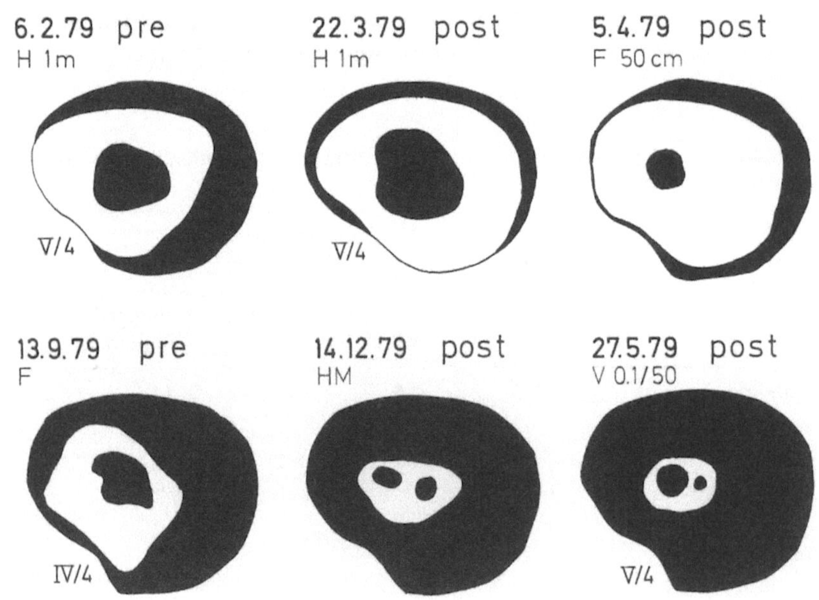

C

Fig. 1 A, C (Caption see opposite page)

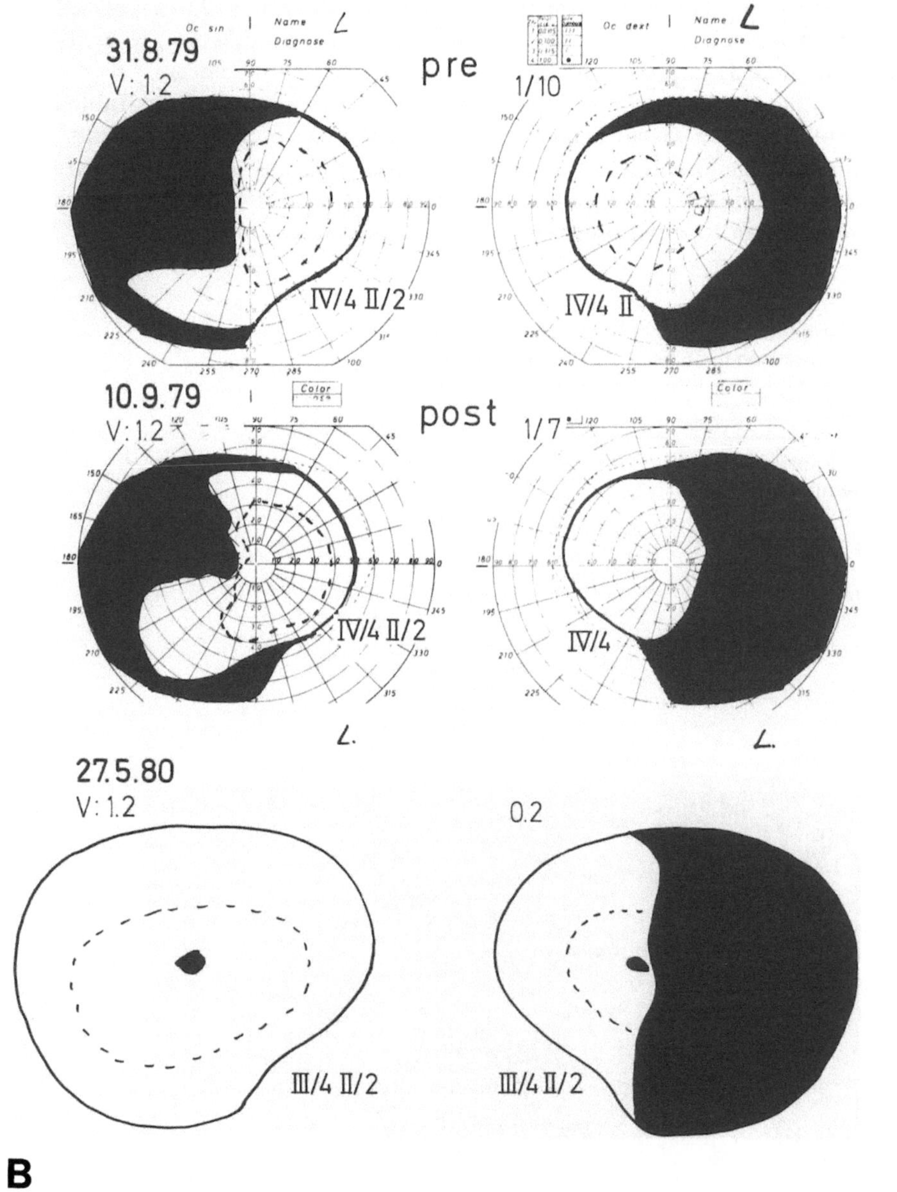

B

Fig. 1 A–C. Follow up of visual defects after optic nerve decompression in 3 pituitary adenomas with suprasellar extension. **A** Improvement of visual acuity and visual field defects after subfrontal removal of the tumor on 18. 9. 1978. **B** Improvement of visual defects to normal on the left eye and slight improvement of visual acuity in the right eye with permanent visual defects due to optic nerve atrophy, after transsphenoidal removal of the tumor on 6. 9. 1979. **C** Improvement of visual function in the right eye after transsphenoidal removal of the tumor on 13. 3. 1979. Impairement caused by the tumor recurrence. Subfrontal approach on 9. 10. 1979. Permanent defects due to optic nerve atrophy

The follow-up examinations of the visual fields show that 23 out of 80 eyes remained unchanged impaired after operative relief of the pressure, whereas five eyes deteriorated, 31 improved, and 21 eyes remained without defects.

Restoration of function in the vision after decompression is listed in Table 2. At the time of operation visual acuity was impaired in 30 eyes of 26 patients with accompanying visual field defects caused by perisellar lesions. After decompression vision remained normal in 19 and unchanged impaired in nine eyes out of 49. Vision improved in 10, deteriorated in five and remained lost in 6 eyes.

Table 2. Restoration of function in vision after optic nerve decompression in 26 perisellar lesions (49 eyes)

Visual acuity	No. of eyes
Unchanged normal	19
Very good improved, normal	4
Improved	6
Unchanged impaired	9
Worse	1
Worse and blind	4
Unchanged blind	6
Total	49

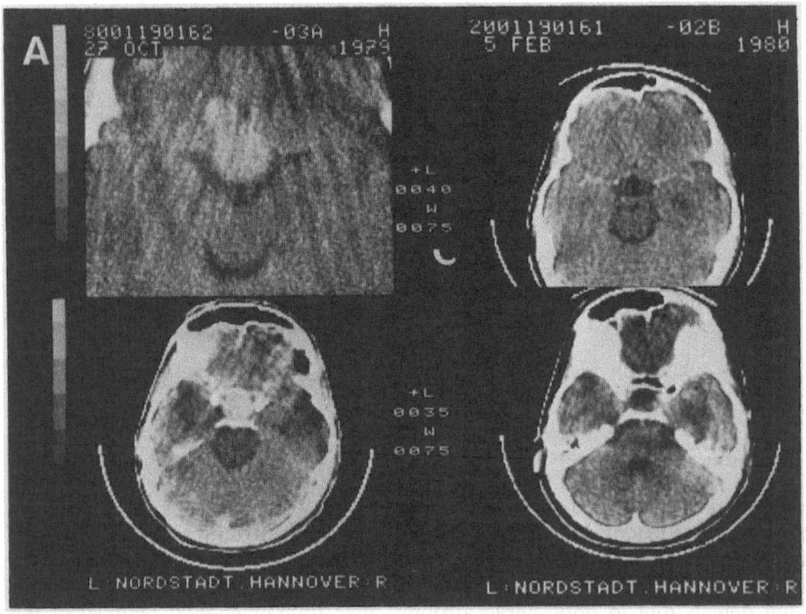

Fig. 2 A, B. Pre- and postoperative CT scan (**A**) and visual defects (**B**) in a 17 year old acromegalic male patient with acute loss of visual function caused by acute hemorrhage into adenoma tissue. Subfrontal decompression and removal on 31. 10. 1979

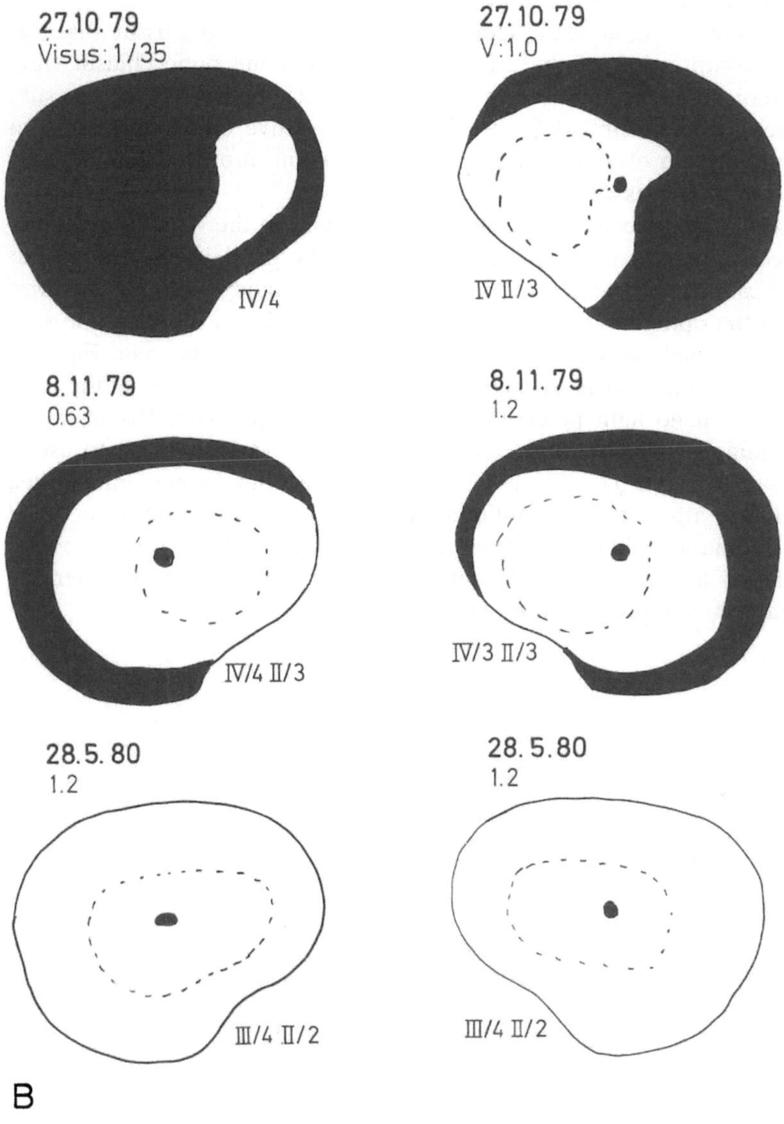

Fig. 2 B. (Caption see opposite page)

Follow-up evaluation of the visual defects reflects the extent on which the optic nerve fibres have been damaged at the time of decompressive operation (Figs. 1, 4, 6).

From our experience and that of others we can say that optic nerves which are merely compressed recover their function after relief of the pressure within a short time period, provided the defects are not too marked or have not been present for too long. Therefore when successful decompression is performed, improvement is usually rapid and dramatic, as it was in a 17 year old acromegalic patient (Fig. 2).

He had an acute loss of visual function that was pronounced in the left eye. The operative findings revealed an acute hemorrhage into the adenoma tissue that had caused massive compression of the left optic nerve and the optic chiasm from below. The tumor could be totally removed and the clot extirpated by the subfrontal approach as demonstrated by pre- and postoperative CT examinations as well as by the follow up of visual defects. Visual function improved immediately and was normal in both eyes after seven months.

Our results were graphically demonstrated as changes in the visual scores after optic nerve decompression in a diagram (Fig. 3). Very good improvement was observed in the case of a mucocele and in two acute traumatic lesions. In the third traumatic lesion the optic nerves had been totally damaged as a result of gun shot injury. The patient died postoperatively from his severe brain damage. Figure 4 shows the follow up in a 47 year old male patient with traumatic lesion of the right optic nerve, who had no light perception at the time of operation. Visual acuity improved immediately after decompression by transethmoidal approach to useful function and was 0.3 after 11 months with an improved but permanent marked visual defect due to atrophy of the optic nerve fibres. It has to be borne in mind that in acute traumatic lesions the fibres rapidly disintegrate and break up into small fragments so that immediate decompression becomes imperative after the diagnosis is established to preserve the visual function.

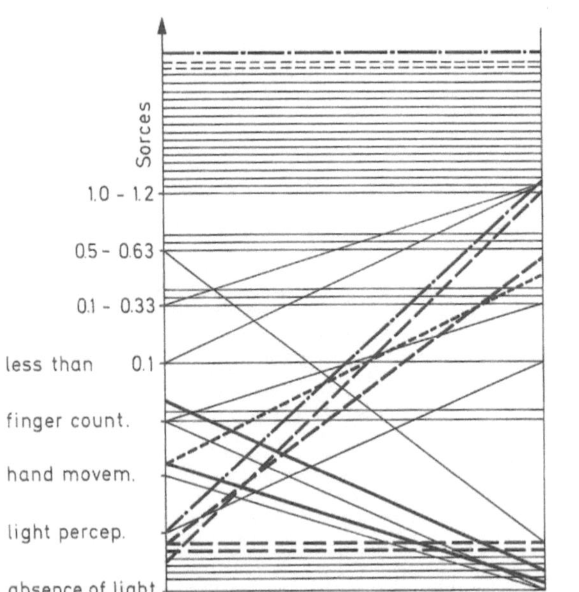

Fig. 3. Changes in the visual scores in 26 patients with optic nerve compression caused by prisellar lesions (49 eyes examined): 19 Pituitary adenomas black lines. 1 Craniopharyngioma black little lines. 1 Meningioma red lines. 3 Traumatic lesions red little lines. 1 Mucocele red dotted lines. 1 Arterial compression red little and dotted lines (see Table 2)

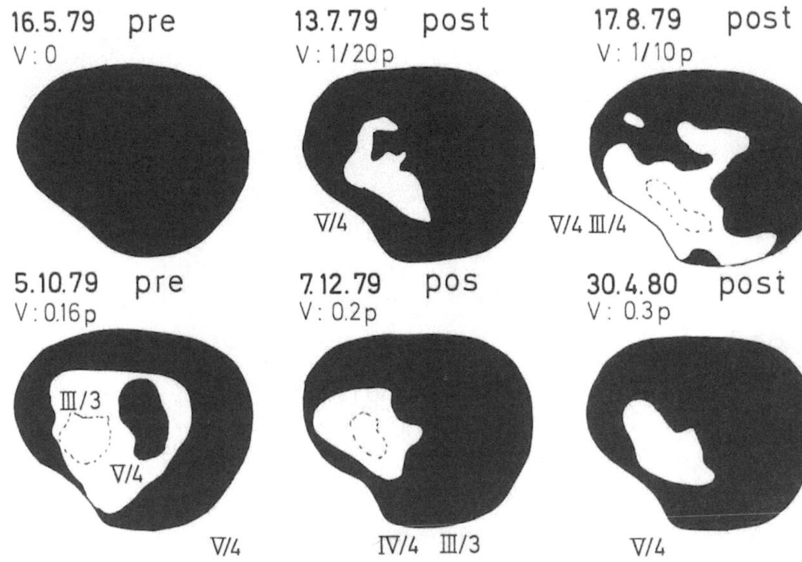

Fig. 4

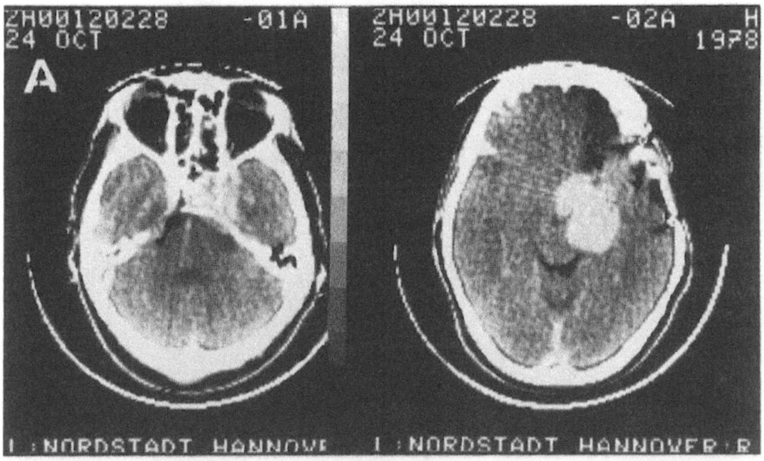

Fig. 5 A

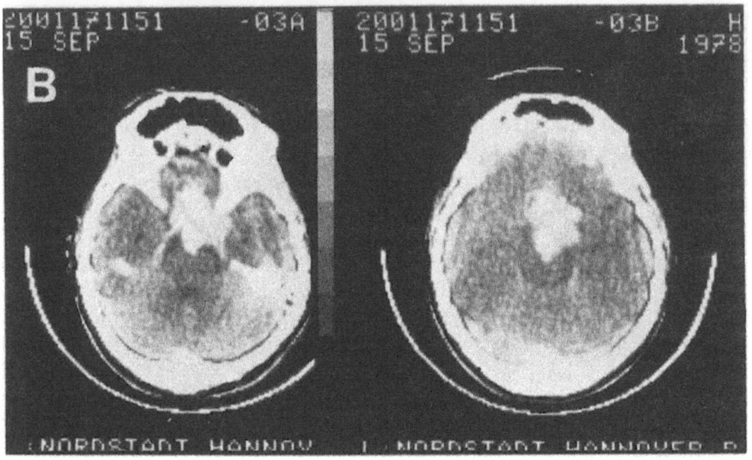

Fig. 5 B

Caption see page 188

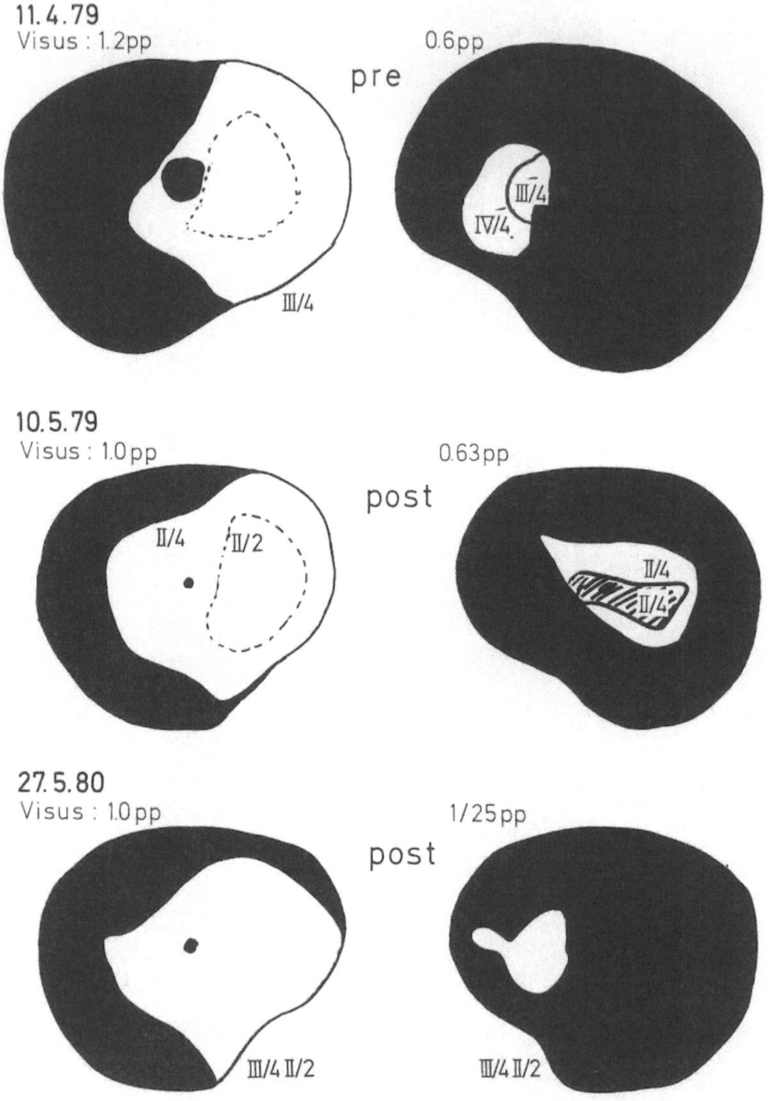

Fig. 6. Follow up of visual defects in a recurrent prolactinoma causing optic nerve and chiasm compression. Subfrontal approach at 20. 4. 1979

Fig. 4. Improvement of visual function after decompression of the right optic nerve by transethmoidal approach at 16. 5. 1979 in a 47 year old male patient with acute traumatic lesion

Fig. 5 A, B. Operative decompression of the optic nerve failed in giant recurrent adenoma (**A**) and suprasellar meningioma (**B**) due to optic nerve atrophy at time of operation

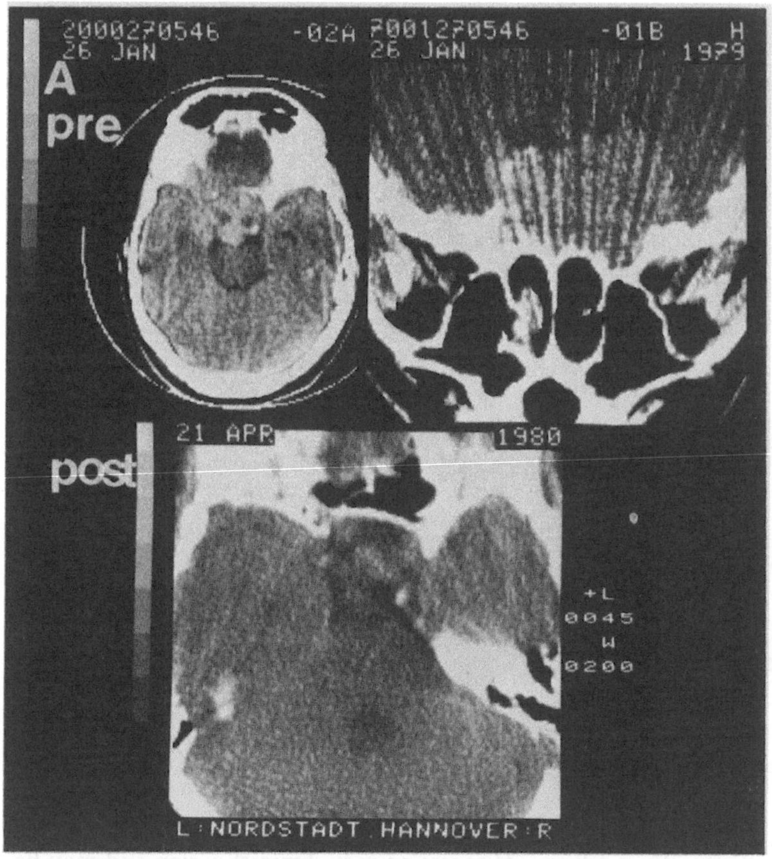

Fig. 7. Giant prolactinoma recurrence (CT 26. January 1979). Impairement of visual function despite the optic nerve decompression and subtotal removal of the tumor on 22. 2. 1979. Improvement of visual acuity 6 months after radiotherapy with good result (CT control 21. 4. 80)

When atrophy has commenced it may progress despite decompression, as happened in a young male who had a meningioma (Fig. 5) with extensive suprasellar extension and three recurrent giant adenomas with optic nerve compression over more than three years (Figs. 1 c, 3, 6, 7).

The follow up of visual defects in one of these recurrent adenomas with pronounced impairment of the right eye is demonstrated in Figure 6. Visual acuity deteriorated in spite of decompressive operation on the right eye from 0.6 to useful function. Moreover, there was an improvement in the left visual field.

This patient, a woman, was operated upon via a subfrontal approach with subtotal removal of the adenoma. The operative findings showed an enormous compression of the stretched right optic nerve that caused the atrophy. After decompression with opening of the optic canal and the dural sheath, one could see a hemorrhagic tight lacing where the nerve was pressed against the bone.

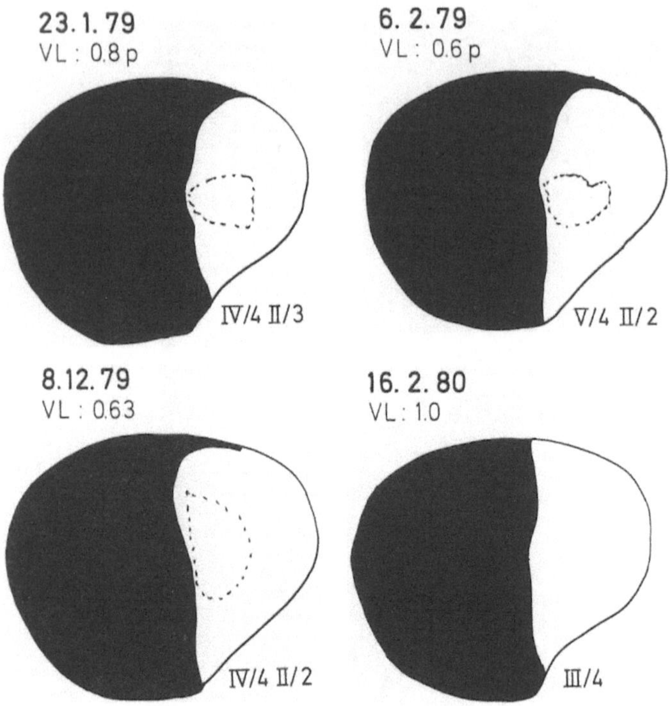

Fig. 7 B. (Caption see opposite page)

If optic nerve atrophy is advanced, operation may diminish vision and may be better left undone in so far, as vision is concerned. In these cases radiotherapy should be considered [1, 2, 5].

A 35 year old male patient developed acute loss of visual function due to adenoma recurrence with tremendous suprasellar extention, as demonstrated by the CT scan (Fig. 7). In spite of decompression of the optic nerves by means of total removal of a recurrent giant adenoma, this patient postoperatively was without useful vision on the left and blind in the right eye. Two years after the first subfrontal approach and 6 months after radiotheraphy that had reduced the tumor mass lesion (Fig. 7) vision improved to light perception on the right with an 1.0 visual acuity on the left eye.

Therefore we want to emphasize that despite an initial loss of visual function following decompressive operation, there can be an improvement in visual acuity up to one year postoperatively, suggesting that the function of some optic nerve fibres could have been preserved.

References

1. Duke-Elder S (1971) System of Ophthalmology. Volume XII Neuro-ophthalmology. Henry Kimpton Publishers, London
2. Jefferson A (1978) The treatment of chromophobe pituitary adenomas by means of trans-frontal surgery, radiation therapy and supportive hormone therapy. In Fahlbusch R, v. Werder K (eds) Treatment of Pituitary Adenomas. Georg Thieme, Stuttgart, p 237–252
3. Ruf H, v Wild K, Neubauer M (1973) Follow-up studies on 33 craniopharyngiomas and 95 cases of chromophobe and acidophil pituitary adenomas after treatment by subfrontal operation. In: Kuhlendahl H, Brock M, Le Vay D, Weston TJ (eds) Modern aspects of neurosurg. IV. Int Congr Series No 306, Excerpta Medica, Amsterdam, p 152–161
4. Samii M, Schürmann K (1978) Operative treatment in relation to location and extension of pituitary adenomas. Results. In: Fahlbusch R, v Werder K (eds) Treatment of Pituitary Adenomas. Georg Thieme, Stuttgart, p 310–316
5. Wild K von, Ruf H (1973) Diagnostic problems and errors in suprasellar meningiomas. In: Kuhlendahl H, Brock M, Le Vay D, Weston TJ (eds) Modern aspects of neurosurg. IV. Int Congr Series No 306, Excerpta Medica, Amsterdam, p 43–47

Oculomotor, Trochlear and Abducens Nerves

(Third, Fourth and Sixth Cranial Nerves)

Angiographic Aspects of the Arterial Supply of the Cranial Nerves

P. LASJAUNIAS [1], L. PICARD [2], C. MANELFE [3], J. MORET [4], and J. ROLAND [2]

Introduction

Following basic arterial anatomic [4, 14, 16, 19] and modern angiographic datas [3], we have focalised our interest on the base of the skull. To study the arterial supply of the cranial nerves, we have used different material, details of which have been extensively presented the past 6 years:

- Anatomical: human adults and embryos, and animals (dogs, chickens, etc), dissected and radiographied.
- Angiographic: from our institution and from other ones in France and abroad; these angiograms were divided into two parts: anatomical (normal aspects) and clinical (complications of embolization).

Our purpose was to give the neuroradiologists a basic and flexible arterial map from which they could understand anatomical variants. From it they can find already described variations, built new ones they will encounter, and predict in each case the theoretical risk of an embolization. The knowledge of these risks does not limit the indications of embolization but the usage of some embolic material. It also transfers some accidents from the personal technical mistake (due to misreading of an information), to the therapeutic risk of a treatment (as it is known in neurosurgery, were it does not rest on the technical aspect but on the topography of a lesion). The recent increasing number of cranial nerve palsies after embolization, has given us exeptional material to demonstrate in detail the angiographic aspects of the arterial supply of the cranial nerves. [5]

Finally, clinical correlation, from these 'experimental' vascular syndromes, showed us that it was conceivable to describe vascular territories at the base of the skull.

It was then possible to reconsider some cranial nerves syndromes [5, 6] thought to be vascular with a negative 'angiographic exploration'.

I. The Extra-Ocular Motor Nerves (IIIrd, IVth, VIth)

(Figures 1, 2, 3)

These nerves belong phylogenetically to a functional entity which includes the VIth (ophthalmic root of the trigeminal nerve) [18].

---

[1] Service de Radiologie, Hopital de Bicêtre, Faculté Paris-Sud 78, Rue du Général Leclerc, 94270 Kremlin-Bicetre/France

[2] Service de Neuroradiologie, CHU, I Rue Foller, 54000 Nancy/France

[3] Service de Neuroradiologie, CHU PURPAN, 31052 Toulouse/France

[4] Service de Radiologie, Fondation Rothschild, 29 Rue Manin, 75019 Paris/France

[5] Presented at the ASNR meeting Los Angeles 1980, and at the French Society of Neuroradiology Toulouse 1979

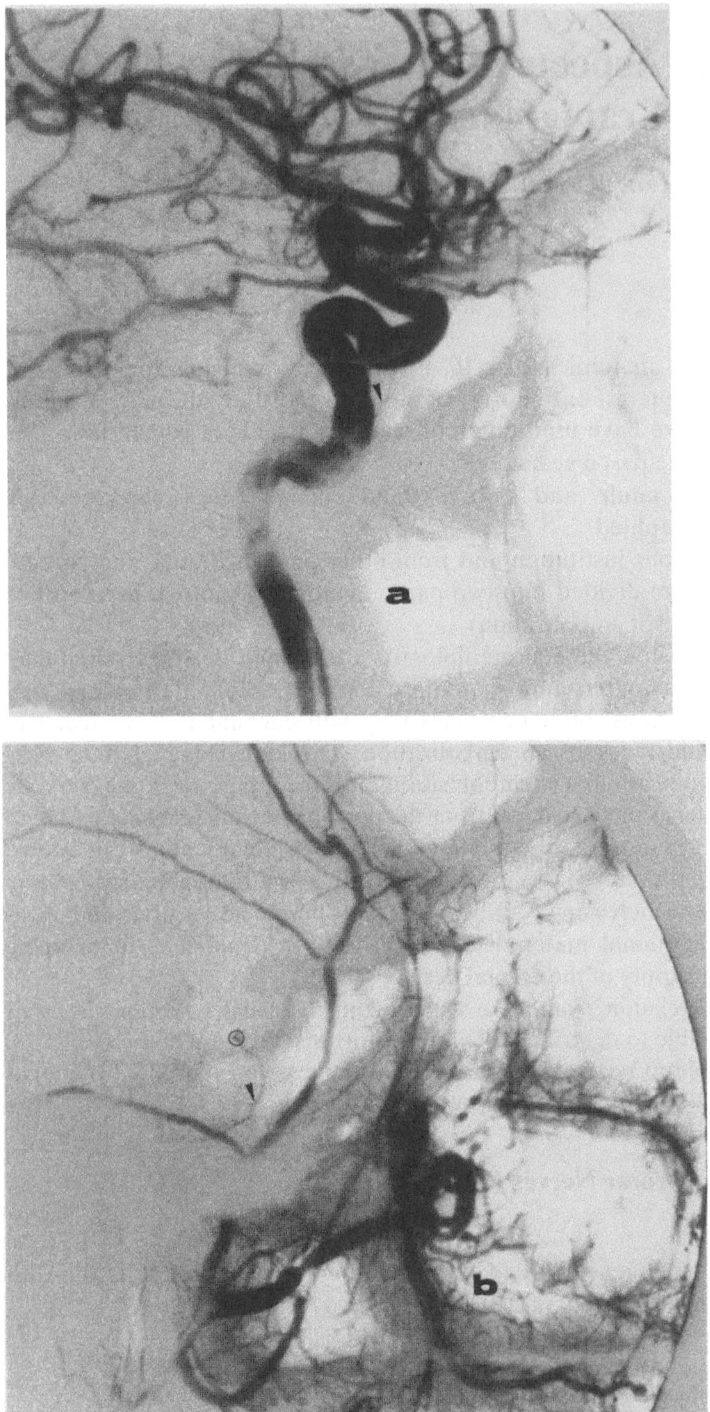

Fig. 1 a, b. Internal carotid **a**, and internal maxillary **b** injections. The infero-lateral trunk (arrow head) is better seen on the maxillary injection. Note the absence of filling of the carotid syphon. The circle represents the origin of the ILT on the internal carotid artery

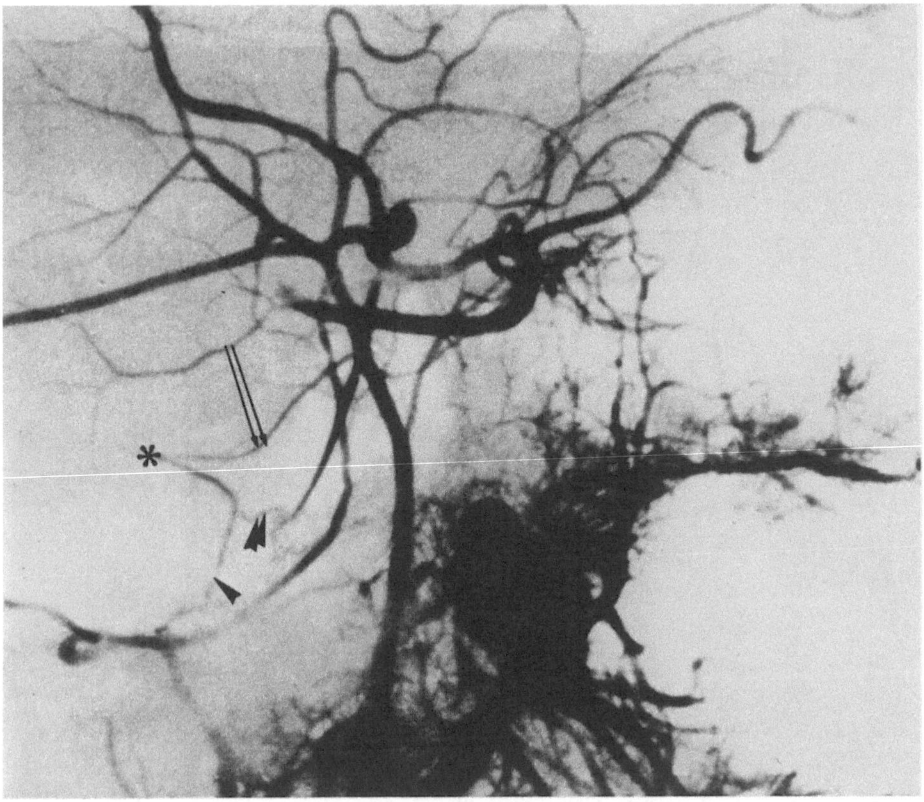

Fig. 2. Selective injection of the internal maxillary artery. The ILT branches are easily identified. – Posterior (*arrow head*) – Antero-medial (*double arrow*), it courses within the ZINN tendon. – Antero-lateral (*double arrow head*). Note the absence of filling of the internal carotid syphon (*asterisk*)

a) – In their *cisternal portion* the nerves are supplied by the basilar system [17]; angiographically speaking, the branches even visible are not routinely recognizable, due to superimpositions.

b) – In their *transdural portion* two groups must be considered: IIIrd and IVth on the cavernous roof, supplied by the marginal tentorial artery regardless of its origin (Table 1).

Table 1. Possible origins of the marginal tentorial artery (IIIrd, IVth)

- C_5 portion of the ICS [a]
- C_4 portion of the ICS [a]
- Accessory meningeal artery
- Middle meningeal artery
- Intra-orbital ophthalmic artery
- Intra-orbital lacrimal artery

[a] ICS Internal carotid syphon

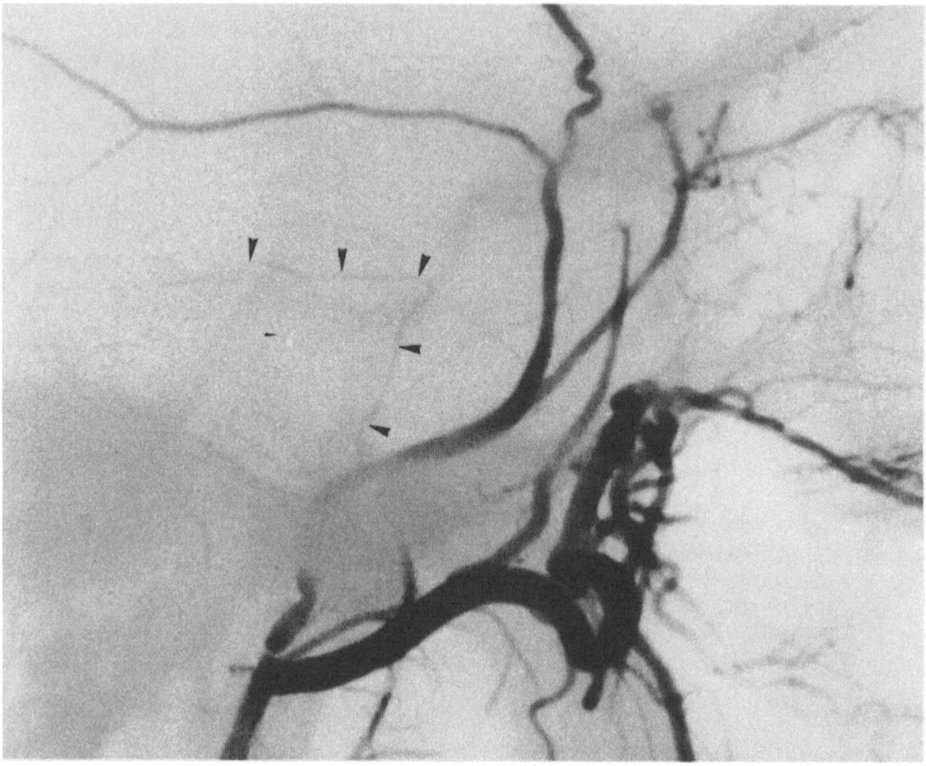

Fig. 3. Selective injection of the internal maxillary artery. Accessory meningeal dominance in the supply of the cavernous area. The artery of the free margin of the tentorium is clearly identified (*arrow head*). It supplies the IIIrd and IVth nerves in their transdural portion

The VIth, supplied by the retro-clival arterial arch between the C_5 collateral of the syphon and the jugular branch of the ascending pharyngeal artery [7, 12].

c) – In their *extradural portion:* IIIrd, IVth, VIth and V_1th belong to the ILT[6] regardless to its type (C_4, accessory meningeal).

d) – In their *transforaminal portion,* two groups can be described:

Within the ZINN tendon where IIIrd, VIth and nasal nerves are supplied by the remnant of the dorsal ophthalmic artery and its variants [10].

Out of the ZINN tendon where the IVth frontal and lacrymal nerves are supplied by the remnant of the orbital branch of the supra-orbital division of the stapedial artery and its variants [15].

Angiographically all the variants of these systems belong either to the intra-cavernous collateral of the internal carotid syphon (ICS), to the intra-orbital ophthalmic system, or to the accessory meningeal artery [8]. As all these arteries are anastomosed, we can choose the best way to visualize them without considering their anatomical origin. For example the intra-cavernous collaterals of the internal

[6] Infero lateral trunk of the internal carotid syphon

carotid artery are poorly seen through internal carotid angiogram even with subtractions and direct magnification. On the contrary selective internal maxillary angiograms as well as the ascending pharyngeal injections visualize them consistently.

We use, when angiography is indicated in *extra-ocular nerve* lesions, the following protocol of injections: internal carotid, internal maxillary, ascending pharyngeal, vertebral (magnified lateral projections).

This procedure is performed under general anesthesia by femoral approach with small catheters (3,7 F to 4,1 F) to allow perfect subtractions of the superselective injections. A good radio-anatomical knowledge permits one to study these films routinely, and find small lesions, non-visualized with CT scanning, often not surgically removable but reachable by endovascular techniques.

II. The Intra-Petrous Facial Nerve

(Figure 4)

The arterial supply has been known for a long time. Recently different groups have reported Bell's palsy after embolization (1, 2, II). Various materials were involved: resorbable, non resorbable, fluid, Gelfoam strips, powder, etc. In fact careful study of the angiographies allows one to identify the facial arch arterial system [7, 9]. It belongs to the middle meningeal system, regardless to its variant (Table 2), since the equivalent vessels course close to the foramen spinosum area (absent in case of non maxillary origin).

As we saw for the extra-ocular nerves, the facial nerve must be incorporated to the supra-tentorial functional group including the V_3th and V_mth. The V_2th root of the trigeminal nerve represents a sort of transition between the two; it remains in most of cases with the V_3th, V_mth and VIIth group for its arterial supply. This trigemino-facial nerve group is supplied by the stapedial and maxillo-mandibular systems. Their remnants and variants are not unquantifiable as they obey a phylogenetic, ontogenetic and hemodynamic logic [7]. The arterial supply of the facial nerve may then be deduced from the angiographic informations even if non-visualized. In some instances the facial arterial arch will be clearly demonstrated thanks to the stylo-mastoid retrograde filling. Previous identification of these

Table 2. Possible origins of the middle meningeal artery

- Internal maxillary artery
- C_4 portion of the ICS [a]
- Basilar trunk
- Carotid branch of the ascending pharyngeal artery
- Intra-petrous ICA [b]
- Intra-tympanic ICA [b]
- Intra-orbital ophthalmic artery
- Intra-orbital lacrymal artery

[a] ICS Internal carotid syphon
[b] ICA Internal carotid artery

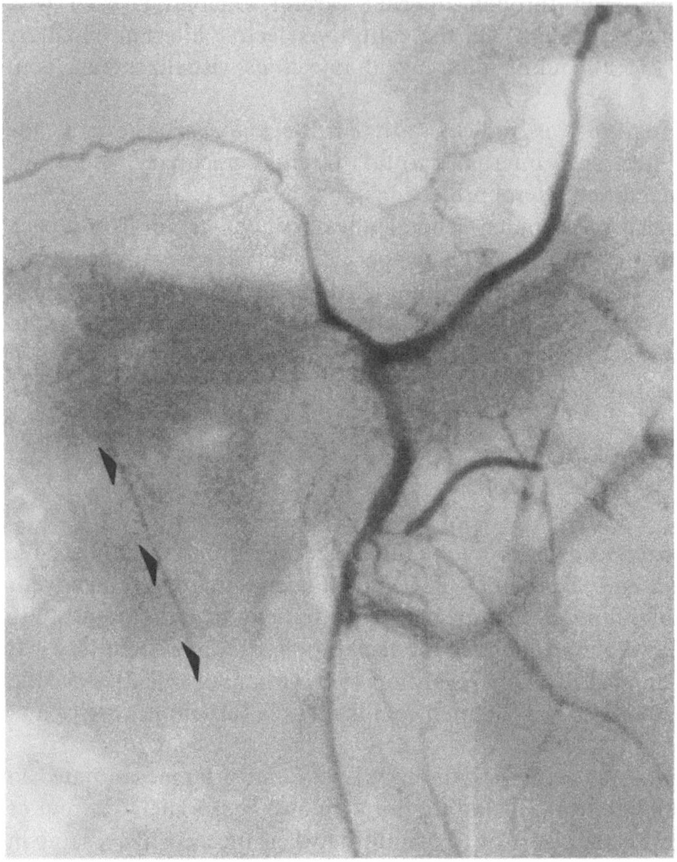

Fig. 4. Selective middle meningeal angiogram. Visualization of the facial arterial arch, particularly in the third portion of the Fallopian acqueduct (*arrow heads*)

branches allows the angiographers to prevent Bell's palsy after embolization, by choosing the most appropriate embolic material. Concerning the clinical aspects of these vascular relationships the common vascular territory, between the trigeminal ganglion as well as V_3 root and the intra-petrous VIIth nerve has to be considered in the discussion of neurological syndromes [6]. The approachability of the nerve by endovascular route is of interest even though presently unused.

Our angiographic protocol of exploration of *the VIIth nerve* is: vertebral (antero-posterior projection), internal carotid (lateral projection), middle meningeal (lateral projection), posterior auricular (depending on the variant, lateral projection).

Fig. 5. Selective vertebral angiogram. Visualization of trans-cranial arterial branch of the ascending pharyngeal artery (hypoglossal) for the XIIth nerve (*arrow head*)

III. The Caudal Cranial Nerves (IXth, Xth, XIth, and XIIth)
(Figures 5, 6, 7)

In their cisternal portion, the supply of these nerves belongs to the vertebro-basilar system [14]; but trans-durally and extra-durally they are supplied by the ascending pharyngeal system [12]. It must be regarded as a metameric system in which the occipital artery represents the cutaneous component and the persistant hypoglossal artery the extreme variant in which the system supplies the central nervous system. It should be then suggested not to name meningeal branches (posterior meningeal, etc) the trans-cranial arteries when they represent 'neuromeningeal' systems.

Anatomically, the ascending pharyngeal artery by its posterior division (neuromeningeal) supplies IXth, Xth and XIth (jugular branch) and XIIth (hypoglossal branch). The meningeal territories may help in their identification, but the visualization of their specific anastomoses constantly identifies them:

- Upward with C_5 group of collaterals of the internal carotid siphon.
- Downward with the third cervical collateral of the vertebral artery.

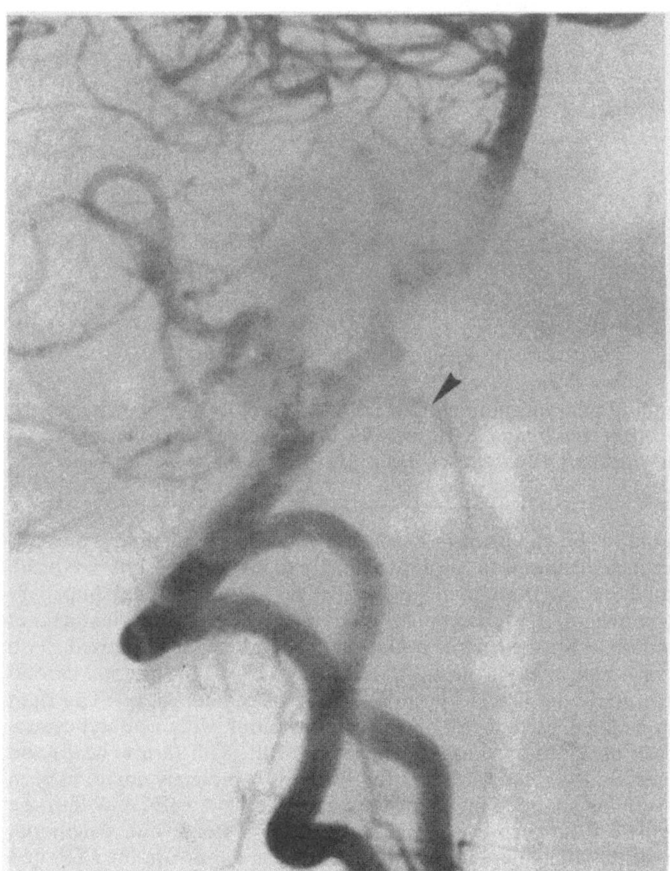

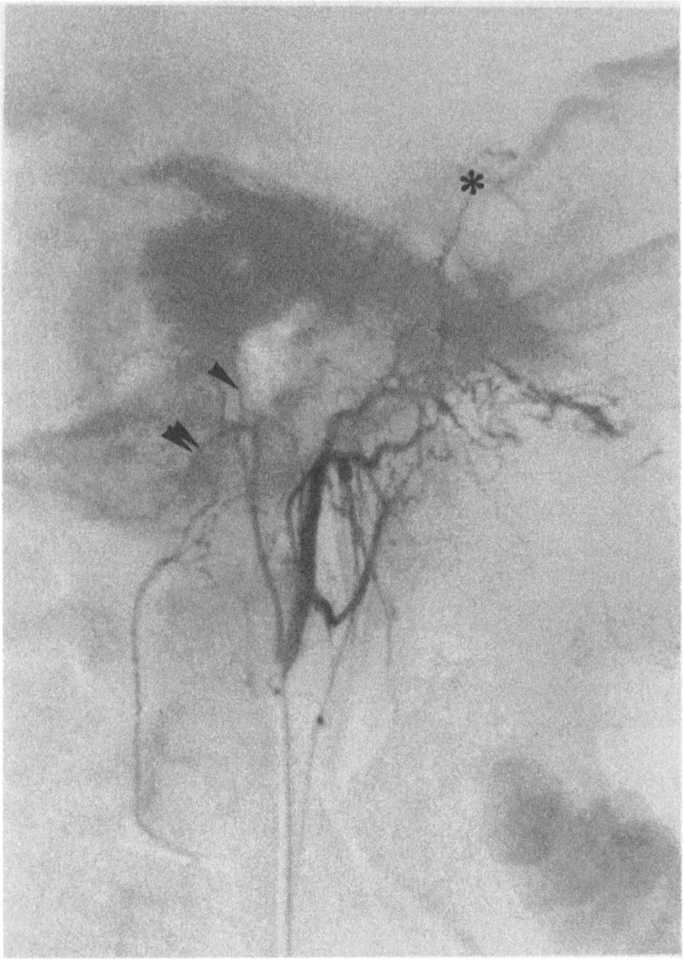

Fig. 6. Selective global ascending pharyngeal angiogram. Visualization of the branches to the IXth, Xth and XIth nerves (*arrow head*), and XIIth (*double arrow head*). Note the cavernous branch of the ascending pharyngeal artery (*asterisk*), it supplies part of the gasserian ganglion

Fig. 7 a–d. Mr. K., 42 years old (to be published *in extenso* in J. of Neuroradiology), presents a spontaneous carotid-cavernous fistula with protopsis and exophthalmous but no bruit. The embolization was carried out in three steps successively: – Both internal maxillary branches (dura-mater) not shown. – Left ascending pharyngeal artery (dura-mater) not shown. Finally, due to incomplete improvement, a last embolization was performed. Two pedicles are still permeable: **a** – Left internal carotid (lateral view) **b** – Right internal carotid (antero-posterior view). Both supply the fistula by the C_5 group of collaterals. **c** – The right ascending pharyngeal artery will be used to fill the cavernous sinus with isobutyl-cyano-acrylate. The branches to reach the sinus are supplying the IXth, Xth, XIth (arrow head) and XIIth (*double arrow heads*) nerves. After embolization, the fistula is completely cured, as seen on CT (*d*). Note the left cavernous sinus, spontaneously dense, due to the IBCA within the venous side (*asterisk*). Complete disappearance of the previous symptoms but, dysphoria, dysphagia and left deviation of the tongue are noted. After 6 months follow up, the IXth and Xth unpairment have returned to normal. The right XIIth nerve remain partially weak

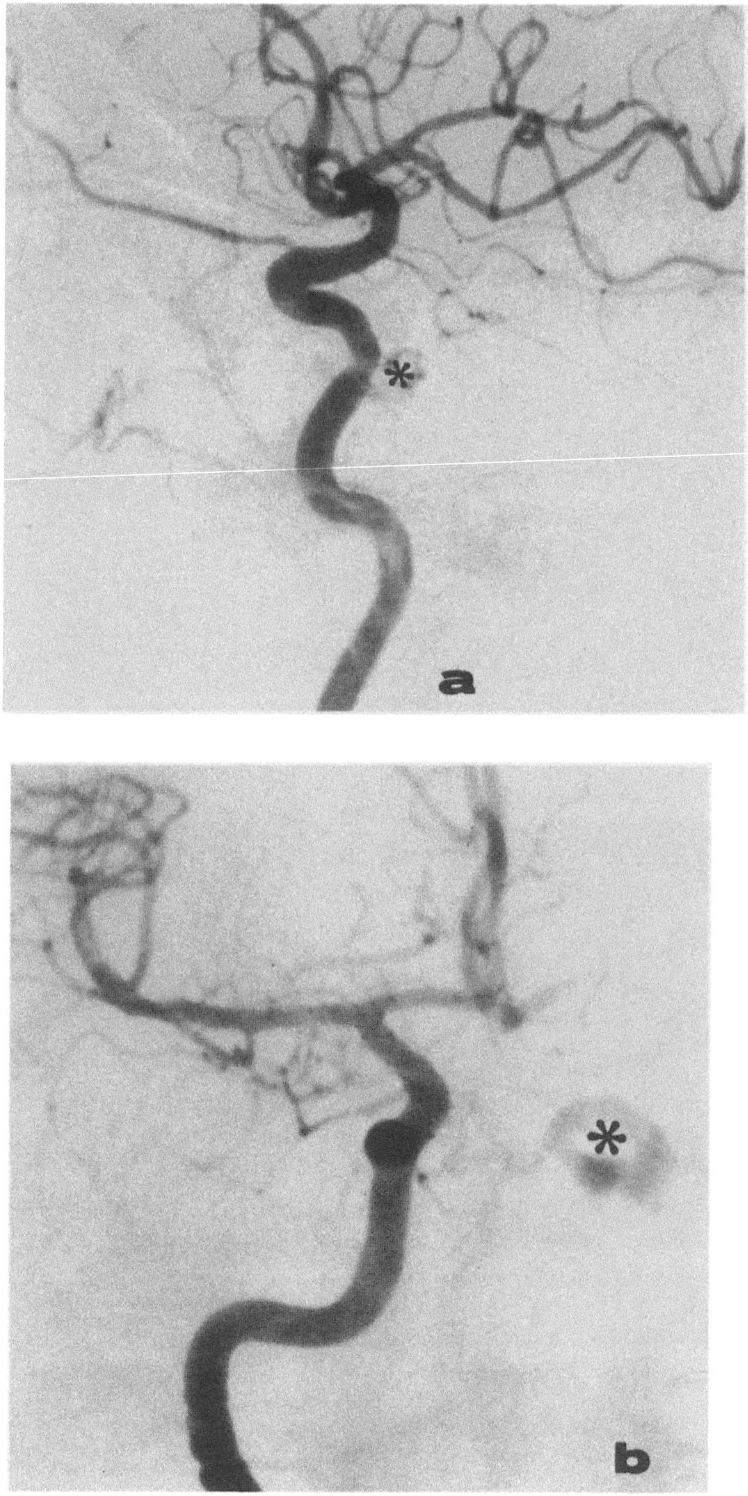
*
a
*
b

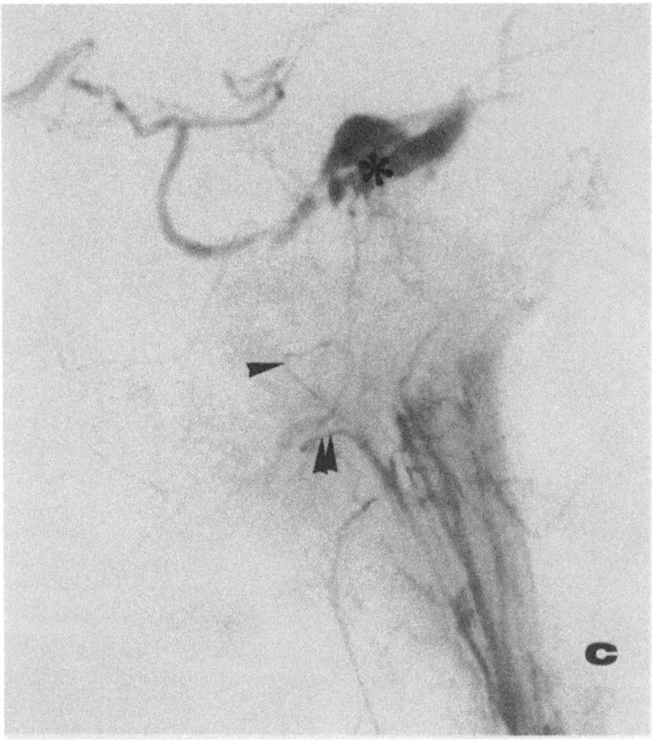

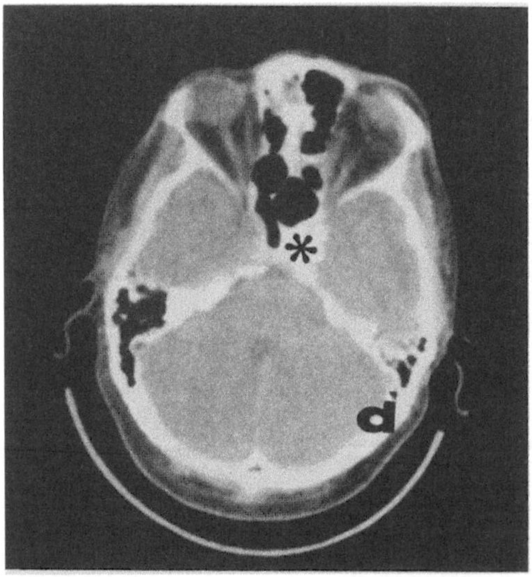

Fig. 7 c, d

Our angiographic protocol to explore *the caudal cranial nerves* is: ipsilateral vertebral, ascending pharyngeal, ascending cervical (depending on the variant) in lateral projection.

It is possible to appreciate the risk of such or such embolization and material. Among the complications reported due to caudal nerves involvement, none was predicted. It should be emphasized that with a basic knowledge most complications may be avoided.

Conclusions

We consider that the numbered percentages of chance for getting such or such variant is not important, if one knows how to recognize a variant when it is present, and how to demonstrate it when suspected.

For that reason, we have devised precise angiographic protocols, from which we explore in detail and in every single case the arterial cartography of a given region.

Concerning the cranial nerves, the study of a strictly intra-cranial system cannot be sufficient as these nerves are trans-cranial structures. Beside this conceptual aspect, for hemodynamic and photographic reasons, the trans-cranial collaterals of external carotid are routinely used to demonstrate the arterial supply of the nerves, for use in either diagnosis or therapy.

References

1. Ahn HA, Kerber CW, Deeb ZL (1980) Extra- and intra-cranial anastomoses in therapeutic embolization recognition and role. AJNR 1:71–75
2. Bentson J, Lasjaunias P, Rand R, Calcaterra T (1978) Some unexpected complications of therapeutic embolization. J Neuroradiol 16
3. Djindjian R, Merland JJ (1978) Super selective arteriography of the external carotid artery, vol 1. Springer Verlag
4. Harris FS, Rhoton AL (1976) Anatomy of the cavernous sinus, a micro surgical study. J Neurosurg 45
5. Lapresle J, Lasjaunias P, Hannabi A (1979) Paralysies de la IIIème paire au cours du diabète et vascularisation du nerf moteur oculaire commun. J Neurol Sci 41:359–367
6. Lapresle J, Lasjaunias P, Fernandez-Manchola I (1980) L'atteinte trigéminale sensitive au cours de la paralysie faciale périphérique essentielle. Nouv Presse Med 9:291–293
7. Lasjaunias P (under press) Cranio-facial and upper cervical arteries (anatomy, normal angiographic aspects), vol 1. Williams and Wilkins. Baltimore
8. Lasjaunias P, Theron J (1976) The accessory meningeal artery: radio-anatomy. Radiology 121:99–104
9. Lasjaunias P, Moret J (1978) Normal and non pathological variations in the angiographic aspects of the arteries of the middle ear. J Neuroradiol 15:213–219
10. Lasjaunias P, Brismar J, Moret J, Theron J (1978) Recurrent cavernous branches of the ophthalmic artery. Acta Radiol [Diagn] (Stockh) 19:553–560
11. Lasjaunias P, Doyon D, Edouard A (1978) Les paralysies faciales périphériques post-embolisation. Rapport sur un cas, discussion, prévention. Ann Otolaryngol Chir Cervicofac 95:595–602
12. Lasjaunias P, Doyon D (1978) L'artère pharyngienne ascendante dans la vascularisation des dernières paires crâniennes (IX, X, XI, XII). J Neuroradiol 5:287–301

13. Lasjaunias P, Manelfe C (1979) Arterial supply for the upper cervical nerves and the cervicocarotid anastomotic channels. Systematization of radiological anatomy. Neuroradiology 19:125–131
14. Libersa C (1951) Contribution à l'étude de la vascularisation artérielle des nerfs crâniens. G. Santai et Fils Edit., Lille
15. Moret J, Lasjaunias P, Theron J, Merland JJ (1977) L'artère méningée moyenne. Son apport à la vascularisation de l'orbite. J Neuroradiol 4:225–248
16. Parkinson D (1964) Collateral circulation of the cavernous carotid artery. Anatomy Canadian Journal of Surgery, vol 7
17. Saeki N, Rhoton AL (1977) Microsurgical anatomy of the upper basilar artery and the posterior circle of Willis. J Neurosurg 46
18. Sarnat HB, Netsky MG (1974) Evolution of the nervous system. Oxford University Press, New York
19. Winkler C (1921) Anatomie du système nerveux. Deuxième partie l'appareil nerveux du N trigéminus et celui du N octavus. De Erven, F. Bohn (eds) Harlem

Ophthalmologic Diagnosis

K. HOFFMANN, Hannover/FRG

Introduction

Disturbances of the ocular motor system with is cardinal symptom of diplopia can have very different and also very serious causes. In any case the diagnosis has to be made with great responsibility. In Table 1 we see an analysis of 907 patients with ocular motor paralysis, which demonstrates the necessity of detailed investigation especially since the group of 'unknown etiology' is the largest one. Table 2 shows the incidence of ocular motor paralysis in tumors of the brain, which is quite high. We must also keep in mind that this symptom can very well be the first evidence of a space-taking intracranial process.

Table 1. Analysis of 907 cases of ocular motor paralysis (Rucker 1958)

	III	IV	VI	III IV	III VI	III IV + VI	
Unknown etiology	95	9	129	14	25	10	282 =→32%←
Tumors	35	3	82	12	13	8	153 =→17%←
Trauma	51	24	57	7	16	13	168 =→18%←
Vascular	63	24	57	6	3		153 =→17%←
Aneurysm	64		19	13	8	8	112 =→12%←
Inflammation	2	4	33				39 =→ 4%←
	310	64	377	52	65	39	907
	34%	7%	42%	6%	7%	4%	

Table 2. Ocular symptoms in 3033 cases of tumors of the brain (Tönnis, Borek 1953)

Papilledema	61%
Optic atrophy (prim.)	15%
Ocular motor paralysis	22%
Visual field defect	38%

(90% of all cases had ocular symptoms)

Clinical Investigation

In analysing the causes of ocular motor disturbances, i.e. the causes of diplopia, it has to be pointed out that we have to think of six muscles in each eye, making 12 muscles altogether. As long as only horizontal motors with horizontal displacement

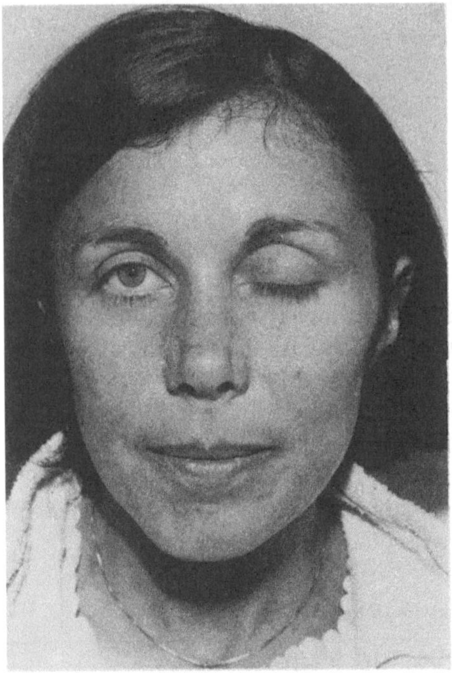

Fig. 1. Ptosis of left eye (partial oculomotor paralysis)

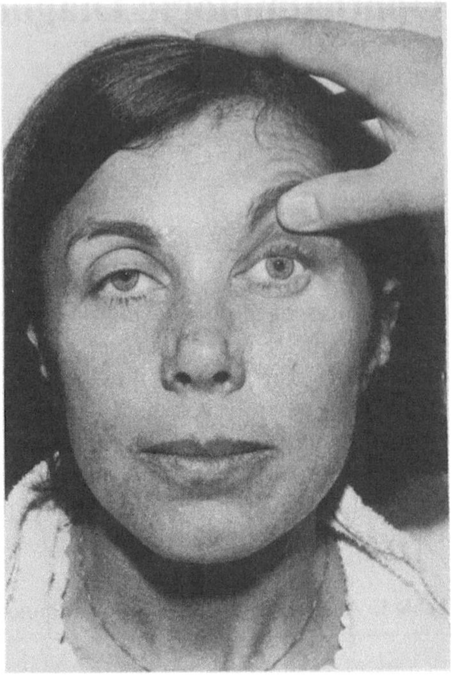

Fig. 2. Slight strabismus divergens paralyticus

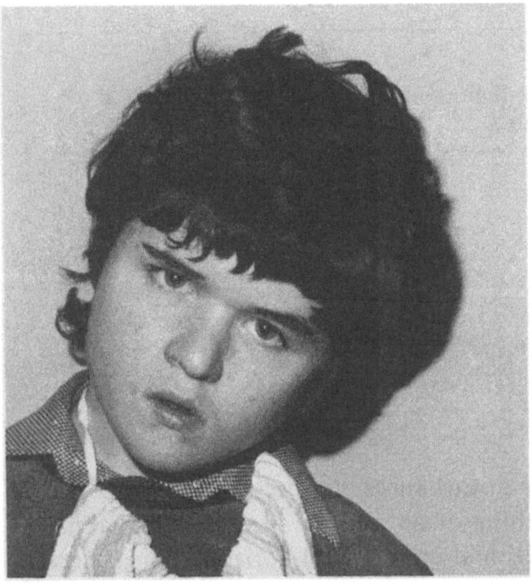

Fig. 3. Head tilting in a patient with trochlear paralysis of the right eye

of double images are involved, the diagnosis of the paretic muscle is usually quite easy. If, however, it is complained of vertical displacement of the double images, vertical or rotating motors are impaired. In these cases the diagnostic procedure is more complicated, as will be demonstrated below.

As usual we should start our clinical investigation with a short medical history, which is not nearly as valuable as it is in optic nerve disease. The patient can give us information concerning the onset and possible periodicity as well as the position of double images. Other diseases such as diabetes, vascular or neoplastic illness have to be sought for.

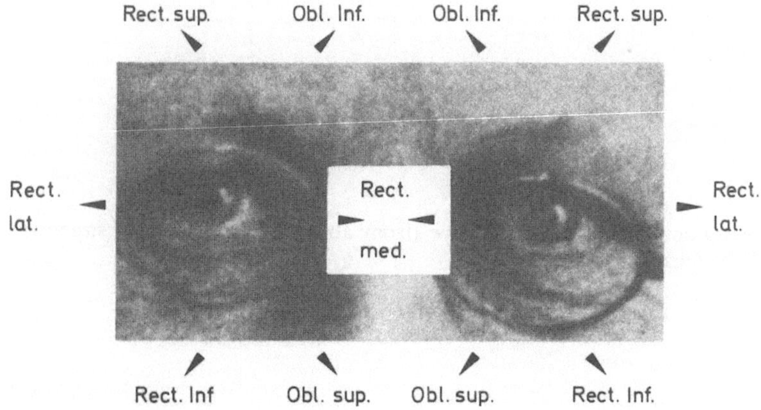

Fig. 4. The action of the extra-ocular muscles

The ophthalmological examination starts with a careful inspection which by itself can give important information: A ptosis has to be noted (Fig. 1) as well as any deviation of the eyes (= squint) (Fig. 2). Diplopia in strabismus convergens suggests palsy of the lateral rectus muscle or disturbance of the VIth cranial nerve. Contrary strabismus divergens, as we know, is suspicious for an impairment of the internal rectus muscle (IIIrd cranial nerve). Strabismus sursumvergens may be the symptom of a palsy of the superior rectus or inferior oblique (IIIrd cranial nerve), strabismus deorsumvergens of the inferior rectus (IIIrd) or superior oblique muscle (VIth cranial nerve). Any kind of head tilting (Fig. 3) or tendency to close one eye in order to avoid diplopia has to be registrated.

In order to rule out concomitant squint, which is caused by a perversion of the sensory stimuli reaching the brain so it cannot command properly coordinated movements, the excursions of the eyes have to be examined. When following a finger outwards from the primary position in the six diagnostic directions, the motility of each muscle can be studied (Fig. 4). As has been mentioned above, the analysis of impaired movement of one eye in horizontal direction is easy. But also gross defects in vertical motility can be analysed without difficulty, as long as we remember the maximum of motility-power of each vertical motor (Fig. 4). These dynamics can be easily understood from the anatomical position of the different muscles within the orbit, which consequently gives the direction of greatest power

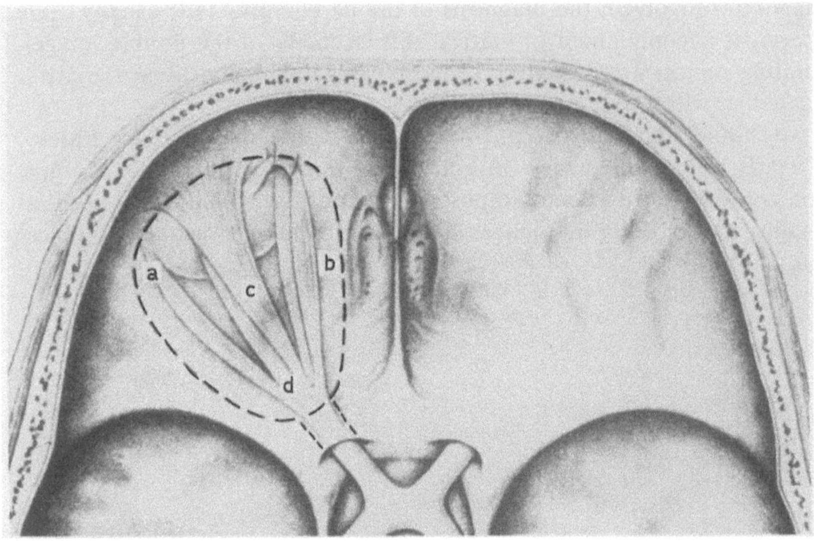

Fig. 5. Anatomy of extra-ocular muscles of left eye (from above). Note course of superior oblique muscle (*b*). (K. Schürmann 1974)

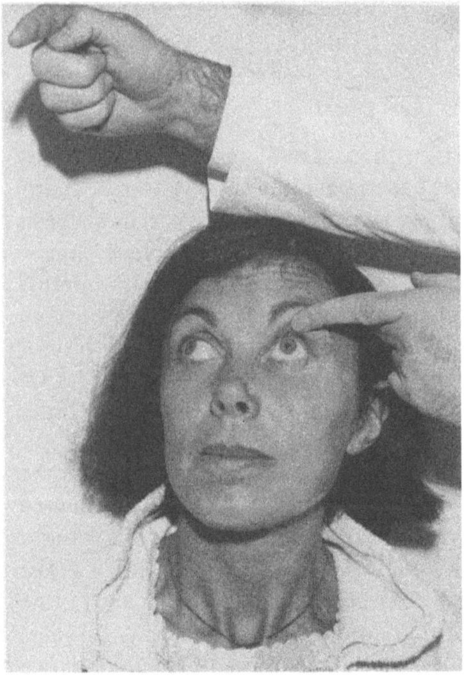

Fig. 6. Dextroelevation shows normal motility of right superior rectus muscle, but impairment of motibility of left inferior oblique muscle

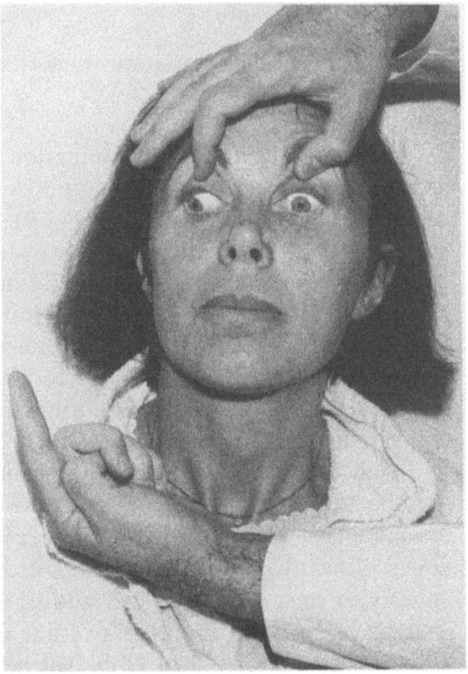

Fig. 7. Dextrodepression shows normal motility of right inferior rectus muscle, but impairment of motility of left superior oblique muscle

of motility (Fig. 5): the superior and inferior recti muscles, having a more divergent course parallel to the direction of the optic nerve, must have their maximum in the upper and lower outward movements of the bulb (Figs. 6, 7). The oblique muscles, however, have a more convergent axis of dynamics. This means their main action of vertical movement of the eyeball develops when the eye is in an inward position (Figs. 6, 7).

In cases of gross defects of ocular motility these investigations may lead to the correct diagnosis concerning the muscles involved. In slight degrees of paresis, however, the 'cover-test' gives more detailed information about the cause of diplopia: The patient is asked to look straight ahead at a test object. While he is

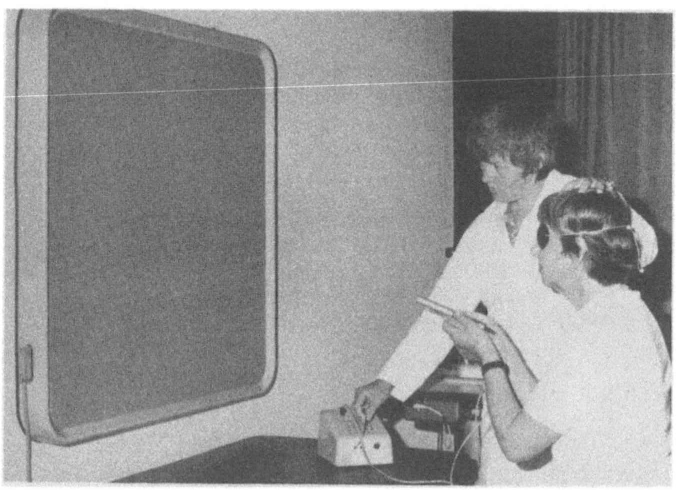

Fig. 8. The projection-test with the Hess-screen, patient wearing red-green goggles

doing so, one eye is covered by an opaque card or a hand of the examiner which is then quickly transferred to the other eye. If neither eye deviates during this procedure a squint can be ruled out. A deviation of one eye behind the cover proves a squint. The deviation of the squinting eye is called primary deviation, that of the non-squinting eye is called secondary deviation. If the deviations of each single eye are equal, the squint is non-paralytic, i.e. concomitant. If the secondary deviation is greater than the primary, the squint is paralytic in origin: trying to move the paretic eye into the intended direction, a greater effort of innervation is necessary and applied. This impulse is involuntarily shared between the two eyes, so that consequently the sound eye moves excessively into the same direction (=secondary deviation). In order to analyze slight degrees of ocular motor paresis, especially when vertical motors are involved, diplopia tests have to be carried out by the ophthalmologist. Although we register the results of subjective demonstration of a deviation, the findings are reproducible and follow-up studies can be more reliable. An even better method of examination is the projection test, for example with the Hess-screen (Fig. 8).

The Causes of Ocular Motor Paralysis

The causes of inconcomitant squint coming from ocular motor palsy can be devided into four parts (Table 3):

1. *Total ocular motor paralysis* or *total ophthalmoplegia* with complete loss of any ocular motor function: complete ptosis, immobile globe, which is slightly proptosed and in divergent position, large dilated pupil without reaction to light, loss of accomodation. If unilateral, the cause of the lesion must be situated in the cavernous sinus or the orbit, since a nuclear defect can never produce a purely one-sided impairment: the trochlear nerve crosses infranuclearly in contrast to the IIIrd and VIth cranial nerve, such a lesion consequently would have to involve the nuclei of these two nerves of one side and of the IVth of the other side of the brain stem. If bilateral, such a lesion would have to affect a widespread area of the brain stem or the cavernous sinus, in any case an extremely serious condition. In so-called external ophthalmoplegia we have the same clinical picture with the difference that pupillary reaction and accommodation are normal. The site of such a lesion has to be localized in the nuclear area.

Table 3. Ocular motor paralysis

I.	Total ocular motor paralysis	
	a) total ophthalmoplegia	bilateral: brain-stem or cavernous sinus unilateral: cavernous sinus or orbit
	b) external ophthalmoplegia	pupillary activity and accommodation normal – nuclear origin –
→ II.	Oculomotor paralysis	
	a) complete oculomotor palsy = involving internal ophthalmoplegia	
	b) partial oculomotor paralysis	1. paralysis of the medial rectus 2. paralysis of the superior rectus 3. paralysis of the inferior rectus 4. paralysis of the inferior oblique
→ III.	Trochlear paralysis palsy of the superior oblique muscle	
→ IV.	Abducent paralysis paralysis of the lateral rectus muscle	

2. *Oculomotor paralysis* has to be differentiated into complete palsy of the IIIrd cranial nerve involving internal ophthalmoplegia, and partial oculomotor palsy. In complete palsy the eyeball can only be moved outwards and slightly downwards. In unilateral cases the site of the lesion must be located in the nerve trunk between the nucleus and cavernous sinus. Beyond this region the IVth and VIth cranial nerve are so close that they are as a rule also impaired. In partial oculomotor palsy the clinical picture naturally can vary depending on the muscles involved. In the patient demonstrated in Fig. 9 we found several external muscles, supplied by the IIIrd cranial nerve, impaired in their function. The causes of partial palsies can be either nuclear or peripheral in the orbit. Fig. 10 shows the etiological factors of oculomotor paralysis.

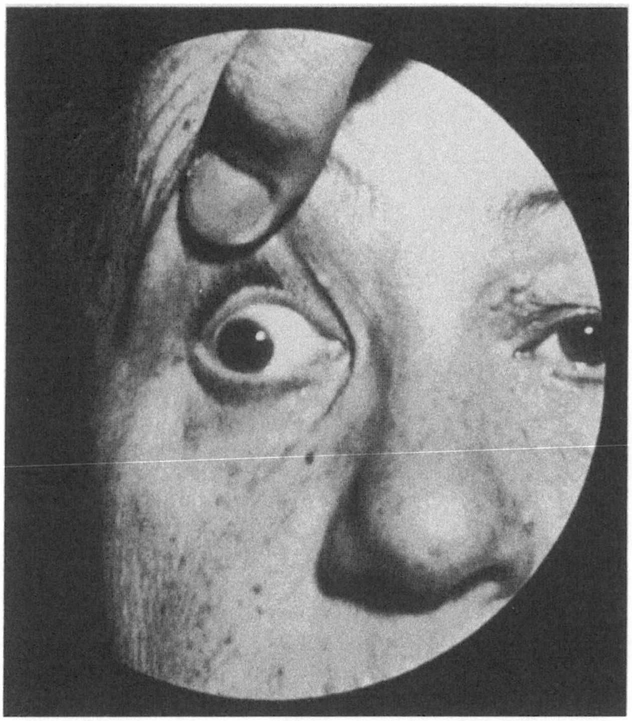

Fig. 9. Patient showing strabismus divergens paralyticus

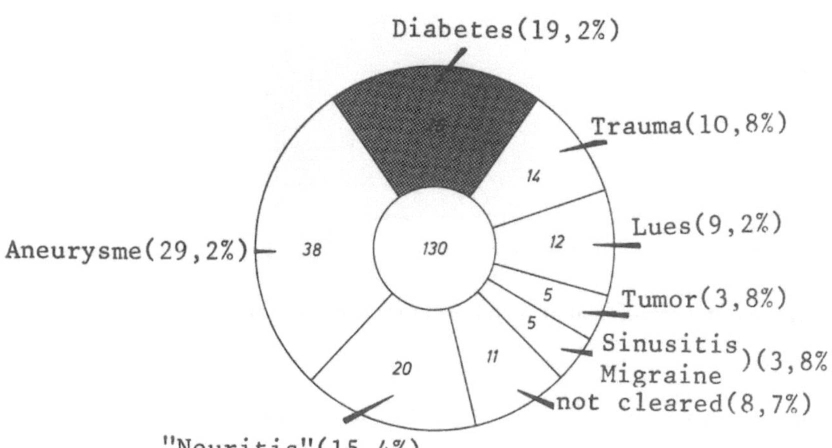

Fig. 10. Etiological factors of oculomotor paralysis (Green, Hackett, Schlezinger 1964)

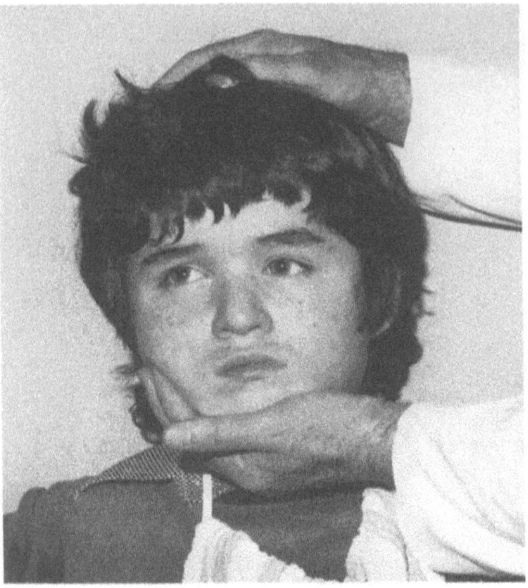

Fig. 11. Same patient as in Fig. 3 with right trochlear palsy. If the tilted head is forced in a straight position, the paretic right eye turns up- and outwards into the direction of the antagonist = superior rectus muscle

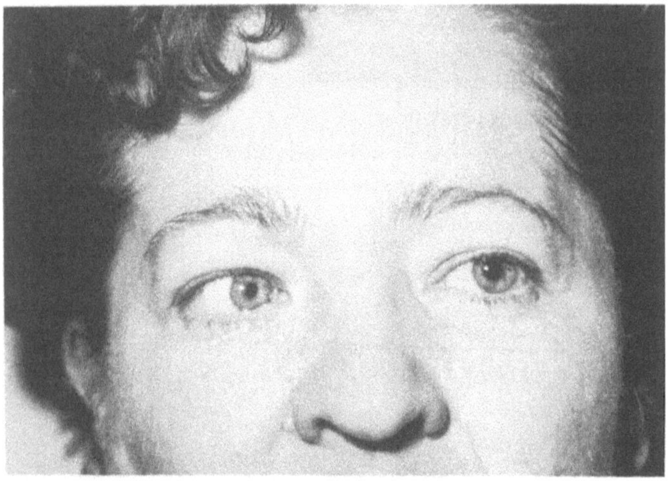

Fig. 12. Patient showing impairment of lateral rectus muscle of left eye

3. *Trochlear paralysis.* As we can see from Fig. 4, the ocular movements in palsy of the IVth cranial nerve are limited when the sick eye looks down- and inwards to the side of the sound eye. In oder to avoid diplopia the patient tilts his head into the direction, into which the palsied muscle should move the eye, that means rotation of the face to the sound side with depression of the chin and tilting of the head to the same shoulder (Fig. 3). If the patient is forced to hold the head straight, the paretic eye moves into the direction where the sound antagonist pulls it (Fig. 11). The etiology of IVth cranial nerve palsy can be seen in Table 1.

4. *Abducent paralysis.* Since a purely horizontal motor is affected, paralytic strabismus convergens results from functional defects of the lateral rectus muscle (Fig. 12). Diplopia shows typical uncrossed displacement with maximum of distance when the patient shows to the palsied side. The compensatory position of the head is consequently a turn to the side of the paretic muscle. An analysis of the causes of VIth cranial nerve paralysis is shown in Fig. 13. Compared with the results in Table 1 published some years earlier it is obvious that diabetic neuropathy seems to be of significant importance, equal to the results of the oculomotor nerve in both statistics.

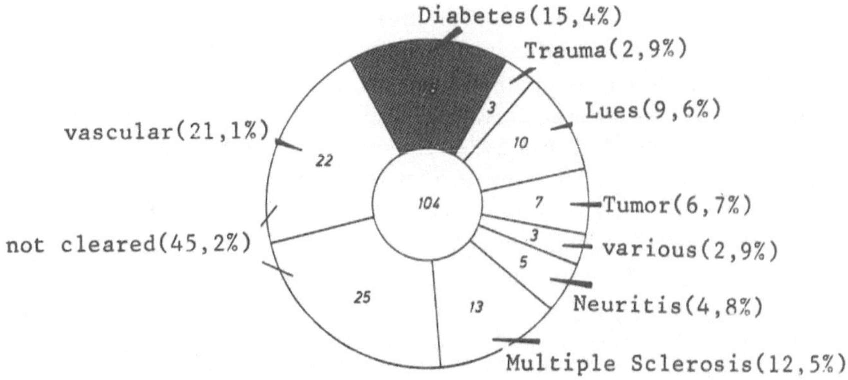

Fig. 13. Etiological factors of abducent paalysis (Shrader, Schlezinger 1960)

References

Green WR, Hackett ER, Schlezinger NS (1964) Neuroophthalmologic evaluation of ocular nerve paralysis. Arch Ophthalmol 72: 154–167

Rucker WC (1958) Paralysis of the third, fourth and sixth cranial nerve. Am J Ophthalmol 46:787–795

Schürmann K (1974) Neurochirurgische Aufgaben in der Orbita. Arch Otorhinolaryngol (NY) 207:253–265

Shrader C, Schlezinger NS (1960) Neuro-ophthalmologic evaluation of abducens nerve paralysis. Arch Ophthalmol 63:84–92

Tönnis W, Borek WF (1953) Großhirntumoren des Kindesalters. Zentralbl Neurochir 13: 72–98

Electrophysiological Diagnosis

A. STRUPPLER, F. ERBEL, and J. PERWEIN, München/FRG

1. Normal Electromyography (EMG) of Extraocular Muscles

The EMG can be relevant to distinguish disorders of central innervation, of extraocular nerves, of the neuromuscular transmission like myasthenia gravis, and of the extraocular muscles, e.g. myopathies.

The motor units of extraocular muscles are composed of only 5 to 10 muscle fibres whereas motor units of limb muscles consist of several hundred fibres. The concentric electrode picks up most of the fibres within one extraocular motor unit.

The action potentials of motor units are normally diphasic. After an initial positive deflection a negative spike potential follows. Some of the unit potentials show three or four phases. Only potentials with more than four phases (polyphasic units) are considered to be pathological. The firing rate of motor units during straight forward gaze is about 50 to 80 imp./sec. The eye is kept in position by active contraction of all eye muscles, each of which develop forces of 10 to 20 g.

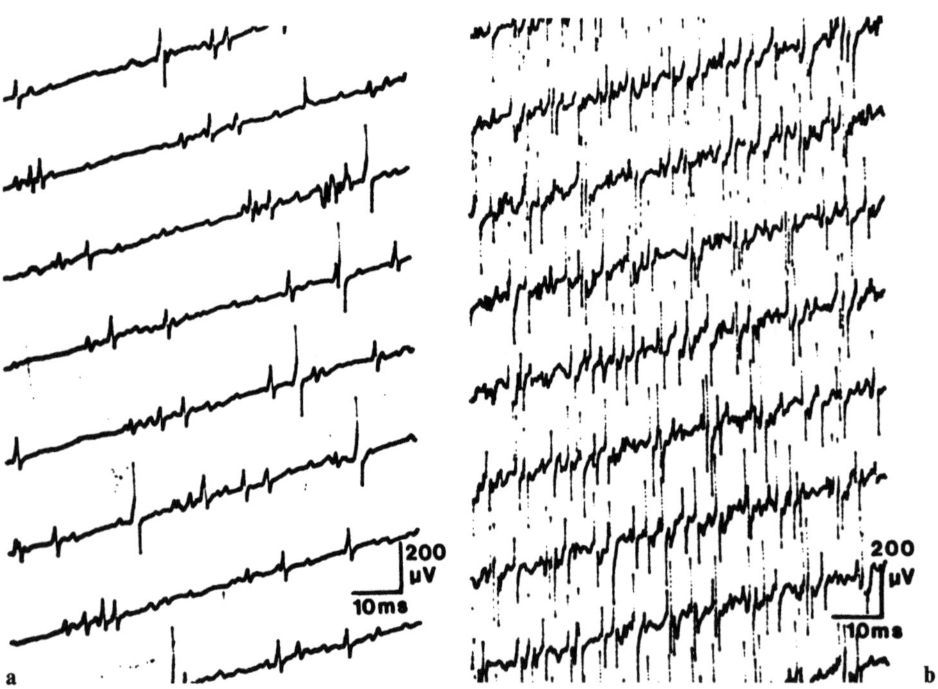

Fig. 1. **a** slight voluntary innervation, **b** moderate voluntary innervation

The eye muscles are only silent during fixation to the opposite direction or during general anaesthesia. During gaze in the direction of the muscle action additional motor units are recruited and the discharge rate is increased to 200–300 imp./sec.

The duration of the action potential is between 1–3 msec dependent upon the electrode position relative to the motor unit. (The amplitude is measured peak to peak highly dependent on the distance of the electrode from the recorded motor unit.)

The EMG can be recorded during eye movements. To investigate saccadic movements the patient is asked to look at small light bulbs which are attached at an arch and separated by angles of 5° in the horizontal and vertical direction. According to which light is illuminated, saccades of 5° or multiples of 5° in either direction can be performed. The movement of the eyes is recorded by two separate EOG's, either each eye in the horizontal plane or one eye in the horizontal and vertical plane.

Recording of the Levator Palpebrae Muscle:

There are two approaches: 1. percutaneously through the upper lid, and 2. through the conjunctiva. The percutaneous method has the advantage that the motility of the eye-bulb is less restricted and local anaesthesia is not necessary.

For the obliquus inferior muscle the percutaneous method is definitely superior to the transconjunctival one. The electrode is inserted through the lower lid right over the zygomatic bone.

Recording of the Recti Muscles:

The electrode is inserted into these four muscles under visual control. We pull the tendinous attachment at the globe foreward with a pincette while the electrode is inserted. The patient should look in the direction opposite to the muscle under investigation. The rectus superior can also be recorded percutaneously.

2. Complications

In a few cases there have been small subconjunctival hemorrhages without serious consequences. (Perforation of the bulb is a very remote danger.) If there is little cooperation, the EMG should not be done, not even following sedation.

3. Indications for Extraocular EMG

3.1. Disorders of central innervation like the Duane Syndrome can only be investigated by EMG, preferably in two antagonistic muscles.

3.2. The extent of a neurogenic lesion as well as normal or false re-innervation can be assessed by repeated EMG investigations. This may be important in neurotraumatology for prognosis and indications to operate.

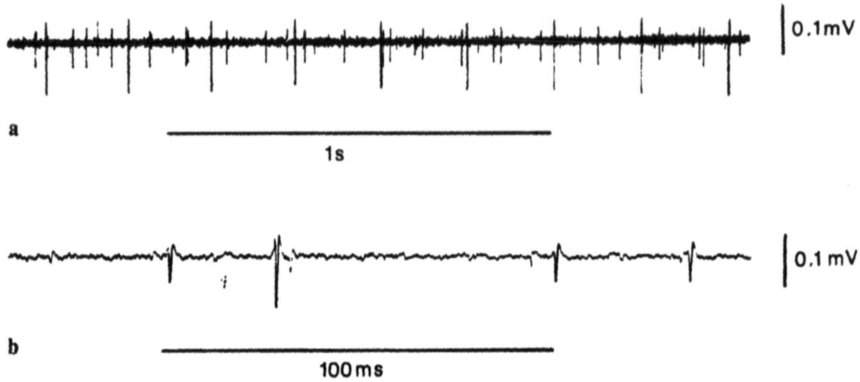

Fig. 2. a slow sweep speed, b 10 times higher sweep speed

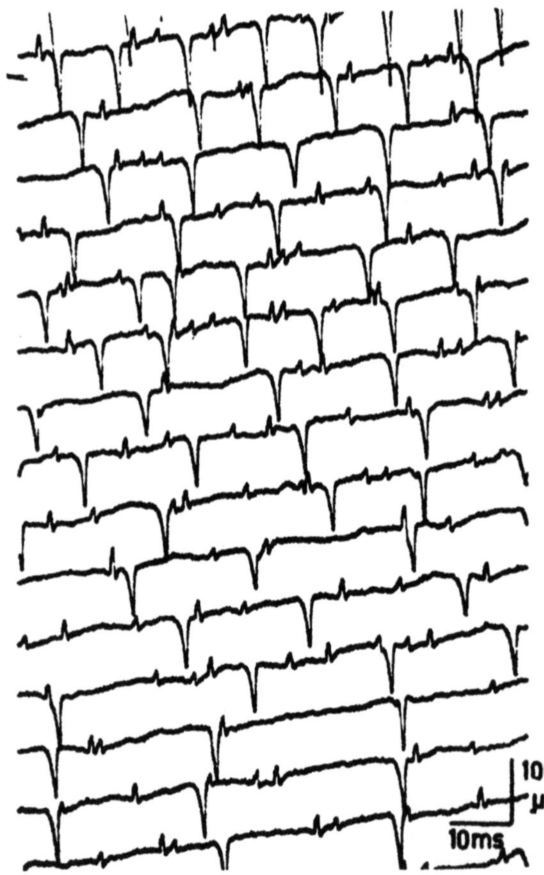

Fig. 3. Pathological spontaneous activity in a patient with 3rd nerve palsy

4. Neurogenic Changes in the Extraocular EMG

The pathophysiological mechanisms of conduction block, degeneration and regeneration are the same as in the limb muscles. The electrophysiological examination is restricted to the EMG since direct nerve conduction studies are not possible.

4.1. Fibrillation

Fibrillations are brief diphasic potentials of about 1 msec duration and 50–200 mikro-V amplitude. Spontaneous discharges of the muscle cell membrane may be due to a decreased resting potential following denervation. Fibrillations normally occur in irregular sequences. Since the motor unit discharges of extraocular muscles are mostly of similar amplitude and configuration, fibrillations are mainly characterized by irregular discharges.

4.2. Positive Sharp Waves

Positive sharp waves have the same significance as in limb muscles and can be seen in neurogenic lesions.

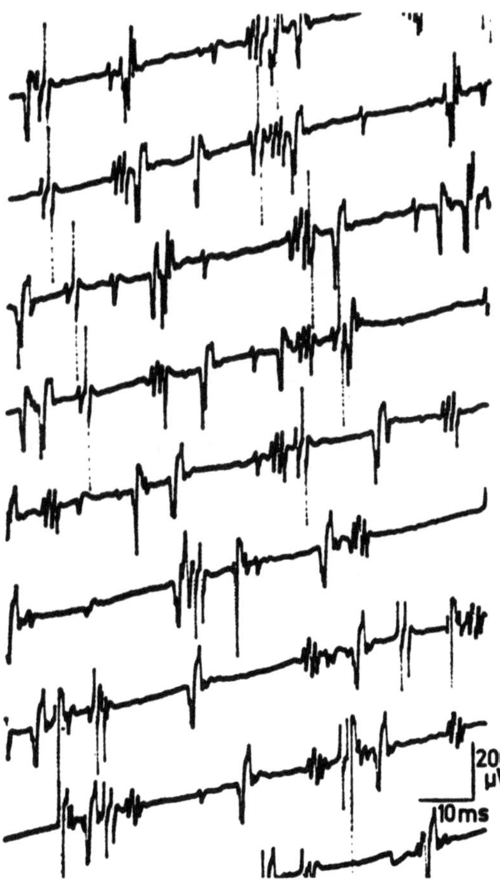

Fig. 4. Note the decreased interference pattern during strong voluntary activation

4.3. Motor Unit Potentials

Motor unit potentials are polyphasic with increased duration and amplitude. These changes are best seen during slight voluntary innervation since the interference pattern does not allow to measure the parameters of motor unit potentials.

4.4. Activity Pattern

Decreased interference as a result of motor axon loss can be noticed only if the paresis is of considerable degree. In severe paresis we can find single oscillations. Only repetitive investigations can answer the question whether the lesion is progressive or whether there is re-innervation. In rare cases following traumatic ocular motor paresis there may be false sprouting into other branches of the same nerve. This can be recorded in simultaneous EMG from different extraocular muscles.

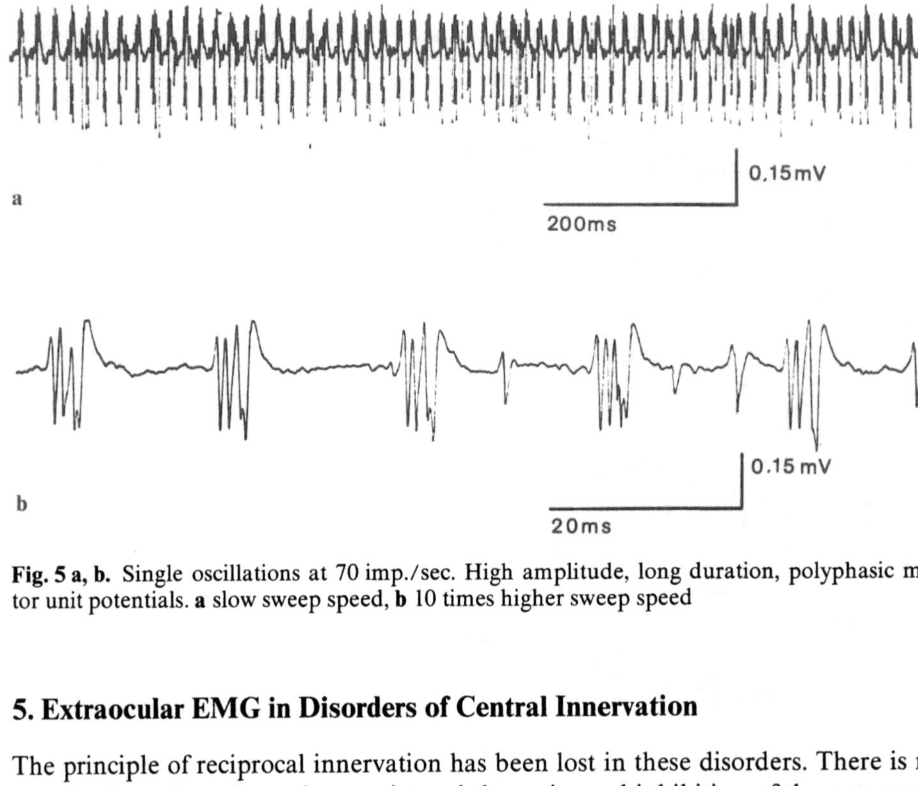

Fig. 5 a, b. Single oscillations at 70 imp./sec. High amplitude, long duration, polyphasic motor unit potentials. **a** slow sweep speed, **b** 10 times higher sweep speed

5. Extraocular EMG in Disorders of Central Innervation

The principle of reciprocal innervation has been lost in these disorders. There is no coactivation of agonist and synergist and the reciprocal inhibition of the antagonist is disturbed. Simultaneous EMG recordings and the electro-oculogram are essential for these investigations.

Overview of the Literature

Breining G (1977) Ocular Electromyography. Electrodiagnosis of Neuromuscular Diseases. 2. Auflg. In: Goudgold J, Eberstein A (ed) Williams and Wilkins Comp, p 264–271

Esslen E (1974) Elektromyographie der Augenmuskeln. Elektromyographie. In: Hopf HC, Struppler A (eds) Thieme Verlag, S 72–84

Esslen E (1977) Electromyography of extra-ocular muscles. Current concepts in clin. neurophysiol. In: Van Duijn et al. (eds), p 141–148

Haupt WF, Fasshauer K, Huffmann G, Kruse H (1978) Besonderheiten and Probleme bei der Elektromyographie der äußeren Augenmuskeln. Nervenarzt 49:422–426

Lennerstrand G, Bach-y-Rita P (1975) Basic mechanisms of ocular motibility and their clinical implications. Pergamon Press, p 9–224

Papst W (1976) Elektromyographie. Die ophthalmologischen Untersuchungsmethoden, Bd. II. In: Straub W (ed) Enke-Verlag, p 692–726

Zett L (1975) Elektromyographie. Neuro-Ophthalmologie. In: Sachsenweger R (ed) Thieme-Verlag, S 198–214

EMG Differential Diagnosis in Case of Abducens Nerve Paresis

M. HEUSER, München/FRG

Introduction

On forced lateral gaze the outer and upper parts of both ears are turned backward tonically:

The Oculoauricularphenomenon (oap)

With surface or concentric needle electrodes (Fig. 1) the EMG is registered simultaneously from the extraocular eye muscles and from the autochthon skin muscles at the back of the external ear (Heuser 1976 a).

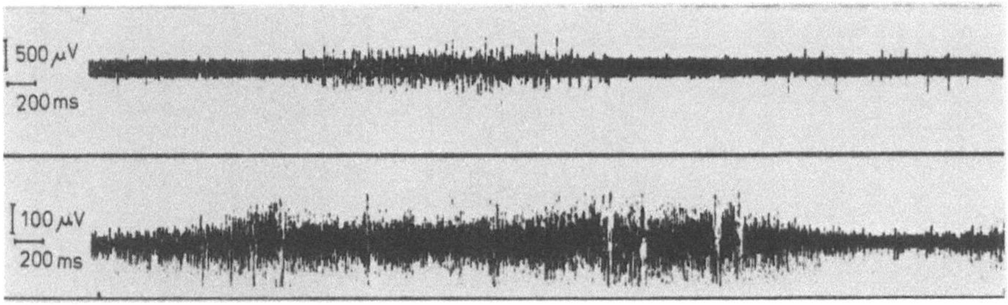

Fig. 1. Polygraphic EMG registration of the *oculoauricular phenomenon* (oap). From a certain degree of innervation of the M. rectus bulbi externus (lower trace) the activation of the M. retroauricularis starts (upper trace)

Results With Discussion

The *oap* in men proved to be a physiologic and constant, automatic and always bilateral interaction between the homolateral abducens nerve and both Nn. faciales with corresponding coinnervation of the Mm. retroauriculares neglected so far.

The obligatory coinnervation of the Mm. retroauriculares in the *oap* and a facultative coinnervation of the Mm. retroauriculares also during involuntary inspiration (Heuser 1976 b) seem to be a phylogenetic relic of the ultrasonic orientation of bats (Fig. 2): 'Bildhör-Mechanismus' (Heuser 1977). Practical diagnostic use of the *oap* is shown – amongst others – for the differentiation between nuclear and peripheral distal pareses of the abducens nerve: In case of medullary, nuclear or internuclear lesions, the *oap* is disturbed, instable, diminished

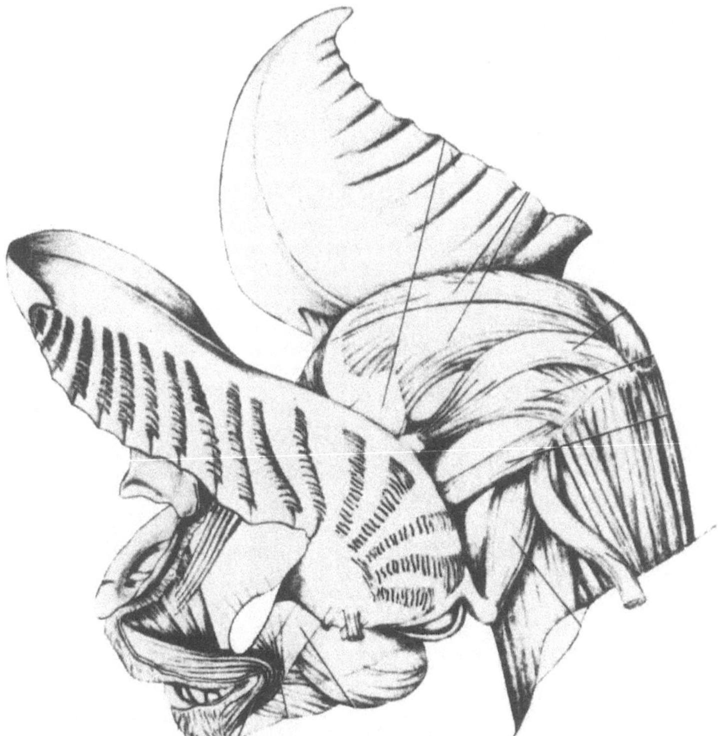

Fig. 2. Elaborate anatomy of the M. retroauricularis in bats (Chiroptera)

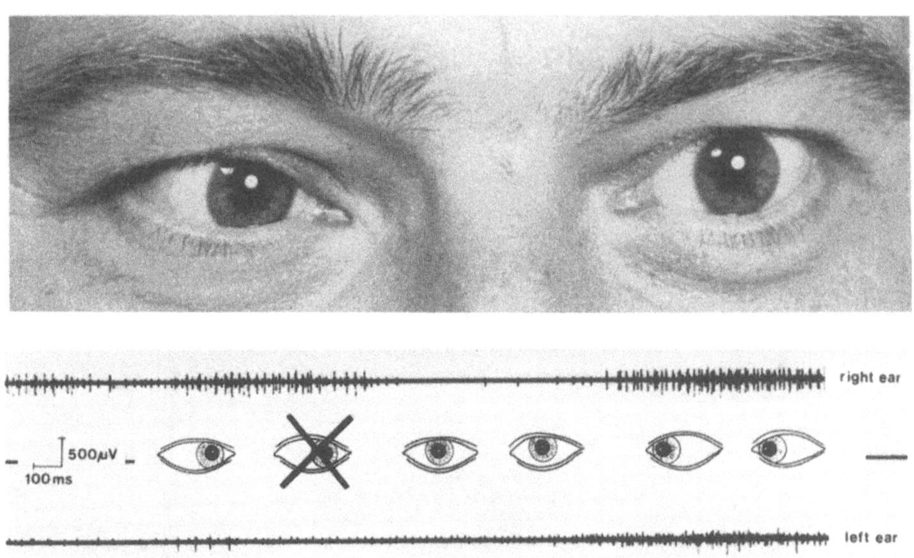

Fig. 3. The oap is disturbed only in nuclear abducens paresis, shown here at the left

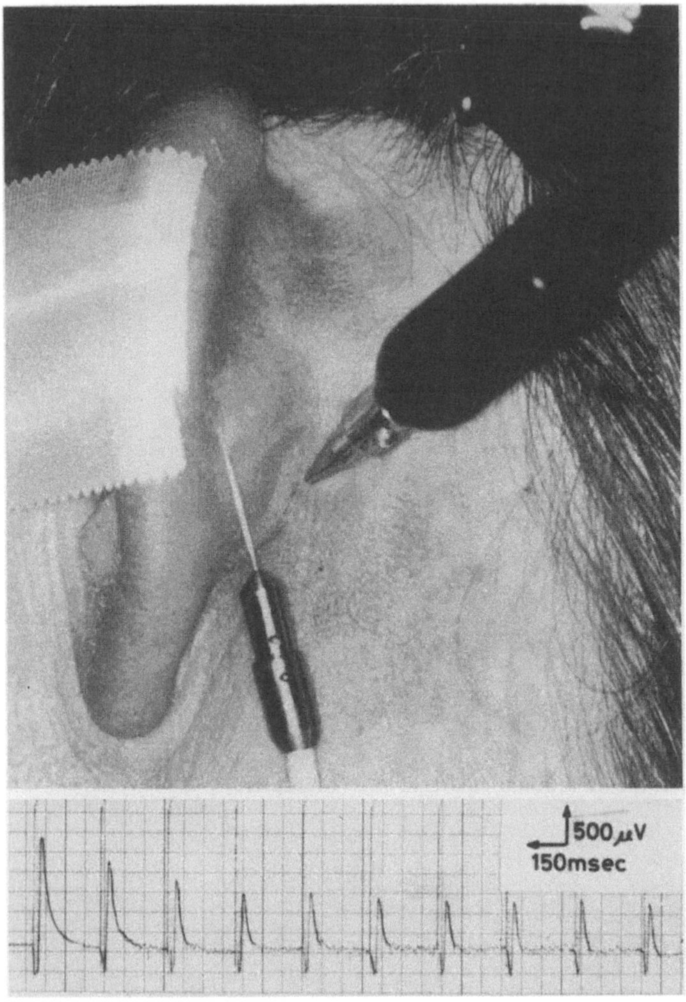

Fig. 4. Myasthenic reaction of the 'exterritorial-eye-muscle' M. retroauricularis

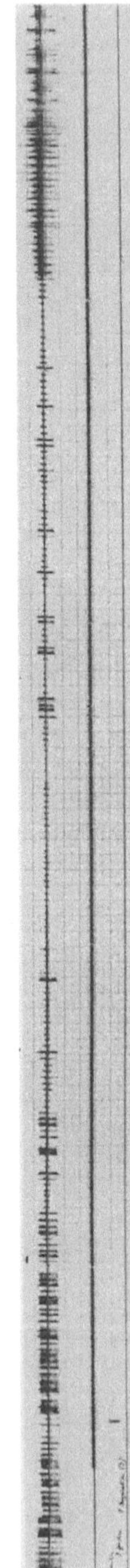

Fig. 5. The varying degree and rhythm of inspiratory coinnervation of the M. retroauricularis between awake, asleep and arousal during a short sleep (appr. 25 min)

or abolished (Fig. 3), whereas in distal neurogenic or myogenic paresis, even in complete paralysis or exstirpation of nerve or muscle the *oap* is bilaterally well preserved (Heuser 1979 a, b). Further diagnostic use will be gained in the various formes of nystagmus, strabismus and facial palsy. The 'exterritorial eye muscle' M. retroauricularis (Fig. 4) offers also a possibility for a Harvey-Masland test in early ocular forms of myasthenic syndromes. – Degree and rhythm of the facultative inspiratory coinnervation of the M. retroauricularis may be used as a reliable indicator to measure the involuntary activation of the somato-motor nervous system (Fig. 5) in 'nervous' muscle tension (Heuser 1976 b).

References

Heuser M (1976) The Oculoauricular Phenomenon. J Neurol 212:95–99

Heuser M (1976) Function and Innervation of the Involuntary M. retroauricularis. J Neurol 213:327–333

Heuser M (1977) The Oculoauricular Phenomenon and Inspiratory Innervation of the M. retroauricularis as a Phylogenetic Relict of Bats (Chiroptera). J Neurol 214:225–227

Heuser M (1979) Elektromyographische Differentialdiagnose bei Abduzensparesen nuklearer oder distalneurogener bzw. myogener Genese. Z EEG-EMG 10:137–139

Heuser M (1979) Ophthalmomimik, Polygraphische EMG-Untersuchung über oculo-faziale Mitbewegungen und Funktionen der autochthonen Ohrmuskeln. Fortschr. Med 97: 2235–2238

Pathomechanism of Oculomotor and Abducens Paresis in Supra- and Infratentorial Processes

K. J. ZÜLCH, Köln/FRG

Oculomotor palsy: The mechanism of the third nerve lesion subsequent to hemilateral increase in volume is clarified and easy to explain: The first step, as far as we can see, is the formation of a 'transtentorial' or 'temporal' pressure cone, the second the 'axial shift' of the lower brain stem, which at the same time puts the third nerve under longitudinal strain (Zülch 1951, 1959; Zülch et al. 1974). During this process the nerve may be strangulated at two locations (Zülch 1959, Figs. 57, 73, 81, 83): a) by the medial plica petroclinoidea (Zülch 1959, Fig. 82) overlying the clivus and covering its edge, in more axial, and the petroclinoidal ligament in lateral shifts. This is the distal involvement of the nerve and the axial shift may be the main cause for it.

The second point of involvement is the crossing of the superior cerebellar artery where the nerve may be squeezed between the posterior and the latter artery (Zülch 1959, Fig. 41). This is the proximal notch observed at the oculomotor nerve in such lesions.

One of the many preconditions seems to be a hemilateral space occupying lesion, the second perhaps a quick progress of the lesion.

It is then the plica or the ligament respectively which provoke the nerve lesion not the 'edge of the clivus' in the sense of Fischer-Brügge (1949).

Abducent palsy: Less well understood is the sixth nerve palsy in supratentorial and infratentorial tumors, which is apparently the most common involvement of an intracranial nerve in space-occupying lesions: In a study of 3000 cases in Tönnis' clinic, Zielinski (1959) found an involvement in two thirds of the cases.

The only reasonable cause was described by Cushing (1910): the sixth nerve has the longest extracerebral intracranial course of all the cranial nerves. This is the general concept discussed for the involvement of the sixth nerve in supra- and infratentorial masses. It is, however, not fully convincing since the shift of the brain stem upwards, for instance, will relieve any longitudinal strain from the nerve.

However, I do not fully understand why in supratentorial tumors the third nerve is sometimes involved – probably particularly in *lateral* and *rapidly developing* space occupying processes – and why and when the abducens, as so frequently observed in the series of Zielinski (1959). Probably a further strain at the entrance in the dural compartment will be the second precondition. This I shall try to explain by the description of the sixth nerve palsy in unilateral or bilateral supratentorial, acute hemispheric edema.

This concept may be proved by the following observation in a 17 year old boy. At operation – antrotomy – of a mastoiditis, a contusion of the facial nerve occurred. Later an attempt was made to decompress the nerve. However, in the first part of the operation the transverse sinus, already relieved of its bony coverings at the first operation, was opened and had to be closed by tamponade. Three days later a homolateral sixth nerve paresis was observed which in the course of two weeks turned into a homolateral paralysis whereas a controlateral paresis of the 6th and a homolateral choked disk of three to four dioptera as well as a contralateral blurred disk occurred three days after the operation. The loss of vision went down to 3/10 of normal! The symptomatology ceased in the next nine months. The papilledema lasted for three months, however, without permanent loss of vision.

In summary: following a tamponade of the right sinus transversus a bilateral involvement of the abducent nerve and a bilateral choked disk – both more so on the side of the lesions – occurred, which disappeared in the course of nine months.

What may be the explanation? The two hemispheres, at least the outer, upper, and middle parts of them – the mantles – are drained by the sagittal sinus which leads in two thirds of cases almost exclusively into the right sinus transversus, less blood going into the left. The ganglia and the brain stem on the contrary are drained by the internal veins via the V. magna Galeni and the sinus rectus predominantly into the left side. In only 10 percent we have an ideal 'confluens sinuum' with equal drainage to both sides. In the remainder of cases there is either a predominance of the left transverse sinus for draining or a mixture between both types (Zülch 1964).

In occlusion of one of the major draining sinuses (and particularly the right transverse sinus!) a transudation edema due to the impeded and partly blocked venous drainage occurs leading subsequently to the papilledema and the abducent paresis. But how and why? Here we can only guess.

The most common cause of sixth nerve paresis is 'transverse sinus thrombosis' after suppurative lesions of the petrous bone. These N. VI palsies after suppurative otitic processes ('Gradenigo's syndrome') are by all probability in the majority not due to the process of permeation of the suppuration, but due to a collateral thrombosis of the lateral sinus. The facts as such have been well known for a long time. Klestadt in 1924 and in 1931 emphasized that his cases with Gradenigo's syndrome were predominantly patients with a right sided sinus phlebitis. Gradenigo, as we all know, had the concept of an inflammation permeating the dura at the tip of the petrous bone and involving the 6th nerve. However, Gradenigo's syndrome also follows merely surgical (non inflammatory) occlusions of the sinus, namely ligatures.

In my opinion it is 1. the enormous intracranial tension pressing on the nerve which probably is strangulated because of a downward, namely 'axial', shift of the brain stem. Again I mention that the abducent is the cranial nerve with the longest extracerebral intracranial course.

Moreover, a second factor probably plays a role: there is a taut cavernous sinus which may lead to a stenosis of the entrance for the sixth nerve into the cavernous sinus, due to the additional amount of blood being forced to flow into the cavernous sinus on a detour via the veins over the clivus. Here the nerve may be additionally strangulated.

References

Cushing H (1910) Strangulation of the nervi abducentes by lateral branches of the basilar artery in cases of brain tumour. With an explanation of some obscure palsies on the basis of arterial constriction. Brain 33:204–235

Fischer-Brügge E (1949) Das „Klivuskanten-Syndrom". Eine durch die Klivuskante hervorgerufene Druckfurche des N. oculomotorius. Zentralbl Chir 74:403

Klestadt W (1924, 1931) Zerebrale Symptomenkomplexe bei otogener Sinusphlebitis. Z Laryng Rhinol 13:83; 21:175

Zielinski HW (1959) Paresen der äußeren Augenmuskeln bei intrakraniellen raumfordernden Prozessen, ein Überblick über die Beobachtungen an über 3000 Fällen. Zentralbl Neurochir 19:235–251

Zülch KJ (1951) Traumatische Störungen der Motorik und Sensibilität und ihre Restitution. Dtsch Z Nervenheilk 166:400–430

Zülch KJ (1959) Störungen des intrakraniellen Druckes. In: Handbuch der Neurochirurgie, Band I/1. Springer-Verlag Berlin Göttingen Heidelberg, S 208–303

Zülch KJ (1964) Neurologische Diagnostik bei endokraniellen Komplikationen von otorhinologischen Erkrankungen. Arch Otorhinolaryngol 183:1–85

Zülch KJ, Mennel HD, Zimmermann V (1974) Intracranial hypertension. In: Vinken PJ, Bruyn GW (eds) Handbook of Clinical Neurology, vol 16. North-Holland Publishing Comp., Amsterdam, pp 89–149

Disturbances of Ocular Movement Due to Cerebral Aneurysm – Based Upon the Experience in 1000 Directly Operated Patients

J. Suzuki, K. Mizoi, and T. Sato, Sendai/Japan

It is well-known that disturbances of ocular movement often arise due to cerebral aneurysm rupture, depending upon the anatomical relationship between the cranial nerves and the aneurysm [8, 12, 15]. Oculomotor palsy is particularly important as a symptom indicating aneurysms at the internal carotid artery (ICA) – posterior communicating artery (PComA) junction or the basilar artery and superior cerebellar artery junction. Furthermore, disturbance of ocular movement, including diplopia and blepharoptosis, are often noticed by the patient himself or his family and the sequential changes in such symptoms are easily followed.

Here we report an investigation of ocular movement disturbances due to aneurysm rupture, based upon our experiences in 1000 directly operated patients.

I. Subjects and Methods

Radical operation was performed upon 1000 patients with cerebral aneurysm at our clinic between 1961 and September, 1975. Excluding all multiple aneurysm cases, records of ocular symptoms were made in 694 patients with single saccular aneurysms. The majority of those patients (86 percent) experienced one to two attacks of aneurysm rupture prior to admission (Table 1).

The correlation between the site of the aneurysm and disturbances of ocular movement were initially investigated, and the cause of the disturbances based upon

Table 1. Site distribution of patients analysed in this study and times of aneurysm rupture in these cases

Site of AN		AComA	ICA	MCA	ACA	VBA	Multiple	Total
No. of cases		346	246	174	49	23	162	1000
No. of analysed cases		276	200	148	47	23	0	694
Frequency of aneurysm rupture	1	154	95	70	26	13		358
	2	83	74	57	16	6		236
	3	27	28	16	4	4		79
	4	8	2	4	1	0		15
	5	4	0	1	0	0		5
	6	0	1	0	0	0		1

AComA: anterior communicating artery, ICA: internal carotid artery, MCA: middle cerebral artery, ACA: anterior cerebral artery, VBA: vertebro-basilar artery angiograms and surgical findings are discussed. A follow-up study was also made of the postoperative recovery of blepharoptosis in the ICA-PComA junction cases, which had the highest incidence of such symptoms. Excepting hospital deaths, subjects for the follow-up study included the 57 patients showing preoperative blepharoptosis. Thirtyone of the 57 patients (54 percent) responded to the postal questionnaire. The follow up varied from one to nine years and 10 months postoperatively.

II. Results

Disturbances of ocular movement were noted in 84 of the 694 patients (12 percent). The highest incidence was seen in the ICA aneurysm cases – i.e., in 70 of 200 patients or 35 percent, followed by vertebro-basilar artery (VBA) patients (four of 23 or 17 percent), anterior cerebral artery (ACA) patients (two of 47 or 4 percent), middle cerebral artery (MCA) patients (three of 148 or 2 percent) and anterior communicating artery (AComA) patients (five of 276 or 2 percent) (Table 2). Disturbances of ocular movement included oculomotor nerve paralysis in 68 patients, abducens nerve paralysis in nine, and the nature of the ocular movement was unclear in seven others.

Table 2. Ocular motor disturbances in patients with ruptured aneurysms

Site of aneurysm / Ocular motor disturbance	AComA 276	ICA 200	MCA 148	ACA 47	VBA 23	Total 694
Total (%)	5 (1.8)	70 (35.0)	3 (2.0)	2 (4.3)	4 (17.4)	84 (12.1)
Oculomotor paralysis	2	62	2	1	1	68
Abducens paralysis	3	2	0	1	3	9
Unknown disturbance	0	6	1	0	0	7

1. Correlation Between Aneurysm Site and Symptoms

a) ICA aneurysms

Seventy of the 84 patients (83 percent) with disturbances of ocular movement were ICA aneurysm cases, 66 of whom had the aneurysm located at the ICA-PComA junction, one on the PComA itself [10] and three at the termination of the ICA. The disturbances were oculomotor nerve paralysis in 62, abducens nerve paralysis in two and unknown disturbance in six. Investigation of the blepharoptosis in the ICA-PComA cases showed onset most frequently on the day of the attack (19 of 60

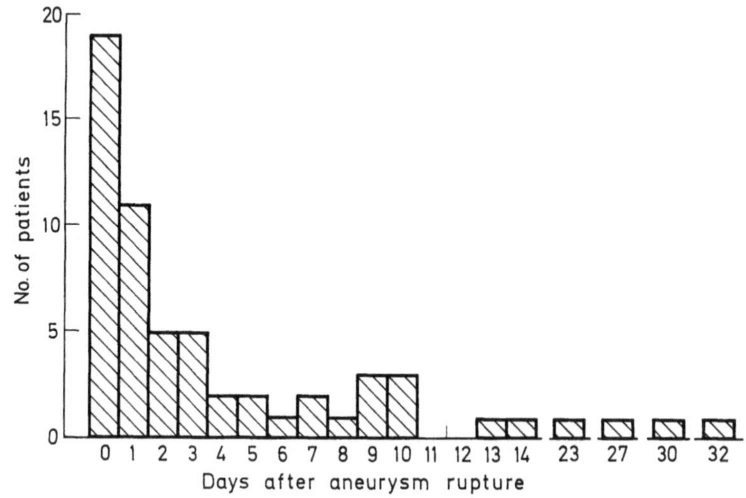

Fig. 1. The onset of unilateral eye-lid ptosis after aneurysm rupture in internal carotid-posterior communicating artery junction aneurysms

patients). Half of these patients (30) presented with ptosis within two days of the attack, but there were also patients in whom the ptosis arose between 23 and 32 days from aneurysm rupture (Fig. 1). Investigation of the correlation between the blepharoptosis and the size and direction of growth of the aneurysm showed that the average size of the aneurysm in the 53 patients with blepharoptosis was 9.4 mm, whereas it averaged 8.1 mm in the 121 patients without this symptom. This finding was, however, not statistically significant (P 0.05). For study of the correlation between the direction of growth of the aneurysm and ptosis, the cases were divided into two groups: those showing growth in directions likely to result in compression of the oculomotor nerve (a posterior-inferior direction or a posterior-inferior-lateral direction) and those with growth in other directions. There was a tendency for blepharoptosis to be more frequent in the former group, but again this result was not statistically significant (Table 3).

Table 3. Correlation between the incidence of eye-lid ptosis and the direction of aneurysm growth in carotid angiograms

		Total no. of cases	Direction of aneurysm growth in CAG		
			Backward, downward & lateral	Backward & downward	Other direction
No. of cases		124	116	27	31
Patients with ptosis	No. of patients	53	37	10	6
	Percent	30.5	31.9	37.0	19.4

b) VBA Aneurysms

Of four such patients, one had oculomotor nerve palsy and three had abducens nerve palsy. In the former patients the aneurysm was at the junction of the basilar artery and the superior cerebellar artery and was found to compress and narrow the oculomotor nerve. All three of the latter patients had bilateral papilledema preoperatively and were found at operation to have extensive adherence of the aneurysm to the subarachnoid membrane and clots in the basal cisterns. The abducens paralysis is thought to have been caused by intracranial hypertension.

c) ACA Aneurysms

Both ACA patients had an aneurysm located at the A_1 portion. One showed abducens paralysis and one showed oculomotor paralysis (Fig. 2), the latter showing so-called megadolichobasilar anomaly [13, 16] on vertebro-basilar angiograms. It is thought that this anomaly of the basilar artery had already brought about a certain degree of compression of the oculomotor nerve, so that when the aneurysm ruptured and subarachnoid hematoma was formed, a rise in intracranial pressure followed. This in turn resulted in still stronger compression of the oculomotor nerve (Fig. 3). In the case of abducens paralysis, a 50 gram hematoma was found in the temporal lobe, which is thought to have brought increased intracranial pressure.

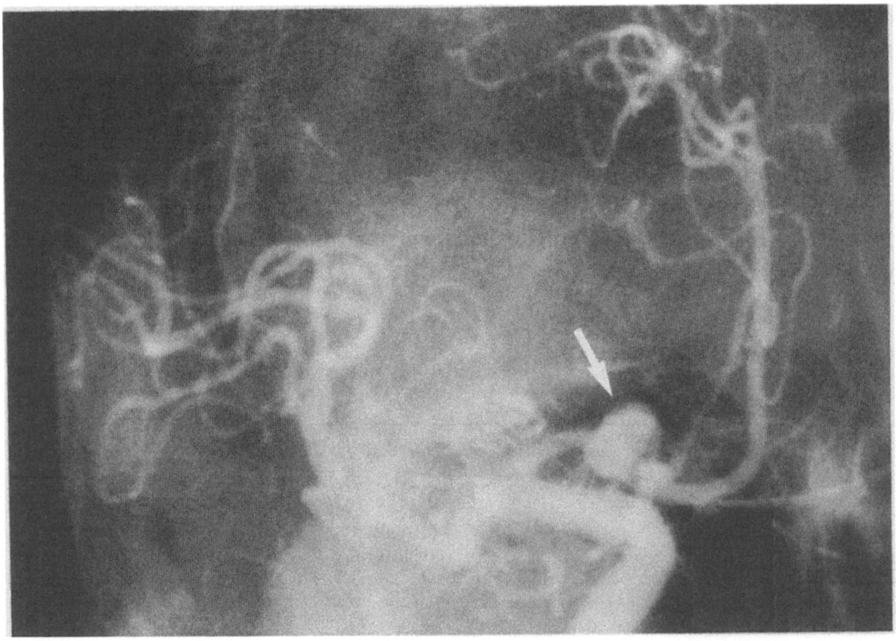

Fig. 2. A-P view of right carotid angiogram in a patient with an aneurysm of the A-1 portion of the right anterior cerebral artery. This patient showed the symptoms of the right oculomotor nerve palsy following the subarachnoid hemorrhage

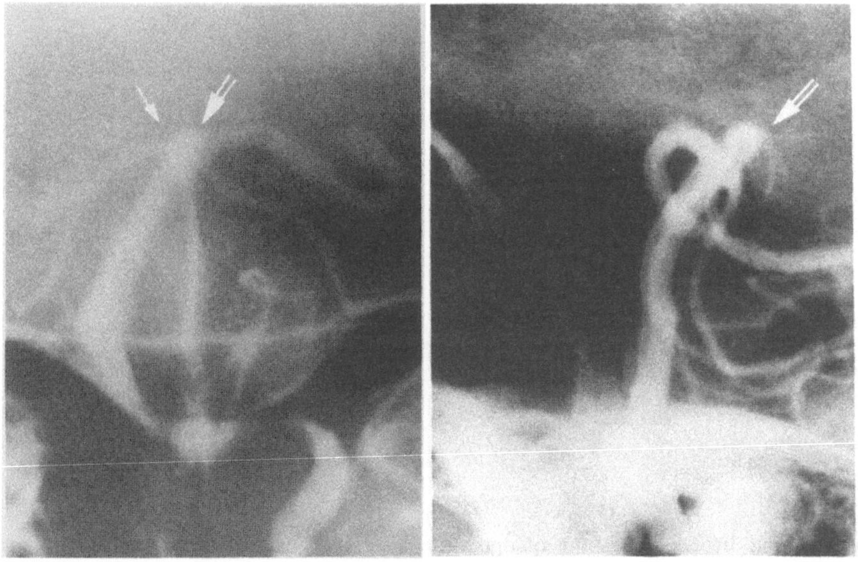

Fig. 3. Left axillary-vertebral angiogram in the same patient as Fig. 2. Note the megadolichobasilar anomaly showing the elongated basilar artery. Single arrow: At this site, the right oculomotor nerve may be squeezed between the right posterior cerebral and superior cerebellar arteries. Double arrow: The terminal portion of the basilar artery

d) MCA Aneurysms

Oculomotor paralysis was found in two patients and unknown disturbance in one case. Both of the former cases had intracranial hematoma in the temporal lobe, which is thought to have been involved in the development of neurological symptoms.

e) AComA Aneurysms

Among these five patients, two had oculomotor paralysis and three had abducens paralysis. One of the former had an intracranial hematoma in the frontal lobe and one had a hematoma in the basal cistern and interhemispherically. One of the latter cases had hematoma in the frontal lobe and subdurally, whereas the other two showed vasospasm in preoperative angiograms, and are thought to have developed symptoms due to ischemic brain edema and intracranial hypertension.

2. Recovery of Blepharoptosis Following Radical Treatment

Disappearance of the ptosis was found in 23 of the 31 patients followed up postoperatively (74 percent). Most patients improved within one month of surgery (eight patients or 35 percent), but one patient showed recovery after two years and four months. With regard to the period from onset of symptoms until

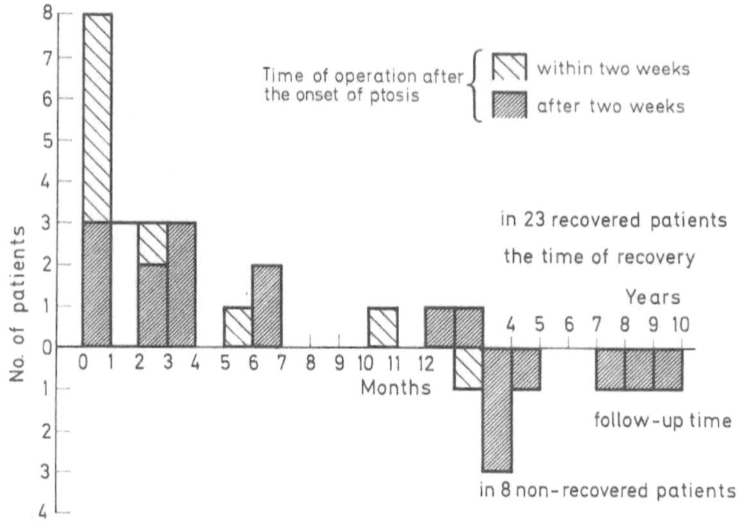

Fig. 4. Correlation between the time of operation after the onset of eye-lid ptosis and its prognosis following intracranial operation upon patients with aneurysms of the internal carotid-posterior communicating artery junction

operation, it was seen that 11 of the 12 patients (92 percent) operated upon within two weeks of onset recovered, whereas only 12 of 19 (63 percent) operated on thereafter showed recovery (Fig. 4).

III. Discussion

According to various reports, the incidence of unilateral oculomotor paralysis in patients with aneurysm at the junction of the ICA and PComA is 34 to 42 percent, making such symptoms an important indicator of the site of cerebral aneurysm [8, 12, 15]. Walsh [17] reported that the oculomotor paralysis in such cases is a complete paralysis, such that nearly all patients show pupillary dilation, disturbances of globe movement and blepharoptosis. In comparison with other reports, the incidence of ptosis in our series, 33 percent, is low.

With regard to the correlation between aneurysm rupture and onset of oculomotor nerve palsy, it was found that most (19 patients) had onset on the day of rupture, and fully 64 percent had onset of ptosis within three days. Green et al. [7] have reported a similar tendency, suggesting that neurological symptoms develop on the day of rupture or soon thereafter in most patients. Previous studies [14, 15, 17] have found no correlation between the incidence of oculomotor paralysis and the size or direction of growth of aneurysms, as determined angiographically. Although we observed a tendency for higher incidence of such symptoms to occur with large aneurysms and when the aneurysm grew in posterior-inferior or posterior-inferior-lateral directions, these findings were not statistically significant.

The development of oculomotor paralysis is thought to occur by two distinct mechanisms. The first is compression of the oculomotor nerve by the aneurysm itself or by surrounding subdural hematoma in an early period following rupture. The second is adherence between the oculomotor nerve and surrounding tissue in the process of absorbance of the subdural hematoma during a relatively late period at least one month from aneurysm rupture [9, 12]. In our series, oculomotor palsy was found in five patients other than those with aneurysm of the ICA or VBA (two AComA, two MCA, and one ACA). Such cases have been found in previous studies [1, 11], and the causal factors of such symptoms remain unclear. Certain abnormalities were found at operation in our patients, but it is uncertain whether or not they constituted the actual cause of the oculomotor palsy. This problem needs further study. Particularly our ACA aneurysm patients showing megadolichobasilar anomaly is of interest [13, 16]. Of course, megadolichobasilar anomaly is known to be associated with various neurological symptoms, but in our case the ocular symptoms arose only subsequent to aneurysm rupture.

Abducens paralysis is known to be a false localizing sign in cases of brain tumor with intracranial hypertension. That is, due to increased intracranial pressure, the entire brain is pushed downward and the abducens nerve is compressed by blood vessels or the brain itself, thus giving rise to ocular symptoms [4, 5, 18]. In fact, most of the patients in our series who showed abducens paralysis also had intracranial hypertension.

Although not discussed above, among the disturbances of ocular movement developing subsequent to aneurysm rupture is gaze palsy, which was found in five of our patients (three AComA, one ICA, and one VBA). These included four patients with internuclear horizontal gaze palsy and one with vertical gaze palsy. It is thought that such symptoms are due to midbrain circulatory disturbances caused by massive hemorrhage into the basal cistern or vasospasm, etc. [16]. There are, however, various problems involved in detailed ophthalmological examination of patients with ruptured cerebral aneurysms, so that many questions concerning causal mechanisms remain unanswered.

Finally, with regard to the recovery of ptosis, it is known that ptosis is the first of the ocular symptoms to show improvement, later followed by improvement in ocular movement disturbances and pupil dilatation [15]. Consequently, our follow-up study of blepharoptosis cannot be said to cover all aspects of ocular disturbances, but it is a useful index for determining the effectiveness of radical operation. Twenty-three of the 31 patients who were followed (74 percent) showed complete recovery of the blepharoptosis. Most previous reports have not dealt with intracranial operation, but rather common carotid or internal carotid artery ligation [3, 14], and functional recovery in those cases has been achieved in 50 to 70 percent. From the point of view of recovery of oculomotor palsy, it is consequently believed that intracranial operation is more effective. It is also apparent from our series that recovery is more favorable in patients who are operated upon within two weeks of onset.

Particularly in light of the reports by Botterell et al. [2], Soni [15], and Grayson et al. [6], in which no case of complete recovery was experienced among patients operated upon after at least 10 days from onset, it is thought that early operation is important.

IV. Summary

Based upon our series of 1000 directly operated cerebral aneurysm patients, we have investigated the relationship between aneurysm and ocular movement disturbances.

1. Excluding cases of multiple aneurysms, 84 patients among the 694 with ocular symptoms (12 percent) were found to have disturbances of ocular movement.

2. Among 200 ICA aneurysm patients, 70 (35 percent) showed such disturbances, followed in order of frequency by VBA, ACA, MCA and AComA aneurysm cases.

3. Investigation of the prognosis of blepharoptosis in cases of aneurysm of the ICA-PComA junction showed that 74 percent (23 of 31 followed patients) recovered, the percentage being higher for those operated upon in an early period following onset.

References

1. Barnett HJM (1968) Some clinical features of intracranial aneurysms. Clin Neurosurg 16:43–72
2. Botterell EH, Lloyd LA, et al. (1962) Oculomotor palsy due to supraclinoid internal carotid artery berry aneurysm. A long-term study of the results of surgical treatment on the recovery of third-nerve function. Am J Ophtalmol 54:609–612
3. Cantu RC, Sonders T, et al. (1969) Effects of carotid ligation on aneurysm-induced oculomotor palsy. J Neurosurg 31:528–532
4. Collier J (1904) The false localizing signs of intracranial tumor. Brain 27:490–508
5. Cushing H (1910) Strangulation of the nerve abducens by lateral branches of the basilar artery in cases of brain tumor. Brain 33:204–235
6. Grayson MG, Soni SR, et al. (1974) Analysis of the recovery of the third nerve function after direct surgical intervention for posterior communicating aneurysm. Br J Ophthalmol 58:118–125
7. Green WR, Hackett ER, et al. (1964) Neuro-ophthalmologic evaluation of oculomotor nerve paralysis. Arch Ophthalmol 72:154–167
8. Hóók O, Norlén G (1964) Aneurysms of the internal carotid artery. Arch Neurol Scand 40:200–218
9. Hyland HH, Barnett HJM (1954) The pathogenesis of cranial nerve palsies associated with intracranial aneurysms. Proc R Soc Med 47:141–146
10. Kamiyama K, Sakurai Y, et al. (1980) Case report: Aneurysm of the posterior communicating artery itself – report of successfully treated cases. Neurol Med Chir (Tokyo) 20:81–84
11. Nakagawa Y, Kuramae T, et al. (1971) An analysis of the intracranial aneurysm in relation to the sites and the neurological manifestations. Clin Neurol (Tokyo) 11:313–319
12. Odum GL (1964) Ophthalmologic involvement in neurological vascular lesion. In: Smith JL (ed) Neuro-Ophthalmology. Springfield, Ill. Charles C Thomas, p 213–216
13. Ohwada K, Iwabuchi T, et al. (1974) The megadolichobasilar Anomaly. Neurol Surg (Tokyo) 2:699–704
14. Raja IA (1972) Aneurysm-induced third nerve palsy. J Neurosurg 36:548–551
15. Soni SR (1974) Aneurysms of the posterior communicating artery and oculomotor paresis. J Neurol Neurosurg Psychiatry 37:475–484
16. Suzuki J, Iwabuchi T (1974) Ocular motor disturbances occurring as false localizing signs in ruptured intracranial aneurysm. Acta Neurochir 30:119–128
17. Walsh FB (1957) Third nerve regeneration. A clinical evaluation. Br J Ophthalmol 41:577–598
18. Wolf E (1928) A bend in the sixth cranial nerve and its probable significance. Br J Ophthalmol 12:22–24

Incidence and Prognosis of Oculomotor Palsy After Subarachnoid Hemorrhage Due to Ruptured Aneurysms of the Posterior Communicating Artery

J. HAMER, Heidelberg/FRG

Introduction

It is well known to every neurosurgeon that oculomotor palsy often occurs with ruptured or unruptured aneurysms at the junction of the internal carotid and the posterior communicating artery. An incidence ranging from 40 to 80 percent has been reported in extensive clinical series (Walker 1956, Pool and Potts 1965). Similar figures have been given in the American Cooperative Study on Subarachnoid Hemorrhage which comprised more than 6000 cases (Locksley 1966 b). However, the neurosurgical literature on recovery from third cranial nerve palsy is surprisingly scanty. In the last two decades, only a few reports, mainly in ophthalmological journals, have been devoted to the problem of regeneration of oculomotor fibers after subarachnoid hemorrhage (Botterell et al. 1962, Cogan et al. 1963, Dailey et al. 1964, Hepler et al. 1967, Kerns et al. 1979). The experience of neurosurgeons has been divergent: In 1947, Jefferson reported on 23 cases which had been treated by external carotid ligation alone, in no instance there was a complete recovery. On the other hand, Botterell et al. stated in 1962 that full recovery of third nerve palsy often occurred if the aneurysm was sucessfully clipped.

The present study contributes more specifically to the questions concerning the relation between time of surgical intervention and duration of recovery, and furthermore the speed of restoration of various oculomotor functions.

Results and Discussion

The present investigation includes 35 patients with an aneurysm at the junction of the internal carotid and posterior communicating artery. 25 patients were females (70%), 10 were males (30%). The female preponderance in internal carotid aneurysms is well known. In the American Cooperative Study, Locksley (1966 a) also reported a ratio of 70 to 30%. 15 patients (43%) had a third cranial nerve palsy: In 11 patients the oculomotor palsy was complete, in four incomplete. In 10 cases, the palsy of the third cranial nerve occurred suddenly, in another five patients it developed progressively within two days and one week. It is noteworthy that four of the latter five cases had suffered no subarachnoid hemorrhage. This sheds some light on the pathophysiology of the oculomotor lesion: Ocular palsies are not due in all cases to hemorrhage *per se.* They may also be produced by dilatation of the aneurysmal sac. Some investigators (Locksley 1966 b, Okawara 1973) have called this the 'warning symptom' prior to rupture. Oculomotor palsy as a preceding warning sign is apparently not uncommon in cases with internal carotid aneurysms. Locksley reported a frequency of more than 80% and Okawara observed it in 70%. In the present series, nine cases suffered subarachnoid hemorrhage, six patients had a third nerve palsy without rupture. Furthermore, the degree of internal and external ocular palsy is not primarily dependent on the pathological cause of compression – either bleeding or aneurysmal dilatation. There was only one incomplete palsy among six cases without hemorrhage, and we did not find a higher incidence of complete palsies in cases with bleeding (see Table 1).

Table 1. Oculomotor palsy associated with ruptured and unruptured intracranial aneurysms

N III palsy *with* SAH
n = 9 : 3 incomplete, 6 complete
N III palsy *without* SAH ('warning symptom')
n = 6 : 1 incomplete, 5 complete

The types of incomplete oculomotor palsy show some peculiarities: We observed 2 cases with sparing of the pupilloconstrictor fibers. This has been also found by some other investigators (Cogan et al. 1963, Dailey et al. 1964, Kasoff et al. 1975). In general, the parasympathetic fibers in the oculomotor nerve are said to be particularly vulnerable to injury, and pupillary sparing in oculomotor palsy is unusual. The pathway of pupilloconstrictor fibers within the third cranial nerve has been investigated by Sunderland (1946) and later by Kerr et al. (1964). According to their anatomical studies, the parasympathetic fibers run peripherally in the dorso-medial arc; some few fibers may also run in the lateral portion of the nerve. Thus, one may argue that the pupilloconstrictor fibers can be spared if the nerve is only displaced laterally and not lifted and pressed against the tentorium.

The restitution of nervous function depends on some important factors which will now be discussed: It should be emphasized that primarily the degree of anatomical lesion, either axonal degeneration or only conduction block, and not the mode of compression (hemorrhage or simply dilatation of the aneurysm) will influence the speed of regeneration. Furthermore, Hyland et al. (1954) and others have shown that there is a lack of correlation between structure and restitution of function in so far as even partial regeneration of fibers may be accompanied with clinically complete recovery. And finally, considering the evaluation of restitution, one should not only differentiate between complete and incomplete recovery, but also between incomplete recovery with residual symptoms which are disturbing for the patients, and recovery with so-called aberrant regeneration. The most frequent and characteristic sign of the latter is the Pseudo-Graefe phenomenon with lid retraction on depression of the ball of the eye. Aberrant regeneration often does not bother patients very much, and it is very common particularly in those cases with delayed restitution as has been shown by Cogan (1963), Hepler (1967), and Kerns (1979).

Table 2 shows the postoperative results: all 15 patients could be followed up. Complete recovery occured in 11 patients. Incomplete restitution of oculomotor palsy was observed in only four cases. Recovery seldom occurs within four weeks, but generally within three months, here in more than half of the cases. The most important role in the quality of regeneration is played by the factor 'time', i.e. the interval between the onset of oculomotor palsy and neurosurgical therapy with clipping of the aneurysm. Only this procedure, as convincingly demonstrated by Botterell (1962) and later by Hepler (1967), will favor full restitution. We observed complete recovery only in those cases which were operated on within three weeks after onset of oculomotor palsy. Beyond this limit of three to four weeks, restitution was delayed over months or even absent. The cases with incomplete recovery fell into this group. Finally, in agreement with other investigators such as Botterell (1962) and Dailey (1964), we observed that the tendency to restitution varies with the different ocular muscle functions. The speed of regeneration was as follows: The levator palpebrae muscle and the rectus medialis showed rapid recovery. Next, there followed the parasympathetic fibers, the M. rectus superior and inferior having the longest regeneration time (see also Jefferson 1947). Thus, patients will have diplopia for some time when ptosis has vanished, and some trouble with accomodation may persist for a while when diplopia subsides.

Table 2. Prognosis of oculomotor palsy after clipping of the aneurysm

Follow-up: n = 15 cases		
complete recovery:		n = 11
incomplete recovery:		n = 4
Time course:		
recovery	within 1 month	n = 2
	within 3 months	n = 9
	within 1 year	n = 4

Conclusions

Oculomotor palsies occurred in about 50 percent of our cases of ruptured and unruptured internal carotid artery aneurysms. The third cranial nerve palsy is often a warning symptom prior to hemorrhage. In at least 70 percent of the cases, complete recovery from ocular paralysis can be expected after clipping of the aneurysm. The results may be improved if the time which elapses from onset of third cranial nerve compression to surgery is kept short. In cases of early operation, i.e. within one to three weeks, recovery generally requires no more than three months. Beyond the period of four weeks, the rate of good functional restitution decreases rapidly.

References

Botterell EH, Lloyd LA, Hoffman HJ (1962) Oculomotor palsy due to supraclinoidal internal carotid artery berry aneurysm. Am J Ophthalmol 54:609–616

Cogan DG, Mount HTJ (1963) Intracranial aneurysms causing ophthalmoplegia. Arch Ophthalmol 70:757–771

Dailey EJ, Holloway JA, Murto RE, Schlezinger NS (1964) Evaluation of ocular signs and symptoms in cerebral aneurysms. Arch Ophthalmol 71:463–474

Hepler RS, Cantu RC (1967) Aneurysms and third nerve palsies. Ocular status of survivors. Arch Ophthalmol 77:604–608

Hyland HH, Barnett HJM (1954) The pathogenesis of cranial nerve palsies associated with intracranial aneurysms. Proc R Soc Med 47: 141–146

Jefferson G (1947) Isolated oculomotor palsy caused by intracranial aneurysm. Proc R Soc Med 40:419–432

Kasoff I, Kelly LD (1975) Pupillary sparing in oculomotor palsy from internal carotid aneurysm. J Neurosurg 42:713–717

Kerns JM, Smith DR, Jannotta FS, Alper MG (1979) Oculomotor nerve regeneration after aneurysm surgery. Am J Ophthalmol 87:225–233

Kerr FWL, Hollowell OW (1964) Location of pupillomotor and accommodation fibers in the oculomotor nerve: Experimental observations on paralytic mydriasis. J Neurol Neurosurg Psychiatry 27:473–481

Locksley HB (1966 a) Report on the Cooperative Study of Intracranial Aneurysms and Subarachnoid Hemorrhage. Section V, part I. Natural History of Subarachnoid Hemorrhage, Intracranial Aneurysms and Arteriovenous Malformations. Based on 6368 cases. J Neurosurg 25:219–239

Locksley HB (1966 b) Natural History of Subarachnoid Hemorrhage, Intracranial Aneurysms and Arteriovenous Malformations. Section V, part II. J Neurosurg 25:321–368

Okawara SH (1973) Warning signs prior to rupture of an intracranial aneurysm. J Neurosurg 38:575–580

Pool JL, Potts DG (1965) Aneurysms and Arteriovenous Anomalies of the Brain. Diagnosis and Treatment. New York, Harper & Row, p 83

Sunderland S, Hughes ESR (1946) The pupilloconstrictor pathway and the nerves to the ocular muscles in man. Brain 69:301–309

Walker AE (1956) Clinical localization of intracranial aneurysms and vascular anomalies. Neurology (Minneap) 6:79–90

Intracranial Compression of the Third, Fourth, and Sixth Cranial Nerves by Tumors

M. SAMII, Hannover/FRG

The pathophysiology of oculomotor and abducens nerves paresis in supratentorial and infratentorial processes has already been described by Professor Zülch. I would like to demonstrate direct compression of the third, fourth, and sixth cranial nerves by different kinds of tumors, which in most cases are located in the region of the tentorial notch.

With the introduction of the operating microscope into microneurosurgery and an increased knowledge of functional anatomical aspects, processes in the region of the tentorial notch became more and more significant.

Fig. 1 shows the different supratentorial approaches to the third, fourth, and sixth cranial nerves:

1. The subfrontal infrachiasmatic approach.
2. The subpterional approach.
3. The subtemporal approach.

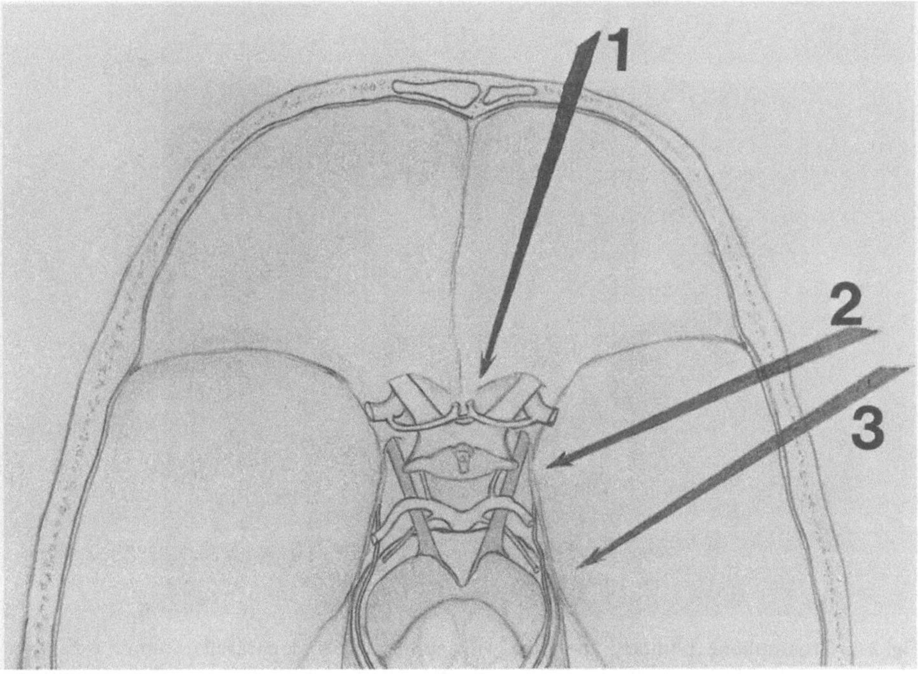

Fig. 1. Different supra-tentorial approaches to the third, fourth, and sixth cranial nerves: (*1*) The subfrontal infrachiasmatic approach. (*2*) The subpterional approach (*3*) the subtemporal approach

We choose the subfrontal, infrachiasmatic approach in patients with suprasellar processes of parasellar and particularly retrosellar extension, provided there is sufficient distance between the anterior chiasmatic angle and the tuberculum sella. This route is especially recommended for pituitary adenomas and craniopharyngiomas. An example of this approach in a patient with third cranial nerve compression on the left side by pituitary adenoma with parasellar extension is demonstrated in Fig. 2 a, b. In this pituitary adenoma it was possible, after enucleation of

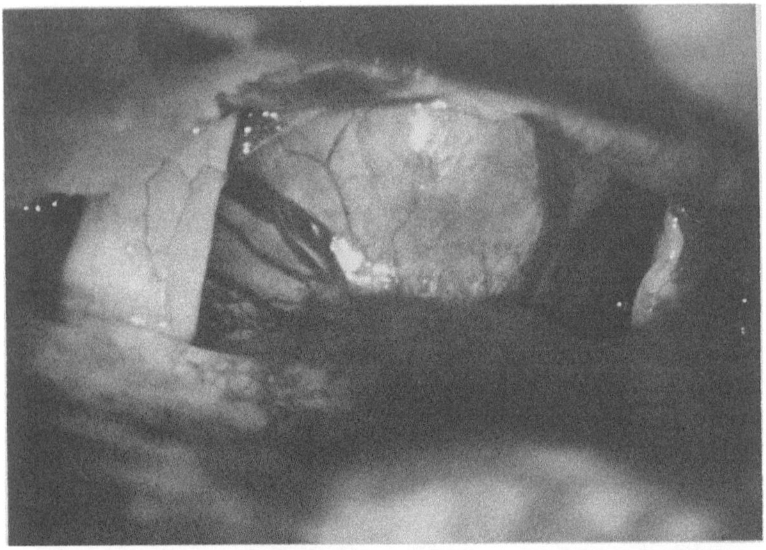

a

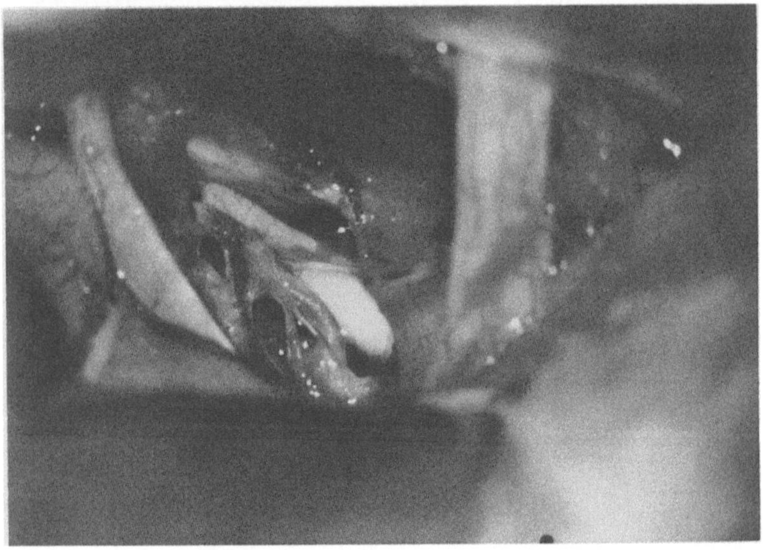

b

Fig. 2 a. Cromophobe pituitary adenoma with suprasellar and parasellar tumor extension. **2 b.** The same patient as Fig. 2 a after total removal of the adenoma with view into the retrosellar prepontine space. Between the decompressed left and right optic nerves the left internal carotid artery, the left posterior communicating artery, and the anterior chorioid artery, the left oculomotor nerve is visible the tumor, to detach microsurgically the severe adhesion of the tumor capsule to the internal carotid artery as well as the anterior chorioid artery and also to decompress the oculomotor nerve.

The pterional approach, modified after Yaşargil, should be recommended for all processes in the region of the anterior and middle third of the tentorial notch, e.g. meningiomas, neurinomas, pituitary adenomas, craniopharyngiomas.

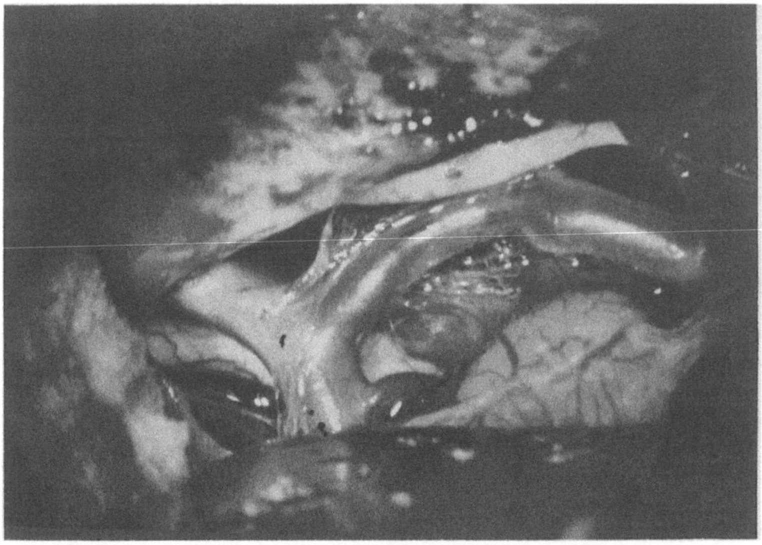

Fig. 3. Microsurgical exposure of the right tentorial notch. The oculomotor nerve is visible between the posterior communicating artery and the tentorial margin

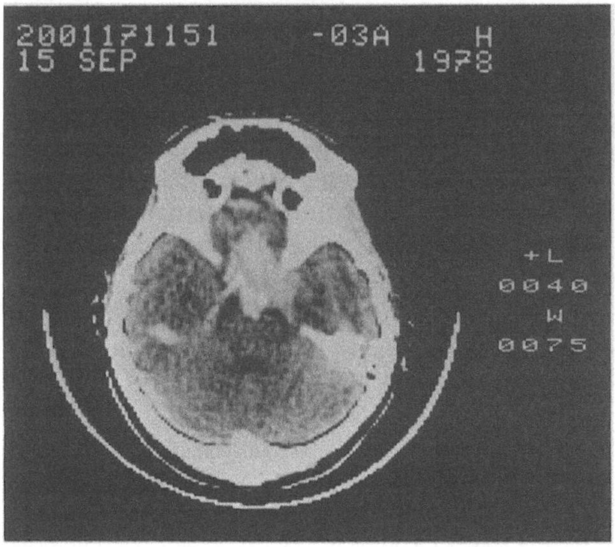

Fig. 4 a. The axial CT shows a meningioma of the diaphragma sellae with suprasellar and right-sided parasellar extension

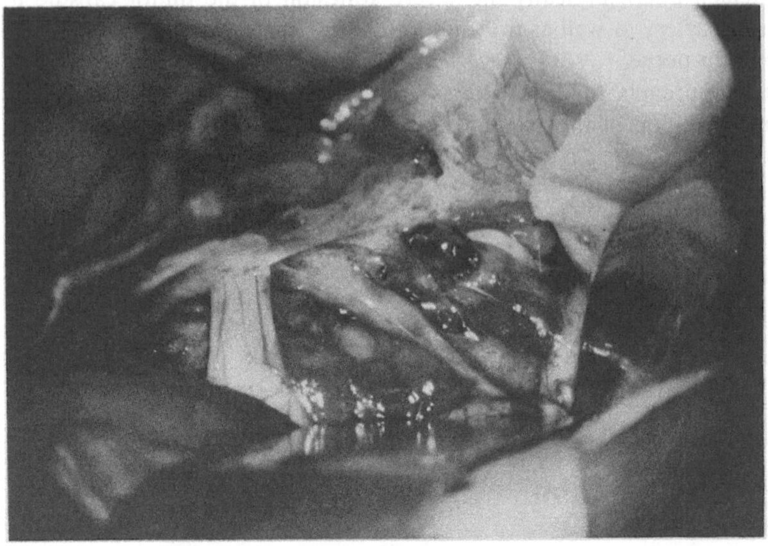

Fig. 4 b. The same patient as Fig. 4 a. Pterional approach on the right side with preparation of the incisura tentorii. The tumor has displaced and pressed up the optic nerve and is growing around and displacing the internal carotid artery. Beyond the tentorial margin, the oculomotor nerve is arch-shaped and displaced in dorsal direction

After a fronto-temporal osteoplastic trepanation with a minimum incision and the removal of the lateral portion of the lesser sphenoid wing one approaches intradurally, along the sphenoid wing edge, in the direction of the anterior clinoid process by stepwise opening the cisterns and successively extracting cerebrospinal fluid. After opening the Sylvian fissure in the basis region, this procedure requires sufficient time in order to render possible pressing apart and slight lifting up of the orbital gyrus on the one side and the temporal pole at the other side by constant CSF drainage and negligible pressure on the brain structures.

After exposure of the optic nerve, the internal carotid artery and the further opening of the cistern along the tentorium cerebellum margin and the posterior communicating artery with its branches, the oculomotor nerve in the anterior third of the tentorial notch is exposed (Fig. 3). Through further preparation in the middle third, along the free margin of the tentorial notch in a dorsal direction, the

Fig. 5 a. Supratentorial and infratentorial neurinoma in the left middle third of the tentorial notch. The ventral part of the tumor is compressing the oculomotor nerve, which is displaced from the dorsal to the ventral direction

Fig. 5 b. The same patient as Fig. 5 a after removal of the supratentorial part of the tumor, the oculomotor nerve is decompressed, the tentorium cerebelli margin is incised and the trochlear nerve dissected

Fig. 5 c. The same patient as Fig. 5 a and b after total tumor removal. From ventral to dorsal exposure of the optic nerve, the internal carotid artery, the posterior clinoid process, the oculomotor, abducens and trochlear nerve as well as the basilar artery

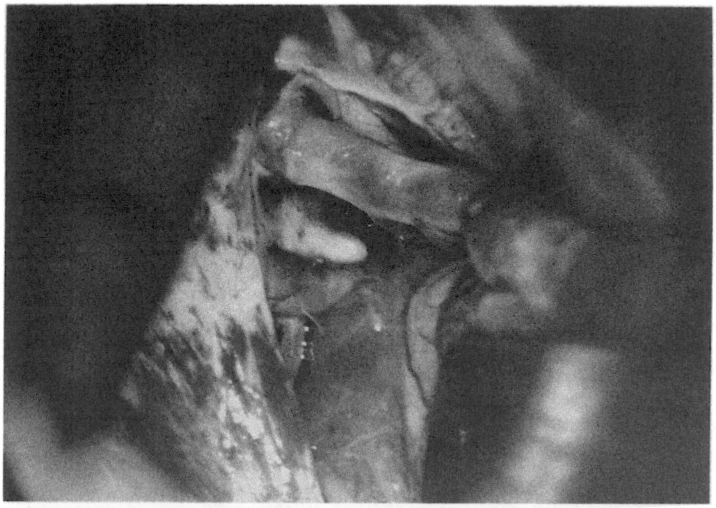

a

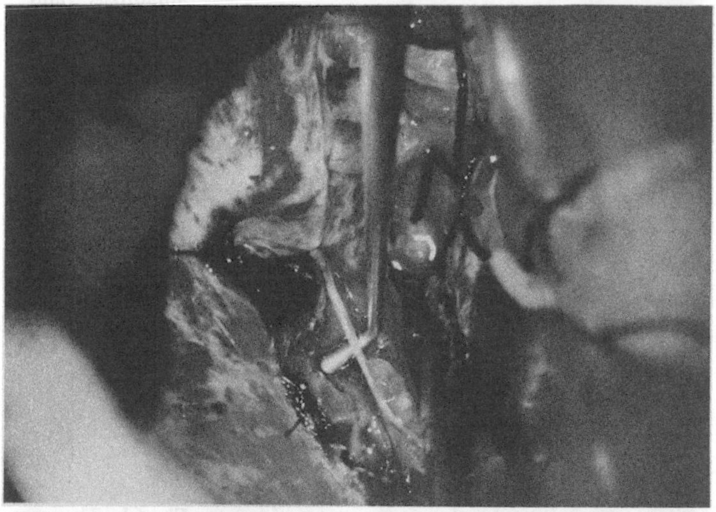

b

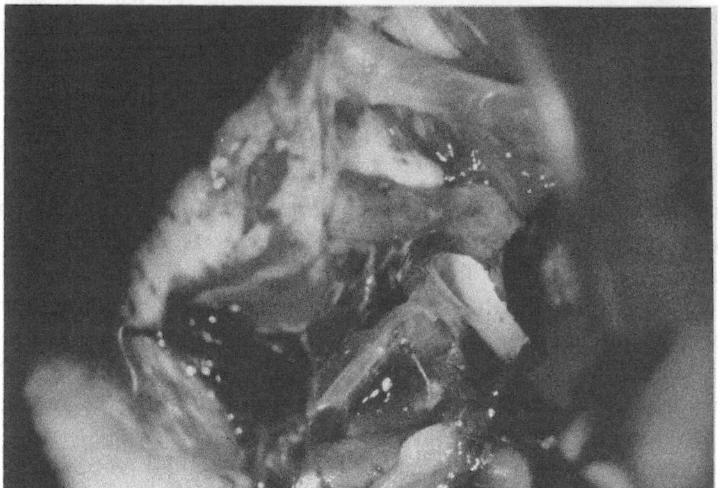

c

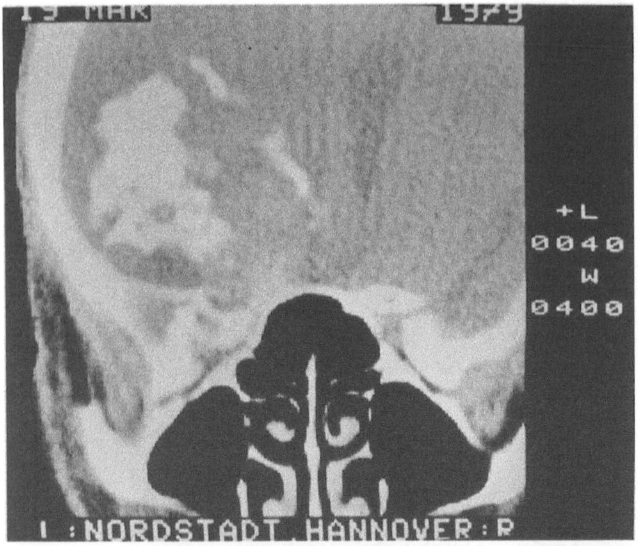

Fig. 6a. CT in coronal section in a patient with a chondroma in the region of the right, middle cranial fossa extending into the tentorial notch with clinical signs of amaurosis and complete ophthalmoplegia as well as occlusion of the internal carotid artery

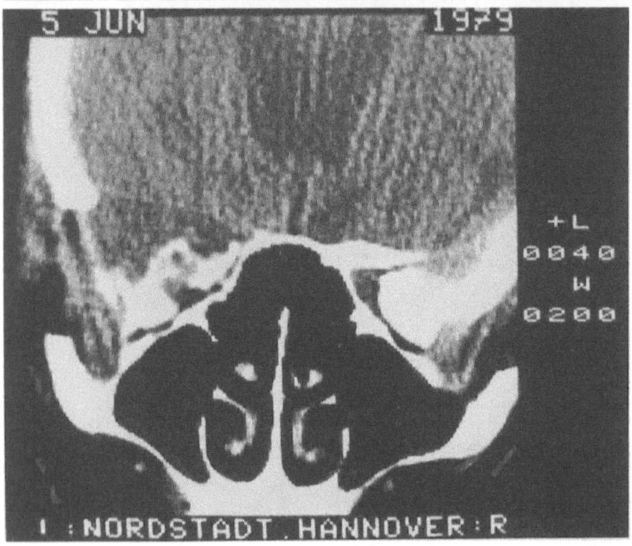

Fig. 6b. The same patient as Fig. 6a. Postoperative CT control after complete tumor removal. Normalized position of the ventricles

trochlear nerve becomes visible. After incision and the suturing up of the tentorium cerebellum margin in the middle third one achieves an excellent view of the infratentorial course of the third, fourth, and sixth cranial nerves.

Severe compression of the third and fourth cranial nerves by a large suprasellar and parasellar meningioma on the right side is demonstrated in Fig. 4a, b. The carotid artery and the oculomotor nerve are displaced from the ventral to the dorsal direction. Partial removal and decompression of the nerves and vessels as well as the brain stem was accomplished in this patient.

Fig. 5a–c demonstrates a neurinoma of the fourth cranial nerve in the middle third region of the left tentorial notch, which extended both supratentorially and

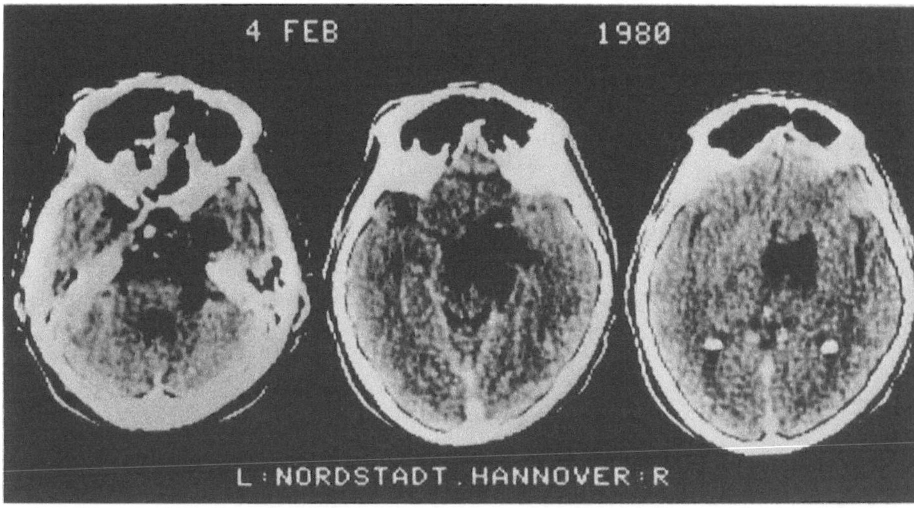

Fig. 7. An extensive dermoid tumor compressing the brain stem and all nerves and vessels in the tentorial notch of the right side as well as in the prepontine region. Despite the tumor compression we found no clinical sign of ocular muscle paresis

infratentorially. Contrary to the last patient, the third cranial nerve is compressed and displaced in the ventral direction. After incision of the margin of the tentorium cerebelli and high suture, removal of the infratentorial tumor portion was also possible.

Fig. 6 a shows a chondroma of relatively rare localisation in the region of the middle cranial fossa with extension into the tentorial notch. The tumor had provoked an occlusion of the internal carotid artery and caused amaurosis on the right side, with internal and external ophthalmoplegia over a period of 15 years. The decompression of the nerve and vessel structures within the tentorial notch allowed complete removal of the partially calcified tumor. Despite the total decompression of the third nerve, a recovery of the function could not be achieved. The postoperative CT scan is demonstrated in Fig. 6 b.

The last patient had a very extensive dermoid tumor (Fig. 7) compressing the brain stem through the bottom of the third ventricle and the oculomotor nerve as well as the vessels of the circle of Willis. The tumor was exposed from the right pterional approach. The optic nerve and the carotid artery were surrounded by the tumor. The arch-shaped internal carotid artery was displaced in a dorsal direction. After total removal of the tumor the right and left sixth cranial nerves were visible and also the basilar and the posterior cerebral artery, as well as the superior cerebellar artery. Despite all this tumor compression there was no clinical sign of ocular muscle paresis in this patient.

Summary

The pterional approach allows for operative treatment of processes in the supratentorial region of the anterior and middle third of the incisura tentorii, with direct compression of the third and fourth cranial nerves. The approach to the infratentorial region of the oculomotor, trochlear, and abducens nerves can be achieved by incising the tentorial margin. In cases of pituitary adenoma with parasellar extension and compression of oculomotor nerve, the decompression can be performed by the subfrontal infrachiasmatic approach. The direct compression of the ocular muscle nerve by different tumor, located in the region of the tentorial notch, are demonstrated in several patients.

Tumor Compression of Oculomotor, Trochlear and Abducens Nerve in Cavernous Sinus and Orbit

K. Schürmann, Mainz/FRG

Starting with intraorbital lesions, we have found in our series of 231 space occupying lesions of the orbit that eye-motility nerve lesions mainly occur in tumors of the dorsal tip of the orbit or near the orbital part of the optic nerve channel as well as near the superior orbital fissure below the sphenoid ridge (Table 1, Pt. 3).

Clinical and neuroradiological diagnostic measures are summarized in Tables 1 and 2.

If the tumor has invaded the muscle cone and nerve elements, the prognosis of function recovery is uncertain or even poor (Table 3). On the other hand, if the tumor causes only displacement of structures, there is hope of functional recovery if microsurgical preparation and isolation of nerves and tendinous insertion is

Table 1. Clinical symptomatology of intraorbital lesions

1 – Unilateral exophthalmos sometimes combined with conjunctival hyperemia and/or chemosis	
2 – Dislocation of the bulb	– lateral – medial – above – below
3 – Diplopia – Motility dysfunction of N. III, IV, VI	
4 – Intraorbital resistance in bulb palpation	
5 – Visual dysfunction	

Table 2. Neuroradiological diagnostic of orbital lesions

1 – Native X-ray	– soft tissue mass – arrosion, destruction of bone walls – bone sclerosis or elucidation (atrophy) – dilatation of the optic canal
2 – X-ray tomography	– more precise identification of bone lesions
3 – Carotid angiography	– Ophthalmic artery, tumor enhancement – Displacement in intracranial lesions
4 – Orbito phlebography	– Characteristic displacements of the superior ophthalmic vein
5 – Subtraction technique by Ziedses des Plantes	
6 – CT – gives best information about *site, size, nature* and *relation to the neighbouring structures* of the lesion	

Table 3.

Prognosis of function recovery of N. II, III, IV, VI the better the more the tumor causes *dislocation* than *invasion* of periorbit and posterior muscle cone within the dorsal tip of the orbit!

Table 4. Symptomatology – M. of the cavum Meckeli and tentorial edge

Characterized by the short distance between the clinoid and the anterior end of the petrous bone (incisural margin):			
Gassero-petrosal tumors		partly supratentorial partly infratentorial	
Homolateral trigeminal paresthesia			N. V
Homolateral oculomotor paresis (ptosis, diplopia)			N. III, IV, VI
Later followed by dysfunction of			N. VII, VIII
Facial paresis, tinnitus, nystagmus, ataxia			
– Cerebello pontine angle syndrome –			
– Brain stem compression –			
Surgical risk	– ICA	supraclinoidal part infraclinoidal-extradural part	
	– PCA, PComA, asca, aica, basilar A.		
	– cavernous sinus, brain stem, BE		
	– opening sphenoid sinus		

successful (Figs. 1, 2, 3, and 4) *. This is the reason why we perform such an extended resection of the surrounding bone of the orbit, as described in the previous paper 'Optic nerve compression by meningiomas'. This means, it is advisable to resect not only the orbital roof but also the lateral and dorsal wall of the orbit as well as the sphenoid ridge, and, if necessary, the anterior clinoid process. The optic nerve channel may be opened, as mentioned before. Furthermore, this extended bone resection enables an optimal overview to be obtained for micropreparation. The larger the tumor, of course, the greater the difficulties in preserving visual and motility function (Figs. 5, 6, and 7)*.

The tumors of the medial part of the middle fossa, compressing the cavernous sinus and the oculomotor, trochlear, and abducens nerve present their own problems (Fig. 8). Tumor compression of the cavernous sinus is followed by congestion of the venous drainage of the orbit with a more or less severe exophthalmos (Fig. 9). In these cases, the visual and eye-motility function can mostly be preserved after removal of the tumor and decompression of the cavernous sinus.

On the other hand, if tumor has invaded the nerve elements, and has caused severe dysfunction or paresis of the nerves, tumor removal is mostly followed by permanent nerve lesion. Of course, there are particular surgical risks if the vessels of the arterial circle of Willis are involved (Table 4).

---

* Figures see separate part at the end of contribution

Surgical Technique

Starting with meningiomas of the sphenoid ridge 'en plaque' which mainly cause compression of the cavernous sinus and serious exophthalmos, we choose a lateral frontotemporal approach. In the first step, the operation is performed extradurally and the sclerotic bone and the bone invaded by tumor masses are resected as far as possible (Fig. 3) in order to preserve the nerve elements and vessels (Fig. 9).

In meningiomas of the inner third of the sphenoid ridge or in meningiomas of the clinoid process, we prefer to approach the tumor in a similar way. This means that in the first step we approach the tumor matrix by an extradural route and resect the sphenoid ridge as far as possible. The aim is to resect as much as possible of the tumor infiltrated bone to diminish the vascularization of the intradural part of the tumor and to attempt a mobilization of the tumor mass.

In a second step, the intradural part of surgery follows. If the extradural part of the intervention has succeeded well, then the intradural part of surgery is facilitated, enabling better isolation of the vessels affected by the tumor. These can be more easily isolated from the periphery to the supraclinoid part of the internal carotid artery or vice versa (Figs. 10, 11, 12, and 13).

To summarize, I should like to point out some banal but essential principles of surgery:

- a sufficient overview may be half the operation
- encircling the tumor mass is under most circumstances the safest measure for its careful and complete removal
- always seek the simplest procedure with the highest effect
- do not hesitate to combine various approaches in *one* procedure
- minimization of surgical risk in elderly patients
- continued consultation of colleagues from neighboring disciplines.

The computer tomograms were kindly made available by Professor Wende, Mainz

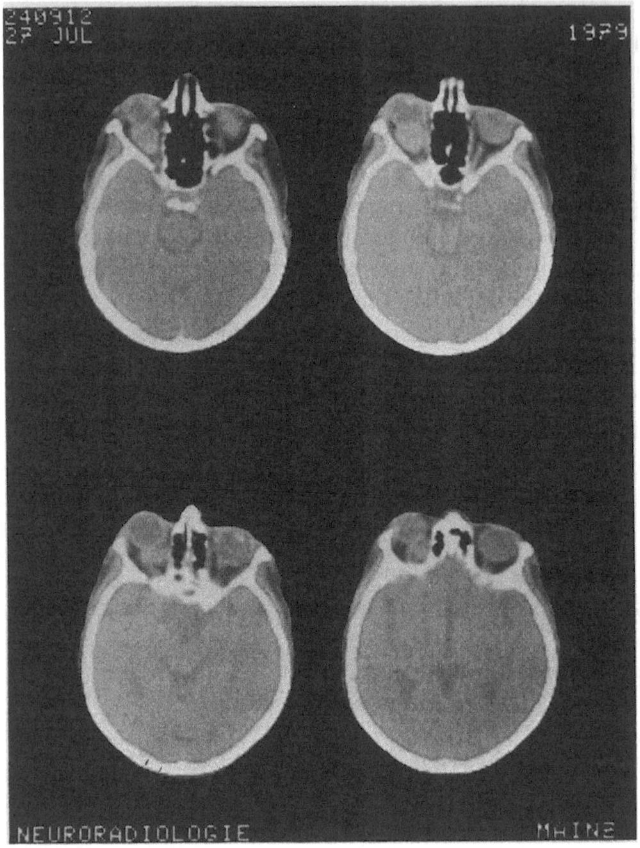

Fig. 1. Axial cranial CT of a 67 year old lady with a hemangioma within the left orbital cavity with tumor extension into the posterior cone of the orbit, but only causing an outside compression and displacement of the muscle cone and nerve elements. Total recovery of nerve function after transcranial removal

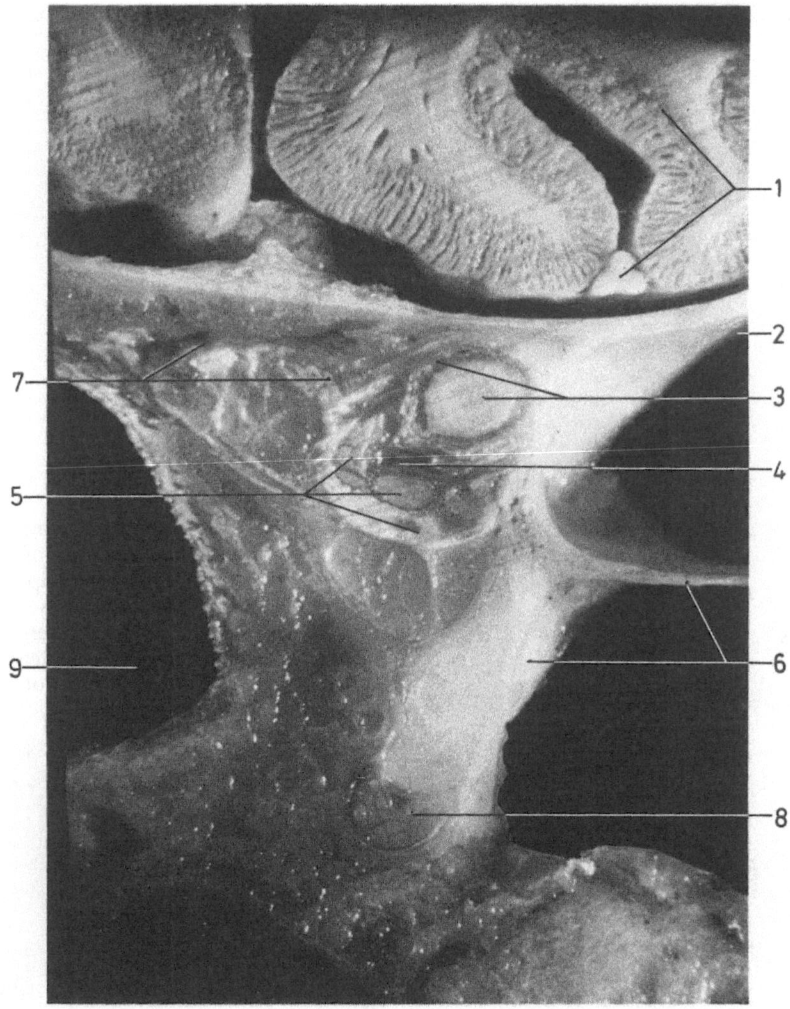

Fig. 2. Anatomical frontal section at the level of the posterior cone of the right orbit. One can realize without difficulties that a space occupying lesion invading the inner circle of the tendinous ring results in a more severe nerve lesion than a process which causes only a displacement from the outside (see text). (I am grateful to Prof. J. Lang, Würzburg, for providing the photograph.)

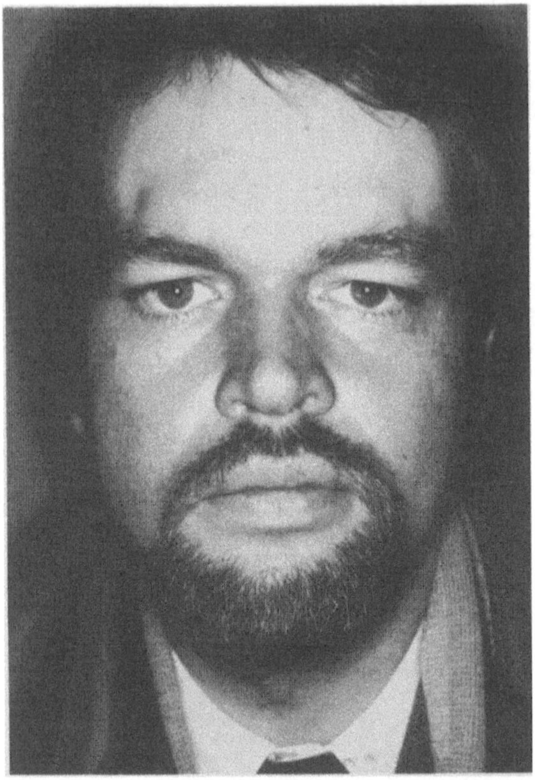

Fig. 3. 29 year old patient six months after total transcranial removal of a small hemangioma of the dorsal tip of the right orbit which caused only an external compression of the posterior muscle cone with the nerve elements situated inside. Complete functional recovery

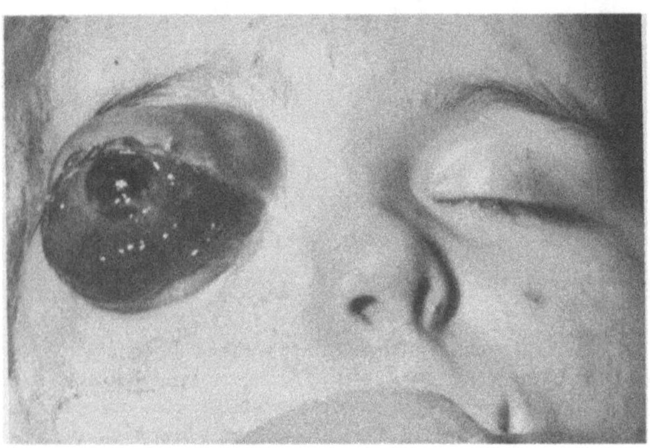

a

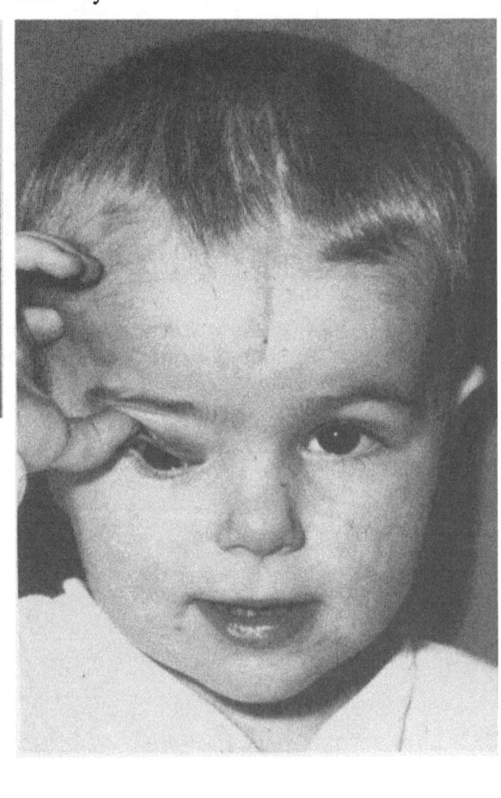

b

Fig. 4 a. 4 year old girl with an extreme exophthalmos, chemosis and N. III, IV, and VI paresis caused by a large hemangioma within the posterior muscle cone and inside of the tendinous ring. **b** The same girl six weeks after transcranial total removal of the tumor. Permanent paralysis of eye motility

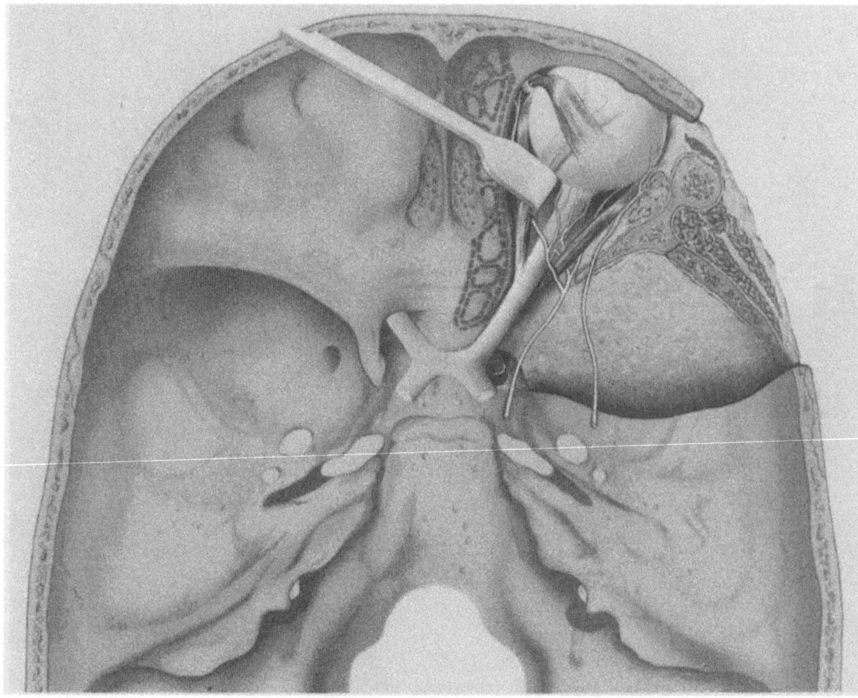

Fig. 5. Extended transcranial approach with resection of the orbital roof, lateral orbital wall and sphenoid ridge in order to obtain an optimal survey, especially of the structures of the posterior cone of the orbit

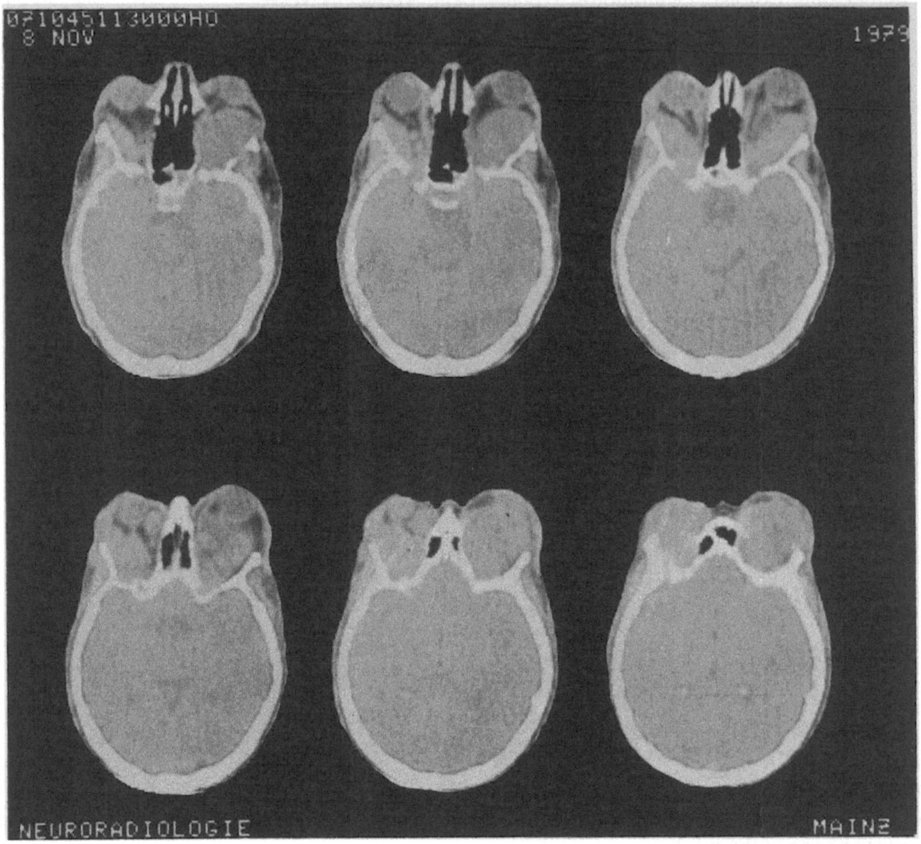

a

Fig. 6 a, b. A 34 year old female patient with a history of Morbus Recklinghausen, with multiple generalized neurofibromas, here bilateral within the orbital cavities. The case history goes back about 17 years. The present bilateral exophthalmos started about 8 to 9 years ago on the right side. During the last four years, a simple orbitotomy was carried out 8 times by an ophthalmosurgeon with an eyebrow skin incision with partial removal of the anterior pole of the tumor mass for 'decompression'. The process proceeded up to the present state shown in the picture (Figs. 6 and 7). Meanwhile the tumor growth proceeded on the left side too. *CT.:* **a** and **b.** Cranial CT in horizontal and coronal sections. Multiple tumor masses within the parasinuses, both orbital cavity as well as along the skull base. Total tumor tamponade of the maxillary sinus with destruction of the anterior maxillary sinus wall. Partial involvement of the ethmoidal cells, total tumor tamponade of the sphenoid sinus with destruction of the right wall. The base of the right middle fossa also shows a bone defect with multiple small tumors. Furthermore, two small tumor nodes in the prepontine cisterna. The largest tumor masses are to be found within the orbital cavities, on the right more than on the left. Elongation of the optic nerves. Bone destruction of the median and lateral orbital wall. Tumor extension bilaterally within the middle fossa

---

Fig. 7 a, b. The same patient as in Fig. 6: **a** Pre-operative state: *right eye:* extreme exophthalmos, dislocation of the bulb anteriorly, laterally and downwards, slight vascular congestion, ophthalmoplegia, blindness. – Hypesthesia in the first and second branch of the trigeminal nerve. *left eye:* exophthalmos, slight congestion of the conjunctive vessels, slight ptosis, motility of the bulb reduced. Visus reduced to 1/35 (9%), concentrical narrowing of visual field to 9°. **b** State six weeks after bilateral surgical removal in two sessions with an interval of 3 weeks. The first operation was done on the left side in order to preserve visual function. Transcranial surgery was done by a very extended transcranial approach, described

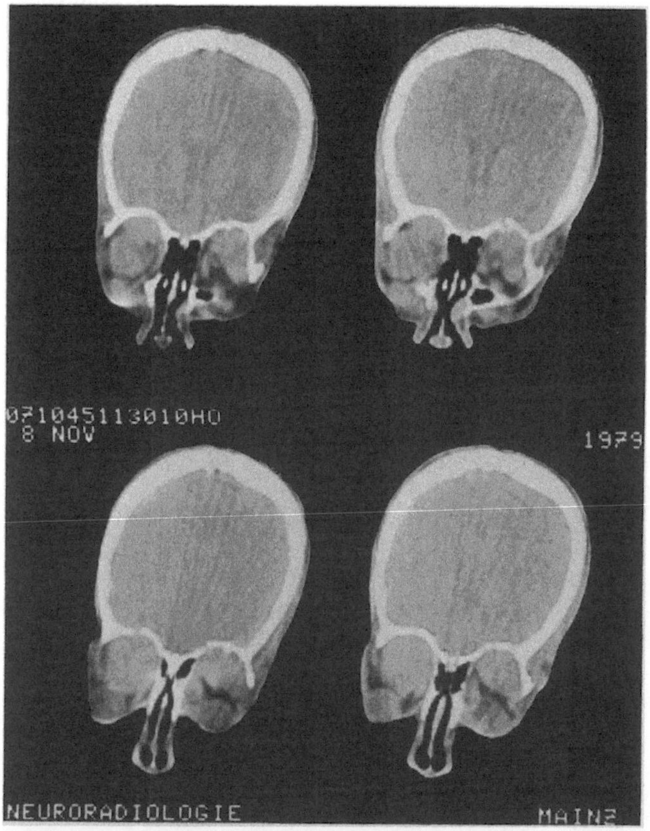

Fig. 6b

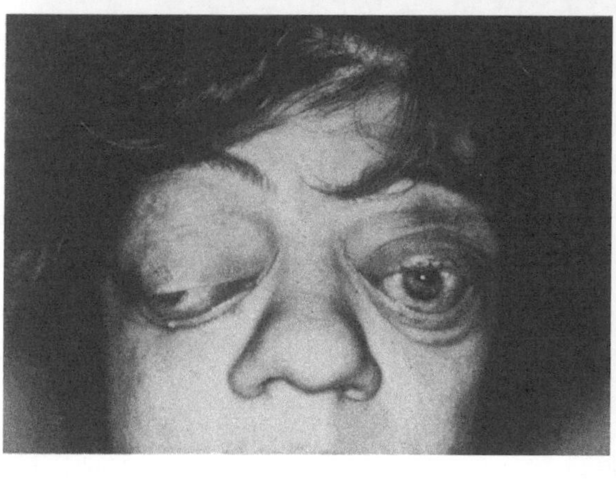

a

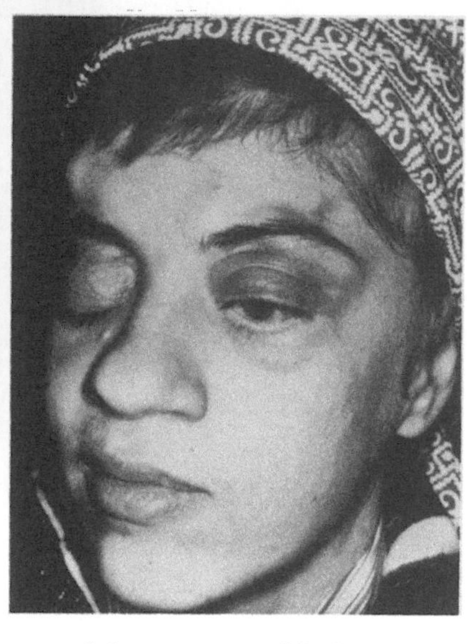

b

Fig. 7a, b

in Fig. 5. Good recovery. *Right eye:* exophthalmos disappeared, but permanent blindness and eye motility paralysis remained. *Left eye:* exophthalmos disappeared, a slight ptosis remained unchanged. However, eye motility and visual function were ameliorated. Visus left: 1/35 (9%), concentrical narrowing slightly wider. In a third stage of surgery, the tumors of the maxillary sinus, sphenoid sinus and ethmoidal cells were removed by the ENT surgeon (Prof. Helms) three weeks after transcranial surgery

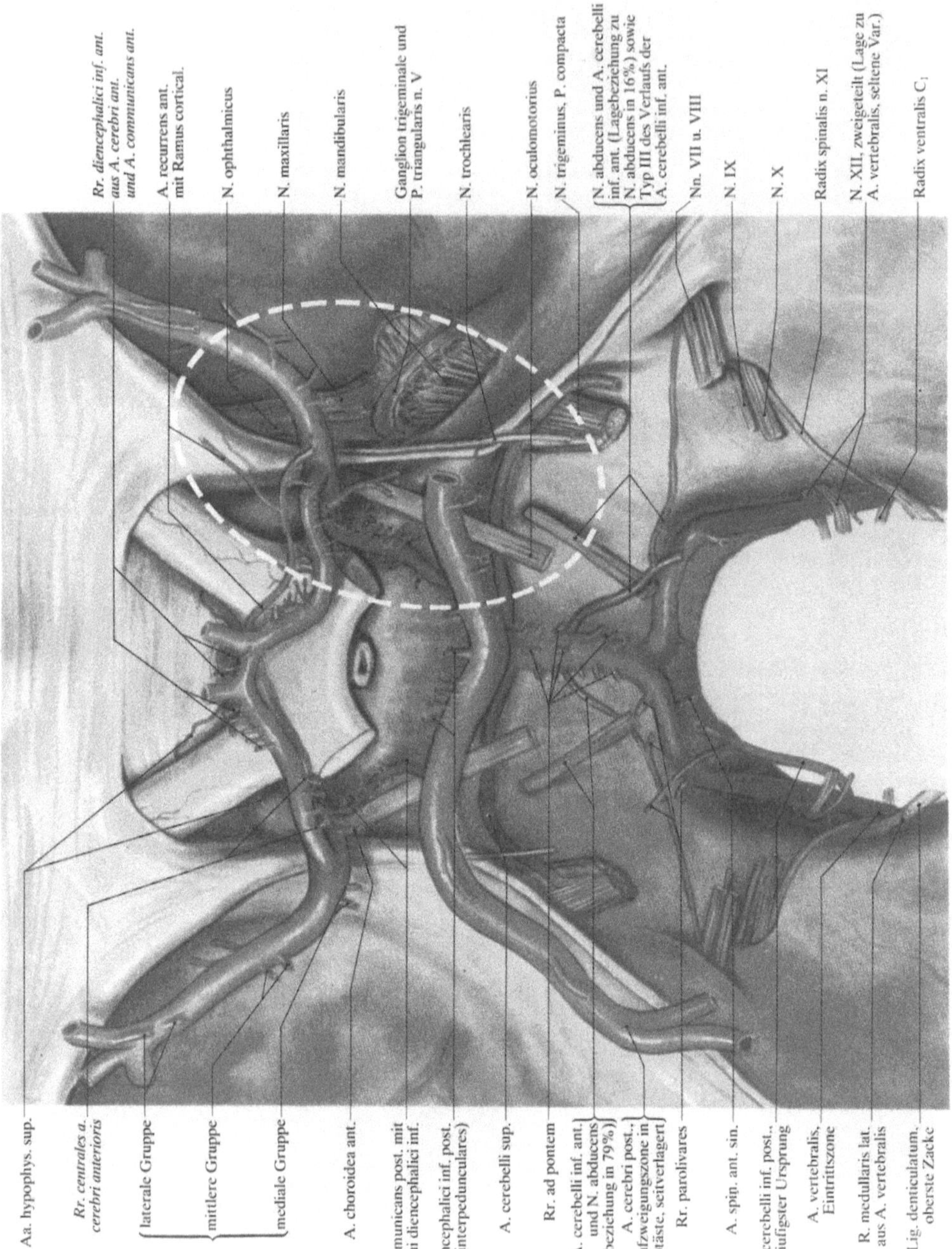

Fig. 8. Anatomical situation of the median part of the middle fossa with the close relation of N. II, III, IV, V, VI and the important vessels. (From T. v. Lanz, Wachsmuth and J. Lang, „Praktische Anatomie", Vol. 1, Kopf, p. 115, Fig. 50, Springer, Berlin Heidelberg New York, 1979)

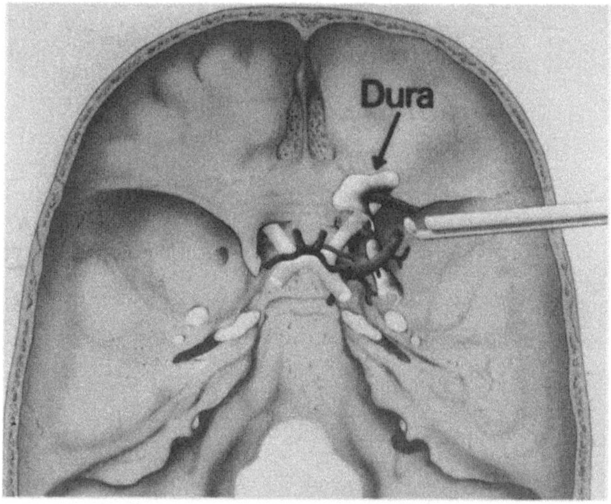

a

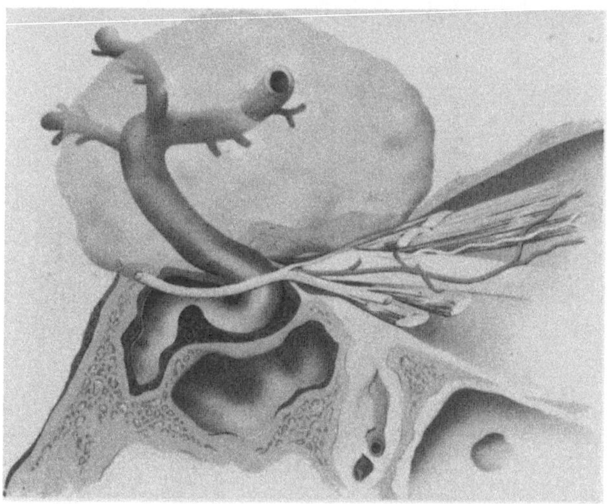

b

2nd step = intradural part of surgery

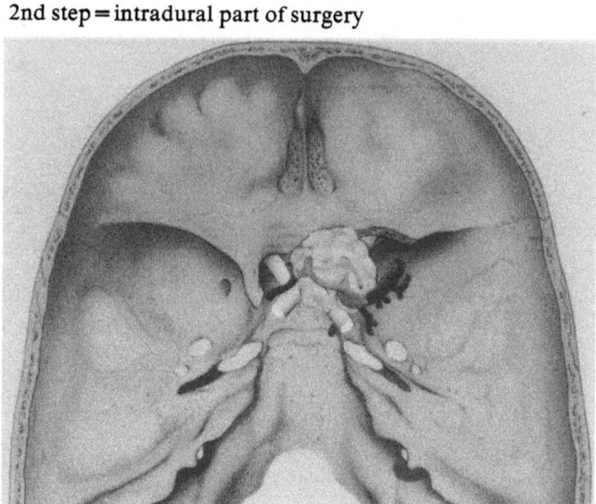

c

Fig. 10 a–c. Preferred surgical technique for the removal of meningiomas of the inner third of the sphenoid ridge, particularly if the tumor has encircled the supraclinoidal part of the internal carotid artery and its main branches, the middle and anterior cerebral artery (see text). **a** In the first step, the dura of the anterior and middle fossa and of the sphenoid ridge and also of the tumor matrix are liberated from the bone as far as possible. **b** lateral view, **c** in the second step, the intradural part of surgery follows with isolation of the tumor involved arteries from the distal periphery to the supraclinoidal part of the internal carotid artery or vice versa

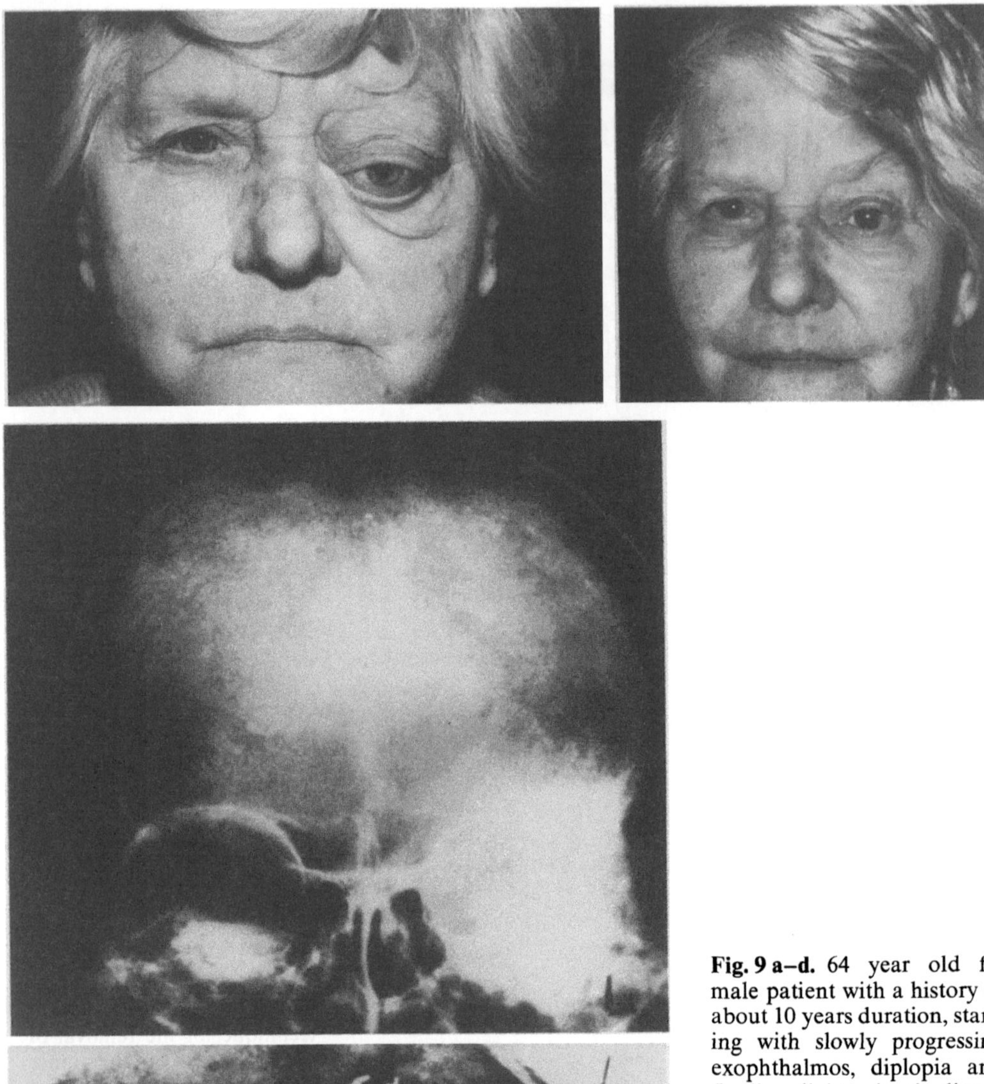

a b c d

Fig. 9 a–d. 64 year old female patient with a history of about 10 years duration, starting with slowly progressing exophthalmos, diplopia and finally slight visual disturbance. Neuroradiological diagnosis: meningioma 'en plaque' of the left sphenoid ridge. **a** preoperative state **b** postoperative state, nearly full recovery after two years. **c** the same patient, *preoperative* X-ray findings: severe bone sclerosis of the orbital roof, the lateral and dorsal wall of the orbit, the sphenoid ridge including the anterior clinoid process. **d** The same patient, *postoperative* X-ray examination: total removal of the tumor and the tumor invaded bone, including the anterior clinoid process and opening of the optic nerve channel

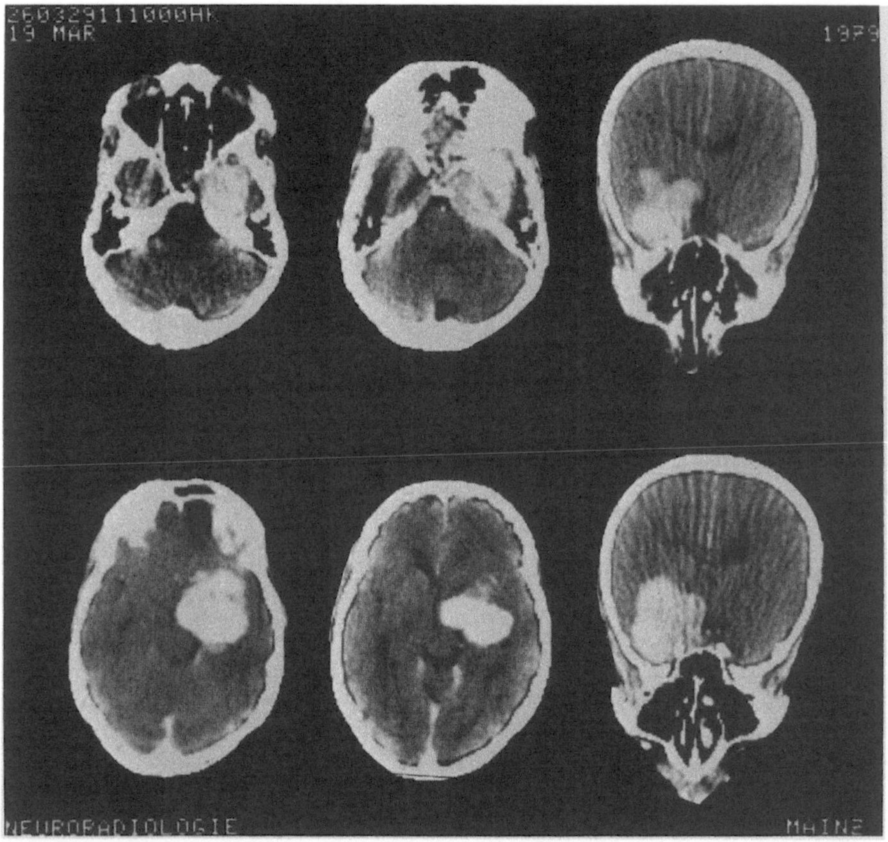

Fig. 11. Cranial CT of a 35 year old patient with a large meningioma of the inner third of the right sphenoid ridge and clinoidal process

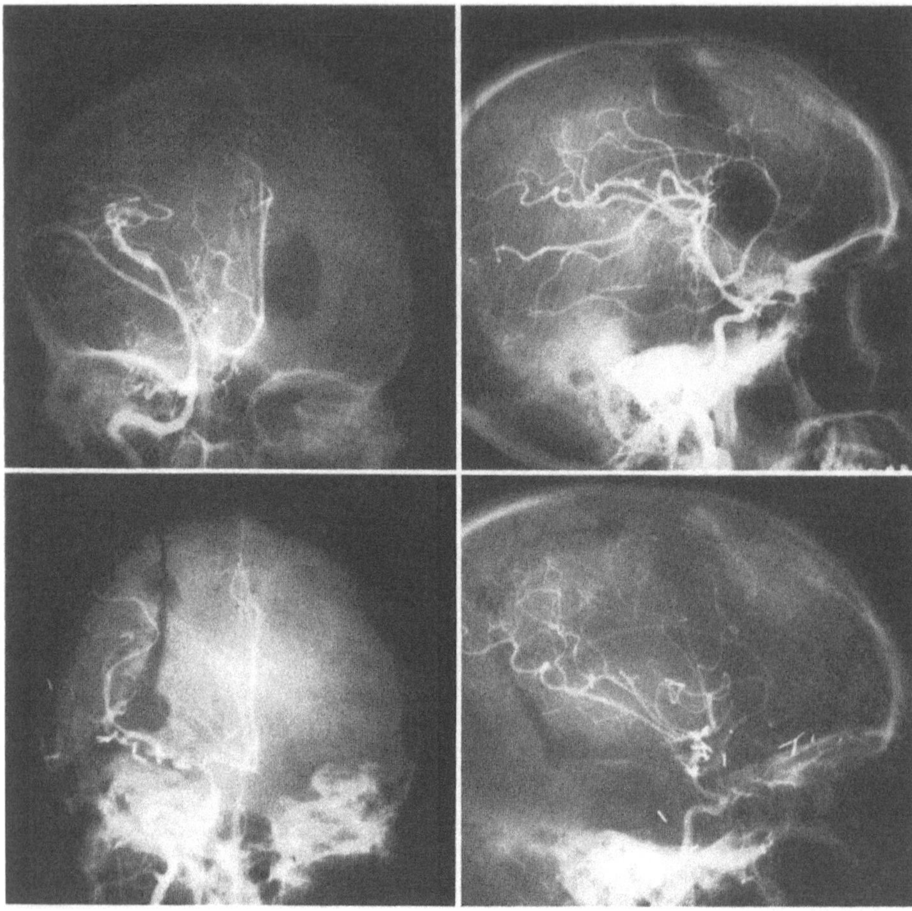

a b c d

Fig. 12 a–d. The pre- and postoperative angiogram of the patient with the large meningioma of the inner third of the right sphenoid ridge. Total removal and preservation of the main vessels succeeded

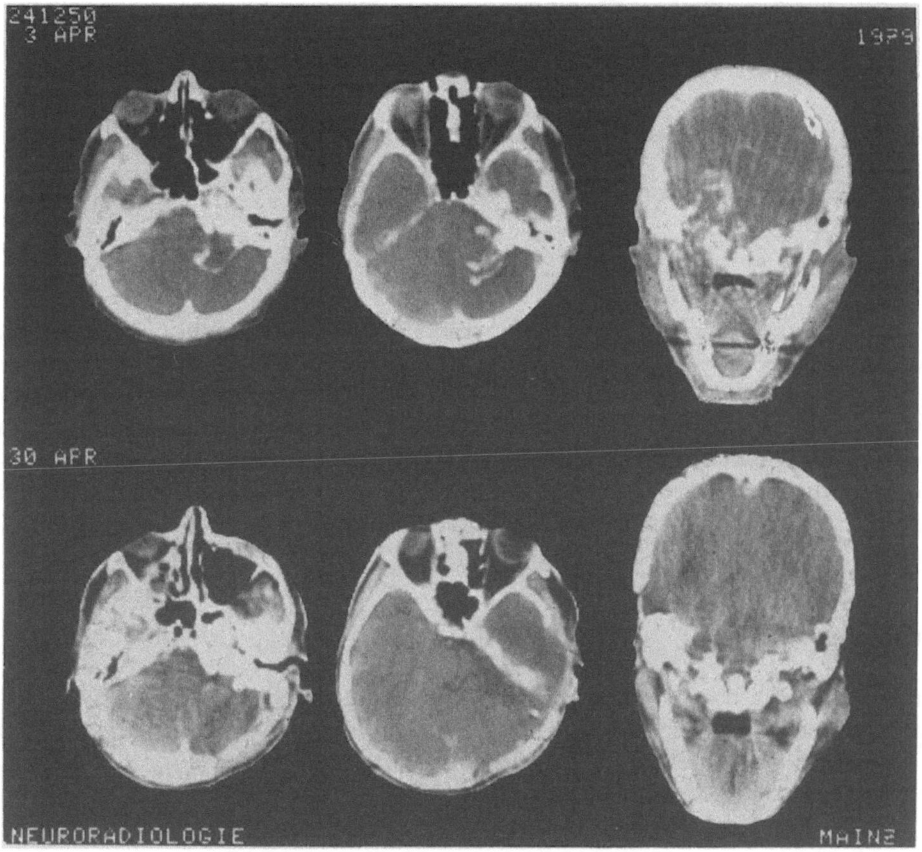

Fig. 13. Cranial CT of a 29 year old male patient with a history of about 10 years duration. Onset with headaches, diplopia (N. VI paresis), paresthesia of the right face (N. V – hypesthesia right), slight facial nerve paresis right (N. VII), hypacousia (N. VIII) and slight N. IX, X, XI paresis. N. XII without affection. *Upper row:* preoperative CT shows a large partially calcified tumor mass within the skull base of the middle and posterior fossa, which also causes a petrous bone destruction and a large intracerebral extension. *Lower row:* post-operative CT shows the successful removal of the large mass. Amazingly, nearly full recovery of the cranial nerve pareses with the exception of the 8th cranial nerve, the cochlear and vestibular parts of which were totally destroyed

Paralysis of the Extraocular Muscles in Tumors of the Sella Turcica Region

M. Schäfer, W.-I. Steudel, and H. Grau, Frankfurt/FRG

Introduction

Palsies of extraocular muscles in sellar tumors are only rarely observed, in contrast to disturbances of visual acuity and the visual field (Walsh 1956, 1969, Symonds 1962, German 1964). As a rule, they depend on parasellar spreading of the tumor (Cairns 1938, Weinberger et al. 1940, Nicola 1972). Computerized tomography (CT) has proved reliable in the diagnosis of hypophyseal processes (Kazner 1978) especially when there is parasellar spreading. The clinical findings are compared with the CT result in eight patients who had sellar processes with ocular muscle disorders.

Material

In the investigation period from June 1974 to December 1979, 112 patients with sellar processes (98 adenomas and 14 craniopharyngeomas) were examined and operated on. There were eight patients with extraocular muscle disorders. CT was performed with the Siretom I (matrix 128 × 128).

Summary of Cases

The clinical results are shown in Table 1: the abducens nerve was affected four times, the oculomotor nerve twice and both nerves in one case; there was complete ophthalmoplegia in one other case. Three patients also had defects of visual acuity and visual fields.

Pituitary tumors with endocrine activity were present in four cases (three prolactinomas and one tumor producing HGH). There were hormonally inactive hypophyseal processes in three cases and one craniopharyngeoma. In four of these eight patients, the extraocular muscle paralysis resulted from a tumor recurrence. The first operation had been performed from two to eight years previously.

Computerized Tomography

Computerized tomography showed parasellar spreading of the tumor to the side of the extraocular muscle disturbance in seven cases (Fig. 1 a, b). No tumor could be demonstrated in the axial CT (Fig. 2 a) in only one patient with microadenoma in which an abducens nerve paresis appeared on the left in the fourth month of pregnancy (case no. 2). However, tomography of the sella revealed a marked excavation of the sellar floor on the paralyzed side (Fig. 2 b, c).

Table 1. Paralysis of the extraocular muscles in patients with a tumor of the sella region. PAL: Pituitary Anterior Lobe; PRL: Prolactin; CT: Computer Tomography

No.	Age Sex	Clinical findings	Endocrinolog. findings	Radiological findings	Histo-pathology	Surgery	Outcome
1	32 F	right N. III-palsy	PRL-excess; partial PAL-deficiency	sellar destruction; CT: right parasellar extension	chromophobe adenoma	transsphenoidal approach	complete recover
2	35 F	left N. VI-palsy; pregnancy	PRL-excess; normal PAL-function	unilateral excavation of sellar floor; CT: normal	chromophobe adenoma	transsphenoidal approach	complete recovery
3	33 F	left Nn. III and VI-palsy; bitemp. hemianopsia	PRL-excess; complete PAL-deficiency	sellar destruction CT: supra and left parasellar extens.	chromophobe adenoma	subfrontal approach	partial recovery
4	22 M	left N. VI-palsy bit. hemianopsia loss of vision	partial PAL-deficiency	small sella; CT: suprasellar tumor extension	craniopharyngeoma	subfrontal approach	complete recovery
5	43 F	left N. III-palsy	partial PAL-deficiency; hormonal substitution	CT: left parasellar tumor extension (recidiv)	chromophobe adenoma	left fronto-temp. approach	partial recovery
6	62 F	right ophtalmoplegia; N. V-palsy loss of vision	complete PAL-deficiency; hormonal substitutio	CT: tumor-recidiv supra- and parasellar (right)	chromophobe adenoma	subfrontal approach; invasive adenoma	no recovery
7	47 F	right N. VI-palsy	partial PAL-deficiency	enlarged sella; CT: supra and right parasellar extens.	chromophobe adenoma	subfrontal approach	complete recovery
8	23 M	left N. VI-palsy; acromegalic	HGH-excess; partial PAL-deficiency	marked sellar destruction; CT: intraparasellar tumor	acidophilic adenoma	transsphenoidal approach tumor bleeding	partial recovery

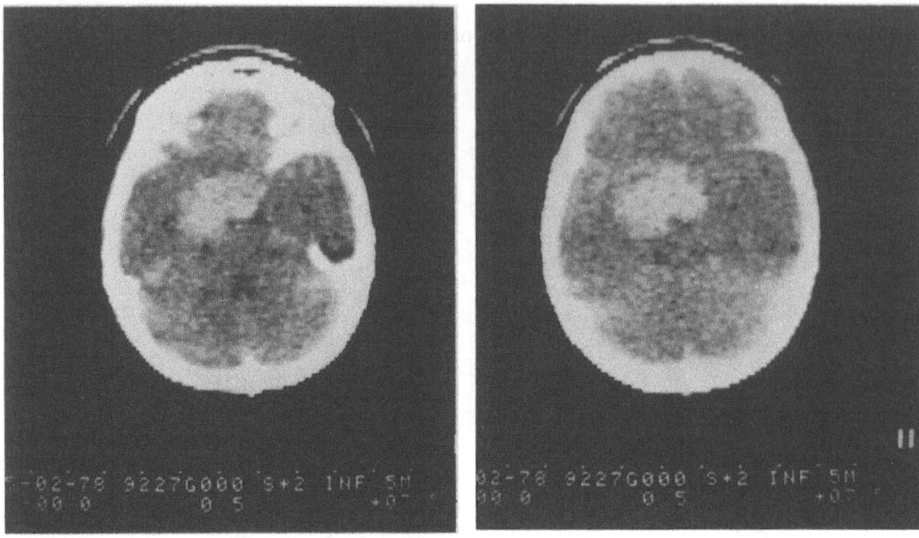

a b

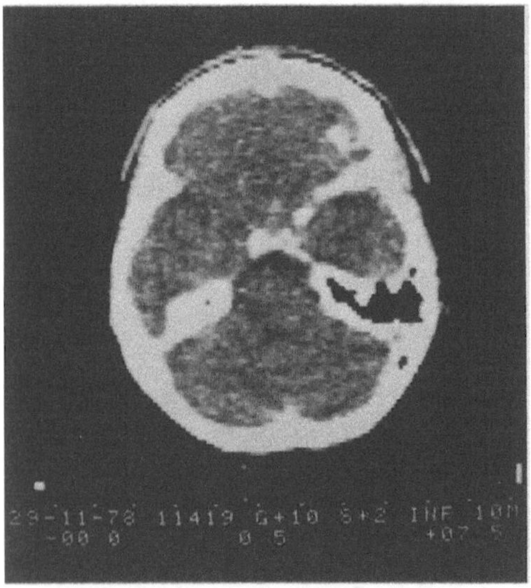

a

Fig. 1a, b. CT (with contrast medium) in a 33 year old patient with a left oculomotor and abducens nerves paresis: marked parasellar spreading of the tumor, especially on the left. After subfrontal surgery, regression of the oculomotor nerve paralysis and the visual field defect

Fig. 2a. CT (with contrast medium) in a 35 year old patient in the fourth month of pregnancy with a prolactinoma and an abducens nerve paralysis on the left; no definite tumor demonstrable. After transsphenoidal operation, regression of the abducens nerve paralysis

Fig. 2b, c. Tomography of the sella (lateral view) of the same patient with marked excavation of the sellar floor on the left

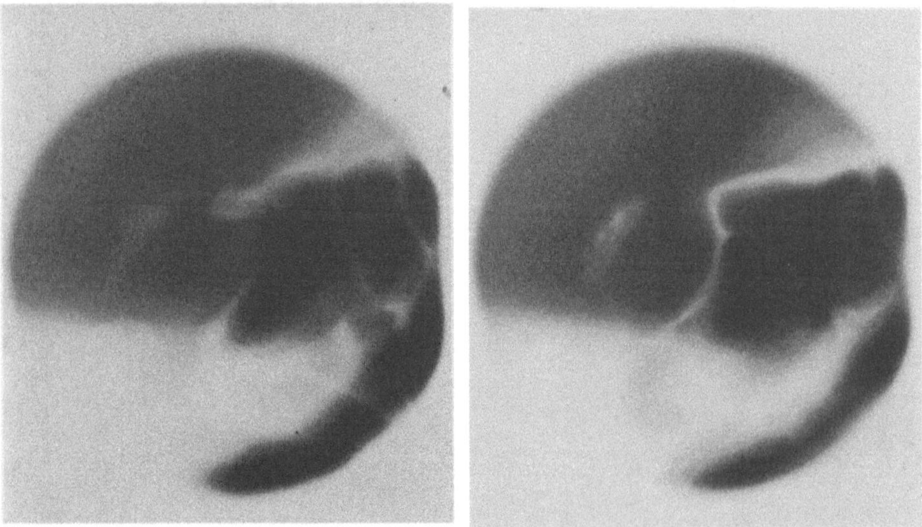

b c

Operation and Clinical Course

We operated via a subfrontal approach in four cases, via a transsphenoidal approach in three cases and a fronto-temporal approach in one case.

Complete regression of the extraocular muscle paralysis was shown in four cases, in two of these after a transsphenoidal operation. A partial recovery of the nerve paralysis occurred three times. A patient with ophthalmoplegia and trigeminal lesion with an extensive invasively growing adenoma showed no improvement.

Discussion

According to Weinberger et al. (1940) the sellar processes in extraocular muscle disorders can be divided into three groups:

1. those in which the nerves to the extraocular muscles and trigeminal nerve were variously affected without there being loss of visual acuity or visual field defects present;
2. those in which the muscle palsies were associated with evidence of chiasmal involvement;
3. those in which there was unequivocal evidence of an intrasellar lesion.

Our results support this suggested classification. In seven of our cases, an equivalent parasellar spreading of the tumor could be demonstrated as cause of extraocular muscle paralysis. Axial CT was negative in only one case, although X-ray tomography showed a clear unilateral excavation of the sellar floor on the paralysed side.

Pathogenetically, an extraocular muscle disorder in sellar processes is attributed to damage to the nerves in the region of the sinus cavernosus. Reference is therefore made to the sinus cavernosus syndrome (Weinberger 1940) or the wall of the sinus syndrome. The lesion is caused by direct ingrowth of the tumor into the sinus cavernosus (Jefferson 1940) or by pressure on the sinus wall (Weinberger 1940). Our results indicate that both mechanisms may come into play. In the patients with a parasellar spreading in the CT and a good postoperative regression of the paralysis, the damage is to be attributable to the effect of pressure on the sinus wall. In extensive invasively growing tumors as shown in the CT, without regression of neurological signs postoperatively, ingrowth of the tumor into the sinus cavernosus can be assumed.

Conclusions

Improvement of extraocular muscle paralysis in sellar processes can frequently be achieved by surgical treatment of the tumor. Analysis of CT-examination is most helpful in choosing the appropriate approach. In invasively growing sellar tumors, the extraocular muscle disturbance cannot be influenced by operation, although decompression of the optic nerves can be achieved.

References

Cairns H (1938) Peripheral ocular palsies from the neurosurgical point of view. Trans Ophthalmol Soc UK 58 (2): 464–482

Chamlin M, Davidoff L (1962) Ophthalmologic criteria in diagnosis and management of pituitary tumors. J Neurosurg 19: 9–18

Foix C (1922) Syndrome de la paroi externe des sinus caverneux. Rev Neurol (Paris) 29: 827–832

German WJ, Flanigan S (1964) Pituitary adenomas, a follow-up study of Cushing series. Clin Neurosurg 10: 72–81

Jefferson G (1940) Extrasellar extension of pituitary adenomas. Proc R Soc Med 33: 433–458

Kazner E, Fahlbusch R, Lanksch W et al. (1978) Computerized tomography in diagnosis and follow-up examination of pituitary adenomas. In: Fahlbusch R, Werder K (eds) Treatment of pituitary adenomas. Thieme, Stuttgart, p 101–114

Lyle TK, Clover P (1961) Ocular symptoms and signs in pituitary tumors. Proc R Soc Med 54: 611–619

Nicola G (1972) Transsphenoidal surgery for pituitary adenomas with extrasellar extension. In: Progress in neurological surgery, vol 6. Karger, Basel, p 142–199

Symonds C (1962) Ocular palsy as the presenting symptom of pituitary adenoma. Bull Hopkins Hosp 82: 72–82

Walsh FB (1949) Bilateral total ophthalmoplegia with adenoma of the pituitary gland. Arch Ophthalmol 42: 646–654

Walsh FB (1956) The ocular signs of tumor involving the anterior visual pathways. Am J Ophthalmol 42: 349–377

Walsh FB, Hoyt WF (1969) Clinical Neuroophthalmology, 3rd ed, Vol 3. Williams, Baltimore, p 2141–2143

Weinberger LM, Adler FH, Grant FC (1940) Primary pituitary adenoma and the syndrome of the cavernous sinus. Arch Ophthalmol 14: 1197–1236

N. VI Palsy in Cerebrovascular Disease

K. J. ZÜLCH, Köln/FRG

An interesting clinical symptom which I would like to discuss here is the involvement of the sixth nerve in cerebrovascular disease. I start the discussion with the history of a patient, aged 59, who was sent to a sanitorium for treatment of his transient ischemic attacks in the territory of the posterior cerebral artery (hemianopia) following cardiac insufficiency subsequent to enormous labile hypertension. One day coming back from a stroll he complained of double vision which was found to be caused by a unilateral sixth nerve paresis. When examined labile hypertension was again noted with extraordinary different values: namely, 220/120 supine, 160/95 sitting and 120/65 standing. This lability could not be sufficiently controlled by drugs and physical therapy. Finally, however, only by the adaptation of a sort of 'a space suit' which pressed mildly upon the lower half of the body a favourable result was achieved: This prevented the rapid fall of blood pressure in orthostasis. After the blood pressure values had normalized the abducens paresis restituted in the course of the following weeks.

A second case, to describe only a few of the many we have observed, was that of a policeman, aged 59, whose job was normally performed in working at a desk in an office. In a course for promotion the stout man was forced to perform physical exercise, which he had never done in recent years, and this for days. One morning during a lecture, one hour after the morning swim, he complained of double vision and subsequently he developed a progressive sixth nerve paresis. In hospital in the following week his mild cardiac insufficiency was treated and his defective brain circulation was supported. Then the double vision began to improve. Again the pathogenesis is not very clear.

Finally a patient aged 46 years with a labile blood pressure had the onset of a sixth nerve paresis suddenly within one day. He was found to have an old occlusion of the right internal carotid and the left vertebral arteries at clinical examination with angiography.

The latter case may give us some hint as to pathogenesis: Are the abducent nuclei in a zone particularly endangered in general circulatory insufficiency (see Fig. 342 of Salamon and Huang, 1976)? Let us say of the type of the endangering of the watersheds or the last fields? Perhaps enhanced in this case by vascular occlusions? But why then does this affect only the sixth and never the third nerve and why only unilaterally? In our third case this concept of the watershed zones has some support by the existing arterial occlusions. But what happens in the many others? Must there be a local stenosing process somewhere in the branches of the basilar or posterior artery supplying that region? I have to leave these questions open as yet and merely point to the fact that we had altogether 28 patients, all with cardiovascular insufficiency and usually labile hypertension.

A merely theoretical question arises at the end: Was this a clear cut abducent paresis or an internuclear paresis mimicing the first mentioned? In the internuclear paresis a nystagmus is obligatory according to the literature, which was lacking in all our cases. In the contrary in some of our cases a mild weakness of the peripheral facial nerve was present pointing to the nucleus of the sixth nerve as region of involvement, around which the facial nerve is sweeping.

Reference

Salamon G, Huang YP (1976) Radiologic Anatomy of the Brain. Spinger-Verlag, Berlin Heidelberg New York

Trigeminal Nerve

(Fifth Cranial Nerve)

Specialized Features of the Trigeminal Nerve and Its Central Connections

L. KRUGER and R. F. YOUNG, Los Angeles/USA

Introduction

The trigeminal nerve is the largest sensory nerve of most mammals. Its central projections dominate the somatosensory system, and trigeminal reflexes are the first to appear in fetal development. A comparison ot the trigeminal nerve with its spinal counterparts reveals a remarkable number of structural specializations which presumably reflect its distinctive functional role. It is the intention of this narrative to briefly survey features of the organization of the V. nerve, ganglion, root and its central brain stem nuclei with some emphasis on those characteristics that should be taken into account by the enlightened clinician.

Accordingly, we shall discuss the gross anatomy of the ganglion and root in terms of its relationships within Meckel's cave and with the petrous ridge and the carotid artery because these have been considered at various times to be possible factors in human trigeminal pathology. Although a review of the peripheral nerve divisions can be evaded due to its accessibility in numerous excellent textbooks, we shall consider the specialized sense organs (e.g. cornea and teeth), the unusual axonal composition, the organization of the Gasserian ganglion, the nature of the coalesced 'sensory' and 'motor' roots, the unique pattern of muscle receptor innervation, the nature of the 'glial dome' of the sensory root and its possible pathological ramifications, the central distribution of the sensory root, and shall conclude with a comprehensive discussion of the several brain stem nuclei in terms of their architecture, recent information concerning their connections, and the experimental and clinical bases for their functional subdivision. Much of the thrust of this review is to identify those areas of ignorance amenable to future investigative efforts.

Trigeminal Sense Organs

The sensory modalities subserving oral and facial function are more complex and specialized than in any other region of the body. In rodents, the complex 'sinus hairs' that serve as exploratory vibrissae are centrally represented (in thalamus and cortex) by a larger volume of neurons than all other structures combined. Reflexes associated with oral-facial receptor stimulation appear earliest in fetal development (Humphrey 1968) and all mammals appear to possess zones of dense cutaneous innervation within the trigeminal territory as might be expected from the large size of the V. nerve compared with other sensory nerves.

Although the receptor population displays essentially the same varieties found in other regions of the body, two specialized structures receiving trigeminal innervation warrant special interest because of their role in pain – the cornea and the teeth. The innervation of the teeth consists principally of sensitive mechanoreceptors located in the periodontal ligament subserving a crucial role in regulating the force and direction of mastication. The function of nerves supplying the dental pulp remains an enigma, for removal of the pulp chamber contents, as commonly performed in modern endodontic procedures, results in no obvious deficit other than elimination of the excruciating pain that can be elicited when the pulp is exposed to any of a wide variety of stimuli that are usually innocuous when applied elsewhere. The enigma lies in the fact that dental pulp receptors appear to be excited only under pathological circumstances, for they are well protected by a dense crystalline coat of enamel. Although both myelinated and unmyelinated axons are present within the pulp chamber, the unmyelinated population must be largely involved in vascular innervation and it is likely that the myelinated axons subserve dental nociceptors whose afferents conduct impulse activity at relatively high velocity. This is most unusual, since the myelinated (delta) nociceptors of the skin differ in several ways including possessing high mechanical thresholds and receptive fields consisting of an array of focal 'pain spots' innervated by axons that penetrate into the basal epidermis (Burgess and Perl 1967, Perl 1968, Kruger et al. 1979). By contrast, the dental pulp nociceptors are activated by minimal mechanical, thermal or chemical perturbations and, when excited, result in a report of throbbing, 'slow' or prolonged pain. Electrical stimulation of the pulp has served as the major tool for studies of trigeminal pain mechanisms (e.g. Matthews 1977, Nord and Young 1975, Sessle and Greenwood 1976, Yokota 1976).

The cornea is also unique, constituting the only integumentary structure innervated solely by unmyelinated (C) afferents (Tower 1943). Although these receptors and the neurons upon which they project in the medulla respond to mild mechanical, thermal and chemical stimuli (Perkins 1961, Mosso and Kruger 1973, Nagano et al. 1975), their excitation results in a rapid 'corneal reflex' and reports of pain in humans; notwithstanding the dubious claim that other sensory modalities are also represented in the cornea (Lele and Weddell 1959) on the basis of human sensory reports. Another specialized feature of the corneal innervation is the invasion of terminals into the epithelial stroma (Hoyes and Barber 1977, Tervo et al. 1979).

Gross Anatomy

The trigeminal ganglion and proximal sensory and motor roots are enclosed in a dural envelope which forms Meckel's Cave. This complex rests in a groove, the trigeminal impression, on the cranial surface of the most medial end of the petrous portion of the temporal bone. Ventromedial to the ganglion, a thin plate of bone (which forms the floor of Meckel's Cave) separates the ganglion and proximal root fibers from the underlying internal carotid artery and the posterior part of the cavernous sinus. Kerr (1963 a) has demonstrated that the bony roof of the carotid canal is often absent and only a thin layer of connective tissue separates the ventral surface of the ganglion from the underlying artery (Fig. 1). Harris and Rhoton (1976) reported that the carotid artery was exposed under some portion of the ganglion, with only a connective tissue separation, in 84% of human cases. Kerr (1963 a) indicated that the relationship between ganglion, root and artery is such

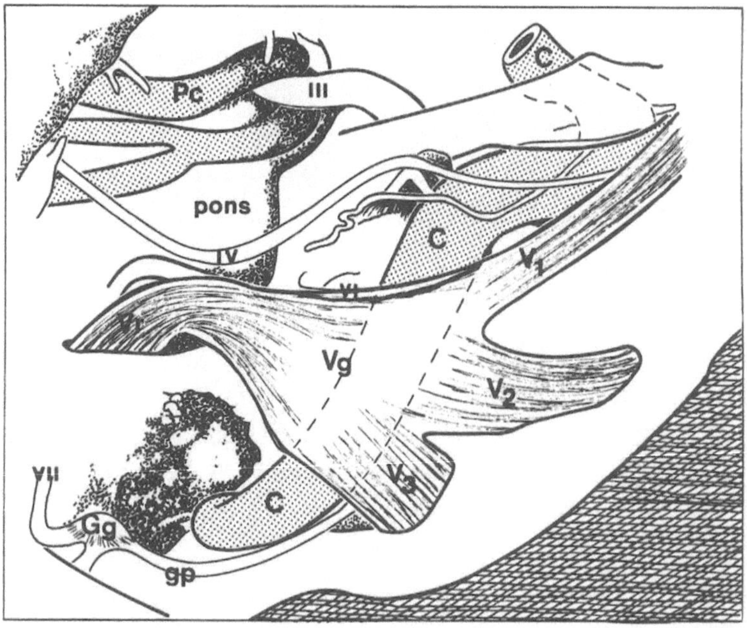

Fig. 1. Diagrammatic representation of gross anatomical relationships between the trigeminal ganglion (*Vg*), root (*Vr*), and the carotid artery (*C*). The petrous portion of the carotid artery (proximal interrupted segment) is inferomedial to the trigeminal root and ganglion and separated from the maxillary (V_2) and mandibular trigeminal (V_3) divisions by a thin plate of bone which is frequently absent, in part or completely. The absence of a bony separation allows direct transmission of arterial pulsations to the trigeminal ganglion through the underlying dura of Meckel's cave. Although the intracavernous portion of the carotid artery (distal to interrupted segment) is in close proximity to the ophthalmic division (V_1), direct transmission of arterial pulsations to the nerve is prevented by intervening venous blood within the cavernous sinus. *III* – oculomotor nerve; *IV* – trochlear nerve; *VI* – abducens nerve; *VII* – facial nerve; *Gg* – geniculate ganglion; *gp* – greater superficial petrosal nerve; *Pc* – posterior cerebral artery. (Drawing after Paullus et al. 1977, by permission)

that contact is possible only between the artery and second and third division fibers, since the first division is located within the walls of the cavernous sinus; the intervening blood acting as a cushion between artery and ophthalmic division. This relationship, particularly when the bony plate is absent, may lead to unintended injury to the carotid artery or cavernous sinus during middle fossa surgical procedures on the trigeminal ganglion or posterior root. Furthermore, Kerr (1963) proposed that prolonged pulsatile contact of the internal carotid artery with the adjacent ganglion and root might induce gradual trauma in the latter and thus might play a role in the etiology of the trigeminal neuralgia syndrome.

The greater superficial petrosal nerve also passes between the trigeminal ganglion and the underlying floor of the trigeminal impression. It is this relationship which results in facial palsy during trigeminal rhizotomy in the middle fossa when attempts are made to separate the dura propria of Meckel's Cave from the overlying temporal dura by blunt dissection. Anterior pressure during this maneuver places

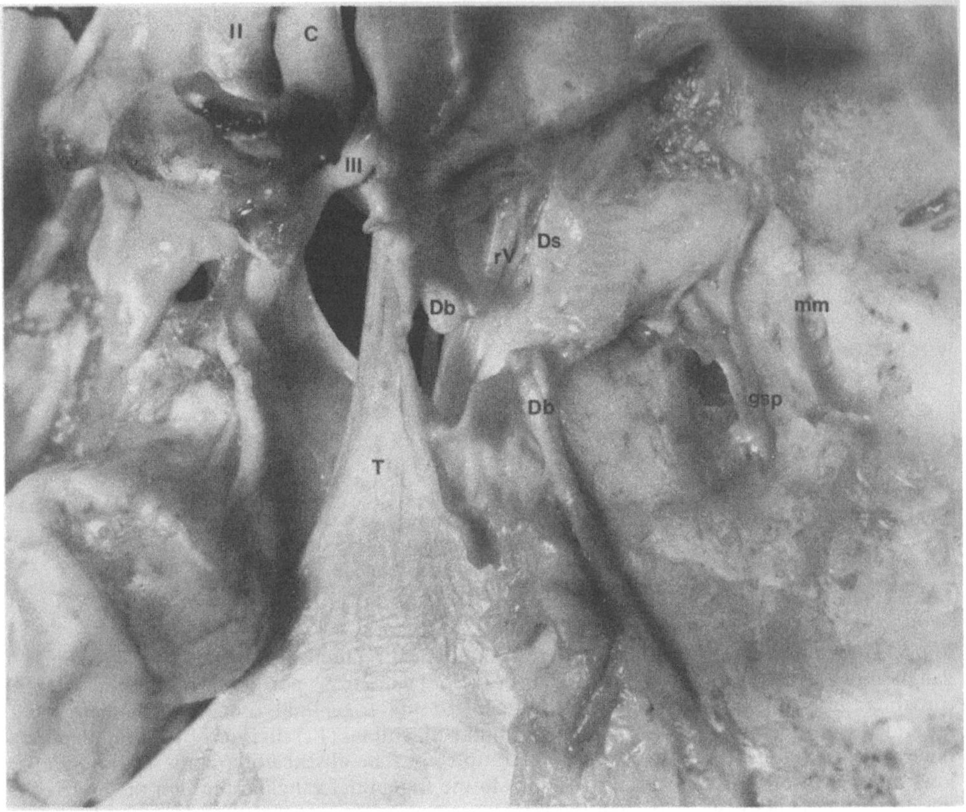

Fig. 2. Relationship between the trigeminal root (*rV*) and dural band (*Db*) which extends from the anterior clinoid process to the anterior surface of the petrous ridge lateral to its apex. In this photograph, the dural band has been transected to reveal the underlying trigeminal root angulated over the petrous ridge as it passes from the middle to the posterior cranial fossae. *Ds* – dural sheath of Meckel's cave; *T* – tentorium; *II* – optic nerve; *III* – oculomotor nerve; *gsp* – greater superficial petrosal nerve; *C* – carotid artery; *mm* – middle meningeal artery. (After Malis 1967, photograph courtesy of Dr. Leonard I. Malis)

traction on the greater superficial petrosal nerve and results in injury to the attached facial nerve near its genu. Such injury can be prevented by sharply incising the connection between the dura of Meckel's Cave and the greater superficial petrosal nerve.

As the sensory fibers pass from the fan-shaped portion of the root just posterior to the ganglion cells, they coalesce to form a flattened, fairly compact bundle with the motor fibers in a separate ventrally located band. As this complex proceeds posteriorly to pass from the middle to the posterior cranial fossa, it is closely confined between the ventrally located petrous ridge and the dorsally placed tentorial edge (Fig. 2). Significant angulation of the root normally occurs at this point and may be aggravated by aging as suggested by Lee (1937) and Olivecrona (1947). Gardner et al. (1956) demonstrated elevation of the petrous ridge and increased angulation of the trigeminal root with aging and suggested (Gardner and Pinto 1953) that compression of the root by this mechanism might be involved in the etiology of trigeminal neuralgia in some patients.

Malis (1967) demonstrated that the dura overlying the sensory root near the free tentorial edge is often specialized to form a separate band (Fig. 2). This band extends from the anterior clinoid process to the anterior surface of the petrous ridge lateral to its apex (Fig. 2) and it forms the roof of the canal which the root fibers traverse as they pass from middle to posterior cranial fossa. Malis (1967) suggested that with aging, as the petrous pyramid elevated, the angle of the dural band changed so as to compress the intervening trigeminal root fibers. He reported excellent results in the relief of trigeminal neuralgia by sectioning this dural band and suggested the band might be a significant factor in tic douloureux.

After entry into the posterior cranial fossa, the trigeminal root fibers pass unimpeded a distance of about 18–26 mm [mean 22 mm] (Gudmundsson et al. 1971) to enter the lateral surface of the pons approximately midway between its dorsal and ventral borders.

Trigeminal Root

The designation, 'trigeminal root', in this discussion will be used to indicate the entire fiber bundle which courses between the trigeminal ganglion and the pons. Classically, the trigeminal root has been divided into the portio major (or sensory root) and the portio minor (or motor root). Dandy (1929, 1932) and later, Jannetta (1967) described the so-called intermediate or accessory root, and Rand (1969) suggested the designation portio intermedia for these fibers. Although specific functional roles have been assigned to these subdivisions, recent evidence suggests that significant functional overlap occurs.

Portio Major

This largest division of the Vth root is identifiable immediately posterior to the Gasserian ganglion and passes to the lateral surface of the pons where the so-called 'fibrous cone' portion of the root is identified. This designation relate to the envelopment of the root at that point with a tough, presumably pia-arachnoidal, covering which clearly separates it from the portio minor and intermediate roots. Gross somatotopic representation of the three major peripheral trigeminal divisions is reasonably well maintained in the portio major, although significant rotational movement and overlap of one division may occur with respect to the others as fibers progress from peripheral to central (Gudmundsson et al. 1971). Specific somatotopic localization does not appear to be maintained within that portion of the portio major representing a particular division (Pelletier 1974), although fibers innervating a particular region do tend to group together. These aspects of somatotopic localization in the sensory root mirror the situation in the Gasserian ganglion. The varied patterns of sparing of facial sensation seen after partial rhizotomy of the portio major (Dandy 1929, 1932) are explicable in terms of the loose somatotopic organization and variable degree of rotation of the sensory root. Thus, a partial section of the root may spare part or all of a single division or, if appropriately placed (Pelletier 1974), spare portions of all three divisions or a variety of combinations of divisions. Since the second and third division fibers are most caudally located, partial root section via the posterior fossa most often results in sparing of sensory loss in the ophthalmic division territory (Dandy 1929). Contrary to Dandy's earlier reports of universal cure of tic douloureux with partial trigeminal rhizotomy, a significant failure rate is seen with this procedure and there is evidence (Otenasek 1971) that Dandy himself abandoned it in favor of complete root section.

Afferent fibers within the portio major comprise the usual spectrum of afferent fiber sizes seen in spinal dorsal roots. Fiber counts in man by Sjoqvist (1938) revealed 140,000 sensory root fibers, but later counts by Belyaev (1963) showed wide variation of myelinated fiber composition; from 76,842 to 150,079 in the sensory root. Recent studies utilizing the electron microscope reveal approximately 125,000 fibers in the human trigeminal sensory root of which about 50% are myelinated (Young 1977) – see Figure 3. Examination of the fiber composition with modern methods suggests that the composition of the roots must be re-evaluated for at least two principal reasons: 1. The gross underestimation of unmyelinated axons in all portions that has been detected with electron microscopy (Young and King 1973, Young 1977) and 2. recent evidence suggestive of 'sensory' fibers in the 'portio minor' (Young and Kruger, in prep.) homologous with the known sensory fibers of spinal ventral roots (Dimsdale and Kemp 1966, Kato and Hirata 1968, Clifton et al. 1976).

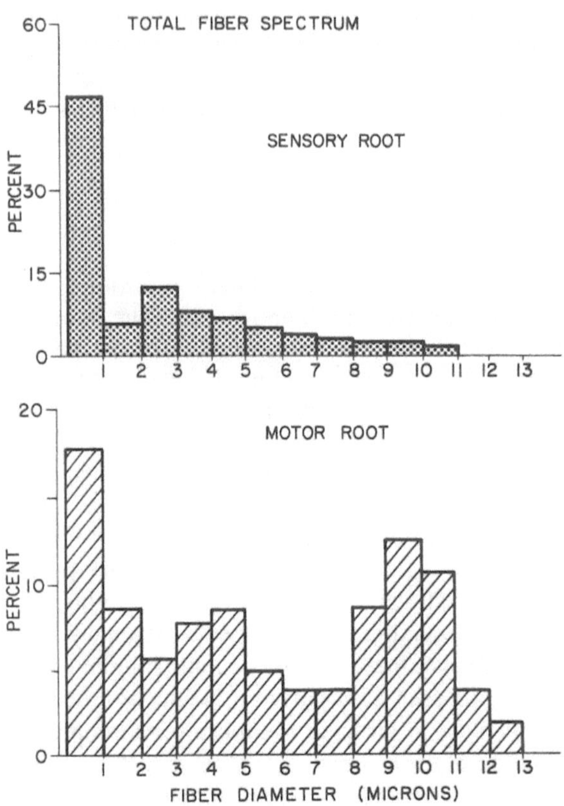

Fig. 3. Fiber spectrum of the human trigeminal motor and sensory roots determined by electron microscopy. All fibers in the size range 0–1 μ and 50% of those in the range 1–2 μ are unmyelinated. (After data from Young 1977 and Young and Stevens 1979)

The proportion of unmyelinated or C-fibers in the trigeminal portio major is considerably reduced compared to dorsal roots, representing about 50% of the total in the former (Fig. 3) and about 80% in the latter in primate, including man (Young and King 1973, Young 1977). This deficiency is compensated for by an increased proportion of medium and large caliber myelinated fibers in the portio major. The functional significance of this difference is unknown. It may be related to the exclusive occurrence of the peculiar pain syndrome of trigeminal neuralgia in the Vth nerve (Darian-Smith 1970) but may also relate to phylogenetic and developmental differences between the spinal and trigeminal roots (Young 1977). Additionally, because of the tapering of axonal diameter (Gerard 1923, Kerr 1966), loss of myelin sheath (Kerr 1966), and slowing of conduction velocity (Wall and Taub 1962) which occurs as primary afferents descend in the spinal V tract, the differences in proportion of unmyelinated fibers in spinal and trigeminal roots is of uncertain significance. Many of the fibers which are myelinated in the trigeminal root, taper and lose their myelin sheath as they descend in the spinal trigeminal tract. It is therefore difficult to correlate the findings relating sensory modality to conduction velocity in cat hindlimb nerves directly to the trigeminal nerve which has not been intensively studied from this point of view. At least one indication of specialization in the trigeminal system can be found in the large diameter myelinated axons innervating the presumptive nociceptors of the dental pulp.

Fibers of the sensory root were believed to bifurcate, as described by Cajal (1911), with a thin ascending branch to the principal nucleus and a thick branch entering the spinal tract that tapers caudally as it innervates various sectors of the spinal nuclei. The search for non-bifurcating root axons to explain the segregation of 'pain' and temperature from tactile modalities could only be identified in fetal and newborn Golgi preparations (Windle 1926), and the possibility of focal nuclear projections has long been doubted. Our recent experience with HRP labeled root fibers suggests that many axons descend without emitting a separate branch to the principal nucleus and this opinion has recently been elegantly and convincingly demonstrated by the intra-axonal labeling of vibrissal afferents by Hayashi (1980).

Although the portio major is usually presumed to be the exclusive route of trigeminal primary afferent fibers, the results of apparent complete transection of the portio major contradict this idea. Dandy (1929) demonstrated that sparing of touch, temperature and occasionally pin-prick sensation was possible over large portions of the face after apparently complete section of the portio major. He also indicated that recurrence of trigeminal neuralgia rarely, if ever, recurred after this procedure in spite of significant sensory sparing. He suggested that the portio major subserved fibers for facial pain perception only and that fibers for innocuous facial sensation traveled in the intermediate root. Recent physiological comparisons of function of the portio major and intermediate root, however, do not support this hypothesis (Pelletier et al. 1974).

Portio Minor

Peripheral axons from motor neuron somata in the trigeminal motor nucleus extend to the muscles of mastication via the portio minor or motor root. The portio minor exits the pons 0.5–4 mm rostral to the portio major (Gudmundsson et al. 1971) and takes a

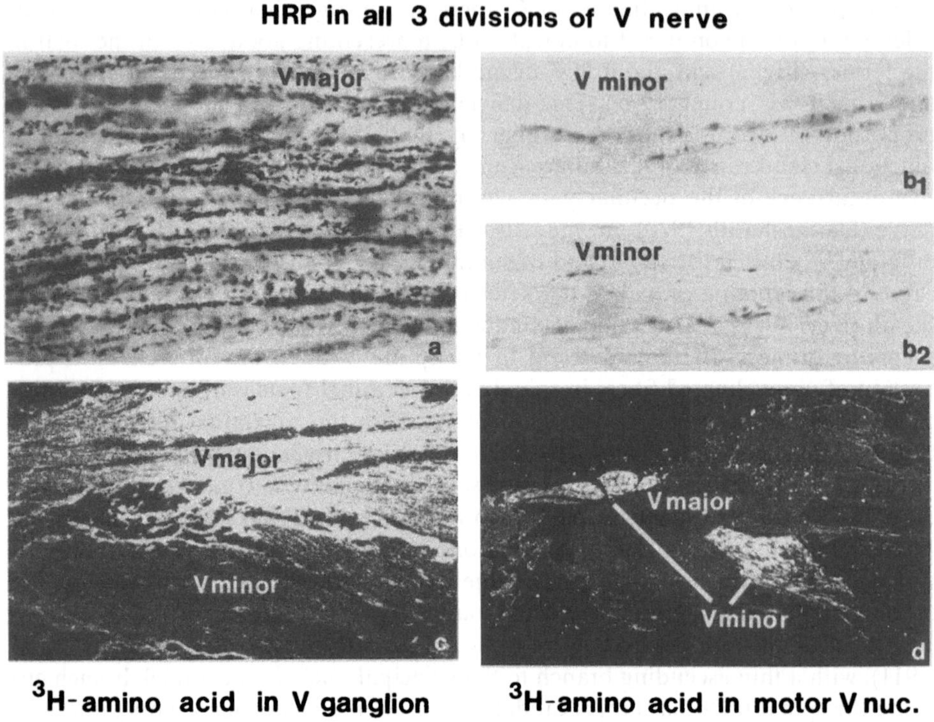

Fig. 4. Labeled axonal transport in the trigeminal root. Exposure of all three divisions of the trigeminal nerve to a solution of horseradish peroxidase (HRP) for 48 hours results in extensive ganglion cell and axonal reaction product in the portio major of the root (a), and a few scant labeled axons in the portio minor (b 1 and 2) suggestive of possible afferent fibers in the 'motor' root. Injection of ^{3}H-leucine and ^{3}H-proline into the Gasserian ganglion results in massive labeled axonal protein in the portio major or 'sensory' root, as expected, and minimal label in the portio minor (c), although apparently above background level in this autoradiograph. Injection of the same radioactive amino acids into the region of the motor nucleus of V results in labeled anterograde transport into the portio minor (d), running diagonally beneath the unlabeled portio major

course diagonally across the ventral aspect of the latter to pass medial to the Gasserian ganglion and join the mandibular division for distribution to the muscles of mastication. The root usually arises from 4–14 separate bundles or rootlets near the pons which join as they run medial and ventral to the ganglion to form a single motor root (Gudmundsson et al. 1971).

Sjöqvist (1938) estimated 8,100 fibers in the human portio minor and later, Belyaev (1963) estimated the myelinated fiber composition to vary from 6,348 to 14,601. Both of these studies utilized the light microscope. Utilizing the electron microscope, estimated total fiber counts of 3,140 to 7,462 have been obtained (Young 1979, Young and Stevens 1979) with 80–88% being myelinated (Fig. 3). The number of neurons in the motor nucleus of V varies from 4,128–11,820 with a coefficient of variation of 28.6% for ten cases (Blinkov and Gleser 1968), thus providing little indication of whether all motor root myelinated axons are derived from motoneurons.

The portio minor has been commonly designated functionally as the motor root and considered to subserve only that function. Several clinicians have suggested a possible sensory function for the portio minor to explain persistent facial sensation after complete section of the portio major (Horsely et al. 1891, Dandy 1929, Adson 1969, Gudmundsson et al. 1971). Pelletier et al. (1974) have demonstrated afferent activity within the portio minor of the Macaque monkey in response to jaw movement or mechanical distortion of the ipsilateral masseter or temporalis muscles. Gudmundsson et al. (1971) identified anastomatic connections between the portio major and portio minor in 47 of 50 human nerves they examined. Electron microscopy has revealed up to 20% of fibers in the human portio minor are unmyelinated and potentially sensory in function (Young 1978). In addition, HRP, applied to exclusively cutaneous trigeminal branches, has been identified in axons of the portio minor in cat, confirming the presence of afferent fibers in this division of the V root (Young and Kruger, in prep.) – see Figure 4. The portio minor, therefore, cannot be considered exclusively motor in function, although the contribution of this root to facial sensation under normal circumstances or after rhizotomy of the portio major is unknown. These relationships in the trigeminal portio minor invite comparison to spinal ventral roots where 13–51% of axons are unmyelinated (Coggeshall et al. 1975) and where both myelinated and unmyelinated axons subserving a sensory function have been physiologically identified (Dimsdale and Kemp 1966, Kato and Hirata 1968, Clifton et al. 1976). It has likewise been suggested that afferent fibers in spinal ventral roots may be responsible for persistent sensation and failure of pain relief after dorsal spinal rhizotomy (Coggeshall et al. 1975). The variability of afferent axon passage from sensory ganglia to central nervous system suggests that in both the spinal nerve system and trigeminal system, the terms 'motor root' and 'sensory root' with specific functional connotations must be applied cautiously.

Intermediate Root

The intermediate or accessory root comprises a variable number of fine bundles – 0–8 (Gudmundsson et al. 1971) – interposed between the portio major and minor. At least one such bundle was identified in 26 of 50 nerves studied by Gudmundsson et al. (1971). The course, termination, and function of nerve fibers composing such bundles is controversial. Most often intermediate rootlets occur as several strands originating from lateral pons parallel to the portio major but not within the fibrous cone which encloses the latter. Most frequently they join the portio major within 12 mm of the pons. In other instances, however, such fibers run from the ganglion to the portio minor or from portio major to minor (Fig. 5). The fiber composition of the intermediate root is unknown since it has apparently never been subjected to light or electron microscopic examination. Pelletier et al. (1974) indicated that the functional characteristics of intermediate fibers were not different from those of portio minor fibers and subserve either pure motor function or could be activated by jaw movement. Sachs and Saunders (1970) had previously reported that fibers passing from ganglion to portio minor or portio major to minor subserved only a motor function. Their conclusion, however, was based solely on gross anatomical features. The recent description of unmyelinated afferent fibers in the portio minor suggests

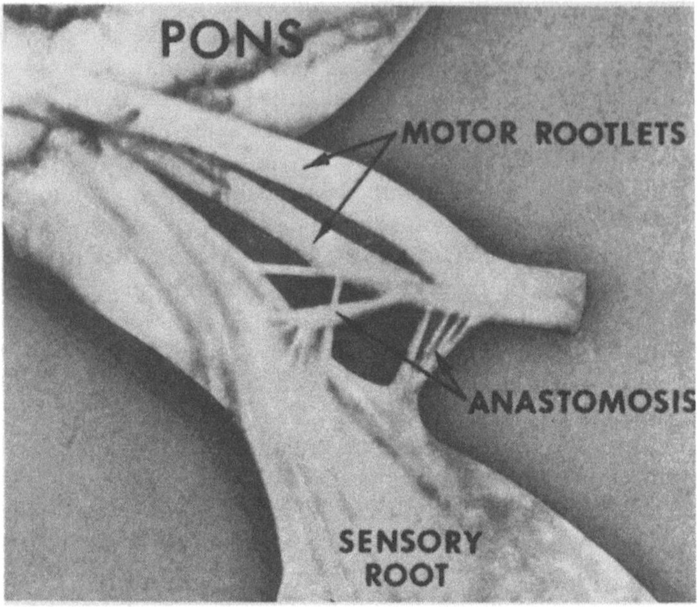

Fig. 5. Anastomotic (intermediate or accessory) fibers between the human motor and sensory trigeminal roots. (From Gudmundsson et al. 1971, by permission)

that such fibers may originate in cell bodies of the Gasserian ganglion and gain access to the portio minor via the anastomotic accessory rootlets. Such afferent fibers coursing to the V brainstem nuclei either directly via the accessory root or via connections between the accessory roots and portio minor most likely explain the preservation of facial sensation seen after 'complete' section of the portio major. Since root electrical impulse activity (Pelletier et al. 1974) is biased in favor of large fiber recording, electrophysiological studies do not exclude a cutaneous sensory or nociceptive function for fine unmyelinated intermediate root fibers which might enter the brainstem via the portio minor. There is no anatomical nor physilogical evidence, however, to support the idea that the afferent fibers in the accessory root subserve a specific sensory modality to the exclusion of other modalities (Dandy 1929, Rand 1980). In summary, intermediate rootlets likely subserve several functions. Some are surely motor fibers separated in part or all of their course from the portio minor. Others are likely sensory fibers separated from the portio major and either enter the brainstem separate from the main sensory root or connect and intermingle with motor fibers in the portio minor. Some of these subserve a proprioceptive function related to jaw or muscle movement and some likely serve a cutaneous sensory function.

Gasserian Ganglion Organization

Even the name of the trigeminal or semilunar ganglion is rather unique for it bears the eponym of Johann Ludwig Gasser, who was not the discoverer but for whom it was named by his admiring student, Anton B. R. Hirsch (1765). The sensory ganglion of the V. nerve is roughly divisible into three major regions associated with each of the main peripheral divisions (Kerr 1963b) and this somatotopic pattern has been confirmed by electrophysiological studies (Kerr and Lysak 1964) although discontinuities in the sequential pattern were observed. A similar pattern of unexpected discontinuities has been noted in experiments in which ganglion cells were retrogradely labeled by applying HRP to individual peripheral nerves. This shows that the neurons supplying each nerve branch are broadly distributed and, rather surprisingly, are separated by substantial number of unlabeled neurons, thus confirming the puzzling pattern of somatotopic discontinuities found in electrophysiological studies. We have noted a similar pattern in spinal ganglia and the geniculate ganglion (after tongue injection) and therefore assume that this is a general rule for sensory ganglia. This 'distributed' arrangement rather than a sharp segregation, which is also reflected in the sensory root, might account for the successful preservation of tactile sensation and corneal reflexes following partial rhizotomies in man (Walker et al. 1956, Jannetta 1967)

Retrograde labeling of the ganglion from the central axons of the sensory root is more homogeneous and complete, but a similar pattern of patchiness can be discerned with retrograde labeling following HRP injection into the separate sectors of the sensory V nuclear complex (Fig. 6). The proportion of labeled cells projecting to

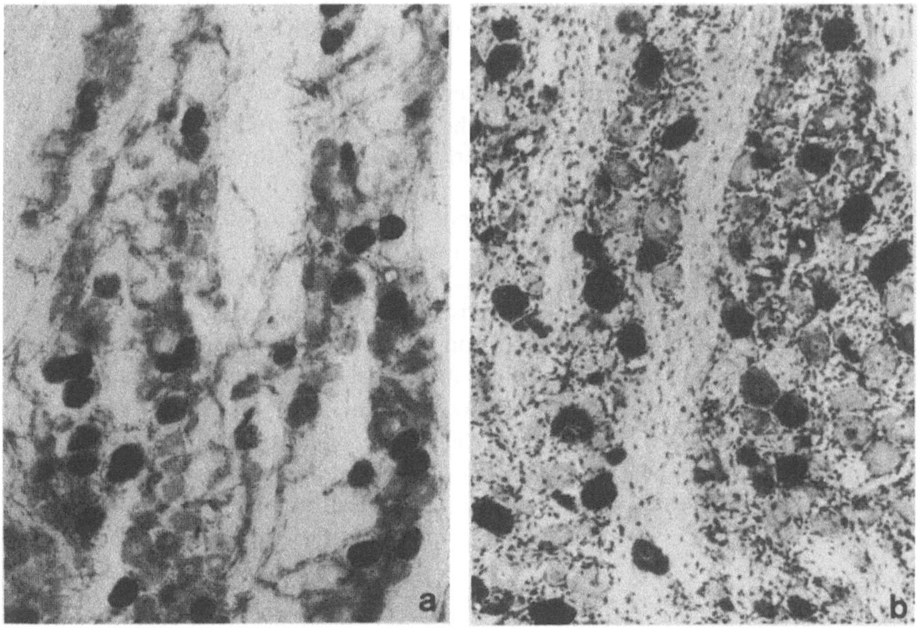

Fig. 6 a, b. Retrograde transport of horseradish peroxidase (HRP) to cat trigeminal ganglion cells following injection of HRP into the principal V nucleus (**a**) and subnucleus caudalis (**b**) revealing non-segregated labeled ganglion cells (black reaction product) among cells that project to other sectors and a lack of ganglion cell size selectivity for each projection. Reaction product is tetramethylbenzidine (**a**) and o-dianisidine (**b**). × 85 the principal V nucleus does not appear to exceed those to subnucleus caudalis and both projection zones receive input from large and small ganglion cells. Differences in nuclear volume and the uncertainties associated with estimating the extent of the enzyme uptake zone preclude reliable quantitative comparisons with this method.

The labeling of Gasserian ganglion cells by injection of tritiated amino acid precursors to protein synthesized in these cells enables tracing of the afferent fibers beyond the roots, into their terminal zones. Thus an anatomical definition of the total sensory V nuclear complex may be secured by normal axonal transport method for comparison with degeneration studies which were based on silver impregnation following root section. The results of such experiments provide an impressive picture of the entire sensory complex (Fig. 8) and present few surprises. They essentially confirm the findings of degeneration studies and the basic architectonic description of the separate components but with sufficient detail to allow photographic illustration at low magnifications.

The Central Peripheral Transition Zone

The lamina cribrosa through which cranial and spinal nerves emerge to form the peripheral nervous system constitutes the 'fibrous cone' of gross anatomical descriptions (Dandy 1932, Jannetta and Rand 1966). Fine structural analysis reveals that the 'glial dome' junction consists of an astrocyte layer with its basal lamina similar to the astrocyte-basal lamina complex at the subpial-brain surface (Maxwell et al. 1969). The axonal transition from peripheral to central myelin occurs at the node of Ranvier (Fig. 7) where the myelin-forming cell changes from Schwann cell to oligodendrocyte. Tarlov (1937) suggested that the transitional lamina or dome was an oligodendrocyte partition, but in the electron microscope, it is evident that astrocyte processes predominate in the central portion of the root (Maxwell et al. 1969).

The occurrence of tumors of cranial nerves is remarkable for its selectivity, being confined primarily to sensory nerves. However, despite the high incidence of Schwannomas found in the VIII. nerve, such tumors are comparatively rare in the trigeminal. Furthermore, some tumors arise from the Gasserian ganglion (Russel and Rubinstein 1977) whereas tumors of other cranial nerve ganglia are extremely rare. It is conceivable that gangliogliomas arising from the trigeminal ganglion are related to the 'islands' of astrocytes (Maxwell et al. 1969) invading the primate Gasserian ganglion and thus account for one peculiarity of V. nerve tumors. Accounts of V. nerve Schwannomas (often designated by other names), fail to provide a clue for explaining the difference in incidence between V. and VIII. nerve (Jefferson 1955, Olive and Svien 1957, Schisano and Olivecrona 1960, Russel and Rubinstein 1977).

The Brain Stem Trigeminal Nuclear Complex

The size, extent and complexity of the nuclei associated with the trigeminal exceeds that of all other cranial nerves, and several aspects of its subdivision remain un-

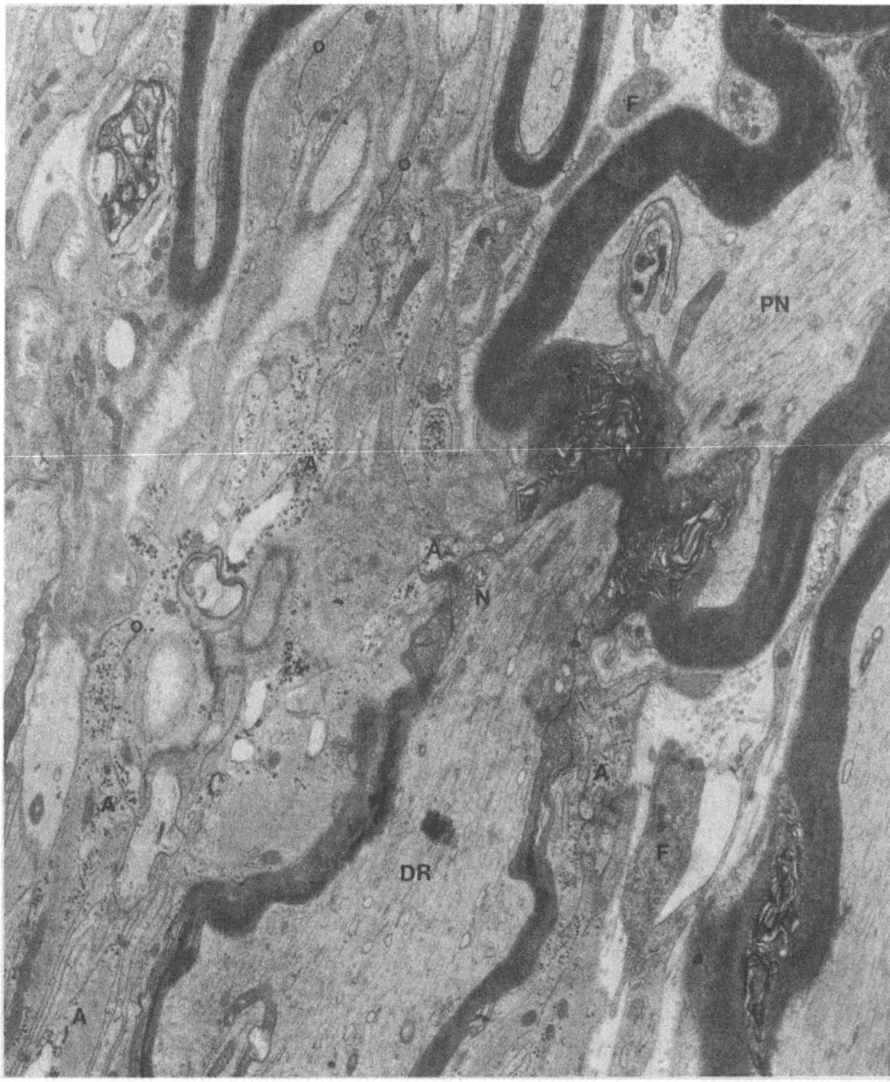

Fig. 7. An electron micrograph of the monkey Gasserian ganglion displaying the glial 'dome' transition from central nervous system (*above*) to peripheral nervous system (*below*), occurring at a node of Ranvier (*N*). Note the diminution in thickness of the myelin sheath as it extends from peripheral to central and the widespread distribution of glycogen-containing astrocyte (*A*) processes displaying numerous zonula occludens (*o*) junctional complexes. The penetration of astrocyte processes among the fibroblasts (*F*) of peripheral nerve extends into the region of ganglion cells. × 14,000 (Modified after Maxwell, Kruger, and Pineda 1969)

resolved. Additionally, the assignment of homologies with precision and clarity has not yet been achieved; thus requiring a description of each component and the pertinent evidence for relegating each to a distinct functional entity.

The sensory trigeminal complex is generally recognized to include the main or principal sensory V nucleus and its extensive caudally contiguous spinal nucleus, the latter commonly divided into subnuclei oralis, interpolaris, and caudalis. In one respect at least, the principal and spinal V nuclei deserve a single functional status because all components serve as recipients of sensitive cutaneous mechanoreceptor inputs from all three trigeminal nerve divisions. Two additional sensory components, the elongate mesencephalic V nucleus and the supratrigeminal nucleus of Lorente de No (1922), apparently lack cutaneous input, but are activated principally by muscle spindle and periodontal ligament afferents suggestive of a proprioceptive function, although each is quite distinct in other important respects (Jerge 1963 a, b). Finally, and perhaps least controversial is the motor nucleus of V, the homolog of the ventral horn of the spinal cord containing the neuron cell bodies of the efferent fibers entering the portio minor of the trigeminal root ultimately to innervate the masticatory musculature.

The supratrigeminal nucleus deserves special consideration although it has often been recognized as only a dorsomedial component of the contiguous principal V nucleus. Its position, at the caudal termination of the mesencephalic V nucleus suggests an involvement in 'proprioceptive' function and this is supported by electrophysiological findings of muscle spindle, articular and periodontal receptor input (Jerge 1963 b). However, recognition of this nucleus may have been obfuscated by a dorsomedial tactile component of the principal V nucleus (Kruger and Michel 1962 a, c) largely devoted to representation of oral structures and which is also known to project upon the ipsilateral thalamus from the study of anterograde and retrograde HRP transport. Separation of the dorsomedial tactile component of the principal V nucleus from the supratrigeminal 'proprioceptive' nucleus is nicely illustrated by Mizuno (1970) and because of its position between the main sensory, motor, and mesencephalic V, it is sometimes called the 'intertrigeminal' nucleus (Taber 1961).

A massive projection to the cerebellum would secure the assignment of the supratrigeminal nucleus as the homologue of the external cuneate nucleus, but retrograde labeling of HRP after large injections of cerebellar cortex is rather sparse (Watson and Switzer 1978, Somana et al. 1980) and apparently does not exceed the projection from the interpolar or principal V nuclei. We are thus forced to the conclusion that the main muscle spindle afferent nucleus and its cerebellar projection remains to be firmly established and that the functional status of the supratrigeminal nucleus remains uncertain, although it may represent a 'proprioceptive' aggregation of 'interneurons' as suggested by Torvik (1957) and Jerge (1963 b). Unfortunately, distinguishing between 'interneurons' and 'sensory neurons' requires establishment of rigorous critieria, but there is some electrophysiological evidence to suggest an 'interneuron' role (Kidokoro et al. 1968) that requires further study in terms of specific afferent supply.

The mesencephalic V nucleus is perhaps the simplest portion of the sensory nuclear groups because there is sound evidence that the neurons of this small, elongate nucleus are ganglion cells largely devoted to supplying the first-order afferents of muscle spindles. However, it can also be argued that it constitutes a most enigmatic specialization of the central nervous system when several details are taken into account. The most unusual feature is the presence of ganglion cells within the neural tube, for all other ganglion cells remain external to the central nervous system and are clearly derived from the neural crest. In addition, the ganglion cells of mesencephalic V deserve the appellation of nucleus because synapses have been observed on these cells in the electron microscope and there are none on spinal or Gasserian ganglion cells (Pineda et al. 1967).

Electrophysiological studies of these neurons (Corbin and Harrison 1940, Jerge 1963a, Stein and Edwards 1978, Nagata and Kruger 1979) reveal characteristics similar to lumbar spinal ganglion cells innervating muscle spindles, displaying typical conduction velocity, a 'silent period' and activation by individual spindles (Jerge 1963a). These cells can be labeled retrogradely when HRP is applied to peripheral nerves or injected into muscles (Batini et al. 1976, Alvarado-Mallart et al. 1975) thus securely establishing that they emit first-order afferent fibers peripherally. However, there are some other unusual problems presented by these 'central' ganglion cells. Some of their axons join the oculomotor nerve to innervate spindles in the extraocular muscles in addition to its trigeminal distribution (Alvarado-Mallart et al. 1975). Another puzzling feature is the existence of Gasserian ganglion cells that also can be labeled with HRP injected into masticatory and extraocular muscles, thus providing two distinct and separated aggregates for afferent innervation of muscle (Batini et al. 1976). It would be interesting to determine whether different receptors are represented in the Gasserian ganglion and mesencephalic V nucleus respectively. Finally, it should be noted that receptors of the periodontal ligament are represented in mesencephalic V (Jerge 1963a). Other 'deep' receptors may also be represented here, but the innervation of the massive temporomandibular joint has not yet been determined. Thus, there is still much to be done before the 'proprioceptive' components of the trigeminal nerve are fully understood.

Several important features emerge from autoradiographic tracing of axonal transport from the Gasserian ganglion. Each of the nuclear subdivisions recognized on cytoarchitectural grounds (Olszewski 1950) can also be distinguished on the basis of afferent innervation pattern (Kruger et al. 1977, Kruger 1979) and remarkably, there is an apparent absence of direct innervation of motor nuclei although further technical refinements may ultimately reveal more extensive connectivity. Taken at face value, currently available results provide an anatomical definition of the sensory V complex that adheres remarkably well to classical descriptions in terms of precise boundaries and even reveals the main subdivisions within the nucleus caudalis (Fig. 8), while excluding contiguous surrounding nuclei. The excellent correlation of electrophysiological mapping of tactile activity with pattern of afferent innervation serves to further define the sensory V complex with reasonable security. By this definition, the motor V and mesencephalic V deserve separate status.

The principal V sensory nucleus is reasonably considered to be the homologue of the dorsal column nuclei and the principal contributory to the trigeminal lemniscus joining the medial lemniscus in a massive projection to the ventrobasal thalamus. Earlier findings of retrograde atrophy of the neurons of principal V nucleus after brain stem lesions (Torvik 1957, Johnson et al. 1968) have been supported in greater detail by demonstration of the retrograde axonal transport of the enzyme horserad-

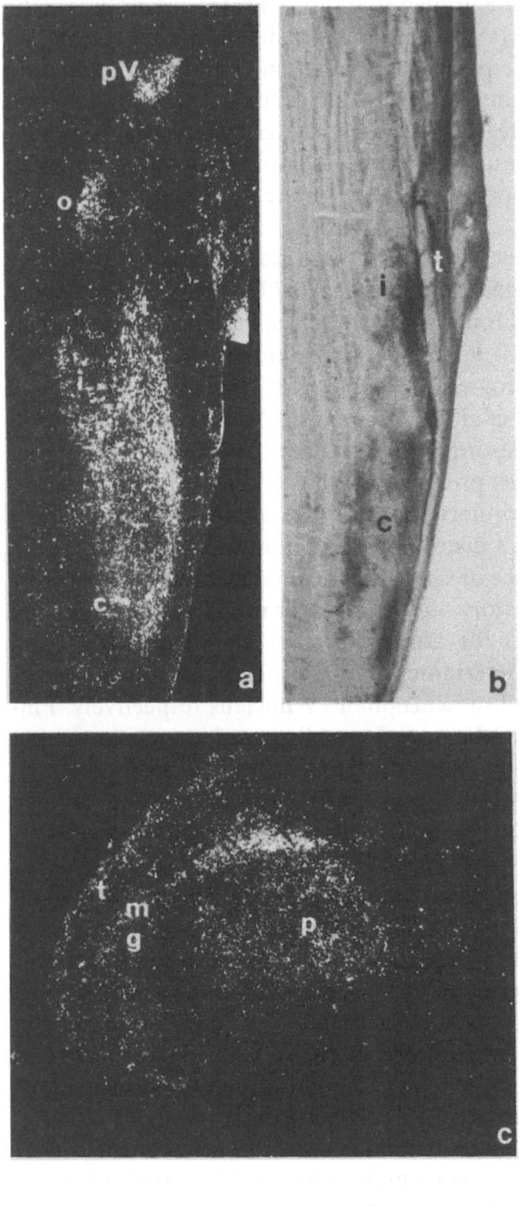

Fig. 8 a–c. Sensory V projection to the cat brain stem sensory trigeminal complex revealed by anterograde transport autoradiography (**a** and **c**) following injection of ^{3}H-leucine and proline into the Gasserian ganglion and following immersion of mandibular and maxillary nerve branches in an HRP solution for tracing the anterograde axonal transport via the trigeminal root and descending tract (*t*) into the spinal nucleus (**b**). Projections can be traced into principal (*pV*), oralis (*o*), interpolaris (*i*) and caudalis (*c*) sectors, displaying a distinctive laminar pattern in caudalis (*c*) with heavy label of the marginal zone (*m*) and nucleus proprius (*p*) and minimal label in the gelatinosa zone (*g*). a × 11, b × 12.5, c × 15

ish peroxidase (HRP) to the vast majority of the neurons of this nucleus (Fig. 9) and additionally has revealed a distinct uncrossed labeled component (Kruger et al. 1977) that projects to the thalamus via the dorsal Wallenberg bundle (Fig. 10) in some, but not all, mammals. It is probable that some neurons emit bifurcating axons projecting to both sides of the diencephalon, but this remains to be determined securely with a double-labeling method.

Electrophysiological mapping studies of single neurons of this nucleus reveals an orderly somatotopic pattern in the several species studied, with the mandibular divi-

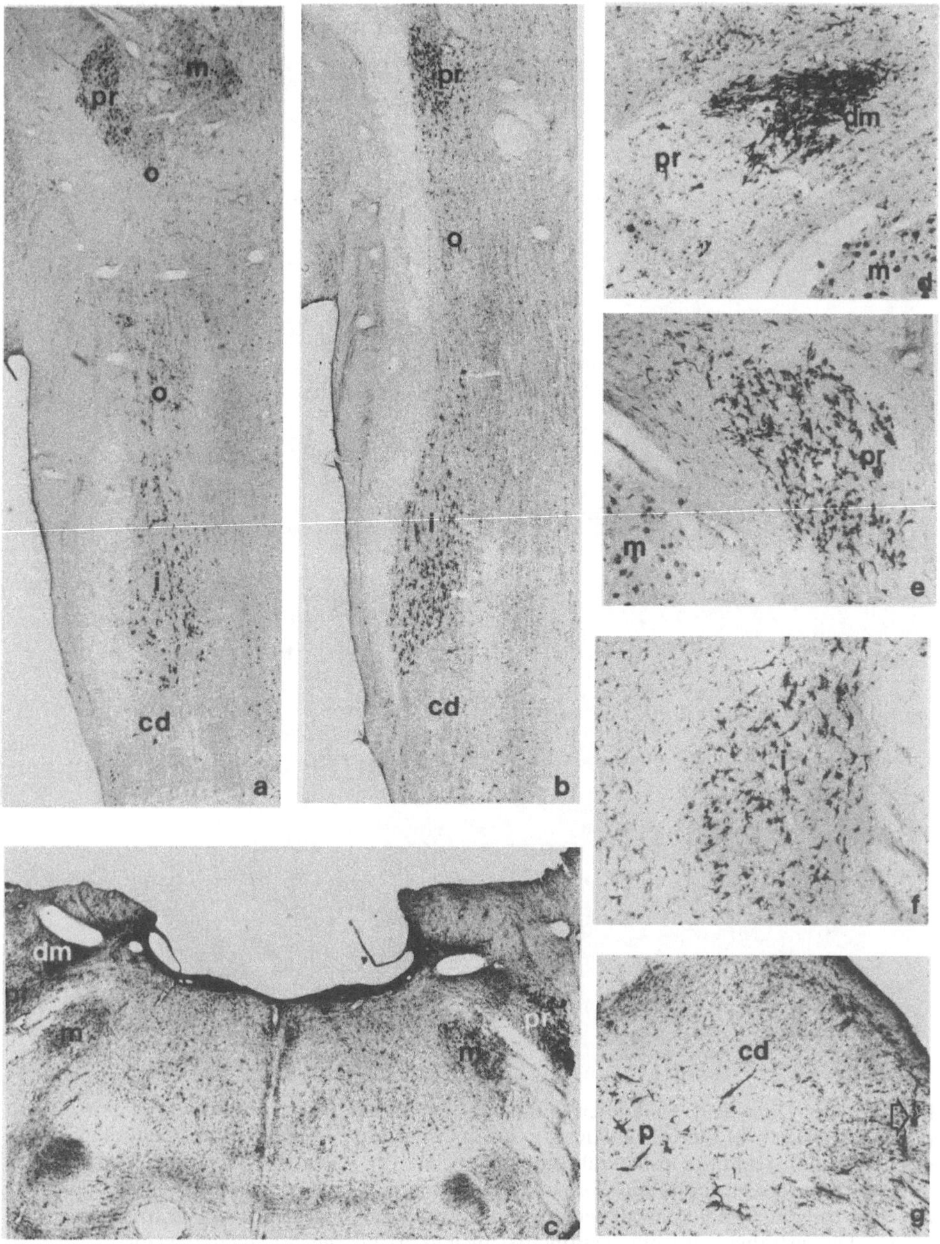

Fig. 9 a–g. Retrograde axonal transport of horseradish peroxidase (HRP) to the sensory V nuclear complex of the cat following HRP injection into the ventrobasal thalamus. In horizontal sections (**a** and **b**), the distinctive pattern of projection from the principal nucleus (*pr*) and interpolaris (*i*) is heavier than the sparse projection from the contiguous nuclei oralis (*o*) and caudalis (*cd*). The principal nucleus projection shown in transverse section in c reveals intense labeling of the main lateral sector of the contralateral principal nucleus (*pr*) on the right and the selective labeling of only the dorsomedial sector (*dm*) on the ipsilateral side overlying the motor V (*m*) nucleus. Higher magnification transverse sections of the ipsilateral dorsomedial sector (in **d**), the contralateral principal nucleus (in **e**), the interpolaris (in **f**) and the selective laminar pattern of the subnucleus caudalis (*cd*) with sparse labeling of marginal neurons (*arrow*) and a few nucleus proprius (*p*) cells (in **g**). a–c × 10, d–g × 25

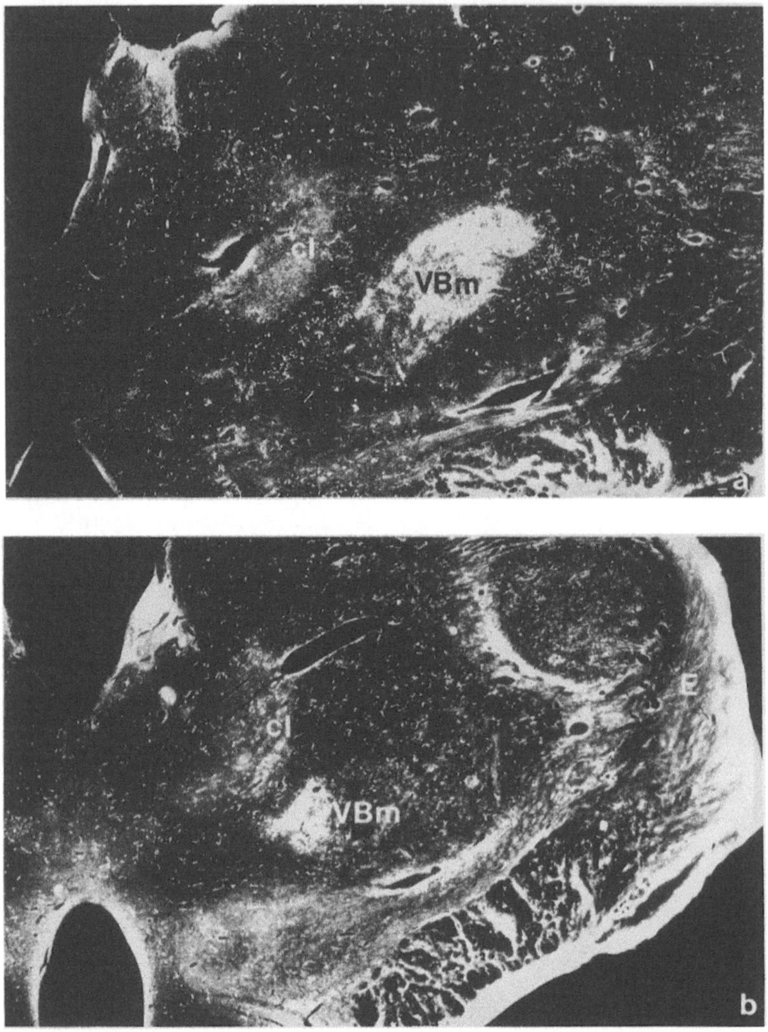

Fig. 10 a, b. Dark-field photomicrographs of anterograde axonal transport of horseradish peroxidase (HRP) to the cat thalamus following injection of HRP into the contralateral nucleus caudalis (**a**) and the ipsilateral principal nucleus (**b**). A massive projection to medial sector of the ventrobasal complex (*VBm*) and centralis lateralis (*cl*) contralateral to the brain stem injection can be found from all sectors of the sensory V complex, with an ipsilateral component demonstrable only from the principal nucleus (**b**) into the most medial sector

sion of V represented dorsad, the ophthalmic division ventrad, and the buccal cavity mediad; a sequence that is distinctly maintained throughout most of the length of the descending spinal nucleus of cat and monkey (Kruger and Michel 1962, Kerr et al. 1968) although an 'onion peel' rostro-caudal sequence has been revealed in the subnucleus (Yokota and Nishikawa 1980). There is persuasive evidence that the input to this nucleus is derived from the large V ganglion cells conducting via large, fast axons subserving the variety of sensitive mechanoreceptors with no contribution from specific nociceptors or thermoreceptors (Kirkpatrick and Kruger 1975) although there is ample evidence that many of the neurons excited delicately by skin contact also discharge following electrical stimulation of the dental pulp (Khayyat, Yu, and King 1975, Nor and Young 1979) and this is supported by a metabolic labeling study employing 2-deoxyglucose (Shetter and Sweet 1979).

The clinical dictum that destruction of the principal V nucleus results in a pure tactile loss is based largely on an unpersuasive early report by Spiller (1915) that remains unsupported by findings in monkeys (Denny-Brown and Yanigasawa 1973) and would be difficult to reconcile with extensive evidence of predominant tactile representation throughout the more voluminous spinal nuclear complex. What remains most puzzling is the relatively small volume of principal V compared with the cuneate and gracile nuclei, especially in rodents in which the trigeminal representation occupies the vast majority of neurons in the thalamic and cortical projection zones.

The spinal V subnucleus oralis constitutes a slender ventral continuation of the principal V nucleus, the functional status of which remains undetermined. It shares with the contiguous principal nucleus a similar somatotopic tactile organization and a projection to the thalamus, although examination of its sparser neuronal population after retrograde HRP labelin (Fig. 9) suggests that its architecture and projection pattern are sufficiently distinctive to deserve separate status on morphological grounds. In some respects, it resembles the less densely populated rostral portions of the cuneate and gracile nuclei and perhaps if it can be subsumed with the principal nucleus, the disparity between the spinal and trigeminal lemniscal components might be reconciled by assigning to each a dense and a sparser region.

The spinal V subnucleus interpolaris is readily recognizable as a distinct entity contiguous with the caudal pole of the subnucleus oralis in the region rostral to the medullary obex. It resembles the rostral components in its tactile somatotopy and in displaying a projection of a substantial proportion of its neurons to the contralateral thalamus (Fig. 9), but differs from the subnucleus oralis in its robust expansion and by possessing a substantial projection to the cerebellum (Cheek et al. 1975). The latter attribute suggests an homology with the external cuneate nucleus (Darian-Smith 1973) but evidence that neurons of the external cuneate receive a dominant muscle spindle input from spinal levels casts serious doubt on this hypothesis. Electrophysiological studies reveal a predominant input from sensitive cutaneous receptors; furthermore, there is evidence of spindle representation in two other nuclei still to be discussed in some detail. Assigning a separate functional role to the distinctive interpolar nucleus remains enigmatic.

The spinal V subnucleus caudalis is the largest and most easily recognized component of the descending spinal nucleus because of its marked resemblance to the dorsal horn of the spinal cord. Although it possesses a dominant tactile input similar to that of the above-mentioned rostral nuclei, there are several distinctive noteworthy features. (1) The pericornual marginal and gelatinosa regions receive a segregated input from specific nociceptors and thermoreceptors (Mosso and Kruger 1973, Price et al. 1976), a condition similar to that found in the lumbosacral dorsal horn (Christensen and Perl 1970, Kumazawa and Perl 1978). (2) Interruption of this portion of the spinal nucleus and tract by the Sjoqvist procedure in man results in a profound hypalgesia and thermanesthesia. (3) The main body or nucleus proprius is the recipient of a predominantly tactile input organized similarly to the rostral components but differs from them in that many of the neurons respond to a wide range of inputs including both low and high threshold afferents. There is evidence to suggest that these 'wide dynamic range neurons' play a role in pain perception (Mayer et al. 1975, Price and Mayer 1975). Additionally, the vast majority of nucleus proprius neurons are not retrogradely labeled after thalamic HRP injection, unlike those of the principal, oral, and interpolar nuclei, although many pericornual neurons project to the thalamus (Kruger et al. 1977, Hockfield and Cobel 1978, Burton and Craig 1979, Fukushima and Kerr 1979, Ciesler et al. 1979, Shigenaga et al. 1979).

It seems reasonable to conclude that the subnucleus caudalis includes the homologue of the spinothalamic tract on anatomical, physiological, and clinical grounds. The fact that the majority of its neurons lack a thalamic projection and possess a tactile function is essentially similar to current information on the dorsal horn.

Defining the ventral limit of caudalis has recently become a special issue because subjacent neurons of the lateral reticular nucleus have long been known to be activated by strong trigeminal stimuli, as well as stimulation of other body regions (Kruger and Michel 1962b, Nord and Ross 1973) and there are some neurons that possess small modality-specific receptive fields (Price et al. 1976) and Yokota and Nishikawa (1977, 1980) have uncovered a somatotopic organization within this nucleus. Some of these cells project to the thalamus and it has been suggested (Nord and Ross 1973, Gobel et al. 1977) that this region is the homologue of the deeper layers of the dorsal horn of the spinal cord despite the lack of direct innervation of this zone by labeled spinal V tract axons. The results to date with labeling of trigeminal afferents (Fig. 8), either by tritiated amino acid injection into the Gasserian ganglion or by applying HRP to peripheral nerves (Kruger 1979, Marfurt 1979, Young and Kruger in prep.), supports the conventional description of the sensory trigeminal complex as the region recipient of first-order trigeminal afferents although an improvement in techniques may reveal innervation of other structures. It is worth noting, however, that although HRP labeling of large peripheral nerves may display innervation of the principal, oral, interpolar, and caudal nuclei as expected (Marfurt 1979), some preliminary evidence for focal accumulation in the rostro-caudal axis (Young and Kruger in prep.) suggests the presence of a hitherto unsuspected rostro-caudal somatotopic pattern within subnucleus caudalis (Yokota and Nishikawa 1980).

The various subdivisions of the sensory trigeminal brainstem nuclear complex were generally assumed to function relatively independently. Primary afferent fibers subserving specific sensory submodalities were believed to synapse on second order neurons in the associated trigeminal brainstem nuclei which, perhaps after relay via one or more interneurons, projected to the appropriate thalamic nuclei. The idea that functionally significant interactions might occur among the nuclear subdivisions originated from the demonstration of an ascending intranuclear pathway originating in nucleus caudalis (Stewart and King 1963) and terminating within the more rostrally located elements of the trigeminal brainstem complex. Inputs to nucleus caudalis have also been demonstrated from the contralateral nucleus caudalis and from presumably non-trigeminal sites such as the upper cervical dorsal roots and the medullary reticular formation (Kerr 1972).

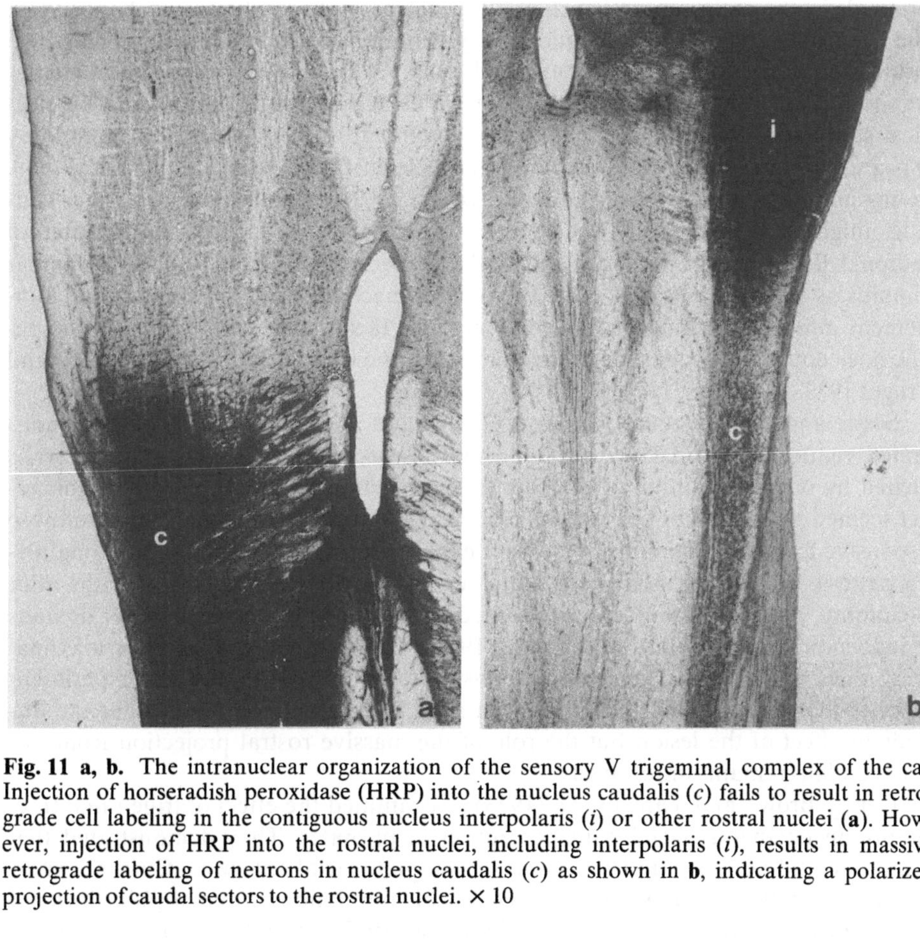

Fig. 11 a, b. The intranuclear organization of the sensory V trigeminal complex of the cat. Injection of horseradish peroxidase (HRP) into the nucleus caudalis (*c*) fails to result in retrograde cell labeling in the contiguous nucleus interpolaris (*i*) or other rostral nuclei (**a**). However, injection of HRP into the rostral nuclei, including interpolaris (*i*), results in massive retrograde labeling of neurons in nucleus caudalis (*c*) as shown in **b**, indicating a polarized projection of caudal sectors to the rostral nuclei. × 10

The intranuclear organization of the sensory V complex is poorly understood and may prove crucial to understanding the role of each of the subnuclei which are extensively interconnected by deep bundles (Gobel and Purvis 1972) and perhaps the spinal V tract. Injection of HRP into the rostral trigeminal nuclei results in extensive labeling of neurons throughout the other portions of spinal V, including a substantial proportion of the neurons within the nucleus proprius of subnucleus caudalis (Fig. 11), i.e. the main population of cells that apparently do not project to the thalamus. The opposite condition can be explored with injections of HRP into the caudalis component with only minimal rostral retrograde labeling (Fig. 11 a), indicating that the direction of interaction is from caudal to rostral, but *not* in the opposite direction. These observations also emphasize that the main projection of caudalis neurons, unlike the other portions, is probably intranuclear and suggests that caudalis must play an important role in modulating the activity of the rostral components upon which it projects.

Electrophysiological studies have demonstrated that nucleus caudalis maintain a tonic presynaptic hyperpolarizing influence on trigeminal primary afferent preterminals in the main sensory nucleus and nucleus oralis (Scibetta and King 1969). The hyperpolarizing influence could be augmented by presumably painful electrical stimulation of the tooth pulp (Young and King 1972), by the application of strychnine to nucleus caudalis (Young and King 1972, Khayyat et al. 1975), and by electrical stimulation of nucleus caudalis (Khayyat et al. 1975). Trigeminal tractotomy appeared to decrease or abolish these internuclear effects (Scibetta and King 1969, Young and King 1972). Such findings gave rise to the hypothesis that nucleus caudalis might subserve facial nociceptive sensation by a specific modulation of neuronal firing in the principal and oralis nuclei which would code a particular stimulus as painful (Khayyat et al. 1975). This mechanism might function to complement information transfer related to noxious facial stimulation carried via specific nociceptive relay neurons in the marginal zone of nucleus caudalis (Mosso and Kruger 1973, Price et al. 1976).

Sessle and Greenwood (1976) and Greenwood and Sessle (1976) have demonstrated reduced neuronal firing in the main sensory nucleus and nucleus oralis elicited by orofacial stimuli after acute trigeminal tractotomy. Interestingly this effect seemed to be greater on neurons responsive to innocuous stimuli than on those responsive to noxious stimuli. In a recent experiment which examined neuronal firing patterns in nucleus oralis and main sensory nucleus one to two months after tractotomy, little effect could be ascertained on neurons responsive to either noxious or innocuous stimuli (Nord and Young 1979). Only a slight reduction in maximal firing rates was noted in neurons responsive to noxious stimuli. This experiment suggests that many of the responses seen after acute tractotomy represent the immediate effect of the lesion but the role of the massive rostral projection from nucleus caudalis remains unresolved.

Denny-Brown and Yanagisawa (1973) re-examined the effect of trigeminal tractotomy on cutaneous facial pain perception in primates. They demonstrated that tractotomy did not result in irreversible or complete facial analgesia. Current experiments also indicate that analgesia to electrical stimulation of dental pulp does not result following tractotomy in cat (Vyklicky et al. 1977), primate (Young and Oleson in prep.) or man (Young in prep.). Review of the results of trigeminal tractotomy in humans reveals that such lesions:

1. produce disturbed but not abolished facial pain and temperature sensation (Rowbotham 1938)
2. tend to spare the central portion of the face near the midline (Kunc 1970) and
3. frequently fail to relieve oral or tonsillar pain (Grant 1955).

Furthermore, facial pain may persist even though significant facial analgesia is present on routine clinical testing (Olivecrona 1942). Although a pattern of analgesia similar to that produced in humans by tractotomy was also observed in monkeys by Denny-Brown et al. (1973), such analgesia could be completely reversed by the administration of strychnine or L-dopa. Similar experiments in our laboratory have confirmed these findings in monkey (Young and Oleson in prep.) and similar observations have been reported in man (Hodge and King 1976). Denny-Brown postulated that tractotomy results in interruption of one of the afferent supplies of the face, namely the trigeminal input to nucleus caudalis. He further proposed that the upper cervical nerve roots act as an important second afferent supply to the face.

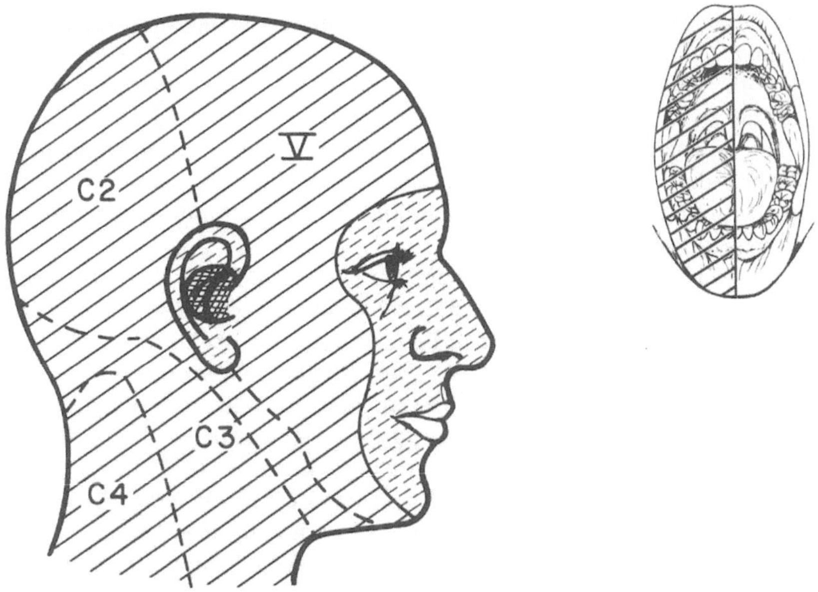

Fig. 12. Afferent supply of the oro-facial and neck regions in human. The oral cavity and paramedien regions of the face (interrupted diagonals) receive exclusive supply from the trigeminal nerve except for IX+X innervation of the pharyngeal region. The majority of skin of the face and neck is supplied from a combination of trigeminal and upper cervical nerve roots as indicated. The pinna and external auditory canal receive supply from the vagal and facial cranial nerves respectively as well as the upper cervical nerve roots

Under the facilitatory influence of strychnine or L-dopa, the synaptic effectiveness of this secondary input may be augmented and results in sufficient central summation to allow input over this single afferent input to be recognized as painful. Only the midline region of the face (Denny-Brown and Yanagisawa 1973) and intraoral structures such as teeth (Young and Oleson in prep., Young in prep.) appear to be exclusively supplied by the trigeminal nerve (Fig. 12). The remainder of the face is supplied by overlapping afferent fibers in the VII. and X. cranial nerves and the upper cervical nerve roots as well as the trigeminal. The *exclusive* afferent supply of an innervated region distinguishes the trigeminal sensory system from the spinal nerve root system since in the latter no exclusive territory is supplied by a single nerve root. In fact, overlapping afferent supply from at least two adjacent rostral and caudal roots characterize the sensory supply of a 'dermatome' on the extremities and trunk (Kirk and Denny-Brown 1970). The intranuclear ascending pathway (Stewart and King 1963) was postulated by Denny-Brown to provide the anatomical framework for interaction between these multiple overlapping somatosensory afferents into the spinal trigeminal nucleus from oro-facial structures. An anatomical substrate for intranuclear interactions within the spinal trigeminal complex is now clearly demonstrable and physiological evidence of such interactions is abundant. However, the significance of such interactions in relation to normal and pathological facial sensory perception remains an important area for further exploration.

The selective distribution of neurotransmitters provides a set of new insights for functional localization and some important clues concerning central trigeminal pain mechanisms. The recency of the several important discoveries and the rapid proliferation of new findings precludes a comprehensive account, but several salient features deserve comment for they provide guidance to an emerging story with important clinical implications.

The discovery of Hokfelt and his collaborators (1975 and 1978) that substance P-like immunoreactivity was restricted to small ganglion cells and only thin sensory fibers distributing principally within the marginal gelatinosa portions of the trigeminal subnucleus caudalis was the first clue. The Hokfelt laboratory (1975) and others (Atwek and Kuhar 1977) also showed that the distribution of met-enkephalin, an endogenous peptide ligand for opiate receptors, had a similar distribution in the same caudalis sector, and Henry and his colleagues (1977) showed that iontophoretic application of substance P excites *only* those neurons that respond to noxious cutaneous stimuli. Activation of low threshold afferents does not effect substance P release, but excitation of A delta and C fibers, which supply nociceptive information, causes a 2.6 fold increase in cerebrospinal fluid substance P (Jessell et al. 1979). It is also known that substance P administration lowers the pain threshold and that its depletion raises the pain threshold.

The release of substance P from the rat trigeminal nucleus caudalis was shown by Jessel and Iversen (1977) to be presynaptically controlled by morphine and opioid peptides in a concentration-dependent, stereospecific, naloxone antagonizable fashion. This led to the proposal (Jessell and Iversen 1977) that enkephalinergic interneurons project presynaptically upon substance P-containing terminals reducing the amount of substance P released. The opioid action is believed to be due to a reduction of calcium ion influx in substance P-containing terminals.

It is perhaps appropriate to end this narrative on this newly unfolding episode in pain research. There is suggestive evidence that an increase in substance P or its receptor sites may account for some cases of causalgia and neuralgia (Henry 1980) and there are many new clues to the mode of analgesic action of opioid agents, including descending as well as afferent control mechanisms. It is exhilarating to close with the thought that despite the extensive information already in hand concerning trigeminal sensory mechanisms, we remain at the threshold of a new era of understanding.

Acknowledgments: Some of the original date presented was supported by grants from the National Institutes of Health (NS-5685, DE-5118 and 5208, CA-16402 and RR-5551), the UCLA Jonsson Comprehensive Cancer Center and the California Institute for Cancer Research. We are indebted to several colleagues for providing material or permission to reproduce their puplished findings, Jane Curtis and Sharon Sampogna for photographic assistance, Anita Roff for preparation and typing of the manuscript and Dr. Lawrence Mallach for computer word processing assistance.

References

Adson AW (1971) Unpublished data cited by GS Baker personal communication, 1969, cited in Gudmundsson K, Rhoton Jr AL and Rushton JG. Detailed anatomy of the intracranial portion of the trigeminal nerve. J Neurosurg 35:592–600

Alvarado-Mallart MR, Batini C, Buisseret-Delmas C, Corvisier J (1975) Trigeminal representations of the masticatory and extraocular proprioceptors as revealed by horseradish peroxidase retrograde transport. Exp Brain Res 23:167–179

Atwek SF, Kuhar MJ (1977) Autoradiographic localization of opiate receptors in rat brain. I. Spinal cord and lower medulla. Brain Res 124:53–67

Batini C, Buisseret-Delmas C, Corvisier J (1976) Horseradish peroxidase localization of masticatory muscle motoneurons in cat. J Physiol (Paris) 72:301–309

Belyaev VI (1968) Absolute number and percentage of medullated nerve fibers of different diameters in the trigeminal and facial nerves. In: Maksimenkov AN (ed) Internal Structure of Peripheral Nerves. Leningrad. (Quoted from Blinkov and Gleser, '68.)

Blinkov SM, Gleser II (1968) The Human Brain in Figures and Tables, Basic Books, Inc., Plenum Press, New York, p. 482

Burgess PR, Perl ER (1967) Myelinated afferent fibres responding specifically to noxious stimulation of the skin. J Physiol (Lond) 190:541–562

Burton H, Craig AD Jr (1979) Distribution of trigeminothalamic projection cells in cat and monkey. Brain Res 161:515–521

Cajal SR (1911) Histologie du système nerveux de l'homme et des vertébrés. 2 vols, p. 986

Cheek MD, Rustioni A, Trevino DL (1975) Dorsal column nuclei projections to the cerebellar cortex in cats as revealed by the use of the retrograde transport of horseradish peroxidase. J Comp Neurol 164:31–46

Christensen BN, Perl ER (1970) Spinal neurons specifically excited by noxious or thermal stimuli: marginal zone of the dorsal horn. J Neurophysiol 33:293–307

Clifton GL, Coggeshall RE, Vance WH, Willis WD (1976) Receptive fields of unmyelinated ventral root afferent fibers in the cat. J Physiol (Lond) 256:573–600

Coggeshall RE, Applebaum MI, Fazen M, Stubbs III TB, Sykes MT (1975) Unmyelinated axons in human ventral roots, a possible explanation for the failure of dorsal rhizotomy to relieve pain. Brain 98:157–166

Corbin KB, Harrison F (1940) Function of mesencephalic root of fifth cranial nerve. J Neurophysiol 3:423–435

Dandy WE (1929) An operation for the cure of tic douloureux: partial section of the sensory root at the pons. Arch Surg 18:687–734

Dandy WE (1932) The treatment of trigeminal neuralgia by the cerebellar route. Ann Surg 96:787–795

Darian-Smith I (1970) The neural coding of 'tactile' stimulus parameters in different trigeminal nuclei. In: Hassler R, Walker AE (eds) Trigeminal Neuralgia. Georg Thieme Verlag, Stuttgart, pp 59–71

Denny-Brown D, Kirk EJ, Yanagisawa N (1973) The tract of Lissauer in relation to sensory transmission in the dorsal horn of spinal cord in the macaque monkey. J Comp Neurol 151:175–199

Denny-Brown D, Yanagisawa N (1973) The function of the descending root of the fifth nerve. Brain 96:783–814

Dimsdale JA, Kemp JM (1966) Afferent fibers in the ventral nerve roots of the rat. J Physiol (Lond) 187:25–26

Fukushima T, Kerr FWL (1979) Organization of trigeminothalamic tracts and other thalamic afferent systems of the brainstem in the rat: presence of gelatinosa neurons with thalamic connections. J Comp Neurol 183:169–184

Gardner WJ, Pinto JP (1953) The Taarnhoj operation: relief of trigeminal neuralgia without numbness. Cleve Clin 20:364–367

Gardner WJ, Todd EM, Pinto JP (1956) Roentgenographic findings in trigeminal neuralgia. Am J Roentgenol 76:346–350

Gerard MW (1923) Afferent impulses in the trigeminal nerve. AMA Arch Neurol Psychiat 9:306–338

Giesler GJ Jr, Menétrey D, Basbaum AI (1979) Differential origins of spinothalamic tract projections to medial and lateral thalamus in the rat. J Comp Neurol 184: 107–126
Gobel S, Falls WM, Hockfield S (1977) The division of the dorsal and ventral horns of the mammalian caudal medulla into eight layers using anatomical criteria. In: Anderson DJ, Matthews B (eds) Pain in the Trigeminal Region. Elsevier Press, New York, pp 443–453
Gobel S, Purvis MP (1972) Anatomical studies of the organization of the spinal V nucleus: the deep bundles and the spinal V tract. Brain Res 85:27–44
Grant FC (1955) Discussion on trigeminal tractotomy. Clin Neurosurg 2:69–70
Greenwood LF, Sessle BJ (1976) Inputs to trigeminal brain stem neurons from facial, oral, toothpulp and pharyngolaryngeal tissues. II. Role of trigeminal nucleus caudalis in modulating responses to innocuous and noxious stimuli. Brain Res 117:227–238
Gudmundsson K, Rhoton AL, Rushton JG (1971) Detailed anatomy of the intracranial portion of the trigeminal nerve. J Neurosurg 35:592–600
Harris FS, Rhoton AL Jr (1976) Anatomy of the cavernous sinus: a microsurgical study. J Neurosurg 45:169–180
Hayashi H (1980) Distributions of vibrissae afferent fiber collaterals in the trigeminal nuclei as revealed by intra-axonal injection of horseradish peroxidase. Brain Res 183:442–446
Henry JL (1980) Substance P and pain: an updating. Trends Neurosci 3:95–97
Henry JL, Hu JW, Lucier GE, Sessle BJ (1977) Responses of units in the trigeminal sensory nuclei to oral-facial stimuli and to substance P. In: Anderson DJ, Matthews B (eds) Pain in the Trigeminal Region. Elsevier/North-Holland Biomedical Press, Amsterdam, pp 295–306
Hirsch, Anton BR (1765) Pars quinti nervorum encephali disquisitio anatomica. Vienna (n.p.)
Hockfield S, Gobel S (1978) Neurons in and near nucleus caudalis with long ascending projection axons demonstrated by retrograde labeling with horseradish peroxidase. Brain Res 139:333–339
Hodge CJ, King RB (1976) Medical modification of sensation. J Neurosurg 44:21–28
Hökfelt T, Ljungdahl A, Steinbusch H, Verhofstad A, Nilsson G, Brodin E, Pernow B, Goldstein M (1978) Immunohistochemical evidence of substance P-like immunoreactivity in some 5-hydroxytryptamine-containing neurons in the rat central nervous system. Neuroscience 3:517–538
Hökfelt T, Elde R, Johannson O, Luft R, Nilsson G, Arimura A (1976) Immunohistochemical evidence for separate populations of somatostatin-containing and substance P-containing primary afferent neurons in the rat. Neuroscience 1:131–136
Hökfelt T, Kellerth JO, Nilsson G, Pernow B (1975) Experimental immunohistochemical studies on the localization and distribution of substance P in cat primary sensory neurons. Brain Res 100:235–252
Horsley V, Taylor J, Colman WS (1891) Remarks on the various surgical procedures devised for the relief or cure of trigeminal neuralgia (tic douloureux). Br Med J 2:1139–1143, 1191–1193, 1249–1252
Hoyes AD, Barber P (1977) Ultrastructure of corneal receptors. In: Anderson DJ, Matthews B (eds) Pain in the Trigeminal Region. Elsevier/North-Holland Biomedical Press, New York, pp 1–12
Humphrey T (1968) The development of mouth opening and related reflexes involving the oral area of human fetuses. Ala J Med Sci 5: 126–157
Jannetta PJ (1967) Gross (mesoscopic) description of the human trigeminal nerve and ganglion. J Neurosurg 26: 109–111
Jannetta PJ, Rand RW (1966) Transtentorial retrogasserian rhizotomy in trigeminal neuralgia by microneurosurgical technique. Bull Los Angeles Neurol Soc 31:93–99
Jefferson G (1955) Trigeminal neuromas with some remarks on the malignant invasion of the Gasserian ganglion. Clin Neurosurg 1: 11–54
Jerge CR (1963a) Organization and function of the trigeminal mesencephalic nucleus. J Neurophysiol 26:379–392
Jerge CR (1963b) Function of the nucleus supratrigeminalis. J Neurophysiol 26:393–402
Jessell TM, Mudge AW, Leeman SE, Yaksh TL (1979) Release of substance P and somatostatin, in vivo, from primary afferent terminals in mammalian spinal cord. Neurosci Abs 5:611

Jessell TM, Iversen LL (1977) Opiate analgesics inhibit substance P release from rat trigeminal nucleus. Nature 268:549–551
Johnson JI Jr, Welker WI, Pubols BH (1968) Somatotopic organization of raccoon dorsal column nuclei. J Comp Neurol 132:1–44
Kato M, Hirata Y (1968) Sensory neurons in the spinal ventral roots of the cat. Brain Res 7:479–482
Kerr FWL (1972) Central relationships of trigeminal and cervical primary afferents in the spinal cord and medulla. Brain Res 43:561–572
Kerr FWL (1966) The ultrastructure of the spinal tract of the trigeminal nerve and the substantia gelatinosa. Exp Neurol 16:359–376
Kerr FWL (1963a) The etiology of trigeminal neuralgia. Arch Neurol 8:15–25
Kerr FWL (1963b) The divisional organization of afferent fibres of the trigeminal nerve. Brain 86:721–732
Kerr FWL, Lysak WR (1964) Somatotopic organization of trigeminal-ganglion neurones. Arch Neurol 11:593–602
Kerr FWL, Kruger L, Schwassmann HO, Stern R (1968) Somatotopic organization of mechanoreceptor units in the trigeminal nuclear complex of the macaque. J Comp Neurol 134:127–144
Khayyat GF, Yu YJ, King RB (1975) Response patterns to noxious and non-noxious stimuli in rostral relay nuclei. Brain Res 97:47–60
Kidokoro Y, Kubota E, Shuto S, Sumino R (1968) Reflex organization of cat masticatory muscles. J Neurophysiol 31:695–708
Kirk EJ, Denny-Brown D (1970) Functional variation in dermatomes in the macaque monkey following dorsal root lesions. J Comp Neurol 139:307–320
Kirkpatrick D, Kruger L (1975) Physiological properties of neurons in the principal trigeminal nucleus in the cat. Exp Neurol 48:664–690
Kruger L (1979) Functional subdivisions of the brainstem sensory trigeminal nuclear complex. Adv Pain Res Ther 3:197–209
Kruger L, Michel F (1962a) A morphological and somatotopic analysis of single unit activity in the trigeminal sensory complex of the cat. Exp Neurol 5:139–156
Kruger L, Michel F (1962b) Physiological excitation of single elements in the trigeminal sensory complex of the decerebrate cat. A reinterpretation of the representation of pain. Exp Neurol 5:157–178
Kruger L, Saporta S, Feldman SG (1977) Axonal transport studies of the sensory trigeminal complex. In: Anderson DJ, Matthews B (eds) Pain in the Trigeminal Region. Elsevier Press, New York, pp 191–201
Kumazawa T, Perl ER (1978) Excitation of marginal and substantia gelatinosa neurons in the primate spinal cord: indications of their place in dorsal horn functional organization. J Comp Neurol 177:417–434
Kunc Z (1970) Significant factors pertaining to the results of trigeminal tractotomy. In: Hassler R, Walker AE (eds) Trigeminal Neuralgia. Georg Thieme, Stuttgart, pp 90–99
Lee FC (1937) Trigeminal neuralgia. J Med Assoc Ga 26:431–436
Lele PP, Weddell G (1959) Sensory nerves of the cornea and cutaneous sensibility. Exp Neurol 1:334–359
Lorente de Nó R (1922) Contribución al conocimiento del nervio trigémino. Libro en honor de Don S. Ramón y Cajal, Móya, Madrid 2:13–39
Malis LI (1967) Structural mechanism of trigeminal neuralgia: petrous ridge compression and its surgical correction. J Neurosurg 26:163–167
Marfurt CF (1979) Somatotopic organization of trigeminal sensory nuclei. Soc Neurosci Abstr 5:710
Matthews B (1977) Responses of intradental nerves to electrical and thermal stimulation of teeth in dogs. J Physiol (Lond) 264:641–664
Maxwell DR, Kruger L, Pineda A (1969) The trigeminal nerve root with special reference to the central-peripheral transition zone: an electron microscopic study in the macaque. Anat Rec 164:113–126
Mayer DJ, Price DD, Becker DP (1975) Neurophysiological characterization of the anterolateral spinal cord neurons contributing to pain perception in man. Pain 1:59–72

Mosso JA, Kruger L (1973) Receptor categories represented in spinal trigeminal nucleus caudalis. J Neurophysiol 36:472–488
Nagata T, Kruger L (1979) Tactile neurons of the superior colliculus of the cat: input and physiological properties. Brain Res 174:19–37
Nord SG, Ross GS (1973) Responses of trigminal units in the monkey bulbar lateral reticular formation to noxious and non-noxious stimulation of the face: experimental and theoretical considerations. Brain Res 58:385–399
Nord SG, Young RF (1979) Effect of chronic descending tractotomy on the response patterns of neurons in the trigeminal nuclei principalis and oralis. Exp Neurol 65:355–372
Nord SG, Young RF (1975) Projection of tooth pulp afferents to the cat trigeminal nucleus caudalis. Brain Res 90:195–204
Olive I, Svien HJ (1957) Neurofibromas of the fifth cranial nerve. J Neurosurg 14:484–505
Olivecrona H (1947) La cirugia del dolor. Archos Neurocirug 4:1–10
Olivecrona H (1942) Tractotomy for relief of trigeminal neuralgia. Arch Neurol Psych 47:544–564
Olszewski J (1950) On the anatomical and functional organization of the trigeminal nucleus. J Comp Neurol 92:401–413
Otenasek FJ (1974) Personal communication 1971, cited in Pelletier VA, Pulas DA, Lende RA, Functional localization in the trigeminal root. J Neurosurg 40:504–513
Paullus WS, Pait TG, Rhoton AL Jr (1977) Microsurgical exposure of the petrous portion of the carotid artery. J Neurosurg 47:713–726
Pelletier VA, Poulos DA, Lende RA (1974) Functional localization in the trigeminal root. J Neurosurg 40:504–513
Perl ER (1968) Myelinated afferent fibers innervating the primate skin and their response to noxious stimuli. J Physiol (Lond) 197:593–615
Perkins ES (1961) Sensory mechanisms and intraocular pressure. Exp Eye Res 1:160–167
Pineda A, Maxwell DS, Kruger L (1967) The fine structure of neurons and satellite cells in the trigeminal ganglion of cat and monkey. Am J Anat 121:461–488
Price DD, Mayer DJ (1975) Neurophysiological characterization of the anterolateral quadrant neurons subserving pain in *M. mulatta*. Pain 1:59–72
Price DD, Dubner R, Hu JW (1976) Trigeminothalamic neurons in nucleus caudalis responsive to tactile, thermal, and nociceptive stimulation of monkey's face. J Neurophysiol 39:936–953
Rand RW (1969) In: Rand RW (ed) Microsurgery. C. V. Mosby, St. Louis, pp 39–49
Rowbotham GF (1938) Treatment of pain in the face by intramedullary tractotomy. Br Med J 2:1073–1076
Russel DC, Rubinstein LJ (1977) Pathology of Tumors of the Nervous System, 4th edition, Williams and Wilkins, Baltimore, p 448
Saunders RL, Sachs E (1970) Relation of the accessory rootlets of the trigeminal nerve to its motor root. A microsurgical autopsy study. J Neurosurg 33:317–324
Scibetta CJ, King RB (1969) Hyperpolarizing influence of trigeminal nucleus caudalis on primary afferent preterminals in trigeminal nucleus oralis. J Neurophysiol 32:229–238
Schisano G, Olivercrona H (1960) Neurinomas of the Gasserian ganglion and trigeminal root. J Neurosurg 17:306–321
Sessle BJ, Greenwood LF (1976) Inputs to trigeminal brainstem neurones from facial, oral, tooth pulp and pharyngolaryngeal tissues: I. Responses to innoxious and noxious stimuli. Brain Res 117:211–216
Shetter AG, Sweet WH (1979) Alterations in regional brain glucose metabolism produced by noxious trigeminal stimulation in the rat. Adv Pain Res Ther 3:337–344
Shigenaga Y, Takabatake M, Sugimoto T, Sakai A (1979) Neurons in marginal layer of trigeminal nucleus caudalis projecting to ventrobasal complex (VB) and posterior nuclear group (PO) demonstrated by retrograde labeling with horseradish peroxidase. Brain Res 166:391–396
Sjöqvist O (1938) Studies on pain conduction in the trigeminal nerve. A contribution to surgical treatment of facial pain. Acta Psychiatr Scand (Suppl) 17:1–139
Somana R, Kotchabhakdi N, Walberg F (1980) Cerebellar afferents from the trigeminal sensory nuclei in the cat. Exp Brain Res 38:57–64

Spiller WG (1915) Remarks on the central representation of sensation. J Nerv Ment Dis 42:399–418
Stein BE, Edwards SB (1978) Hysteresis and multimodal convergence in cells of mesencephalic V. Exp Neurol 59:396–403
Stewart WA, King RB (1963) Fiber projections from the nucleus caudalis of the spinal trigeminal nucleus. J Comp Neurol 121:271–286
Taber E (1961) The cytoarchitecture of the brainstem of the cat. I. Brainstem nuclei of cat. J Comp Neurol 116:27–69
Tarlov IM (1937) Structure of the nerve root. I. Nature of the junction between the central and the peripheral nervous system. Arch Neurol Psychiat 37:555–583
Tervo T, Joó F, Huikuri KT, Toth I, Palkama A (1979) Fine structure of sensory nerves in the rat cornea: An experimental nerve degeneration study. Pain 6:57–70
Torvik A (1957) The ascending fibers from the main trigeminal sensory nucleus: An experimental study in the cat. Am J Anat 100:1–15
Tower SS (1943) Pain: definition and properties of the unit for sensory reception. Res Publ Assoc Reserv Ment Dis 23:16–43
Vyklicky L, Keller O, Jastreboff P, Vyklicky L Jr, Butkuzi SM (1977) Spinal trigeminal tractotomy and nociceptive reactions evoked by tooth pulp stimulation in the cat. J Physiol (Paris) 73:379–386
Walker AE, Miles FC, Simpson JR (1956) Partial trigeminal rhizotomy using suboccipital approach; experiences in the treatment of trigeminal neuralgia. Arch Neurol Psychiat 75:514–521
Wall PD, Taub A (1962) Four aspects of trigeminal nucleus and a paradox. J Neurophysiol 25:110–126
Watson CRR, Switzer RC, III (1978) Trigeminal projections to cerebellar tactile areas in the rat. Origin mainly from N. interpolaris and N. principalis. Neurosci Lett 10:77–82
Windle WF (1926) Non-bifurcating nerve fibers of the trigeminal nerve. J Comp Neurol 40:229–240
Yokota T (1976) Trigeminal subnucleus caudalis neurons excited by tooth pulp stimulation. Adv Pain Res Ther 1:171–176
Yokota T, Nishikawa N (1980) Reappraisal of somatotopic tactile representation within trigeminal subnucleus caudalis. J Neurophysiol 43:700–712
Yokota T, Nishikawa N (1977) Somatotopic organisation of trigeminal neurons within caudal medulla oblongata. In: Anderson DS, Matthews B (eds) Pain in the Trigeminal Region. Elsevier Press, New York, pp 243–257
Young RF (in prep.) Effect of trigeminal tractotomy on dental sensation in man
Young RF (1978) Unmyelinated fibers in the trigeminal motor root: possible relationship to the results of trigeminal rhizotomy. J Neurosurg 49:538–543
Young RF (1977) Fiber spectrum of the trigeminal sensory root of frog, cat and man. In: Anderson DJ, Matthews B (eds) Pain in the Trigeminal Region. Elsevier Press, New York, pp 137–147
Young RF, King RB (1973) Fiber spectrum of the trigeminal sensory root of the baboon determined by electron microscopy. J Neurosurg: 65–72
Young RF, King RB (1972) Excitability changes in trigeminal primary afferent fibers in response to noxious and non-noxious stimuli. J Neurophysiol 35:87–95
Young RF, Kruger L (in prep.)
Young RF, Oleson TD (in prep.) Behavioral response to dental pulp stimulation in primate – effect of trigeminal tractotomy
Young RF, Stevens R (1979) Unmyelinated axons in the trigeminal motor root of human and cat. J Comp Neurol 183:205–214

Neurophysiological Diagnosis of Trigeminal Nerve Function

R. DENGLER and A. STRUPPLER, München/FRG

Introduction

The fifth cranial nerve arises from the pons with a portio major containing sensory fibers and a portio minor with motor efferents and proprioceptive afferents supplying the chewing muscles. Motor as well as sensory function may be evaluated by appropriate clinical neurophysiological tests. Valuable information can thus be added to clinical examination since investigation of the trigeminal nerve often fails to give accurate results. Particularly interesting are these tests in the large number of patients with facial pain when clear discrimination between the idiopathic and the symptomatic type is desirable. In this study methods testing the motor and sensory function of the trigeminal nerve will be described as they are in use in our clinical lab. In addition some new approaches to improve the neurophysiological diagnosis of the trigeminal system will be mentioned.

Methods and Results

Methods Testing Motor Function

1. Electromyography

A lesion in the motor portion of the nerve along the way from the pons to the muscles of mastication causes partial or complete conduction block and will finally lead to denervation in the associated muscles. This can be easily detected by means of conventional needle electromyography. The criteria sought for are essentially the same as in the examination of other skeletal muscles, i. e. pathological spontaneous activity, polyphasic motor unit potentials of increased duration and loss of interference pattern at maximal volitional innervation (Rupprecht 1974).

Figure 1 shows an EMG recorded in both masseter muscles during brisk jaw closing in a patient suffering from a malignant osteolytic process in the left medial cranial fossa. Clinical examination revealed minor left-sided abducens palsy, weakness in the left chewing muscles and questionable dysesthesia in the area of the left third trigeminal branch. As illustrated, on the right side an interference pattern, whereas on the left side a single unit discharge pattern is recorded. Additionally (not illustrated) fibrillation potentials were detected in the left masseter muscle.

Careful examination of one or two muscles bilaterally (m. masseter and temporalis) will be sufficient to obtain reliable data concerning denervation. The investigation of additional chewing muscles or polygraphic recordings may be helpful to study various problems in detail such as temporomandibular joint dysfunction

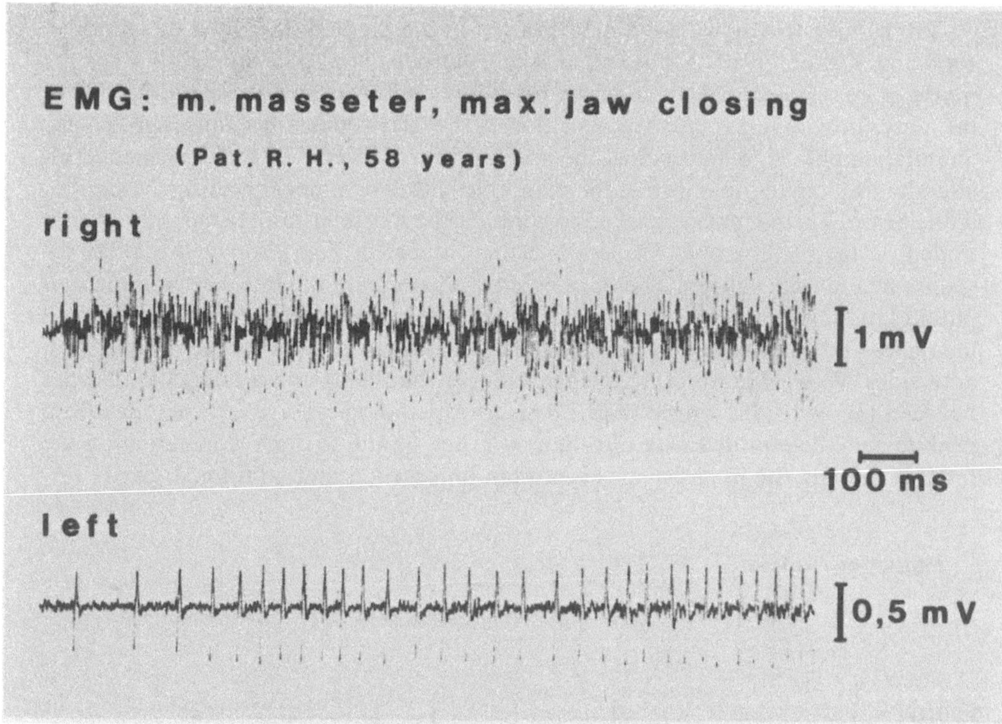

Fig. 1. EMG-records of both masseter muscles in a patient with a left-sided trigeminal lesion (see text). On maximum jaw closing consecutively tested at either side a full interference pattern is achieved on the right, whereas on the left only one unit fires with a frequency of up to 50/s

and malocclusion (Munro 1972b, Munro 1975) or dyscoordination of the chewing muscle activities following intrinsic brain stem lesions (Jelasic and Freitag 1978) or tetanus (Struppler et al. 1963).

Finally we want to stress that an EMG of at least the masseter muscle should be performed in all patients presenting a sensory disorder or pain in the area of the third trigeminal branch because of its close anatomical vicinity to the motor portion.

2. Masseter Reflex

The masseter reflex is a typical stretch reflex elicited by a tap to the chin. The reflex pathway is monosynaptic as has been demonstrated by Szentogothai (1948). Ia-afferents arising from the muscle spindles of the mandibular elevators pass via the motor portion to the associated cell somata in the trigeminal mesencephalic nucleus. The central processes of these cells form synapses at the motoneurons predominantly in the ipsilateral trigeminal motor nucleus. Thus, the afferent as well as the efferent limb of this reflex arc runs in the trigeminal motor portion (McIntyre a. Robinson 1959). Unilateral or bilateral alterations of the masseter reflex which can be determined as follows below, point to a lesion in the motor portion or the associated brain stem structures.

For routine testing we use a modification of the method described by Goodwill 1968 and Kimura 1970. A pair of surface electrodes is placed bilaterally over the masseter muscle near the angle of the mandible and over the corresponding side of the nose, providing symmetrical positions. The electrodes are connected via differential amplifiers to an oscilloscope and a print recorder. The reflex is elicited bilaterally by a tap to the centre of the mandible with a hammer triggering the oscilloscope beam. The patients are asked to contract the masseter muscles slightly as controlled on the oscilloscope. The upper pair of traces in Fig. 2 shows the reflex response of a normal subject. The parameters evaluated are the latencies and the amplitudes of the reflex responses. Consecutive trials in one individul reveal variations in latency and amplitude, but a rather stable ratio when comparing the responses on both sides. We regard absolute latencies longer than 9 ms and a latency difference between the two sides longer than 1.0 ms as a pathological sign. Amplitudes from peak to peak determined with our method range from 0 to 5 mV depending on the force of the tap, the intensity of the pre-tap innervation and additional, partly for-

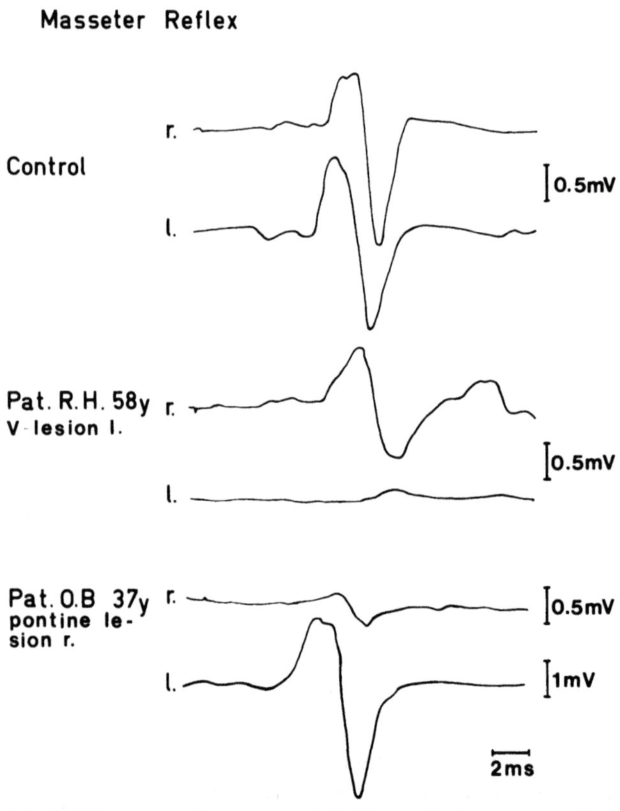

Fig. 2. Masseter reflexes recorded bilaterally by means of surface electrodes. The upper pair of tracing shows a normal response right (*r*) and left (*l*). The medial pair of tracings was taken from the patient described in fig. 1. On the left side a pathological response is recorded with a prolonged latency and an amplitude near to zero. The lower tracings show the reflex of a patient with a right-sided intrapontine vascular malformation. The right response is markedly decreased. Note that the amplification right is twofold compared to left

tuitous factors such as bi- or unilateral dental prostheses. Thus, absolute amplitude values apper to be not too meaningful. Comparing the responses on both sides we take unilateral absence or a difference of more than 70 percent (larger amplitude set 100 percent) as a sign of a motor trigeminal lesion. These criteria are in good agreement with those applied by Kimura et al. 1970, and Ongerboer de Visser a. Goor 1974.

The medial traces in Fig. 2 illustrate the reflex responses of the same patient as in Fig. 1. As has been expected, no response was recorded on the left side.

The lower traces in Fig. 2 show the bilateral masseter reflex in a patient suffering from right-sided intrapontine vascular malformation. The clear decrease of the response on the affected side is probably caused by an intrapontine involvement of the efferent path, since electromyographically denervation signs have been detected.

We regard the masseter reflex as a valuable measure for screening and follow-up of patients. It is routinely performed in all patients with disorders of the trigeminal nerve as well as of other cranial nerves or the brain stem. In pathological cases additional needle electromyography should be performed to distinguish between a central and a peripheral disorder.

Methods Testing Sensory Function

1. The Orbicularis Oculi Reflex (OOR)

A measure to evaluate sensory function seems necessary particularly in the trigeminal system since clinical examinations often fail to give unequivocal results. Unfortunately the tests used to investigate peripheral nerve function can not be applied to the trigeminal system for anatomical reasons. Therefore other somewhat more complicated approaches have to be choosen. A method which can provide objective data concerning the sensory trigeminal function is the OOR.

Since Kugelberg's electromyographical analysis in 1952 an increasing literature has dealt with this subject. As far as the clinical application is concerned the OOR has been predominantly used in the investigation of brain stem lesions (Kimura 1971, Shahani a. Young 1972, Ongerboer de Visser a. Kuypers 1978) or of disorders of the facial nerve (Schenck a. Manz 1973, Kimura et al. 1976). A study selectively dealing with the use of the OOR in trigeminal disorders was published by Kimura et al. in 1970 and Ongerboer de Visser a. Goor in 1974. The OOR is a trigeminofacial reflex consisting of an early and a late response (see Fig. 3). It is usually elicited by unilateral electrical stimulation of the supraorbital nerve and recorded from the lower eyelid bilaterally. The early ipsilateral component is relayed through the pons via an oligosynaptic pathway involving the trigeminal main sensory and the facial nucleus (Kimura 1970, Hiraoka a. Shimamura 1977). The late component appears to pass through the spinal trigeminal complex and projects to the ipsilateral and contralateral facial nuclei via a polysynaptic pathway in the lateral and medial bulbar reticular formation (Ongerboer de Visser a. Kuypers 1978).

The OOR appears to be a sensitive test to detect peripheral and central sensory trigeminal disorders, provided an additional lesion of the efferent path can be ruled out.

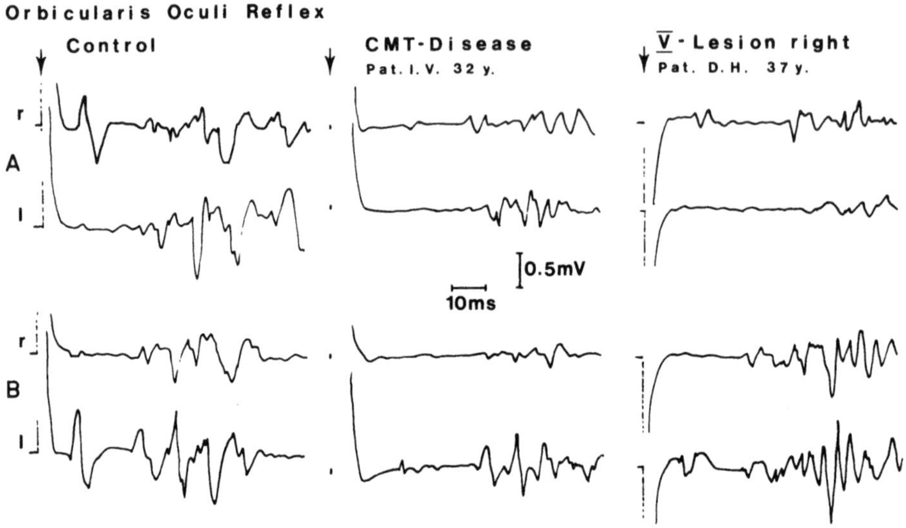

Fig. 3. Orbicularis oculi reflex recorded bilaterally by means of surface electrodes. Arrows indicate the stimulation of the right (**A**) and the left (**B**) supraorbital nerve. On the left side a normal OOR is illustrated. The medial tracings show bilaterally delayed early and late responses in a patient suffering from Charcot-Marie-Tooth disease. On the right on OOR of a patient with a right-sided trigeminal lesion is presented. A pathological delay and a reduction of the late components following right-sided stimulation can be recognized

Stimulation and recording techniques will be briefly described. The supraorbital nerve is stimulated with a bipolar electrode with the cathode placed over the foramen supraorbitale. Constant current pulses (2 to 20 mA, 0.1 ms) are applied with a frequency of 0.1 Hz to avoid habituation of the late response. At least five trials are carried out on either side using the same stimulus strenght. The responses are recorded bilaterally placing a pair of surface electrodes over the palpebral part of the lower eyelid and the corresponding side of the nose. The potentials are amplified and displayed as described for the masseter reflex. Routinely the distal conduction velocity of the facial nerve and the amplitude of the directly evoked responses of the lower eyelids are measured to discover a possible additional lesion in the efferent path.

Figure 3 shows a normal OOR on the right. The parameters evaluated are the latencies of the ipsilateral and contralateral responses. In Table 1 the control values of our lab are listed. The amplitudes, however, are rather variable, particularly of the late responses, which are in fact desynchronized motor unit potential trains. Thus, at the moment, we only regard an absence or a repeatedly reproduced clear decrease of a component as a pathological sign. Generally speaking, peripheral trigeminal lesions may show prolonged latencies and diminished or even absent amplitudes of the ipsilateral and contralateral responses evoked by stimulation on the affected side. In this context the evaluation of the bilateral late responses is of particular importance.

In the medial column of Fig. 3 the OOR of a patient suffering from the hypertrophic type of Charcot-Marie-Tooth disease is illustrated. Decreased conduction

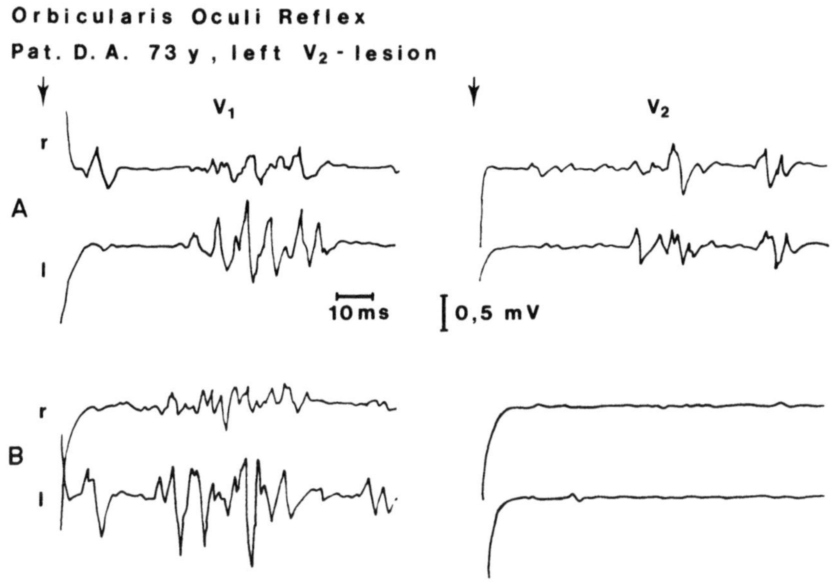

Fig. 4. Orbicularis oculi reflex recorded bilaterally by means of surface electrodes. Arrows indicate stimulation right (**A**) and left (**B**). Stimulation of the supraorbital nerves (V_1) evokes normal responses. Following stimulation of the infraorbital nerves (V_2) on the right side a normal OOR, on the left side no response is recorded

velocity in the trigeminal as well as in the facial nerve accounts for the clearly prolonged latencies. On the left Fig. 3 shows the OOR of a patient with a slight right-sided facial hypesthesia of unknown origin. Ipsilateral and contralateral responses were delayed when stimulating the right side as compared with stimulation on the left side.

The OOR can also be evoked by stimulation of the infraorbital and mental nerve. In this case a careful search for the best stimulation site is necessary since no unequivocal anatomical landmarks can be felt by palpation and the tissue layers between the electrode and the nerve are thicker than at the supraorbital site. This may be one of the reasons why, to our knowledge, these stimulation sites have not been used for diagnostic purposes. In all cases with a suspected disorder of the second or third trigeminal branch we evoked an OOR from the intraorbital and mental nerve

Table 1. Orbicularis oculi reflex

Latency (ms) of the early (R_1) and late response (R_2) in 25 normal subjects

	mean ± SD	limit	difference right-left	limit of difference
R_1	11.4 ± 0.9	13.3 (14)	0.3 ± 0.6	1.5
R_2-ipsilateral	31.6 ± 3.2	38.1 (40)	0.3 ± 1.9	4.3 (5)
R_2-contralateral	32.4 ± 3.0	38.5 (40)	0.5 ± 2.1	5.0
R_2-difference between ipsi- and contralateral			0.8 ± 1.6	4.1 (5)

respectively using a small stimulation electrode. Regarding the latencies, the same criteria are used as in supraorbital stimulation, mainly comparing the second components evoked by stimulation on either side. The amplitudes are frequently smaller and sometimes not elicitable also in normals, in particular from the mental nerve. Thus, only a unilateral absence is considered to be pathological. Fig. 4 shows the OOR of a patient who has previously undergone avulsion of the left infraorbital nerve for trigeminal neuralgia. There was still pain and slight hypesthesia in the associated area. Whereas the OOR stimulated from both supraorbital and the right infraorbital nerves appear to be normal, no response was obtained from the left infraorbital nerve.

Finally, idiopathic trigeminal neuralgia should be considered briefly. In agreement with Kimura et al., 1970, and Ongerboer de Visser and Goor, 1974, we did not find definite alterations of the OOR in cases of idiopathic trigeminal neuralgia with the typical anamnestic and clinical signs. It should be mentioned, however, that sometimes in patients with the idiopathic form we got the impression of even more accentuated responses on the affected side (see Struppler and Dobbelstein 1963). But such alterations concerning the activity of the responses still escape exact quantification. At present we are making an attempt to accurately quantify the OOR responses, but are still in an experimental phase.

New Approaches

1. The Jaw Opening Reflex (JOR)

Hoffmann and Tönnies, 1948, were the first to demonstrate the constant occurence of the jaw opening reflex in man. Following unilateral stimulation at various intraoral and perioral sites the volitional EMG-activity in both masseter muscles is suppressed for one or two short periods (Munro 1971, Godaux a. Desmedt 1975). The oligosynaptic reflex arc involves the second or third trigeminal branch, the main sensory trigeminal nucleus, the nucleus supratrigeminalis and the bilateral trigeminal motor nuclei (Munro 1975). Since it is a pure trigemino-trigeminal reflex it may provide a means to study central and peripheral trigeminal disorders.

Figure 5 on the right shows a normal jaw opening reflex stimulated unilaterally at the lower lip and recorded with needle electrodes in the masseter muscles. About 15 ms after the stimulus a period of nearly complete suppression of the EMG activity lasting about 20 ms can be observed. A second silent period can be seen after about 60 ms.

The medial column of Figure 5b shows the JOR of a patient with a left sensory and motor trigeminal lesion (same patient as in Fig. 2b). The EMG was recorded in the right normal masseter muscle only. Consistent with a left-sided lesion of the third trigeminal branch the JOR is elicited by stimulation on the right, but not on the left lower lip. On the left of figure 5 the IOR of the same patient (O. B.) as in Figure 2 is illustrated. Following left-sided stimulation a normal IOR is seen in the left, but not in the partially paretic right masseter muscle. After right-sided stimulation the IOR is missing bilaterally. Obviously, this reflex pattern points to a right central interruption of the reflex arc.

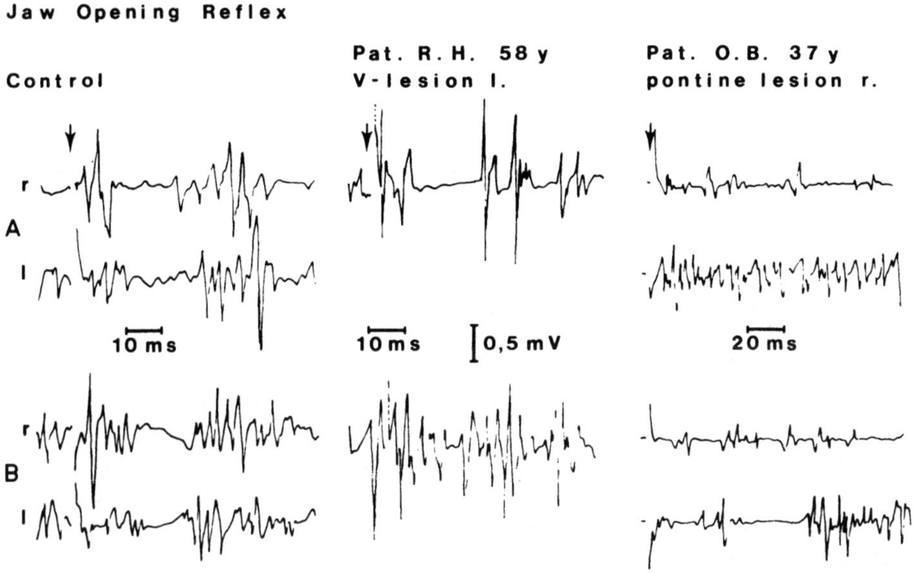

Fig. 5. Jaw opening reflex recorded bilaterally with concentric needle electrodes. Arrows indicate the stimulation at the right (**A**) and the left (**B**) lower lip. On the left a normal IOR is illustrated with the typical silent periods (see text). In the middle the IOR of the patient described in fig. 1 is presented. Recording from the right masseter only, since in the left only one unit was found in the previous EMG. Stimulation on the right side evoked on IOR whereas from the left side no silent period was elicitable. On the right the IOR of the patient O. B. described in fig. 2 is illustrated. Stimulation on the right side fails to evoke an IOR on either side. On left-sided stimulation a silent period in the left masseter is elicited whereas the moderately paretic right masseter continues firing

At present we are testing whether the IOR can be applied in the diagnosis of lesions of the second and third trigeminal branches. We hope that parameters can be established which allow diagnostic conclusions also in cases with rather discrete clinical symptoms.

2. Somatosensory Evoked Potentials

Stöhr and Petruch, 1979, and Bennett and Jannetta, 1980, have reported on somatosensory evoked potentials following trigeminal stimulation. At present the method seems still to be in an experimental phase. Further studies must reveal whether this method is appropriate for routine examination of trigeminal disorders.

Discussion

Concerning trigeminal motor function, neurophysiological tests are available which can add valuable and often superior information to the results of the clinical examination. If these tests are applied, lesions of the trigeminal motor protion can hardly be overlooked. In addition, pathological results obtained in patients suffering from pain in the trigeminal area point to a symptomatic neuralgia and justify further diagnostic steps.

Sensory trigeminal function is more difficult to be tested neurophysiologically. The methods routinely used in the investigation of peripheral nerves cannot be applied to the trigeminal nerve. Brain stem reflexes, where either the afferent limb only (OOR) or both, the afferent and the efferent limb (masseter reflex, IOR), run in the trigeminal nerve, can be a valuable tool.

The OOR provides appropriate information in peripheral and central sensory trigeminal disorders. Diagnostic conclusions can be drawn not only in clinically obvious trigeminal lesions but also in slightly or questionably affected cases. As has been described, this method can also be applied to investigate the major three branches selectively. This may be important in patients with lesions distal to the semilunar ganglion. A major clinical goal is to discriminate between the idiopathic and symptomatic type of trigeminal neuralgia since further diagnostic steps and treatment may be different. A normal OOR does not exclude a symptomatic origin. An altered reflex pattern, however, points to an essential lesion of the nerve and requires further careful examination. In idiopathic trigeminal neuralgia no definite reflex changes can be observed.

The complex brain stem distribution of the OOR pathway and the fact that the efferent limb runs in the facial nerve causes alteration of the diagnostic parameters following lesions of these structures. A pure facial nerve disorder can be easily distinguished (Kimura et al. 1976) by the reflex pattern, and even a combined trigemino-facial lesion can be analysed by careful studying the reflex responses. In conditions where the peripheral nerves may be affected as well as the central brainstem connections such as in cerebello-pontine angle tumors a statement as to what extent the trigeminal system is involved may be possible when adding the results of the EMG and the masseter reflex investigations. The possibility of localizing intrinsic or extrinsic brain stem lesions accurately shall not further be considered in this context.

The major advantages of the described tests are: 1. that they provide objective data, 2. that they can be frequently repeated in the follow up of patients in an average EMG lab, 3. that they are free of hazards and do not produce essential discomfort. They can be used as screening examinations before further, more complicated diagnostic measures are planned. In particular, when combined and repeated, these tests are able to provide information regarding disturbed trigeminal function early in the course of the disease when clinical examination alone may fail to give unequivocal results.

In our laboratory, new approaches to improve accuracy of the neurophysiological examination in the trigeminal system comprise the exact quantification of the OOR components and an attempt to apply the jaw opening reflex in clinical studies. Another hopeful approach appears to be the investigation of trigeminal evoked somatosensory potentials.

Conclusions

Clinical neurophysiological tests to investigate the motor and sensory function of the trigeminal nerve are available. Since they are easily performed in an average

EMG lab and free of complications, they are highly appropriate for screening and follow-up examinations. They should be applied in every patient suspected of having a trigeminal disorder since they are superior to clinical examination alone, particularly when used in combination. Further steps to improve the neurophysiological diagnosis in the trigeminal system seem to be necessary.

References

Bennett MH, Jannetta PJ (1980) Trigeminal evoked potentials in humans. Electroencephalogr Clin Neurophysiol 48:517–526

Godaux E, Desmedt JF (1975) Exteroceptive Suppression and Motor Control of the Masseter and Temporalis Muscles in Man. Brain Res 85:447–458

Goodwill CJ (1968) The normal jaw reflex: Measurement of the action potential in the masseter muscles. Ann Phys Med 9:183–188

Hiraoka M, Shimamura M (1977) Neural Mechanisms of the Corneal Blinking Reflex in Cats. Brain Res 125:265–275

Hoffmann P, Tönnies JE (1948) Nachweis des völlig konstanten Vorkommens des Zungen-Kieferreflexes beim Menschen. Pfluegers Arch 250: 103–108

Jelasic F, Freitag V (1978) Inverse activity of masticatory muscles with and without trismus: a brainstem syndrome. J Neurol Neurosurg Psychiatry 41:798–804

Kimura J (1970) Alteration of the Orbicularis Oculi Reflex by Pontine Lesions. A Study in Multiple Sclerosis. Arch Neurol 22: 156–161

Kimura J (1971) Electrodiagnostic Study of Brainstem Strokes. Stroke 2:576–586

Kimura J, Rodnitzky RL, Van Allen MW (1970) Electrodiagnostic Study of Trigeminal Nerve. Neurology (Minneap) 20:574–583

Kimura J, Giron LT, Young SM (1976) Electrophysiological Study of Bell's Palsy. Arch Otolaryngol 102: 140–143

Kugelberg E (1952) Facial Reflexes. Brain 75:385–396

McIntyre AK, Robinson RG (1959) Pathway for the jaw jerk in man. Brain 82:468–474

Munro RR (1972b) Electromyography of the masseter and anterior temporalis muscle in subjects with potential temporo-mandibular joint dysfunction. Aust Dent J 17:209–218

Munro RR, Basmaijan JV (1971) The jaw-opening reflex in man. Electromyography 11:191–206

Ongerboer de Visser BW, Goor C (1974) Electromyographic and reflex study in idiopathic and symptomatic trigeminal neuralgias: latency of the jaw and blink reflexes. J Neurol Neurosurg Psychiatry 37: 1225–1230

Ongerboer de Visser BW, Kuypers HGJM (1978) Late blink reflex changes in lateral medullary lesions. An electrophysiological and neuroanatomical study of Wallenberg's syndrome. Brain 101:285–294

Ruprecht EO (1974) Das EMG des partiell denervierten Muskels. In: Hopf HC, Struppler A (eds) Elektromyographie. Thieme Stuttgart, 39–47

Schenck E, Manz F (1973) The blink reflex in Bell's palsy. In: Desmedt JE (ed) New Developments in Electromyography and Clinical Neurophysiology, Vol. 3. Karger, Basel, p 678–681

Shahani BT, Young RR (1972) Human orbicularis oculi reflexes. Neurol 22: 149–154

Stöhr M, Petruch F (1979) Somatosensory evoked potentials following stimulation of the trigeminal nerve in man. J Neurol 220:95–98

Struppler A, Dobbelstein H (1963) Elektromyographische Untersuchung des Glabellareflexes bei verschiedenen neurologischen Störungen. Nervenarzt 34:347–352

Struppler A, Struppler E, Adams R (1963) Local Tetanus in Man. Arch Neurol 8: 162–178

The Pathophysiology of Trigeminal Neuralgia

P. J. JANNETTA and M. H. BENNETT, Pittsburgh, Pa/USA

Twenty years ago, it could be said with some veracity that, 'With all reference to the opinions of distinguished men who have advanced theories concerning the etiology of trigeminal neuralgia (TN), so far as we are aware, no pathological lesion has been established as the causative factor' [28]. This was so despite the work of Dandy concerning frequent abnormalities of the dorsal root of the trigeminal nerve, most commonly vascular but occasionally neoplastic or otherwise. Dandy's ideas and observations on trigeminal neuralgia took some buffeting at the hands of Stookey and Ransohoff, the authors of the above quotation. He now appears to be vindicated. Dandy sectioned the nerve in treatment of TN. He did not and possibly could not treat it definitively except by removing the occasional tumor. He had few immediate heirs to continue his work. He had no magnification techniques to aid visualization. He had no photographs to share with others. No one outside his own circle verified his observations.

By 1962, however, James Gardner [7, 8] had made his own observations in 18 patients who had recurrent TN. He was able to operate in the cerebellopontine angle safely. He noted some blood vessels and tumors but again, sectioned the nerve in treatment.

More recently, starting in 1966, many others have shown abnormalities of the dorsal root entry zone in patients with TN and, using magnification techniques, some have treated TN by mobilizing the vessel away from the nerve and holding it away with a small implant [11–15]. On this basis, a concept of pathophysiology can be formulated based on some experimental and pathological evidence.

In 1965, Beaver, Moses, and Ganote [1] showed ultrastructural abnormalities of myelination in nerves of patients with TN. These changes, verified almost immediately by Kerr [17, 18] consisted of focal areas of hypermyelination, hypomyelination, overgrowth of myelin into great axis cylinders and sometimes, totally disrupted myelin.

Saunders et al. [26] demonstrated electromyographic evidence of denervation on the affected side in the temporalis and masseter muscles in seventy percent of patients with TN. Earlier, physiological experiments in cats by King and Cowhers studied the electrophysiologic effects of the injection of alumina cream (an intense epileptogenic scar forming agent) into the trigeminal ganglia. These animals were oversensitive to stimuli in the ipsilateral trigeminal sensory distribution. King found delayed high voltage activity in the peripheral trigeminal nerves of these cats, arising from the caudal nuclei and conducted centrifugally. These cats appeared hypersensitive and although King was careful to state that this was not TN, others stated that it was, and that TN was therefore, due to epilepsy in the brainstem nuclei. Others, more recently, have found disorders in the dorsal root reflex in tic.

The occurrence of sclerotic plaques, tumor and vascular cross compression at the root entry zone [7, 11–16, 23, 24, 29] may, in TN patients, produce the forces leading to or contributing to ongoing degenerative changes seen in the fifth nerve and ganglion [1, 17, 18]. Most theories on the etiology of classical TN place the primary lesion peripheral to the brainstem and abnormal function of the primary afferents is presumed. Short circuiting of nerve impulses from large fibers with abnormal myelin structure to unmyelinated fibers ('crosstalk') [7, 16] has been suggested as a mechanism by which the pain signaling system is activated during an attack. Calvin et al. [4] have proposed that extra impulses generated at the sites of altered myelin may start reflected and then reverbatory impulses in the large primary afferents. The large fiber activity is thought, in turn, to produce presynaptic depolarizations in A fibers, activating reverberations and thus abnormal activity in the pain signaling system. In the above theories, no abnormality of the central components of the trigeminal system is assumed (stated or implied) and its activity simply reflects the abnormal activity of the pain-signaling afferents.

While especially appealing as an explanation for many of the characteristics of TN, the present theories do not clearly treat some long standing observations on trigeminal system function. First, the activation of large primary afferents (touch, tooth tap) inhibit the response to presumed pain-provoking tooth pulp stimulation [19, 27]. Secondly, activation of only the large primary afferents by electrical stimulation is relatively ineffective in triggering a pain attack in TN patients [20]. And, abnormal (epileptiform) activity and changed synaptic relationships in the trigeminal system follows experimental deafferentation [3, 30]. It is not known whether a changed afferent 'message' would prevent the expression of such normal inhibitory function or whether secondary central nervous system changes occur as a result of long term changes of the input in TN. In addition, partial deafferentation of the trigeminal system has been shown in experimental animals to produce functional changes at thalamic levels [3] and the animals showed altered behavioral responses to previously innoccuous stimulation of the face area. It is not unreasonable to propose that a reduced input occurs with compression of the trigeminal root entry zone and that the largest fibers are most affected [9]. Considering the effects of long term changed input, known to occur in other modalities, one might expect secondary central nervous system changes in response to trigeminal root compression. For instance, sensory deprivation has been shown to produce behavioral, anatomical and physiological changes [5, 6, 10, 22, 25, 31].

Although highly variable, trigeminal sensory and motor abnormalities have been seen in TN [21, 26]. In a recent report, Bennett and Jannetta [2] have shown increased trigeminal threshold and evoked potential latencies in a group of TN patients. However, the abnormalities correlated more with the reversibility of the pain state following microvascular decompression than with the presence of the pain state. Overall, the results were consistent with the expected effects of root compression, but normal electrophysiological findings were also seen. In every patient with classical TN and normal electrophysiological measures, the pain state was relieved following vascular decompression (5/5). It would appear that the critical measure produced by compression and consistent with the pain state has not been identified. By the time objective measures of compression are evident, the pain state has long been established.

With age, arteries elongate gradually and even may dilate as arteriosclerosis develops. Also, the brain shrinks slightly and sags caudally starting as early as the third decade of life. The many arteries at the base of the brain may loop and may, by chance, impact the root entry zone of the trigeminal nerve, causing pulsatile compression at the area of the nerve where the central myelin (oligodendrocytes) joins with the peripheral myelin (Schwann cells) and where defects in the myelin are seen. Scattered axis cylinders and their myelin become abnormal and their myelin enter into what appears to be a dynamic process of abnormal conduction (disordered root reflex, crosstalk, reflected impulses, reverberations, slowed conduction, threshold changes and the pain state) and widespread degeneration and regenerating going on simultaneously in different axis cylinders. One can almost imagine the artery elongating and the nerve accommodating until the vessel is deeply impacted into the nerve and loss of function develops.

Despite what we know, there is much more to learn. We must have an effective physiological chronic animal model to clarify the many unknowns in this disabling symptom called trigeminal neuralgia. We must continue to search for the physiological correlates of the pain state. This is now on the horizon. Hopefully, new information will be forthcoming to clarify the remaining questions.

References

1. Beaver DL, Moses HL, Ganote CE (1965) Electron microscopy of the trigeminal ganglion. III. Trigeminal neuralgia. Arch Path (Chicago) 79:571–582
2. Bennett MH, Jannetta PJ (1980) Evoked potentials in trigeminal neuralgia. Presented at the American Association of Neurological Surgeons Annual Meeting, New York
3. Black RE (1974) A laboratory model for trigeminal neuralgia. Adv Neurol 4:651–658
4. Calvin WH, Loeser JD, Howe JF (1977) A neurophysiological theory for the pain mechanism of tic douioureux. Pain 3:147–154
5. Dews PB, Wiesel TN (1970) Consequences of monocular deprivation on visual behavior in kittens. J Physiol (Lond) 206:437–455
6. Ganz L, Fitch M (1968) The effect of visual deprivation on perceptual behavior. Exp Neurol 22:614–637
7. Gardner WJ (1962) Concerning the mechanism of trigeminal neuralgia and hemifacial spasm. J Neurosurg 19:947–958
8. Gardner WJ, Sava GA (1962) Hemifacial spasm: A reversible pathophysiologic state. J Neurosurg 19:240–247
9. Gasser HS, Erlanger J (1929) The role of fiber size in the establishment of a nerve block by pressure or cocaine. Am J Physiol 88:581–591
10. Glass JD, Crowder JV, Kennerdell JS, Merckangas JR (1977) Visually evoked potentials from occipital and precentral cortex in visually deprived humans. EEG and Clin, Neurophysiol 43:207–217
11. Jannetta PJ (1967) Arterial compression of the trigeminal nerve at the pons in patients with trigeminal neuralgia. J Neurosurg 26:159–162
12. Jannetta PJ (1977) Observations on the etiology of trigeminal neuralgia, hemifacial spasm, acoustic nerve dysfunction and glossopharyngeal neuralgia. Definitive microsurgical treatment and results in 117 patients. Neurochirurgia (Stuttgart) 20:145–154
13. Jannetta PJ (1976) Microsurgical approach to the trigeminal nerve for tic douloreux. Prog Neurol Surg 20:180–200
14. Jannetta PJ (1977) Treatment of trigeminal neuralgia by suboccipital and transtentorial cranial operation. Clin Neurosurg 24:538–549
15. Kempe LG, Smith DR (1969) Trigeminal neuralgia, facial spasm, intermedius and glossopharyngeal neuralgia with persistent carotid-basilar anastomosis. J Neurosurg 31:445–451

16. Kerr FWL (1967) Evidence for a peripheral etiology of trigeminal neuralgia. J Neurosurg 26:168–174
17. Kerr FWL (1967) Pathology of trigeminal neuralgia: Light and electron microscopic observations. J Neurosurg 26:151–156
18. Kerr FWL, Mill RH (1966) The pathology of trigeminal neuralgia: Electron microscopic studies. Arch Neurol 15:308–319
19. Khayyat GF, Ya YJ, King RB (1975) Response patterns to noxious and non-noxious stimuli in rostral trigeminal relay nuclei. Brain Res 97:47–60
20. Kugelberg E, Lindblom V (1959) The mechanism of the pain in trigeminal neuralgia. J Neurol Neurosurg Psychiatry 22:36–43
21. Lewy FH, Grant FC (1938) Physiopathologic and pathoanatomic aspects of major trigeminal neuralgia. Arch Neurol Psychiat 40:1126–1134
22. Lund JS, Lund RD (1972) The effects of varying periods of visual deprivation on synaptogenesis in the superior colleralus of the rat. Dr Res 42:21–32
23. Petty PG, Southby R (1977) Vascular compression of lower cranial nerves: Observations using microsurgery, with particular reference to trigeminal neuralgia. Aust NZ J Surg 47:314–320
24. Revilla AG (1962) Tic douloureux and its relationship to tumors of the posterior fossa. J Neurosurg 19:947–958
25. Riesen AH (1975) The developmental neuropsychology of sensory deprivation. Academic Press, N.Y., p 303
26. Saunders RL, Krout R, Sachs E Jr (1971) Masticator electromyography in trigeminal neuralgia. Neurology (Minneap) 21:1221–1225
27. Sessle BS, Greenwood LF (1976) Inputs to trigeminal brain stem neurones from facial, oral, tooth pulp and pharyngolaryngeal tissues: I. Responses to innoccuous and noxious stimuli. Brain Res 117:211–226
28. Stooky B, Ransohoff J (1951) Trigeminal neuralgia: Its history and treatment. C.C. Thomas, Springfield, IL, p 91
29. Waga S, Morekawa A, Kojima T (1979) Trigeminal neuralgia: Compression of the trigeminal nerve by an elongated and dilated basilar artery. Surg Neurol 11:13–16
30. Westrum LE (1974) Electron microscopy of deafferentation in the spinal trigeminal nucleus. Adv Neurol 4:53–60
31. Wiesel TN, Hubel DN (1963) Single-cell responses in striate cortex of kittens deprived of vision in one eye. J Neurophysiol 26:1003–1017

Symptomatic Trigeminal Neuralgia

F. REGLI, Lausanne

In the great majority of patients trigeminal neuralgia is idiopathic; i.e. usually no underlying anatomical cause can be identified after a thorough search. This idiopathic form is characterized by: brief paroxysms of severe pain confined to one or more divisions of the trigeminal nerve, lack of objective evidence of motor or sensory deficit of the involved nerve, common occurrence of trigger zones and trigger mechanisms and unpredictable remissions and exacerbations of pain.

Only in a small percentage of patients trigeminal neuralgia is shown by a careful study to be symptomatic and related to verified lesions. This form of neuralgia is classified according to the side of the lesion. Four groups can be considered: A. Trigeminal lesions by a brain stem disease. B. Trigeminal lesions by a disease outside the brain stem but in the intracranial space. C. Trigeminal lesions by an extracranial disease. D. Trigeminal sensory neuropathy. For each of these groups we present some characteristic diseases.

A. Trigeminal Lesions by a Brain Stem Disease

Although brain stem vascular syndromes, tumors and syringomyelia can cause a trigeminal neuralgia, the most typical disease of this group associated with a trigeminal neuralgia is multiple sclerosis (Olafson et al. 1966, Harris 1950, Rushton and Olafson 1966). Approximately two percent of patients with trigeminal neuralgia have multiple sclerosis and one percent of patients with multiple sclerosis have trigeminal neuralgia. Therefore trigeminal neuralgia due to demyelinating disease is 300 times more frequent than in a nonselected population. Except for the combination with a trigeminal neuralgia the onset and the course of multiple sclerosis in these patients is similar to those seen in other patients with multiple sclerosis. In about 80 to 90 percent of cases symptoms of multiple sclerosis preceed trigeminal neuralgia by several years. In about half of these patients the neurological examination reveals the presence of signs showing brain stem or cerebellar involvement. In 10 to 20 percent of the cases the trigeminal neuralgia preceeds symptoms of multiple sclerosis for some months. At the beginning some relationship can be found between exacerbations of the demyelinating disease and the episodes of trigeminal neuralgia. In a later phase the progression of multiple sclerosis is independent of the trigeminal neuralgia.

The mean age of onset of trigeminal neuralgia in patients with the combined disease is 45.2 to 5 years below the mean age of patients with trigeminal neuralgia alone. Both are represented in the same proportion. The neuralgia is bilateral in about 11 percent of the cases with combined disease and in four percent of the cases of idiopathic trigeminal neuralgia, therefore the bilateral form is also quite rare in patients with multiple sclerosis. The pain has in the combined form the same characteristics as in the isolated one, although some patients can experience paresthesias at the beginning. Seldom do patients display any objective sensory or motor disturbance of either trigeminal nerve at the examination. Some authors assume that the pain irradiation is confined to one or more divisions of the trigeminal nerve, while other authors assume that the lancinating pain paroxysms can irradiate also to the territories of the facial, glossopharyngeal and vagus nerves. The first hypothesis seems more appropriate: in no instance has a combination of multiple sclerosis and glossopharyngeal neuralgia been reported in the literature.

In the few reports of postmortem examination of cases with both multiple sclerosis and trigeminal neuralgia, plaques have been found at the point of emergence of the trigeminal nerve, but they can also involve the sensory nucleus or the descending root. It should be stressed, that in other postmortem examinations plaques with similar localisation produced only paresthesia but no paroxysmal pain burst. As for the other paroxysmal phenomena in multiple sclerosis the neuralgia is probably caused by transverse spreading: ephatic activation of axons within a partially demyelinated lesion. Generally patients with trigeminal neuralgia and multiple sclerosis respond to treatment of the neuralgia in a manner similar to that of patients who have trigeminal neuralgia alone.

B. Trigeminal Lesions by a Disease in the Intracranial space

It is not necessary to describe all the classical basal skull syndromes with involvement of the fifth nerve. The less known Raeder paratrigeminal syndrome should be mentioned because it represents not infrequently the first manifestation of a severe disease of the internal carotid artery. In 1924 Raeder reported five cases with paralysis of the ocular sympathetic pathway associated with a lesion of the ophthalmic branch of the fifth nerve. Owing to its important localizing value the recognition of this syndrome is of great diagnostic interest. In fact it can only be caused by a middle cranial fossa lesion located to a well-defined area, the paratrigeminal space lying between the medial border of the gasserian ganglion and the short vertical segment of the internal carotid between the anterior foramen lacerum and the carotid siphon. The two neurological signs of this syndrome are:

1. A partial Horner's syndrome with ptosis, myosis, enophthalmia, ocular hypotonia, hyperemia of bulbar conjunctiva, excess tearing but without anhydrosis of the face. The diagnosis of paralysis of the ocular sympathetic system can be substantiated by instillation of a one percent cocaine solution in the conjunctival sac (no dilatation of the pupil). The absence of anhydrosis shows clearly that the lesion involves the third or postganglionic neuron which ascends in the sympathetic plexus about the internal carotid artery, except for the sudomotor fibers mediating facial sweating, which accompagny the external carotid artery and thus remain extracranial. Anhydrosis will occur only with lesions proximal to the origin of the external carotid artery.

2. Lesion of the ophthalmic branch of the fifth nerve: this is characterized by a supraorbital pain. The pain can be very intense in short paroxysms or may have a burning character. At the examination the sensory disturbance with paresthesia or hypesthesia can be very mild with a slight sensory impairment of the cornea. The onset of symptoms is mostly sudden, but a progressive course is also known.

Concerning the etiology, Raeder's syndrome can be separated into two groups. The first group is a symptomatic group with parasellar cranial nerve involvement: a neoplasma in the anterior part of the middle cranial fossa, an infectious focal disease or a trauma are the most important causative factors.

The second group includes cases of Raeder's syndrome with neuralgia but without parasellar cranial nerve palsies. The pathogenesis of this group was not known before these cases were systematically subjected to angiographic studies, revealing frequently multiple pathological conditions of the internal carotid artery: calcification of the distal portion of the carotid artery (Boniuk and Schlezinger 1962), obstruction of the distal portion of the carotid artery (Castaigne et al. 1978), a dolichocarotid artery (Toussaint 1959), a fibromuscular dysplasia (Lederman and Salanga 1976, Cohen et al. 1975), a dissecting aneurysm (Cohen et al. 1975, West et al. 1976), a subcranial carotid aneurysm (Davis et al. 1968), and a thrombosis of the cervical carotid artery (Charbonnel et al. 1957, Castaigne et al. 1978).

We observed recently a similar case: a 55 year old man was asymptomatic until October, 1979, when he suddenly experienced a slight pain in the right orbital region and a dropping of the right upper eyelid. Visual acuity was normal, there was a severe ptosis of the right upper eyelid with a mild myosis, enophthalmia and anhydrosis of the face on the right side. Except for a slight hypoesthesia on the right side of the forehead the rest of the neurological examination was normal. By Doppler ultrasound-sonography the flow on the right supraorbital artery was reversed. Three weeks later a right carotid angiography showed a complete occlusion of the internal carotid artery 1 cm above the carotid bifurcation. Five months after the acute onset the Horner syndrome was still present while the cutaneous sensation of the face was normal.

The pathogenesis of this vascular Raeder's syndrome is most likely explained by ischemia of the vasa vasorum of the carotid artery wall as well as by ischemia of the fibers of the ophthalmic branch of the fifth nerve.

C. Trigeminal Lesions by Extracranial Diseases

The peripheral divisions of the fifth nerve mediate sensation from an extensive cutaneous territory and a large area of mucous membranes. It is concerned in transmission of pain caused by a large variety of traumatic, inflammatory and neoplastic lesions of the face, eye, ear, nose, paranasal sinus, oral cavity, tongue, and teeth (Selby 1975). The supratrochlear, supraorbital, and infraorbital nerves are frequently involved in craniofacial trauma, but the result is more often anesthesia than pain. Partial regeneration of the injured nerve may cause a constant pain confined stictly to the distribution of the nerve. Involvement of peripheral branches of the trigeminal nerve may result from primary or metastatic malignant tumors of the face, mouth, tongue, and paranasal sinuses: in some situations such a pain can be precipitated by a trigger mechanism. Neuritis of the infraorbital nerve secondary to maxillary sinusitis can cause pain that continues long beyond the cure of the sinus infection but is never paroxysmal.

Pain of dental origin though often not precisely localized to the offending tooth, only very rarely extends to involve the whole dermatome of the mandibular or maxillary division. Trauma to alveolar branches occurring during complicated extractions of impacted wisdom teeth or during excision of dentigerous cysts may cause protracted facial neuralgia. This pain in general is constantly of burning quality and associated with unpleasant dysesthesia. Seldom some dental illness like a pulpitis, an acute periodontitis can produce a paroxysmal pain by a trigger mechanism (intraoral trigger points) similar to that operating in genuine trigeminal neuralgia. It is well known (Mumford 1978) that people with idiopathic trigeminal neuralgia sometimes have teeth unnecessarily extracted. It is less well known that pain which seems to be due to idiopathic trigeminal neuralgia is occasionally due to dental causes. For this reason it is suggested that such cases should be given very careful dental and oral examination before the commencement of drug therapy or surgery.

D. Trigeminal Sensory Neuropathy

Idiopathic trigeminal sensory neuropathy is a sensory disturbance of one or more of the peripheral branches of the fifth cranial nerve of commonly unknown etiology. The disorder was first mentioned by Harris in 1935. Attention has been directed to the benign and reversible nature of this condition in the last fifteen years (Blau et al. 1974, Eggleston and Haskell 1972, vom Brocke and Regli 1974, Horowitz 1974, Gibbin and Griffith 1978). The patients complain of a sudden numbness affecting part or the whole of one side of the face. The sensory disturbance is noticed spontaneously on awakening or while shaving, touching or washing the affected area. The symptoms are confined in the second or in the third division or both divisions simultaneously. All three divisions are rarely affected together. Pain is not an initial feature. Only a few patients experience a burning sensation or, when touching, a tingling.

Examination reveals an impaired sensation to pinprick and touch, either partial or complete. In some cases there is only a subjective sensory difference. In no case the corneal reflex is lost, and the masseter, temporals and pterygoid muscles contract normally. The neurological and general examinations are within normal limits except for a slight vestibular imbalance or a partial facial paresis in rare cases. X-ray investigations are normal. Seldom is the recovery only partial with residual sensory symptoms like paresthesia. Paroxysmal trigeminal neuralgia does not appear to be a common sequel to sensory trigeminal neuropathy, although some patients suffer severe facial pain.

In view of the anatomical distribution of numbness, the absence of pain and the occasional presence of an impaired taste, it seems likely that the trigeminal nerve is affected peripheral to the gasserian ganglion. This idiopathic neuropathy presents some analogy with Bell's palsy and with the benign and transient impairement of function of the abducens nerve. Most of the authors postulate a virus as the cause of trigeminal idiopathic neuropathy like herpes, cytomegaly, Epstein-Barr or zoster-varicella. Evidently the diagnosis of benign trigeminal sensory neuropathy is primarily one of exclusion. A symptomatic form can be observed with diabetes mellitus, sarcoidosis, a connective tissue disease or a chemical agent. Multiple sclerosis must be excluded as well, because facial numbness is the presenting complaint in two to three percent of patients with multiple sclerosis. The absence of pain and the sudden onset facilitate the differential diagnosis with a space-occupying lesion of the middle cranial fossa or a post-nasal carcinoma.

Conclusion and Summary

These examples show that many causes inside and outside the skull can involve the trigeminal nerve and produce a symptomatic trigeminal neuralgia. This neuralgia is characterized in most cases by a permanent pain and objectively by deficits in one or more of the usual methods of facial sensory testing like pinprick, light touch, and temperature. A symptomatic neuralgia can manifest itself not infrequently with pain paroxysms and trigger mechanisms similar to the genuine trigeminal neuralgia. All patients with suspected symptomatic trigeminal neuralgia require a complete neurological examination and a precise X-ray investigation. Often an otolaryngological opinion or a dental consultation may be helpful in differentiating some of the causes of a symptomatic trigeminal neuralgia.

References

Blau JN, Harris M, Kennett S (1969) Trigeminal sensory neuropathy. N Engl J Med 281:873–876

Boniuk M, Schlezinger NS (1962) Raeder's paratrigeminal syndrome. Am J Ophthalmol 54:1074–1084

Castaigne P, Brunet P, Ribadeau-Dumas JL, Rouques C, Thomas-Lamotte P (1978) Syndrome de Raeder et pathologie de la carotide interne. A propos de 3 observations. Rev Otoneuroophthalmol 50:43–48

Charbonnel A, Duverger A, Colas J, Baron A (1957) Le syndrome paratrigéminal de Raeder. A propos d'un cas. Rev Otoneuroopthalmol 29:81–87

Cohen DN, Zakov ZN, Salanga VD, Dohn DF (1975) Raeder's paratrigeminal syndrome. Am J Ophthalmol 79:1044–1049

Davis RH, Daroff RB, How WF (1968) Hemicrania, oculosympathetic paresis and subcranial carotid aneurysm: Raeder's paratrigeminal syndrome (group 2). J Neurosurg 29:94–96

Eggleston DJ, Haskell R (1972) Idiopathic trigeminal sensory neuropathy. Practitioner 208:649–655

Gibbin KP, Griffith IP (1978) Idiopathic sensory trigeminal neuropathy. J Laryngol Otol 92:915–923

Harris W (1935) Paroxysmal neuralgic tic as a sequel of trigeminal neuritis. Br Med J 1:1112–1114

Harris W (1959) Rare forms of paroxysmal trigeminal neuralgia and their relation to disseminated sclerosis. Br Med J 2:1015–1019

Horowitz SH (1974) Isolated facial numbness. Clinical significance and relation to trigeminal neuropathy. Ann Intern Med 80:49–53

Law WR, Nelson ER (1968) Internal carotid artery aneurysm as a cause of Raeder's paratrigeminal syndrome. Neurology (Minneap) 18:43–46

Lederman RJ, Salanga V (1976) Fibromuscular dysplasia of the internal carotid artery. A cause of Raeder's paratrigeminal syndrome. Neurology (Minneap) 26:353

Mumford JM (1978) Role of the dentist in trigeminal neuralgia. Pain 5:83–92

Olafson RA, Rushton JG, Sayre GP (1966) Trigeminal neuralgia in a patient with multiple sclerosis. An autopsy report. J Neurosurg 24:755–759

Raeder JG (1924) Paratrigeminal paralysis of oculo-pupillary sympathic. Brain 47:149–158

Rushton JG, Olafson RA (1965) Trigeminal neuralgia associated with multiple sclerosis. Report of 35 cases. Arch Neurol 13:383–386
Selby G (1975) Diseases of the fifth cranial nerve. In: Dick PJ, Thomas PK, Lambert EH (eds) Peripheral Neuropathy, Saunders, Philadelphia chap. 26
Toussaint D (1959) Contribution à l'étude du syndrome de Raeder ou syndrome paratrigéminal du sympathique oculaire. Acta Neurol Belg 7:892–914
Vom Brocke I, Regli F (1974) Die idiopathische Trigeminusneuropathie. Schweiz Med Wochenschr 104:1029–1031
West TET, Davies RJ, Kelly RE (1976) Horner's syndrome and headache due to carotid artery disease. Br Med J 1:818–820

Percutaneous Controlled Thermocoagulation of Gasserian Ganglion in Trigeminal Neuralgia. Experiences with 1000 Cases

J. Siegfried, Zürich

From February 1972 to June 1980, we operated 1000 cases of trigeminal neuralgia by applying the technique of percutaneous coagulations within the Gasserian ganglion and the use of temperature control [15, 16]. Immediate clinical results and follow-up studies have been widely published by many groups, including ourselves [12, 13]. We therefore do not propose herewith to submit a detailed report on our clinical results of these 1000 cases. Nevertheless, our extensive experience qualifies us to:

1. emphasize the value of this method;
2. define the indications;
3. advise on the performance of the operation;
4. comment on the mechanisms of trigeminal neuralgia.

1. The Value of Percutaneous Controlled Thermocoagulation of Gasserian Ganglion in Trigeminal Neuralgia

Any neurosurgical method for the treatment of pain is of substantial value when:

a) The operation is safe and does not create stress for the patient;
b) the rate of success is high;
c) the rate of relapse is low or acceptable;
d) the rate of complications is low and acceptable.

a) The percutaneous approach to the Gasserian ganglion introduced by Härtel creates little stress or hazard, can be performed on very old patients and with the patient practically ambulatory throughout. In our series of 1000 cases, we have had no mortality, and the oldest patient was 94 years old. Hospitalization lasts from one to three days, depending on the patient's living and social conditions. In a single case the patient was kept in hospital for one week, and this was due to a slight infection of the cerebro-spinal fluid which was not accompanied by neurological symptoms with the exception of a meningismus. With the aid of a barbiturate acting for only a brief period (for instance Brietal or Brevital, Lilly), the operation is not painful for the patient. Lateral and submento-vertex X-ray views confirm the position of the electrode in the Gasserian ganglion through the foramen ovale, and the electrical stimulation which elicits a non-painful sensation of itching or tingling in the field of projection of one, two or sometimes three divisions of the trigeminal nerve is helpful for the best localisation of the electrode. The percutaneous thermocoagulation of the Gasserian ganglion is a safe method.

b) The rate of success immediately following the percutaneous controlled thermocoagulation of the Gasserian ganglion for 'idiopathic' trigeminal neuralgia (tic douloureux) is very high. The rate of short-term success in our whole series reached 98 percent during the postoperative months. Recurrence of pain in the first postoperative days, mainly during the first or the second day but occasionally up to 12 days, was observed in 20 cases (two percent); all these cases were immediately reoperated upon with success. This brief recurrence of pain was observed nearly always in the cases of elderly patients in whom short general anaesthesia is often followed by a prolonged drowsy state. When the patient is not sufficiently awake to give adequate information about pin-prick and touch sensation, thermocoagulation may be prematurely ended if the surgeon is not patient enough. Technical impossibility to introduce the electrode within the foramen ovale was never encountered.

c) The rate of recurrence of pain must be evaluated after a long period of follow-up. Here we report on the results of cases operated on and followed up during periods from five and a half to eight years. From February 1972 until October 1974, 228 operations were performed on 208 patients. In seven patients the effect of the thermocoagulation was not sufficient, with recurrence of pain in the first few days up to 10 days postoperatively (3.8 percent). The operation was repeated in almost all patients because the patients were still hospitalized, and the results were good. Of these 208 patients (110 females and 98 males), 135 were interviewed directly or by means of questionnaires in spring of 1980. We were unable to reach 16 patients. Thirty four did not answer and 23 had died in the meanwhile, all of them at an advanced age. Four patients were younger than 40 years at the time of the operation. The oldest was aged 89 years. The great majority of patients were between 60 and 80 years of age. The neuralgia was localized on the right side 122 times and 86 times on the left. The root of the trigeminal nerve most frequently affected was the second (Table 1). At the time of the operation, patients had suffered from tic douloureux for an average of 7.3 years. The treatment which had previously been carried out is shown on Table 2. Of the 135 patients whom it was

Table 1. Division of trigeminal nerve involved in the series of 208 patients followed from five and a half to eight years

	Number	%
V_1	5	2.4
V_2	70	33.7
V_3	45	21.6
V_1, V_2	15	7.2
V_2, V_3	65	31.3
V_1, V_2, V_3	8	3.8
	208	100.0

Table 2. Treatment applied to the series of 208 patients followed from five and a half to eight years before percutaneous controlled thermocoagulation of Gasserian ganglion

Carbamazepin (Tegretol®)	95.2%
Phenytoin or Clonazepam (Rivotril®)	7.2%
Alcohol-injections	24.5%
Retrogasserian root section	11.5%
Suboccipital operations	1.5%

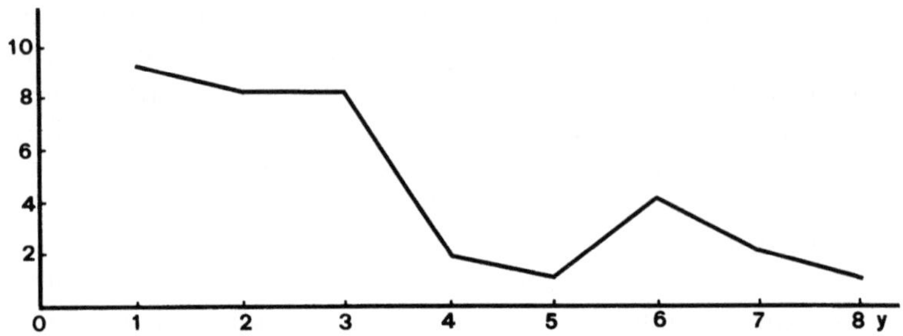

Fig. 1. Number of recurrences of pain over the years in the series of 135 out of 208 patients followed up to eight years

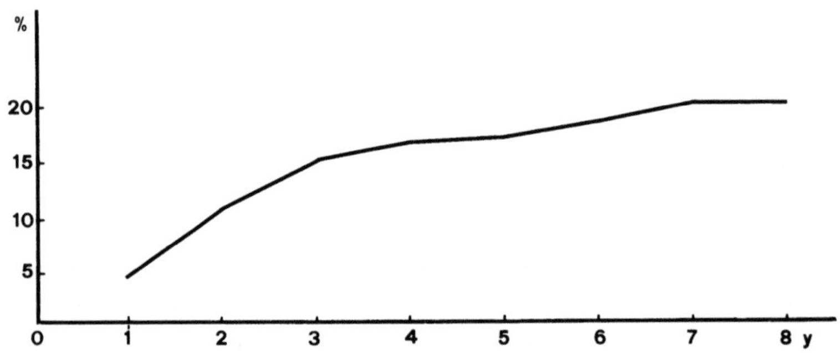

Fig. 2. Percentage of recurrence of pain over the years in the series of 135 out of 208 patients followed up to eight years

possible to follow for five to seven years, 34 were suffering from recurrent pain. However, in three cases the pain originated in another root on the same side, in three more cases on the opposite side, which gives a real recurrence rate of 20.7 percent. Of the 34 patients involved, 24 wished to be reoperated on by the same technique and were afterwards pain-free. One was operated on in another clinic by another method. In 5 cases, the recurrence of pain was so minimal that they preferred therapy with low dosages of carbamazepine, which was effective. The frequency of recurrence of pain is decreasing over the years (Fig. 1), but the percentage of relapse of pain of all patients operated on rises slowly in the course of time (Fig. 2).

The cause of recurrence of pain can be directly related to the degree of postoperative elimination of the pain sensation in the prior painful territory (hypalgesia/analgesia). Patients who after the operation have only a slight hypalgesia will most certainly suffer recurrence of pain. When analgesia is complete, even with slight hypesthesia, the recurrence of pain is improbable. No relation between the recurrence of pain and age of the patient or duration of the neuralgia has been found. Strangely enough, the number of males showing recurrence of pain was double that of females so affected.

A recurrence rate of five percent after one year and of 21 percent after five to seven years appears acceptable because the operation causes no mortality and no severe morbidity and can be repeated easily. No other clinical studies have indicated a rate of recurrence after five years and more, but our experience seems to confirm the results obtained with a large series by Sweet, who reports a relapse rate of 22 percent [17].

d) The rate of complication. Subjective complications due to objectively measurable sensory disturbances and objective neurological function deficits must also be considered. All complications are summarized in Table 3.

Transitory difficulties with ocular motor function from two days to six months occured in five patients.

In 28 patients who had first division pain, the analgesia obtained suppressed the corneal reflex, and slight keratitis occured in eight without long-lasting effects. Analgesia without total loss of touch sensation (pinprick appreciated as touch) is the goal of the operation and could be achieved in a majority of cases. However, a slight or moderate diminution of touch sensation is very common postoperatively and lasts from a few weeks to a few months. Almost 75 percent of the 135 patients

Table 3. Overall complications in the series of 135 out of 208 patients followed up to eight years

	Short-term	Long-term (5½ to 8 years)
Ocular palsy III palsy : 3 IV palsy : 1 VI palsy : 1	5 (3.7%)	0
Keratitis	8 (5.9%)	all cured
Anesthesia/Hypesthesia dolorosa	5 (3.7%)	4 (3.0%)
Dysesthesia of cornea		6 (4.4%)
Overall disturbances of sensitivity		36 (26.7%)
Masseter weakness	33 (24.4%)	2 (1.5%)

Table 4. Disturbances of touch sensitivity in the series of 135 out of 208 patients followed up from five and a half eight years

	Total	Not disturbing	Disturbing
Paresthesias	23 (17.0%)	15 (11.1%)	8 (5.9%)
Hypesthesias	49 (36.3%)	34 (25.2%)	15 (11.1%)
Paresth. + Hypesth.	17 (12.6%)	8 (5.9%)	9 (6.7%)
Anesth./Hypesth. dol.	4 (3.0%)		4 (3.0%)
No disturbances	42 (31.1%)	42 (31.1%)	
	135 (100%)	99 (73.3%)	36 (26.7%)

of this series followed from five and a half to eight years mentioned some sensitivity disturbances and more than 25 percent were complaining to some extent about these disturbances. These may be paresthesias, hypesthesia, a combination of both or anaesthesia/hypesthesia dolorosa (Table 4). The four patients affected by hypesthesia or anaesthesia dolorosa were old.

Masseter weakness is often seen immediately after the thermocoagulation. This is due probably to some slight mechanical lesion of the third division at the level of the foramen ovale by the introduction of the electrode or from thermocoagulation for third division pain by an extension of the Gasserian lesion into the post-ganglionic area. However, this slight postoperative weakness of the operated sides disappears rapidly and in only two cases was still present after a few years.

2. Indications

Surgical indications for trigeminal neuralgia exist:

a) when the neuralgia is typical (tic douloureux);
b) when medical therapy fails to achieve long-term control;
c) when medical therapy is not well tolerated;
d) when medical therapy is effective only with relatively high dosages of drugs and must be administered without interruption.

Besides the classical form of tic douloureux (still known by us as 'idiopathic trigeminal neuralgia', our definitions below), a symptomatic trigeminal neuralgia, particularly in cases of multiple sclerosis, is considered a good indication for operation. Atypical facial pain should not be treated surgically.

An analysis of the last 25 cases we have operated upon this year showed that 115 teeth were removed (4.6 per patient) and that more than 56,500 tablets of carbamazepine were swallowed (an average of 2,260 per patient). Under these circumstances, it seems that an earlier indication for surgery in the majority of the cases would have been beneficial for the patients.

3. Technical Considerations

The objective of percutaneous controlled thermocoagulation of Gasserian ganglion is to achieve an analgesia of the division which is affected by the disease without anaesthesia or marked hypesthesia. Unfortunately, this result cannot be obtained with certainty. In animal experiments it can be carried out under constant conditions, with temperatures from 60 to 65 °C maintained for 60 seconds; this abolishes the A-delta and C fibres components with little or no alteration of the earlier components of the compound action potentials [1, 3]. In human conditions, on the other hand, the differential critical range of temperature is greater. There are many reasons for this discrepancy: larger or smaller quantities of spinal fluid cooling the tip of the electrode, tip of the electrode in the border of the ganglion, variability in the consistence of the Gasserian ganglion. Measurements of the temperature at the tip of the electrode within the ganglion and the intensity of current over the past few months have so far shown that no consistent direct relation-

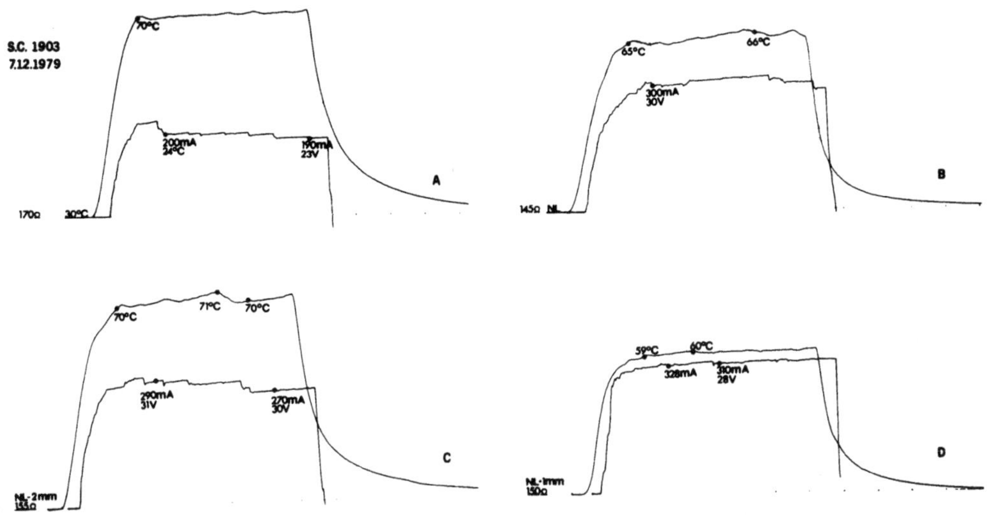

Fig. 3. Example of the measure of four different coagulations of Gasserian ganglion in the same patient (top curve: temperature, bottom curve: milliamperes and volts, Ω: impedance, *NL*: new positioning of the electrode)

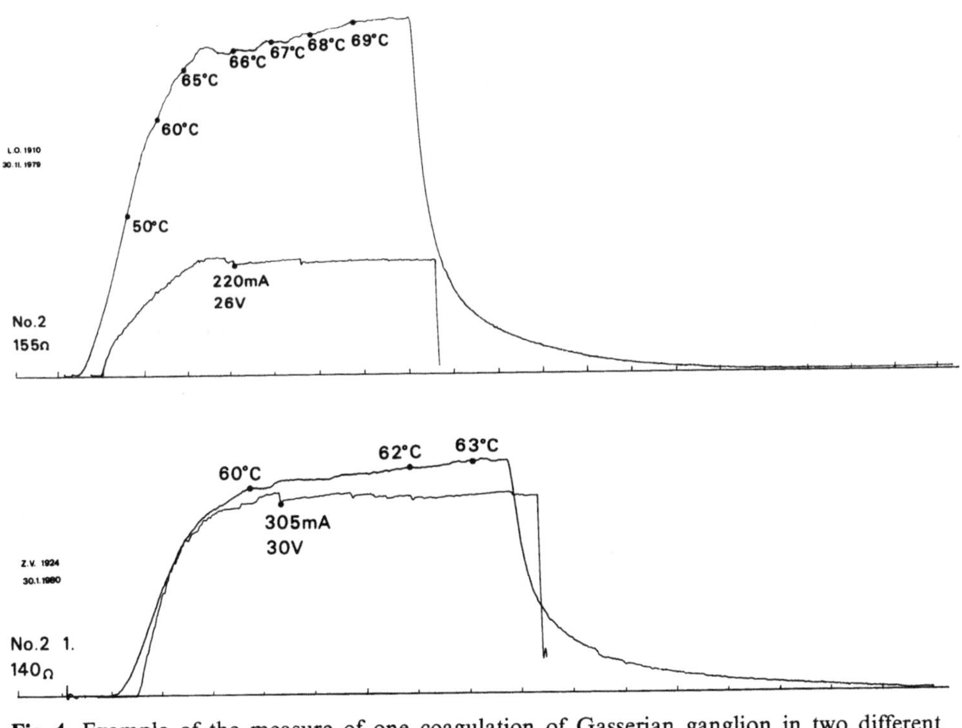

Fig. 4. Example of the measure of one coagulation of Gasserian ganglion in two different positions

ship exists between these two parameters (Figs. 3 and 4), but promising studies are in progress. For these reasons, the neurosurgeon must proceed carefully in successive coagulations until an analgesia is obtained. However, when the patient is not sufficiently awake after the brief anaesthesia or not cooperative enough to give adequate informations about pin-prick and touch sensation, evaluation of sensitivity is difficult. The neurosurgeon may then terminate coagulation prematurely, as a result of which recurrence of pain may be possible over the years. Conversely, the surgeon may cause excessive coagulations, whereupon anaesthesia or hypesthesia dolorosa may appear. It is certainly preferable to accept a recurrence of pain than to risk an anaesthesia dolorosa, and we are increasingly convinced that this should be our policy.

4. Comments on Mechanisms of Trigeminal Neuralgia

By almost daily contact over many years with patients suffering from trigeminal neuralgia, the data obtained from their pain descriptions, the careful neurological examinations, the follow up of cases operated on or conservatively treated led us to formulate some comments on this very particular affliction.

Three main aspects of facial pain can be distinguished:

a) Idiopathic trigeminal neuralgia or tic douloureux;
b) Symptomatic trigeminal neuralgia;
c) Atypical facial pain.

Our comments will be restricted to the analysis of trigeminal neuralgia or tic douloureux and ignore all other varieties of facial pain. Nevertheless, trigeminal neuralgia in multiple sclerosis merits some attention, since the clinical symptoms of pain attacks due to multiple sclerosis are very similar to those of idiopathic trigeminal neuralgia. Trigeminal neuralgia in cases of multiple sclerosis is considered as symptomatic, but in a series of 25 consecutive cases, in contrast to trigeminal neuralgia due to organic lesions which is usually accompanied by neurological symptoms, trigeminal neuralgia of multiple sclerosis has shown no such symptoms [14]. Autopsy studies of multiple sclerosis patients with trigeminal neuralgia frequently show one or multiple plaques of sclerosis somewhere in the central sensory part of the trigeminal nerve. However, such plaques have also been described without the appearance of trigeminal neuralgia and patients were also suffering from trigeminal neuralgia without a plaque being discovered [2, 4, 5, 6, 18]. In case of peripheral or central mechanical compression, neurological symptoms may be expected for this kind of symptomatic neuralgia such as sensory disturbances; our series of 25 cases of multiple sclerosis with typical neuralgia did not show any sensory deficit or other neurological symptoms of trigeminal nerve at the time of the examination. This is also true for the 1000 cases of trigeminal neuralgia we have operated on and who had not previously been subjected to surgical procedures. We were unable to find any mild sensory loss in the pure trigeminal distribution or differences in corneal reflex, in contrast to the findings of Jannetta [7]; a vascular cross-compression as causation of trigeminal neuralgia would give more frequent neurological symptoms.

Since classical trigeminal neuralgia (tic douloureux) has no neurological detectable symptoms and since compression of sensory nerves, such as the dorsal root, causes long lasting pain, a pure peripheral mechanical compressive causation does not seem to be an absolutely satisfactory pathogenesis. Nor can this causation explain the trigger points and the limitation of pain to the area of a single cranial sensory nerve, not even of one root of this V. nerve, and generally always the same one. Finally, post-mortem brain examinations older individuals reveal a large number of tortuous arterioles that impinge on and groove the cranial sensory and motor roots without, in the vast majority of instances, producing any clinical evidence of their irritation or impairment [9].

Among several other theories on the pathogenesis of trigeminal neuralgia, the epileptiform aspect of the pain attack is worth discussing. Is trigeminal neuralgia (paroxysmal facial pain) a localized epileptic after-discharge? The character of pain (sudden onset, short duration, trigger mechanisms) and the therapeutical effect of antiepileptic drugs appear to favour this hypothesis. Kaemmerer observed in 12 patients out of 18 with tic douloureux a spike-and-wave component, particularly after activation with Metrazol (2 cc) given intravenously. Some patients were also photosensitive, so a flickering light induced spike-and-wave components [8]. An interesting contribution is the one of Nashold who reported on a woman suffering from unbearable facial pain on the right side [11]. Her spontaneous paroxysms, which were accompanied by epileptiform discharges in the left lower brain stem (tegmentum), could be induced by means of electrical stimulation with a chronically implanted electrode in that area and abolished by coagulation in the mesencephalic tegmentum and subthalamus. The neurons of the mesencephalon seemed to be hyperexcitable, like the neurons of the cortex and the scar formation in Jackson's epilepsy. This led Nashold to believe that tic douloureux can be the expression of focal epileptiform discharges accompanying disorders of the mesencephalon.

The clinical observations that a refractory period exists (once the paroxysm is over there is a period during which further stimulation of the trigger point will not elicit pain) are strong evidence that complex central factors are involved in the mechanisms of pain in trigeminal neuralgia [9].

The etiology of trigeminal neuralgia remains an enigma. As an example, the two different aspects of a possible pathogenesis presented here, namely, a peripheral locus and a central locus, both seem acceptable. This shows that much remains to be done before a satisfactory explanation of paroxysmal neuralgia is achieved. It may be concluded, like Kerr did in 1967 in a workshop on trigeminal neuralgia, that perhaps one might bring the central and peripheral theories together by suggesting that the lesion is peripheral but the mechanisms central [10]. However, the reverse could also be suggested.

Summary

Clinical experiences of 1000 cases of trigeminal neuralgia operated on by the method of percutaneous controlled thermocoagulation of Gasserian ganglion provide certain signs concerning the value of this treatment, its indication as well as directives concerning the manner of conducting the operation. It also permit to make some comments on the causation of the disease. The favourable long-term results are reported and the indications specified. A single valid theory explaining the mechanisms of trigeminal neuralgia apparently is impossible to establish yet, the similarity of paroxysmal pain to an epileptic fit is particularly emphasized by the author.

References

1. Broggi G, Siegfried J (1977) The effect of graded thermocoagulation on trigeminal evoked potentials in the cat. Acta Neurochirurgica Suppl 24: 175–178
2. Daum S, Vogein-Rappoport M, Gruner J, Foncin JF (1960) Sclérose en plaques révélée à l'âge de 64 ans par une névralgie trigeminale. Etude anatomo-clinique. Rev Neurol (Paris) 102:500–503
3. Frigyesi TL, Siegfried J, Broggi G (1975) The selective vulnerability of evoked potentials in the trigeminal sensory root to graded thermocoagulation. Exp Neurol 49: 11–21
4. Garcin R, Godlewski St, Lapresle J (1960) Neuralgie du trijumeau et sclérose en plaques. A propos d'une observation anatomo-clinique. Rev Neurol (Paris) 102:441–451
5. Guillan G (1924) Rapport sur la sclérose en plaques. Etude clinique, anatomo-pathologique et pathogénique. Rev Neurol (Paris) 1:648–683
6. Huhn A, Daniels L (1973) Die Syntropie von Encephalomyelitis disseminata und Trigeminusneuralgie. Fortschr. Neurol Psychiatr 41:477–496
7. Jannetta PJ (1977) Treatment of trigeminal neuralgia by suboccipital and transtentorial cranial operations. Clin Neurosurg 24:538–549
8. Kaemmerer E (1970) Discussion. In: Hassler R, Walker AE (eds) Trigeminal Neuralgia. Thieme, Stuttgart, p 120–121
9. Kerr WFL (1970) Peripheral versus central factors in trigeminal Neuralgia. In: Hassler R, Walker AE (eds) Trigeminal neuralgia. Thieme, Stuttgart, p 180–187
10. Kerr FWL (1970) Discussion. In: Hassler R, Walker AE (eds) Trigeminal Neuralgia. Thieme, Stuttgart, p 189
11. Nashold BS jr, Wilson WP (1966) Central pain. Observations in man with chronic implanted electrodes in the midbrain tegmentum. Confin Neurol 27:30–44
12. Siegfried J (1975) Results of percutaneous controlled thermocoagulation in 300 cases of trigeminal pain. Adv Neurosurg 3:287–296
13. Siegfried J (1977) 500 percutaneous thermocoagulations of the Gasserian ganglion for trigeminal pain. Surg Neurol 8: 126–131
14. Siegfried J, Lindenberger J (1980) Trigeminal neuralgia in multiple sclerosis. Therapeutical considerations. Il dolore 2 (in press)
15. Siegfried J, Vosmansky M (1975) Technique of the controlled thermocoagulation of trigeminal ganglion and spinal roots. Advanced Technical Standards Neurosurgery 2: 199–209
16. Sweet WH (1969) Pain, vol 1, Ch. C. Thomas, Springfield, p 184–197 and 603–609
17. Sweet WH, Wepsic JG (1974) Controlled thermocoagulation of trigeminal ganglion and rootlets for differential destruction of pain fibers. J Neurosurg 40: 143–156
18. Van Gehuchten P (1962) Sclérose en plaques et névralgie du trijumeau. Rev Neurol (Paris) 106:257–265

Vascular Decompression in Trigeminal Neuralgia

P. J. JANNETTA, Pittsburgh, PA/USA

Early work by Dandy [3–6] and Gardner [7] concerning vascular compression and other abnormalities of the root entry zone of the trigeminal nerve form the basis for our current concepts of the etiology and definitive treatments of this disabling symptom called trigeminal neuralgia (TN). Dandy [3–6], starting in 1932, noted abnormalities of the dorsal root in a progressively larger percentage of his patients with TN. This innovative surgeon sectioned the portio major at the brainstem in these patients. He was able to treat TN without giving complete numbness by preserving fascicles which he described and called 'accessory sensory fascicle' during the nerve section. In the 5.6 percent of patients where an extra-axial tumor was the cause of the TN, he removed the lesion as treatment. He did not treat the TN by vascular decompression. Indeed, it was impressive that he was able to see vascular compression by 'normal' (although perhaps elongated) arteries and veins in 60 percent of the patients. Gardner [7] further elaborated upon abnormalities of the dorsal root of the trigeminal nerve and lucidly elaborated upon the pathophysiological mechanisms involved. Others more recently described gross lesions such as aneurysms, tumors and other abnormalities in the cerebellopontine angle of patients with TN. Despite these publications, there was little or no acceptance of this concept until recently. Many reasons for this lack of acceptance may be given: Some of them may include: relatively primitive technology, lack of verification by others, inadequate documentation of findings and rare definitive treatment. However, with the development of safer operative and anesthetic techniques for surgery of the cerebellopontine angle, the use of microsurgical techniques, photographic and videotape documentation of findings and definitive treatment, the concepts of root entry zone abnormality as the etiology of TN and microvascular decompression as therapy have had wide acceptance in recent years.

Preoperative Evaluation of the Patient With Tic Douloureux

The History

The physician with a clear understanding of the symptom-complex of TN, including severe lancinating unilateral face pain of sudden onset and offset, usually of brief duration, more common in women than men, more common in older patients, more common on the right than the left, and much more common in the lower and mid face than the upper face in distribution, will not miss the diagnosis. Special points of interest concerning the history include the observation that the patient with TN, even of many years duration, can almost always remember a multitude of details about the first attack of pain. He will recall the time of day, the circumstances of the attack, what the weather was like, what he was doing at the time, etc. This is in distinct contrast to other types of facial pain. On questioning, the patient will state that the pain is superficial rather than deep in the jaw or head. He may recognize an 'aura' or 'strike', a fraction of a second when he knows he is going to have an attack just before it begins. Attacks awakening patients from sleep are uncommon.

A six percent incidence of tumors and arteriovenous malformations is noted in our series. Only about half the patients had the diagnosis established preoperatively. The examiner should pay careful attention to symptoms which may reflect the presence of a cerebellopontine angle tumor. Despite such care, neoplasms will be missed. Two of our six patients with multiple sclerosis causing the tic douloureux had the diagnosis established for the first time during the immediate preoperative period: another situation which must be recognized.

In addition to the attack of pain, the panic over the threat of the next attack in these patients must be emphasized. The patient who suffers from TN for a prolonged period may develop constant burning pain in the face, a symptom which is rarely discussed in the literature. Occasionally, this type of pain may supervene totally. Carbamazepine, in several of our patients, has abolished tic douloureux only to bring about constant burning pain which then regressed with concurrent recurrence of tic after cessation of the drug.

A 'trigger point' is frequently noted. It is usually located in the area of distribution of the pain, but may be located well outside the distribution. Trigger points have a tendency to exacerbate and remit and to change in location, but are usually located around the snout. Stimulation of a trigger point will commonly not cause an attack for a brief period after an attack of tic, the so-called 'refractory period'.

The Physical Examination

It is commonly stated that the patient with tic douloureux has no abnormalities on physical examination. This is frequently true, but we have found that the ipsilateral corneal reflex was decreased preoperatively in many cases of first division TN. In several of these patients, the corneal reflex was decreased over only the upper half above meridian of the globe. Similarly, we have noted a decrease in the corneal reflex in the lower half below meridian in several patients who had V_2 TN. Mild hypesthesia or hypalgesia is noted in 25 percent or more of patients [13] with careful testing. We have noted such abnormalities in about 30 percent of our patients [10, 11]. Frank weakness of the temporo-masseter muscles has been noted on physical examination in just two patients of a large series although jaw opening is uneven in many patients.

Special Laboratory Examination

Plain roentgenography of the skull including a basal view an lumbar puncture are obtained. Computerized tomography with contrast is performed with particular attention to be paid to the posterior fossa. Complete otovestibular testing is performed in all patients. We have performed many angiograms in patients with lower facial tic douloureux and have been able to identify a downward sweep of the ipsilateral superior cerebellar artery as it comes around the pons. This may be helpful evidence that such is the etiologic factor preoperatively but the neutral-vascular relationships are otherwise not clearly helpful. Tortuous or looping vessels noted on angiography have not otherwise proved to be helpful in denoting which vessel is causing the syndrome in tic douloureux or several other cranial nerve compression syndromes which we are evaluating and treating at the University of Pittsburgh. We do not feel that routine angiography is indicated.

Indications for Operation

The procedure to be described below appears, in our hands, to be indicated in patients with intractable tic douloureux who are in reasonably good health, and who are not responding to diphenylhydantoid and carbamazepine [10, 11]. Almost all our patients have had a course of carbamazepine which has been stopped for one reason or another. It is unfortunate that the elderly frail patients appear to be more sensitive to the side effects and complications of carbamazepine. The procedure is contraindicated in the very elderly and in those who are in poor health, but the usual older person in generally good health appears to tolerate the procedure easily. A prior unsuccessful procedure, or a recurrence, is no contraindication to operation.

Operative Technique

The patient is prepared 12 hours preoperatively with dexamethasone, 10 mg intramuscularly. This is continued postoperatively in a dose of 4 mg every six hours for 48 hours and then discontinued. The patient is anesthetized, intubated and placed in the contralateral decubitus position with the neck on mild stretch, the chin flexed to two fingerbreadth from the sternum and the head rotated a few degrees to the ipsilateral side using a three point pin fixation headholder. An axillary roll is put into place and the patient held to the table with straps and tape across the hips (Fig. 1).

The ipsilateral posterior side of the head from midline to the ear and from just below the vertex to the hairline is shaved in the operating room. A vertical incision approximately six or seven cm long is made, two cm medial to the mastoid process with about one third of the incision above the superior nuchal line. The incision is placed lateral enough to avoid the greater occipital nerve. The incision is carried directly to the calvarium except caudally where further dissection of the deeper muscles is performed with the electrocautery. Periosteal elevators are used to separate the nuchal muscles, fascia, and pericranium away from the calvarium. A

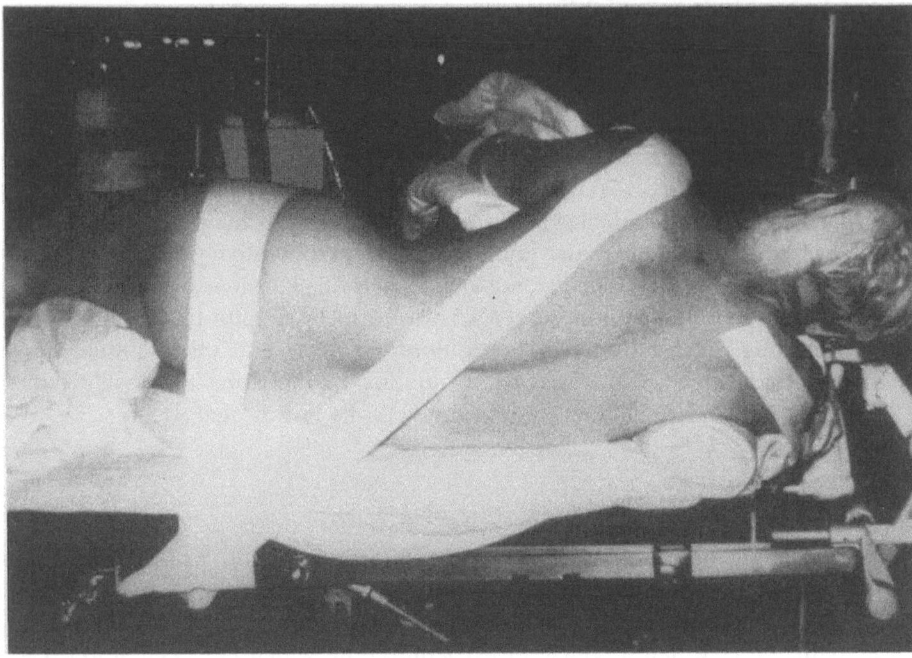

Fig. 1. The lateral decubitus position. Note that the patient is tightly held in position so that position is stable on lateral rotation of the table, and that head and neck relationships are the same as in the lounging position. (Reprinted from J. of Neurosurgery, 47:321–328, 1977)

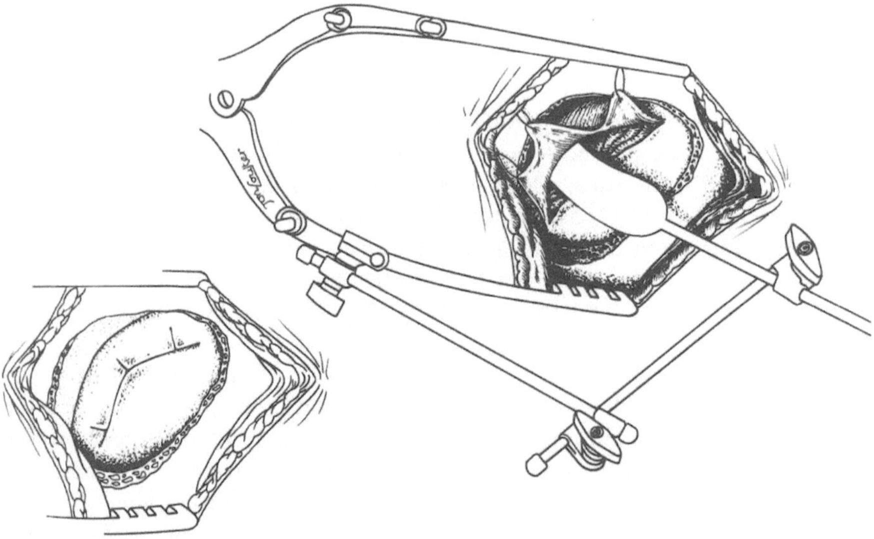

Fig. 2. Retractor blade connected with two connecting rods to post of angulated Weitlaner retractor. We now use a narrower blade than is shown in this photograph

self-retaining angulated Weitlaner retractor with posts is placed[1]. The posterior aspect of the mastoid eminence is partially cleared. The electrocautery blade on cutting current is helpful in separating the attachments of the nuchal line to the calvarum.

A craniectomy about 4.0 cm in size is then performed high and lateral in the posterior fossa exposing the horizontal portion of the lateral sinus and extending to the sigmoid sinus laterally. Any open mastoid air cells are waxed heavily after this dissection. The dura mater is incised about three or four mm under the lateral sinus and extending inferolaterally for several centimeters. The supralateral dura mater flap is incised to the lateral sinus and the dura sutured to the galea, tenting the lateral sinus up and away. More bone may be rongeured supralaterally at this point if exposure is not adequate. It is important to achieve this supra-lateral exposure and the short time necessary to obtain the exposure is well worth it. The retractor, connected by two rods to a post of the Weitlaner retractor which has been clamped to the drapes using a gauze sponge through the handles, is then put into place over a piece of rubber glove cut to size. A narrow blade is used and no cerebellar retraction is used at this point. The retractor is placed superficially over the lateral aspect of the superior surface of the cerebellum (Fig. 2).

The Zeiss surgical microscope with a 250-mm focal length objective is then used for the remainder of the procedure. Minimal retraction is necessary to find the superior petrosal vein which is usually shaped like an inverted 'Y'. Using sharp dissection, the arachnoid is opened over the vein which is then coagulated with Bipolar coagulation. A set of microsurgical instruments with bayonet shaped handles is used for this and the remainder of the intracranial dissection[2]. Valsalva maneuver is performed after partial and after complete section of the vein, as it is easy to miss some of the anterior limb of the 'Y' in coagulating.

After the superior petrosal vein is divided, the retractor is placed more deeply, again over the rubber dam which prevents trauma to the cerebellum. The arachnoid is opened anteromedial to the vein, giving an excellent view of the trigeminal nerve. The trochlear nerve may be seen before the trigeminal nerve is clearly visualized and is easily avoided. The dissection is too cephalad if the trochlear nerve is in the center of the field. The trigeminal nerve lies obliquely coursing from Meckel's cave to the pons just anteromedial to the superior petrosal vein. A variable degree of sideward tilt of the operating table may be necessary at this point and subsequently to give a good line of sight to the trigeminal nerve. The retractor, with joints only partially tightened, can be moved about gently and gradually as dissection continues. The retractor must not be allowed to slip down over the side of the cerebellum onto the seventh and eighth cranial nerves or significantly compress the cerebellum. The arachnoid is next dissected from the trigeminal nerve. It may be adherent both to the nerve and to the artery compressing and distorting the nerve. The arachnoid must be separated from the trigeminal nerve for most of the length of the dorsal root. After some experience, the vascular-trigeminal nerve relationship can usually be appreciated before the arachnoid is open.

---

[1] V. Mueller, Chicago, IL, USA
[2] V. Mueller, Chicago, IL, USA

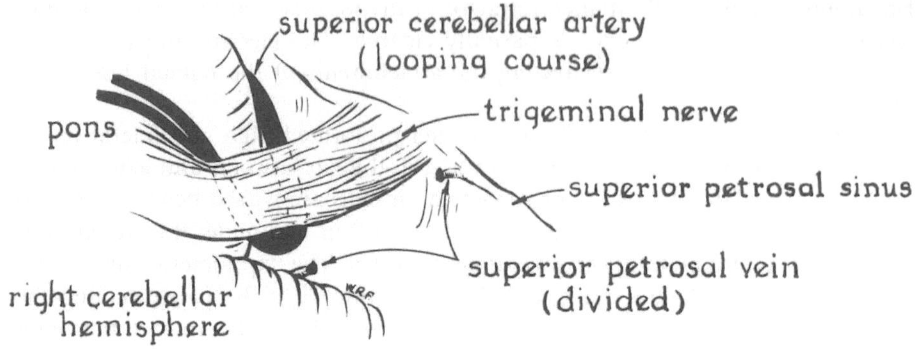

Fig. 3. Right trigeminal nerve, lower facial tic douloureux supracerebellar route

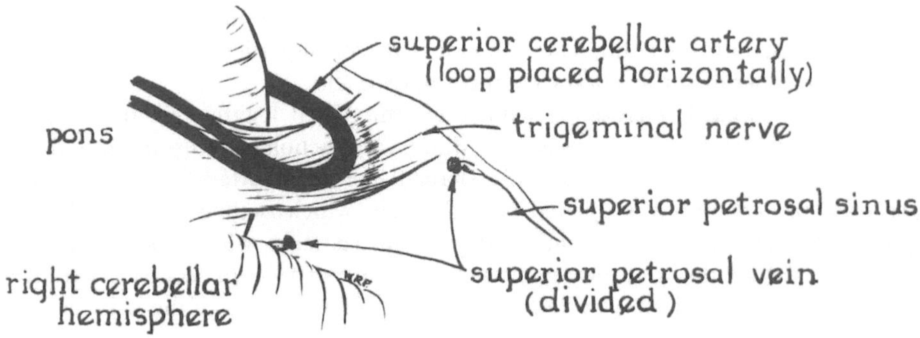

Fig. 4. Right trigeminal nerve, lower facial tic douloureux after compression, supracerebellar route

The most common situation in lower facial tic douloureux is that the superior cerebellar artery is found coursing cephalad around the pons and then bifurcating, with the medial and lateral branches impinging upon the anterosuperior aspect of the entry zone of the nerve, the motor-proprioceptive fascicle side, as it loops back to the brain stem and cerebellum (Fig. 3). After sharp and blunt dissection of the widely opened arachnoid from the nerve and the visible part of the artery, the arterial loops are gently teased out from between the trigeminal nerve and the pons (Fig. 4). The loops are usually longer in older patients and especially in those with long-standing tic douloureux. They must be manipulated carefully. The arterial loops may be quite adherent to the nerve or easily separable. Perforating branches to the pons have accommodated in length to the loop and will not tear with gentle manipulation of the vessels over the trigeminal nerve.

In first division tic douloureux, a vessel is seen compressing the inferolateral portio of the trigeminal nerve entry zone at the pons at the portio major side. The superior cerebellar artery has a normal horizontal loop in this case. The most common cause of isolated V_2 neuralgia is compression by the trigeminal vein coursing alongside the nerve. This may run parallel to the nerve.

One or several small implants of teflon felt are placed between the vessel and the nerve at the brain stem. The Valsalva maneuver is performed several times under control of the anaesthetist to see if the relationships are stable. It is easy to decompress a large bridging vein. The teflon felt may be shredded and rolled for easy placement. A large piece of gelfoam is placed over the arachnoid opening. This appears to decrease postoperative headache, which is much milder and of briefer duration in the lateral position as in stress upon the patient in general. The retractor is removed and the dura closed with interrupted and running sutures of 4-0 silk over gelfoam. The incision is closed in layers and a small dry dressing applied. Postoperatively, the head of the bed is kept elevated about 10°. The patient is usually able to return from the neurosurgical continuous care unit to the floor on the morning of the first postoperative day. Postoperative care is routine as for any intracranial neurosurgical procedure. Mild analgesics are given for incisional pain.

Postoperative Course and Operative Results

If the trigeminal nerve is manipulated at operation, the patient awakens pain-free. If the nerve is not traumatized during the dissection, the patient may have TN for a few days to several weeks postoperatively. The attacks may not begin for several days after operation if trauma to the nerve has been minimal. The pain is usually well controlled with small doses of diphenylhydantoin. Common self-limited postoperative morbidity has consisted of temporary postoperative headaches much like after a pneumoencephalogram, especially if the patient is operated upon in the sitting position.

Operative Findings and Results

Abnormalities on the root-entry zone of the trigeminal nerve in 411 patients are collated in Table 1. As our experience grows, we are finding progressively more multiple vessels causing TN.

In the contralateral-lateral decubitus position, which is the position in which most patients find relief from their pain, an arterial loop may be away from the nerve for a mm or more. All vessels should be treated. Retraction of the cerebellum may move a blood vessel away from the nerve. A bridging superior petrosal vein

Table 1. Microvascular decompression in trigeminal neuralgia

Operative findings:	
Arterial	242
Aneurysm	1
Venous	57
AVM	1
Mixed arterial/venous	96
Tumor	15
No pathology	1
Unrecorded	1

Table 2. Microvascular decompression in trigeminal neuralgia

Result of Operation		No.	Percent	
Well after MVD [a, b]		343	83.5	83.5%
No pain on Rx		38	9.3	92.8%
Occasional mild pain, No Rx		2	0.5	93.3%
Frank recurrence		22		
relief after RFL	17		4.1	97.4%
persistent severe pain	5		1.2	98.6%
Deceased		5	1.2	99.8%
postop				
suicide				
accident		1	0.2	100.0%
Status unknown				
Total		411		100.0%

[a] MVD: Microvascular decompression
[b] repeat operation necessary in 15 patients

may be causal of the TN. Coagulation and division of this vein without careful prior inspection of relationships may cause a 'negative' exploration. It must be emphasized that the neurovascular compression in TN may be extremely subtle. We have seen two patients in whom the compression was caused by a vessel under the ala of the cerebellum and one in whom we found no abnormality, and, as we began a portio major selective section, came upon a large intrinsic vein running outward inside the nerve. The root entry zone of the trigeminal nerve extends quite distally in the lateral aspect of portio major, so a vessel quite distally located on the side of the nerve may be causal. Tumors most commonly cause TN by causing vascular compression, usually pushing the nerve against a blood vessel.

Results of operation are collated in Table 2. Quality of survival is excellent in the vast majority of patients as they remain free of pain with no numbness or paresthesias to remind them of their prior syndrome. This author admits to some bias regarding quality of survival with this procedure versus a destructive operation. Others [1, 2] without a vested interest, have compared procedures and state strongly that microvascular decompression is the procedure of choice in TN.

Table 3. Microvascular decompression in trigeminal neuralgia

Complications:	
Cranial nerve deficit	23
Aseptic meningitis	21
Intracranial hematomas	4
Mortality	4
Bacterial meningitis	3
Pneumonia	2
CSF rhinorrhea	2
Pulmonary embolism	2

Complications are tabulated in Table 3. The major cranial nerve deficits consisted of some hearing loss (less than five percent of patients) or some persistent trigeminal distribution numbness. Of the four deaths, two ocurred in tumor patients, on AVM who suffered a hemorrhagic brain stem infarction, one acoustic diagnosed by CT scan in a woman with chronic lymphatic leukemia admentted for a radiofrequency lesion in whom an uneventful procedure was followed by a postoperative stroke. Two deaths occurred without tumors, the first in a 79 year old woman operated upon in the modified sitting position, who developed a stroke postoperatively, and the second in a woman aged 63, who suffered a hemorrhagic infarction of the brain stem and cerebellum from a rather hard implant which compressed the superior cerebellar artery. We have had no intracranial hematomas or mortality in over 300 more recent operations. The aseptic meningitis groups are patients who have had a self-limited postoperative headache syndrome with meningismus and mildly increased intracranial pressure with some white cells in the cerebrospinal fluid but no infarction.

Discussion

The concept of neurovascular compression as the common cause of trigeminal neuralgia has become generally accepted in recent years. The early reports of Dandy [3–6] and Gardner [7] have been well supported. Jannetta [9] reported his experience with vascular findings in 1967, but at this time, he had performed only one microvascular decompression for TN (with Rand [8]), although he had done a similar procedure for hemifacial spasm previous to this experience. The next verification of the vascular etiology and of the treatments by vascular decompression was by Petty in 1976 [15]. Petty and others have continued to report their expanding series [16]. Apfelbaum compared percutaneous radiofrequency trigeminal neuralgia (RFL) with microvascular decompression and in 1977 published a large series where the quality of survival and results were clearly superior to the destructive procedure [1]. It must be remembered that RFL is well indicated in many patients, the frail and elderly, and we have performed this operation, the best of the destructive procedure in the above group plus a few patients who have developed recurrent pain after vascular decompression. Becker [2] has stated that vascular decompression is the treatment of choice in TN and Loeser [14] has compared it formally with RFL. Recently, Lazar [12], Weidmann [18], and Rhoton [17] have published their experiences with microvascular decompression.

Neurovascular compression of the root entry zone of the trigeminal nerve can now be clearly stated as causal of the vast majority of cases of trigeminal neuralgia. As our operative experience in relieving this compression grows, the results of operation should improve so that relief of the pain with little or no sequellae is a standard goal.

References

1. Apfelbaum RI (1977) A Comparison of Percutaneous Radiofrequency Trigeminal Neurolysis and Microvascular Decompression of the Trigeminal Nerve for the Treatment of Tic Douloureux. Neurosurgery 1:16
2. Becker DP (1978) What's New in Neurological Surgery. American College of Surgeons Bulletin, January, p 23
3. Dandy WE (1925) Section of the Sensory Root of the Trigeminal Nerve at the Pons. Bull Johns Hopkins Hosp 36:105–106
4. Dandy WE (1929) Operation for Cure of Tic Douloureux; Partial Section of the Sensory Root at the Pons. Arch Surg 18:687–734
5. Dandy WE (1932) Treatment of Trigeminal Neuralgia by the Cerebellar Route. Ann Surg 96:787–795
6. Dandy WE (1945) Surgery of the Brain. A monogram. In: Lewis (ed) Practice of Surgery Vol 12, Prior, Hagerstown, p 167–187
7. Gardner WJ (1962) Concerning the Mechanism of Trigeminal Neuralgia and Hemifacial Spasm. Neurosurg 19:947–958
8. Jannetta PJ, Rand RW (1966) Transtentorial Subtemporal Retrogasserian Neurectomy in Trigeminal Neuralgia by Microsurgical Technique. Bull Los Angeles Neurol Soc 31:93–99
9. Jannetta PJ (1967) Structural Mechanisms of Trigeminal Neuralgia: Arterial Compression of the Trigeminal Nerve at the Pons in Patients with Trigeminal Neuralgia. J Neurosurg 26(II):159–162
10. Jannetta PJ (1976) Microsurgical Approach to the Trigeminal Nerve for Tic Douloureux. In: Krayenbuhl H, Maspes PE, Sweet WH (eds), Progress in Neurological Surgery. Vol 7 S. Karger, AG, Basel, Switzerland (Pain – Its Neurosurgical Management), p 180–200
11. Jannetta PJ (1977) Treatment of Trigeminal Neuralgia by Suboccipital and Transtentorial Cranial Operations. Clin Neurosurg 24:538–549
12. Lazar ML (1978) Trigeminal Neuralgia: Recent Advances in Management. Tex Med 74:45
13. Lewey FH, Grant FC (1938) Physiopathologic and Pathoanatomic Aspects of Major Trigeminal Neuralgia. Arch Neurol Psychiat 40:1126–1134
14. Loeser JD (1978) What To Do About Tic Douloureux. JAMA, vol 239, No 12, p 1153
15. Petty PG (1976) Arterial Compression of the Trigeminal Nerve at the Pons as a Cause of Trigeminal Neuralgia. Inst Neurol Madra Proc 6:93
16. Petty PG, Southby R (1977) Vascular Compression of Lower Cranial Nerves: Observations using Microsurgery, with Particular Reference to Trigeminal Neuralgia. Aust NZ Surg 47:314
17. Rhoton AL (1978) Microsurgical Neurovascular Decompression for Trigeminal Neuralgia and Hemifacial Spasm. J Med 65:425
18. Weidmann MJ (1979) Trigeminal Neuralgia. Med J Aust 2:628

Critical Remarks on Different Surgical Methods in Trigeminal Neuralgia

H. Penzholz and A. Kühner, Heidelberg/FRG

Of the classical methods for surgical treatment of trigeminal neuralgia, partial retroganglionic root resection according to Spiller and Frazier have retained their place, as have partial percutaneous electrocoagulation of the Gasserian ganglion according to Kirschner or its modern variant, thermocoagulation according to Sweet (1974). A new method is vascular decompression of the nerves in the posterior cranial fossa with the microsurgical technique according to Jannetta (1976). There are many indications that here one has found a method of curing this condition by eliminating its cause. For this reason alone it deserves special attention.

It therefore appeared to be of interest to compare and contrast the advantages and disadvantages of the various methods of treatment, also taking into account the long-term results.

Material and Results

In the ten-year period 1969 to 1978, 500 patients were operated upon in Heidelberg for idiopathic trigeminal neuralgia: 155 with temporal operation according to Frazier, 190 with electrocoagulation according to Kirschner and (since 1975) 155 with thermocoagulation according to Sweet (1974). 350 patients could be followed up for a long period of time.

The main advantage of the percutaneous methods according to Kirschner and Sweet is the brief stay in hospital and the minimal surgical mortality and morbidity.

The thermolesion is a substantial improvement of electrocoagulation, especially since it damages the non-myelinated fibers for pain conduction to a greater extent than the epicritic afferents (Sweet 1974). Excruciating dysesthesia or even anesthesia dolorosa therefore occurs more rarely. We saw it in nine percent of the patients after electrocoagulation, but only in four percent of patients after the thermolesion. Other undesired secondary lesions, e.g. of the masticatory musculature or of the corneal reflex are rarer after thermolesions.

Unpleasant postoperative dysesthesias extending to anesthesia dolorosa are the most serious consequences of destructive interventions in the central trigeminal pathways. However, even if they do not occur, the sensitivity defect necessary to eliminate twitch is felt to be disturbing by many patients. Many complain that they could only chew on the healthy side, that they had no feeling in their mouth on the operated side and that they did not notice when fluid dropped from the corner of the mouth when they were eating. Complaints about disturbances of hearing or ear symptoms were expressed by some patients. These are probably due to concomitant damage to motor pathways serving the musculus tensor veli palatini.

On the other hand, patients with severe sensory deficits are better protected from twitch relapses than patients with slight sensory deficits. Such relapses are more frequent after percutaneous interventions than after open temporal operation. They are most frequent in the first postoperative years. However, even later the danger of their occurring never disappears completely. With a four year follow-up period, 23 percent of the patients treated with temporal operation, 43 percent of those with electrocoagulation, and 44 percent of those with thermolesion had a recurrence of twitch. In further follow-up over ten years, these figures rose to 27 percent for the Frazier operation, and to 55 percent for electrocoagulation.

The argument is only partly correct that a twitch recurrence is not so serious for patients operated upon percutaneously, because this operation can be readily repeated at any time and with just as little risk. Optimal placing of the thermoprobe is often especially difficult in precisely such patients. This then applies to reoperated patients to and equal or even greater extent.

Finally, the risk of surgical mortality cannot be entirely dismissed even with percutaneous operations. Thus, out of 350 percutaneously operated patients, we lost one patient with rapid meningitis, and another patient operated upon several times developed a carotid-cavernous fistula.

The euphoria of experiencing abrupt elimination of intolerable pain by means of a relatively harmless percutaneous operation is sobered by these observations. One can understand why many neurologists hesitate to advise their patients to undergo operation.

In the light of these facts, efforts to improve possibilities of operation further are understandable and justified. The statement of Jannetta (1976) that vascular or tumorous radicular compressions can be demonstrated in the cerebello-pontine

Table 1. Abnormalities of the root entry zone of the trigeminal nerve in 17 patients with typical trigeminal neuralgia (Tic douloureux alone)

			Result of decompression		
Abnormality	certain	suspect	excellent	partial	none
Blood vessel					
Artery s. c. a. [a]	10		9	1	
Artery s. c. a.		3	2	1	
Vein	2		2		
Artery and vein		1			1
Arachnitis	1			1	
	13	4			
Total	17		13	3	1

[a] s. c. a.: Superior cerebellar artery

angle more frequently with modern microneurosurgery than was earlier the case (Dandy 1934) awakens increasing interest on the part of the neurosurgeon. The idea that one can cure this condition solely by eliminating a compressive noxa without destructive measures performed on the trigeminal tract is fascinating.

It can be assumed that the technique of microvascular decompression of the posterior trigeminal root in the cerebellopontine angle will be familiar to you (Jannetta 1976). We have applied it in 23 selected patients in the last two and a half years: in 17 patients with trigeminal tics alone and six further patients with additional chronic pain components. Especially the latter group mostly involved patients who had already undergone one or several percutaneous operations on the ganglion without lasting freedom from pain (Tables 1 and 2).

The most frequent finding was the visible compression of the trigeminal by/or contact with a pathologically elongated loop of the superior cerebellar artery. Figure 1 a–c shows an especially frequent form of arterial compression and its microsurgical elimination. Of our 17 patients with typical neuralgia, ten patients had such or similar arterial compressions, as did three out of the six patients with atypical chronic pain components. We found contacts between artery and nerve in three of the typical and one of the atypical cases. Venous compressions become more distinct with intraoperative compression of the jugular vein, and mostly require coagulation of such veins. We found this variant of vascular compression in two of our typical cases. One of our atypical cases involved a compression by an extremely thickened petrosal vein with an angiomatosis tentorii which could not be demonstrated angiographically.

The etiological significance of an arterial contact without discernible compression is difficult to appraise. With demonstration and successful elimination of

Table 2. Abnormalities of the root entry zone of the trigeminal nerve in 6 patients with 'atypical' trigeminal neuralgia (Tic douloureux permanent or 'burning' pain)

			Result of decompression		
Abnormality	certain	suspect	excellent	partial	none
Blood vessel					
Artery s. c. a.		1		1	
Artery and Arachnitis	3		1 R [a]	2	
Neoplasms					
Angioma	1 [b]		1		
No abnormality	1				1
	5	1			
Total	6		2	3	1

[a] R = Recurrence of tic douloureux 1 year later after a car accident: prothesis had slipped: reoperation.

[b] Cerebral panangiography before operation had been normal!

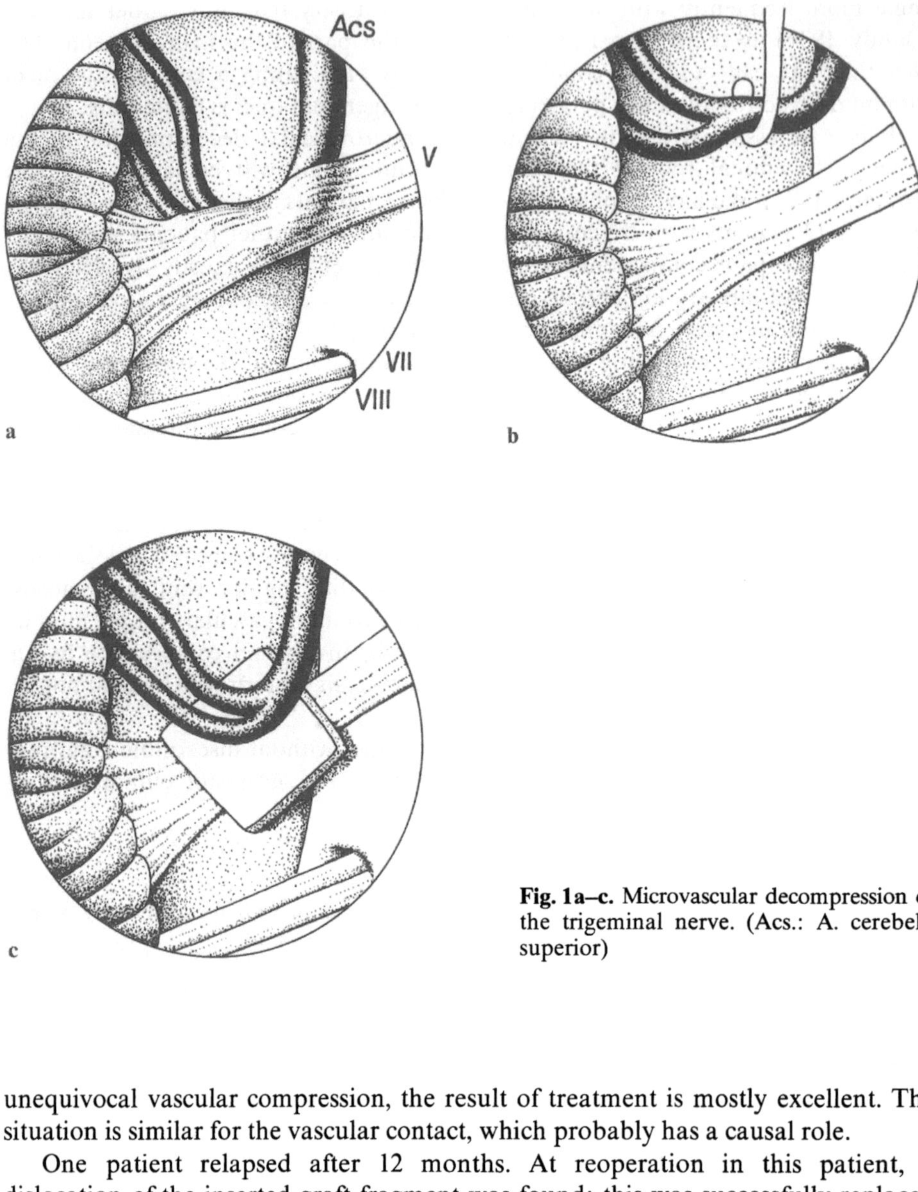

Fig. 1a–c. Microvascular decompression of the trigeminal nerve. (Acs.: A. cerebelli superior)

unequivocal vascular compression, the result of treatment is mostly excellent. The situation is similar for the vascular contact, which probably has a causal role.

One patient relapsed after 12 months. At reoperation in this patient, a dislocation of the inserted graft fragment was found: this was successfully replaced in position.

The majority of cases attained lasting freedom pain and symptoms.

In one patient, we saw the undesired side effects of an unilateral loss of hearing and facial paresis: these nerves had probably suffered traction or pressure damage from being displaced with the spatula. In addition, a few patients suffered postoperatively from disturbances of balance and moderate ataxia which completely regressed after four to eight weeks at the latest. In two cases, there were transient trochlear paresis. So far we have not observed further complications, in particular no potentially fatal complications.

The number of vascular compressions and contacts we found thus largely corresponds to that reported by other authors (Apfelbaum 1977, Haines and Jannetta 1980).

Discussion

We regard our experience with microvascular decompression of the trigeminal nerve as encouraging so far. If we were not as yet able to achieve the even better results of other authors, this is mainly attributable to typical starting difficulties. The operation requires dexterity, much surgical experience and perfect mastery of microsurgical technique. It requires very clean dissection at a considerable depth through a small trepanation opening. Pressure with the spatula on the cerebellum, pons and adjacent cranial nerves must be avoided just as meticulously as injuries to arterial vessel branches to the brain stem. The sitting position substantially facilitates microsurgical work in the cerebellopontine angle. However, it is associated with the danger of air embolism.

Preoperative insertion of a central atrial venous catheter and continuous monitoring with the Doppler instrument is therefore indispensable during the entire operation. The most important danger sites are the deep veins of the neck between muscles and ligaments, the emissarium mastoideum and the sinus durae matris. Even tiny injuries to the wall of venous tracts can lead to dangerous air aspiration. Frequent jugular compressions during the critical phases of the trepanation up to opening of the dura enable even very tiny lesions to the wall of veins to be detected. In very old patients with endangered circulation, the threat of a serious fall in blood pressure must also be considered and met by inclining the operation table or other appropriate measures. When anesthesiological monitoring is inadequate, the operation should preferentially be performed with the patient on his side with upper part of the body elevated.

Conclusions

The controlled percutaneous thermocoagulation of trigeminal ganglion still seems to be one of the most advisable methods to treat trigeminal neuralgia, especially in very old patients and by bad general condition. The new concept of microvascular trigeminal decompression in the posterior fossa according to Jannetta with elimination of the tic without an additional neurological deficit is fascinating. However, this method requires optimal microneurosurgical and anesthesiological conditions. Then it is hardly likely to be more dangerous than other operations, which have been common up to now.

References

Apfelbaum RJ (1977) A comparison of percutaneous radiofrequency trigeminal neurolysis and microvascular decompression of the trigeminal nerve for the treatment of tic douloureux. Neurosurgery 1: 16–21

Dandy WE (1932) The treatment of trigeminal neuralgia by the cerebellar route. Ann Surg 96:787–795

Haines StJ, Jannetta PJ, Zorub DS (1980) Microvascular relations of the trigeminal nerve. An anatomical study with clinical correlation. J Neurosurg 52:381–386

Jannetta PJ (1976) Microsurgical approach to the trigeminal nerve for tic douloureux. Prog Neurol Surg 7:180–200, Karger Basel

Penholz H (1976) Die neurochirurgische Behandlung der Trigeminusneuralgie. Langenbecks Arch Chir 342 (Kongreßbericht 1976):117–125

Sweet WH, Wepsic JG (1974) Controlled thermocoagulation of trigeminal ganglion and rootlets for differential destruction of pain fibers. J Neurosurg 39:143–156

Alteration of Sensibility in Trigeminal Neuralgia Before and After Selective Section of the Root by Posterior Approach

S. MINGRINO and G. SALAR, Padova/Italy

Introduction

The interest for our study originated from Dandy's initial observations after juxtapontine section of the trigeminal root for tic douloureux in 1929. He described the accessory fibers between the principal sensory root and the motor root, whose preservation after section of the major sensory root could explain touch sensory sparing of the face. Similar observations were reported by Jannetta and Rand (1967) and by Provost and Hardy (1970) after microsurgical section of the major trigeminal root and preservation of the intermediate or accessory fibers. They reported disappearance of pain associated with thermo-analgesia but touch sensory sparing particularly in the territory of the first branch.

In the present work sensibility of the face was carefully evaluated in normal subjects and in patients affected by trigeminal neuralgia before and after selective section of the major trigeminal root.

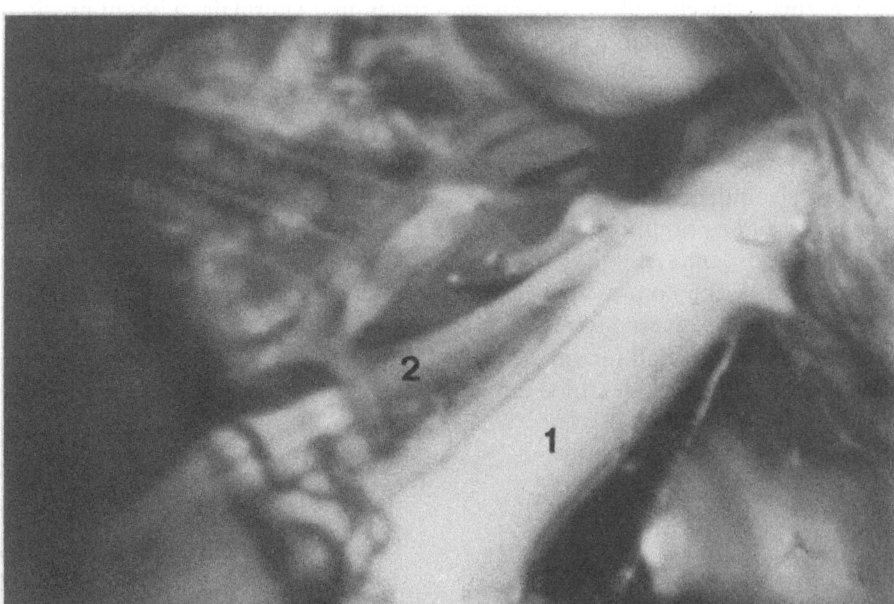

Fig. 1. *1* = Major root; *2* = Accessory fibers

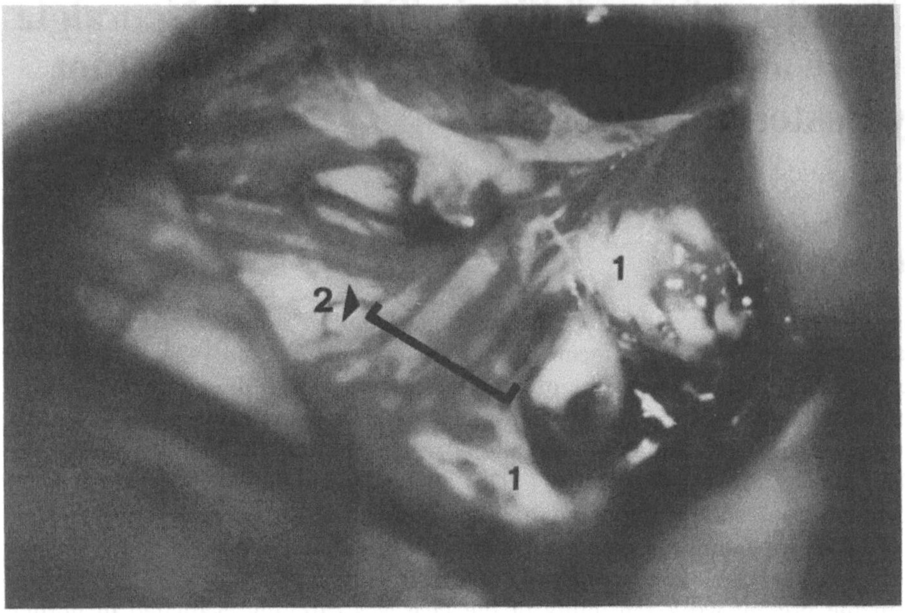

Fig. 2. *1* = Major root sectioned; *2* = Accessory fibers spared

Material and Method

Twenty normal subjects and 14 patients with trigeminal neuralgia, without previous surgical or alcohol treatment were examined.

Touch sensory examination was performed according to the technique of Von Frey modified by Semmes et al., with a battery of ten nylon wires of different calibers. The strength necessary to bend each wire was tested on a scale, and its logarithm was assumed as the corresponding value. Threshold resulted from the average of six independent examinations with the battery of wires used alternatively in ascending or descending sequence according to their caliber.

Thermic and pain sensibility was evaluated in a simple way, by comparative examination with the contralateral site. The type of response could be: normal, impaired or absent. Juxtapontine section of the trigeminal root was performed in nine cases through a small lateral suboccipital craniectomy, under the microscope the major root was easily identified and sectioned while motor and accessory fibers were spared.

Results

Normal subjects had a threshold of 1.38 with a standard deviation of 0.07. No significative difference in the territories of innervation of the right and left sides was found.

Table. 1. Preoperative abnormal touch sensibility 8/14 (57%)

	Painful sites	Non-painful sites	Contralateral corresponding sites
Range	1.46 – 2.62	1.19 – 2.01	1.29 – 1.64
Average	1.88	1.54	1.40

Table 2. Juxtapontine rizothomy

No. cases 9

		Branches		
		I	II	II
Touch sensibility		3.36	3.62	3.71
Pain sensibility	absent	7	8	8
	impaired	2	1	1
	normal	–	–	–
Thermic sensibility	absent	8	8	9
	impaired	1	1	–
	normal	–	–	–

Table 3.

Corneal reflex				Average I branch touch sensibility
		No. cases	Percentage	
Juxtapontine rizothomy	absent	5	55.5	3.93
	impaired	4	44.5	2.62
	normal	–	–	–

In eight of the 14 patients with trigeminal neuralgia (57 percent) preoperative examination revealed that the sites of pain had a higher threshold (Table 1) than non-painful sites. It is interesting to note that only four of the patients (28 percent) presented an alteration of the sensibility on routine examination.

The motor activity was studied by electromyography and was normal. After operation the sensory threshold on the operated side was much higher in all three areas (Table 2), however, in the first branch there was a significantly lower value ($p < 0.05$). Five of the patients (56 percent) had complete touch, pain, and thermic anesthesia with loss of the corneal reflex. In the other four patients (Table 3) touch sensibility was partially spared in the territory of the first branch with the corneal reflex present, although hypoactive; there was associated partial sparing of the sensibility of the second branch in a case and of the third branch in another case. Pain sensibility was also partially spared in the first and second branch in a case and in the first and third branch in another case; thermic sensibility was partially spared in the first branch in a case and in the second branch in another case.

Discussion

Instrumental examination reveals sensory alterations in about half of the patients while clinical findings were positive in only 28 percent of the cases. This last value is similar to the 25 percent reported by Lewy and Grant in 1934.

Selective section of the major sensory root provokes partial sparing of sensibility in only 44 percent of the cases. The sensibility preserved has the following characteristics:

1. It is mainly spared in the territory of the first branch.
2. Touch is the most frequent type of sensibility spared.

Table 4. Correlation between anatomical and clinical data

	Percentage		
	I	II	III
Intermediate fibers (Gudmundsson et al.)	74	15	11
Spared touch sensibility after juxtapontine rizothomy cases 6/9	66 (4)	17 (1)	17 (1)

These clinical results are in agreement with the anatomical study in humans by Gudmundsson et al. (1971), who found that intermediate fibers are predominantly motor in a proportion of four to one. Only 54 percent of their cases had intermediate sensory fibers which distributed mainly in the first branch (Table 4). In addition, our results do not confirm the hypothesis that intermediate fibers transport touch sensation and the major root pain and thermic sensation (Dandy, Jannetta, and Rand). Also experimental observations exclude this type of sensory specialization, as Emmons and Rhoton (1971) found that selective section of intermediate fibers provoked degenerative changes in the nucleus principalis as well as in the trigeminal spinal nucleus of monkeys.

References

Dandy W (1929) An operation for the cure of tic douloureux. Partial section of the sensory root at the pons. Arch Surg 18:687–734

Emmons WF, Rhoton AL Jr (1971) Subdivision of the trigeminal sensory root. J Neurosurg 35:585–591

Gardner WJ (1968) Trigeminal neuralgia. Clin Neurosurg 15:1–50

Gudmundsson K, Rhoton AL, Anderson DE (1971) Detailed anatomy of the intracranial portion of the trigeminal nerve. J Neurosurg 35:592–600

Jannetta PJ, Rand RW (1967) Gross mesoscopic description of the human trigeminal nerve and ganglion. J Neurosurg 26:101–111

Lewy FH, Grant FG (1938) Physiopathologic and pathoanatomic aspects of major trigeminal neuralgia. Arch Neurol Psychiat 40:1126–1134

Ley A, Montserrat L, Bracci F, Ley A Jr (1975) Clinical and electrophysical studies on sensory conduction mediated by the accessory rootlets of the human trigeminal nerve. J Neurosurg 42:513–521

Pelletier VA, Poulos DA, Lende RA (1974) Functional localization in the trigeminal root. J Neurosurg 40:504–513

Pertuiset B, Philippon G, Fohanno D, Khalil M (1972) Traitement microchirurgical de la névralgie faciale essentielle par neurotomie retrogassérienne sélective transtentorielle. Rev Neurol (Paris) 126:97–106

Provost J, Hardy J (1970) Microchirurgie du trijumeau: anatomie fonctionelle. Neurochirurgie 16:459–470

Semmes J, Weinstein S, Ghent L, Teuber HL (1960) Somatosensory changes after penetrating brain wounds in man. Harvard University Press, Cambridge

White JC, Sweet WH (1955) Pain. Its mechanism and neurosurgical control. Charles C. Thomas, Springfield, p 433

Reconstruction of the Trigeminal Nerve

M. SAMII, Hannover/FRG

New indications for the surgical treatment of a traumatized trigeminal nerve have recently evolved (Samii 1972). Severe facial injuries may be accompanied by lesions of different branches of the trigeminal nerve, most commonly at the forehead in the area of the frontal branches or in fractures of the mandible where the inferior alveolar nerves are located. Fractures of the base of the skull or intracranial space-occupying processes may lead to a lesion of the trigeminal nerve with partial or total loss of sensation in one part of the face and paralysis of the masticatory muscles. Radical tumor extirpation of the lower jaw often requires the resection of the inferior alveolar nerv. The consequence is loss of sensation in the region of the mucosa, the lip, and the chin. Transection of the frontal nerve caused by an incised wound produces hypesthesia in the region of the forehead which is of relatively minor significance. Trigeminal neuralgia resistant to any therapy may also appear owing to the formation of a neuroma and is of greater clinical importance (Fig. 1 a). The technique of neurolysis has been successful only in rare cases. Dissection of the trigeminal nerve in this region in order to re-establish the continuity of the nerve through an end-to-end suture or a nerve graft can be performed (Fig. 1 b). As a result, not only is the pain relieved but also the restoration of sensation can be observed.

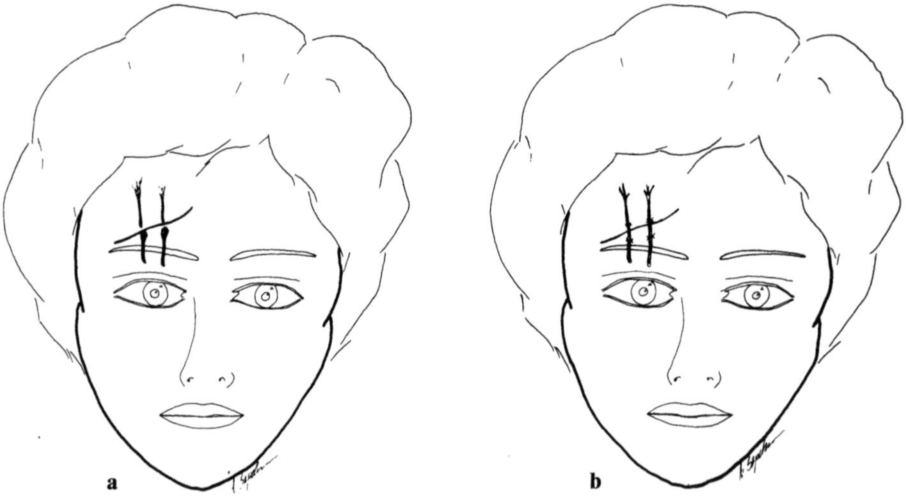

Fig. 1 a, b. Transection of the frontal nerve caused by an incised wound in the region of the forehead with development of neuroma and trigeminal neuralgia (**a**). Resection of neuroma and reconstruction of the continuity of the frontal nerve through a nerve graft (**b**)

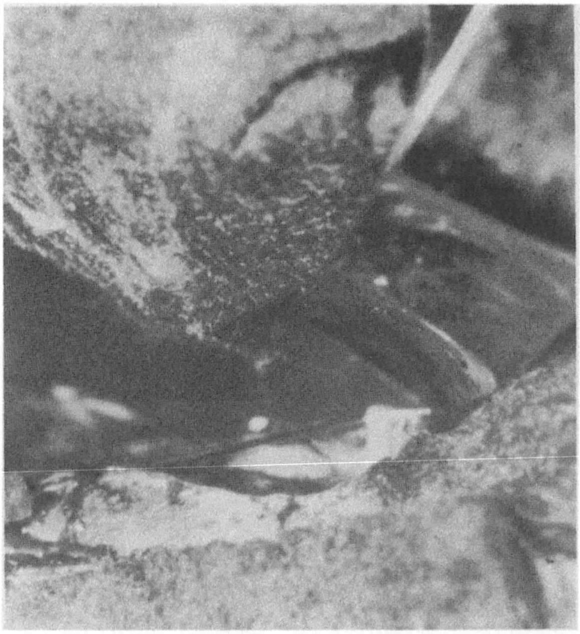

a

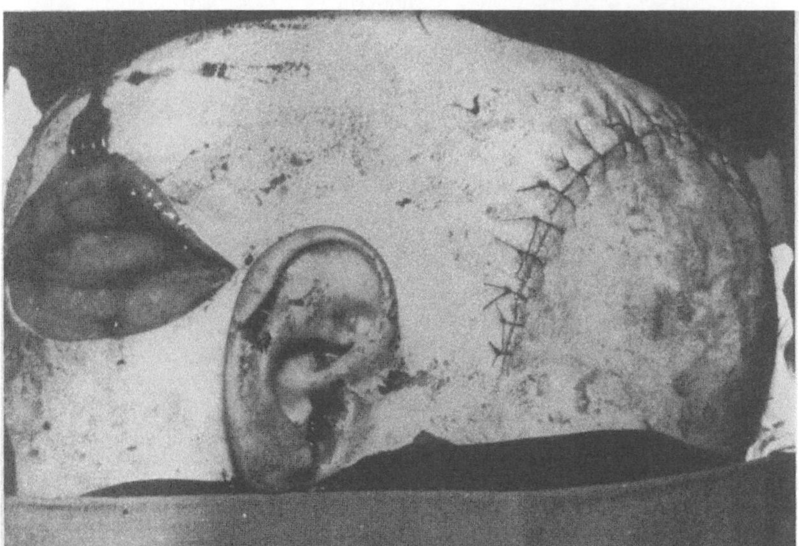

b

Fig. 2a, b. Transfrontal orbitotomy. Exposure of the ophthalmic nerve in a patient with retroganglionic trigeminal lesion (**a**). After suture of a 17 centimeter long autologous nerve graft between the ophthalmic nerve and the major occipital nerve, the right sided frontal craniotomy is closed again. The nerve graft is still visible behind the ear (**b**)

The loss of function of the ophthalmic nerve constitutes a special problem and can have serious consequences. Ceratitis neuroparalytica can lead to ulcer of the cornea and even to blindness as a result of sensory and trophic disorder of the cornea. Disorders of the ophthalmic nerve occur in connection with retroganglionic injury or after operative treatment of trigeminal neuralgia, which may result in a complete loss of sensation. In this case restoration of sensation in the cornea must be the surgical goal. A direct surgical approach to intracranial damage of the

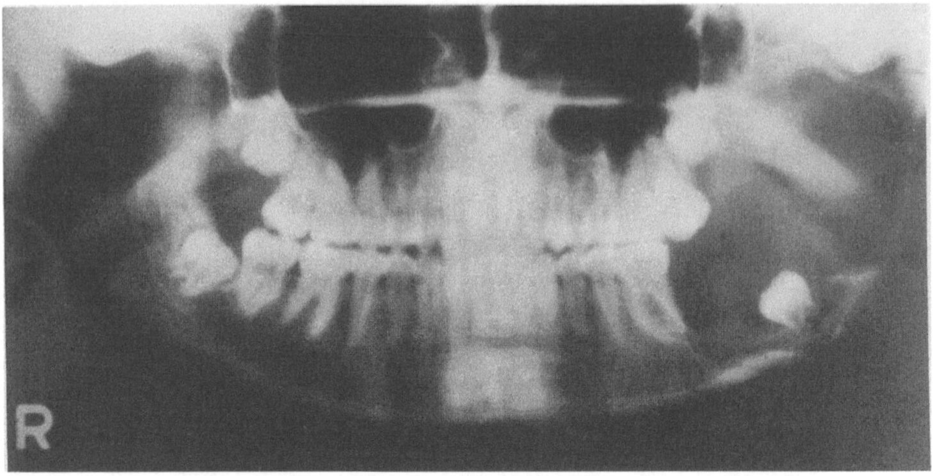

a

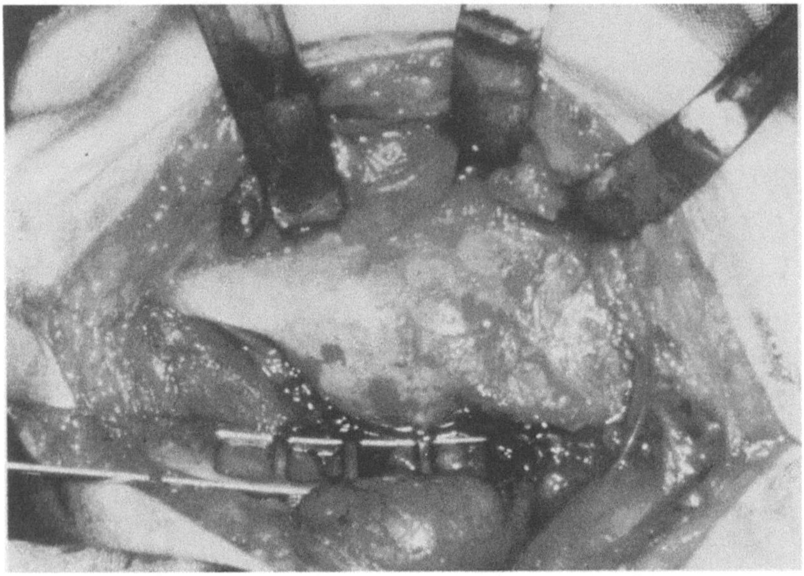

b

Fig. 3a, b. X-ray of the lower jaw of a cystic adamantinoma on the left side (**a**). Exposure of the left lower jaw tumor (**b**)

trigeminal nerve was previously technically impossible. The only possible method of reconstruction is an anastomosis between the ophthalmic nerve and cutaneous nerve. The major occipital nerve seems to be most suitable, as it is of the same diameter as the ophthalmic nerve and participates, as does the major ophthalmic nerve, in the sensory innervation of the galea. Also the auricularis magnus nerve has every suitability for a donor nerve. After exposure of the major occipital nerve an osteoplastic frontal craniotomy is performed. The anterior cranial fossa is exposed epidurally, the roof of the orbit is opened and, through an incision of the

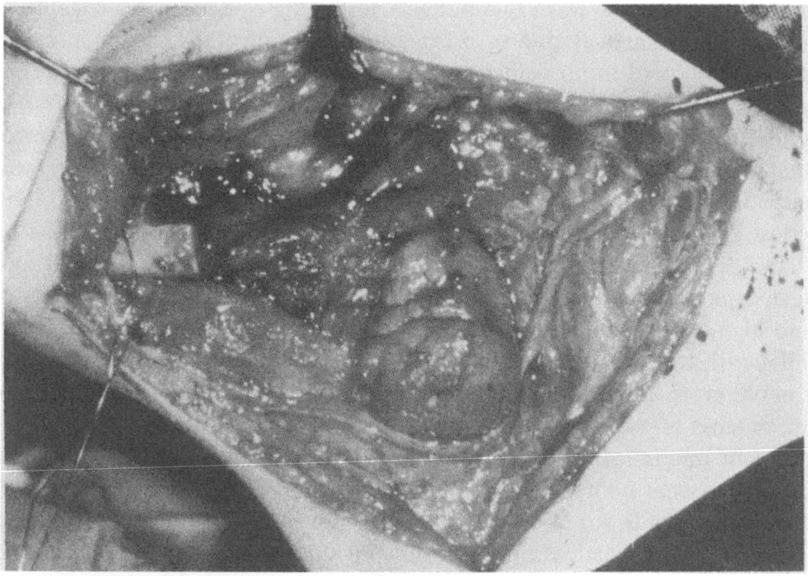

c

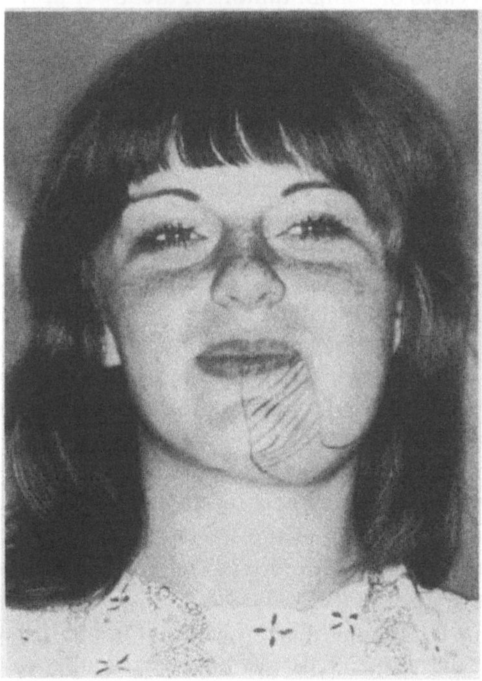

d

Fig. 3c, d. Total removal of the lower jaw along with the inferior alveolar nerve. Bridging of the defect by means of a 12 centimeter long autogenous nerve graft (**c**); (**d**) the same case as Fig. 3a, 3b, and 3c. Postoperative loss of sensation in the region of the lower lip, the mucosa and the chin. Six months later, complete return of sensation

periorbital capsule, the ophthalmic nerve is exposed (Fig. 2a) and transected proximally. The peripheral stump of the ophthalmic nerve is then anastomosed with a sural nerve graft. The transplant is led out of the skull and anastomosed with the major occipital nerve in the subgaleal layer. The craniotomy is closed (Fig. 2b). To present, three patients have been operated upon with this technique. Disorders of the ophthalmic nerve occured in two patients following operation for trigeminal neuralgia and in the other was due to retroganglionic injury after trauma. In all three patients we observed improvement of the trophic disorder of the cornea, but not full recovery of sensation.

Resection of the inferior alveolar nerve is often unavoidable during surgery of benign or malignant tumors of the mandible. An example is a 15 year old girl with a cystic adamantinoma of the whole ascending branch of the left mandible (Fig. 3a, b). For the reconstruction of the inferior nerve after resection of the lower jaw, it is advisable (Samii 1972, Hausamen et al. 1973) to mark and cut the proximal and distal nerve stumps at the mandibular and mental foramina. Thereafter, the tumor resection and the osteoplastic reconstruction may be performed. The tumor is removed along with the inferior alveolar nerve, and the nerve defect is bridged by means of a nerve graft 12 cm in length (Fig. 3c). Anesthesia of the affected side of the lower lip, mucosa and the chin (Fig. 3d) is sometimes a serious problem for the patient because of uncontrolled drooling and difficulty in drinking. Ulceration of the lower lip may appear when the anesthetic lip is traumatized between the teeth while chewing. Although in some patients this may not be irritating, others seem to suffer tremendously from this loss of sensation. For this reason all attempts should be made to preserve this nerve, at least in cases of benign tumors of the lower jaw.

We introduced this technique in 1971 at the Clinic for Oral and Maxillo-facial surgery of the University in Mainz, in cooperation with Professor Scheunemann and Hausamen. In 19 patients reconstruction of the inferior alveolar nerve was performed. Thirteen patients could be examined postoperatively with the follow up between one to eight years. Complete recovery of sensation could be achieved in two young patients aged eight and 15 years old. In the other cases there was a satisfactory improvement in the involved areas (Schmidseder and Nissen 1979).

The course of the peripheral part of the lingual nerve in the floor of the mouth is of special interest. After leaving the pterygomandibular space, the lingual nerve establishes very close contact with the mandible at the level of the third molar. Its branches are to be found under the mucosa before they enter the tongue. The nerve supplies the sensory innervation of the anterior two thirds of the tongue and the floor of the mouth, as well as the lingual side of the mandibular gingiva. In addition, it sends out the afferent parasympathetic fibres for the submandibular and sublingual glands. The lingual nerve can be traumatized by careless extraction of the lower third molar, by improper intraoral incision of a sublingual abscess and by injuries with drills during preparation of cavities of the lower molars. Fig. 4a and b demonstrate an example of reconstruction of the lingual nerve in a case of traumatic lesion following extraction of the wisdom teeth.

Furthermore the lingual nerve may have to be sacrificed in cases of tumor of the floor of the mouth which have invaded the nerve. This can also be reconstructed (Fig. 5). Reconstruction of the lingual nerve may be successful if performed near its trunk and proximal to its divisions in the floor of the mouth. If an extraoral approach is used to resect the mandible, identification of the proximal and peripheral stumps and performance of nerve grafting do not present any special problem. The intraoral approach to the nerve stumps of the pterygomandibular space and in the floor of the mouth is also not particularly difficult.

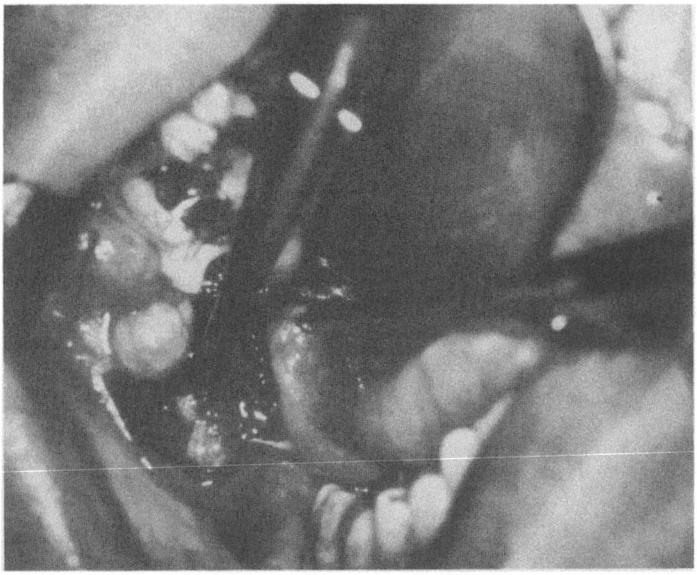

a

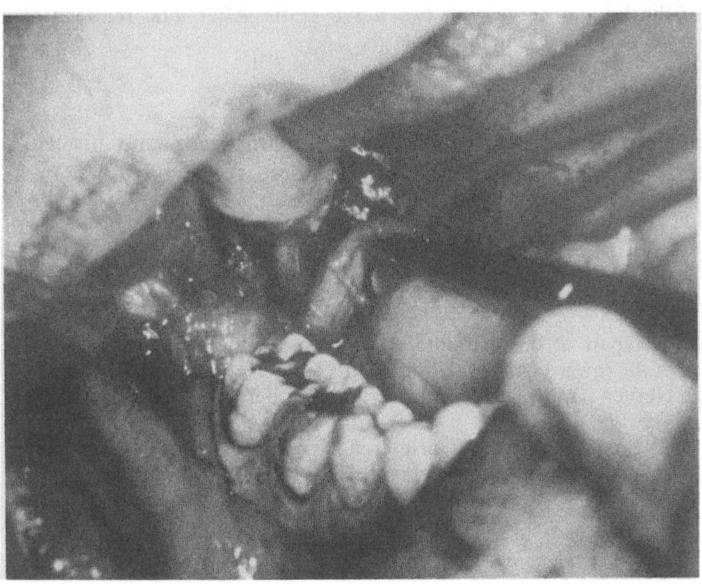

b

Fig. 4a, b. Lesion of the lingual nerve after extraction of the right wisdom tooth (**a**). The lingual nerve has been reconstructed by means of a nerve graft (**b**)

In contrast, nerve grafting is technically difficult in patients with full dentition because of the very narrow surgical field. Because of the superficial course of the lingual nerve, the transplant has to be bedded directly underneath the mucosa and exact wound closure is all important. We have been disappointed by the results in

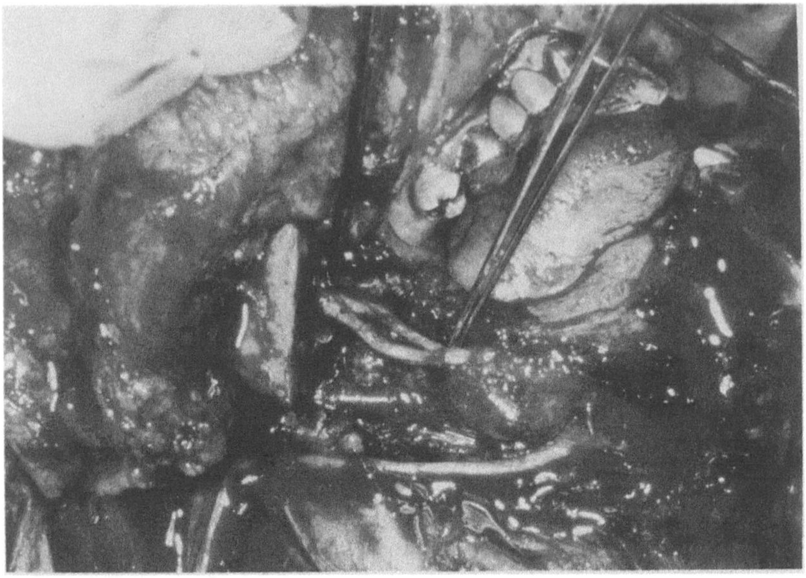

Fig. 5. Reconstruction of the lingual nerve with two nerve grafts. After total removal of a large tumor of the floor of the mouth and the mandible

four patients operated upon together with Professor Scheunemann and his team. Despite an optimal anatomical reconstruction of the nerve the sensation of taste could not be achieved.

References

Hausamen JE et al. (1973) Repair of the mandibular nerve by means of autologous nerve grafting after resection of the lower jaw. J Maxillofac Surg 1:74–78

Samii M (1972) Autologe Nerven-Transplantation im Trigeminusbereich. Med Mitt (Melsungen) 46:189–194

Schmidseder R et al. (1979) Spätergebnisse der primären Nervenrekonstruktion im Kiefer- und Gesichtsbereich. Kiefer-Gesichtschir Supplement Heft 11–116

Trigeminal Paresthesias in Cervical 5/6 Disk Involvement

K. J. ZÜLCH, Köln/FRG

One interesting, not well described phenomenon is the occasional occurrence of paresthesias and even hypesthesias in the cheek and temple in cases of cervical disk degeneration.

We have first noticed this in the case of a lady aged 39 years suffering from a right-sided neurological hemisyndrome for four years, together with a mild cervical pain. She was always diagnosed as a case of multiple sclerosis or amyotrophic lateral sclerosis, particularly because of an apparently permanent sort of Lhermitte's sign, which turned out to be a root paresthesia in certain positions of the neck, entirely restricted to the left C 6 root.

For years she severely complained of the afore mentioned permanent paresthesias of the three branches of the trigeminal nerve sparing the submandibular area. After a C 5–6 Cloward operation the paresthesias ceased immediately and permanently the very same afternoon of the day the operation was performed.

A second patient with similar symptoms, 69 years of age, was also immediately releaved of his facial paresthesias on the day of the operation. We found the same symptom briefly mentioned and without discussion in Verbiest's general report (1970) as also in Elvidge and Li's (1950) paper. However, in the latter the symptoms were bilateral and only in a very restricted territory. In Ch. Zülch's dissertation (1975) discussing the cases of chronic cervical myelopathy of A. Stender's clinic in West-Berlin she found four cases similar to this observation out of a total number of 49 patients. In all these cases the motor division of the trigeminal nerve was found completely intact, however, in our last patient the corneal reflex was almost abolished.

In man, Sjöqvist (1957, p. 6) demonstrated the end of the spinal trigeminal root at the lower edge of the third cervical segment. In textbooks (I. S. Wechsler 1958, A. Brodal 1959) it is stated that it can still be found at the second segment. If these are the data then the problem arises that either the sequelae of the lesion must go as far as the first or second cervical segment or else the descending tract goes actually further downwards to extend down to the 5th cervical segment.

I seem to remember that Foerster's personal teaching – I do not know whether on the base of such observations – was that the descending trigeminal tract went further down, namely to C5.

I have gone through textbooks and anatomical descriptions of the descending root and never found any extension assumed below C2.

I may mention a last possibility, namely that the main cervical arterial supply usually passes at the intervertebral foramen C 5/6. But to construct here a vascular mechanism seems hardly possible.

Therefore, I cannot give any decent explanation of this symptom but summarize the phenomenon as such: that not unfrequently facial paresthesias and even neurological deficits are observed in the trigeminal area in cases of chronic cervical myelopathy C 5/6 which disappear after corresponding operations either by the Cloward procedure or by posterior laminectomy.

References

Brodal A (1959) The cranial nerves. Blackwell Scientific Publications, Oxford

Elvidge AR, Li CC (1950) Central protrusion of cervical intervertebral disc involving descending trigeminal tract. Arch Neurol Psychiat 63:455–466

Sjöqvist O (1957) Surgery of the Cranial Nerves. II. Physiology. Sensory Innervation of the Head and Face. In: Handbuch der Neurochirurgie, Band VI, Springer-Verlag, Berlin Göttingen Heidelberg, pp 4–7

Verbiest H (1970) La chirurgie antérieure et latérale du rachis cervical. Neuro-chirurgie 16, Suppl. 2. Masson & Cie, Paris

Wechsler IS (1958) A textbook of clinical neurology with an introduction to the history of neurology. 8. Edition. W. B. Saunders Comp, Philadelphia London

Zülch Ch (1975) Ergebnisse der cervicalen Myelolyse bei akuter und chronischer Myelopathie. Doktor-Dissertation, Universität Berlin

Facial and Vestibulocochlear Nerves

(Seventh and Eighth Cranial Nerves)

Facial and Vestibulocochlear Nerve, Topographic Anatomy and Variations*

J. LANG, Würzburg/FRG

The facial nerve (second branchial arch nerve) innervates all the mimic muscles, the muscle stapedius, the posterior belly of the digastric muscle, and the stylohyoid muscle. Related to it, the intermedius nerve innervates the external acustic meatus, the posterior inferior part of auricle, and a part of the skin above the mastoid process (Hunt Zone). This nerve probably contains proprioceptive fibers from the mimic muscles. The sensory fibers of facial nerve carry taste sensations from the anterior two thirds of the tongue towards the central nervous system. In addition, the parasympathethic-secretory fibers of the lacrimal gland, the nasal, palatine, pharyngeal, lingual, as well as of the submandibular and sublingual glands run through the nerve partially over the intermedius segment.

Nucleus of Facial Nerve

The information regarding the size of the facial nerve nucleus varies considerably. In general it is assumed that the nucleus has a length of 4 (2–5.6) mm. According to Vraa-Jensen, 1942, who has done remarkable basic investigations, the largest rostro-caudal expansion is given as 3–3.5 mm and the transverse expansion as 2.5–3.0 mm.

The nucleus is located inside the reticular formation, a large part of it in pons and a smaller part in the region of medulla oblongata. In its neighbourhood the nucleus ambiguus lies caudally; the motoric trigeminal nucleus rostrally; the trapezoid corpus ventrally; the nucleus of the tractus spinalis n. trigemini and parts of reticular formation dorsolaterally. Section of the ramus temporofacialis in the face region of a dog showed that cellular damage occurred in the posterior and central parts of the nucleus. Section through the ramus cervico-facialis resulted in chromatolysis of the cells of the lateral nuclear region. The ramus auricularis posterior, according to the findings of the author, emerges from the mediomedial nucleus group. That of the stapedius muscle from the medial and dorsal nucleus region. The nuclear regions responsible for the parasympathetic innervations are the superior and inferior salivatory nuclei.

The sensory mucous-membrane fibers of facial nerve together with those of the glossopharyngeal nerve, of the vagus nerve, and a few fibers of the trigeminal nerve pass through the solitary tract to its nuclear region in the rostral part. The sensory fibers in facial nerve reach the rostral part of the nucleus tractus spinalis n. V.

* Supported by DFG

Intracerebral Pathway

From 25 to 60 μm large-cell stem neurites, converge fan-shaped, ascend dorso-medial through the reticular substance against the bottom of rhombic fossa (pars prima), and bend directly underneath the ground of the ventriculus quartus around the nucleus of abducent nerve. The bending point is called genu nervi facialis. The fibers then course laterally, posteriorly, and caudally (pars secunda), as well as lateral to the stem nucleus of the facial nerve and lateral to the spinal tract of trigeminal nerve. In the region of the cerebellopontine angle the nerve leaves medial to the statoacoustic nerve as an oval bundle of fibers from the brain stem. In our investigations, the exit zone lies, on the average, 11.8 (9.5–14.5) mm lateral to the median line. A few fibers often pierce through the transverse fibers of the pons. The elliptical cross-section of the nerve is on the average 1.8 (1.0–2.0) mm, and its cross-sectional area about 1.2 mm^2. The intracisternal path up to the porus acusticus internus is 15.5 (10.5–19.5) mm. According to several researchers, the nerve contains between 4,000 and 14,000 fibers, most of which are 7 to 10 μm (3–14) thick. Some authors however, maintain that the intracisternal path up to the porus is 10 to 13 μm long (Pulec and House 1964). Up to the fundus meatus acustici there is additional distance of 5 to 6 mm in length.

Vestibulocochlear Nerve

The vestibular part of the nerve traverses rostral and medial to the cochlear part towards the piercing point in the central nervous organ. This is located in adults, according to our investigations, 13.93 (8.5–20) mm paramedial and 1.36 (0.5–2.0) mm lateral to the facial nerve exit. The anterior and superior (pars vestibularis) fibers group enter through the medial cerebellar peduncle. The posterior and inferior (pars cochlearis) enter that zone where the caudal cerebellar peduncle disappears under the middle cerebellar peduncle. Between the exit regions of the facial and vestibulocochlear nerves, the so-called lingula acustica is intercalated, which corresponds largely to the lower cochlear nucleus. The long diameter of the whole oval nerve is on the average, 3.05 (2.0–5.0) mm, the small diameter 1.2 (1.0–2.5) mm. Occasionally, the vestibular radix (superior) at the entrance into the nervous central organ can be differentiated as a single bundle from the cochlear radix (inferior). In such cases, the cochlear section runs, as otherwise inside the whole nerve, more dorso-caudal; the vestibular part above and forward. The distance between the nerve perforations into the nervous central organ and porus acusticus internus, as determined in our investigations, is 13.93 (8.5–20.0) mm.

Nervus intermedius

Earlier researchers pointed out that the proximal segment of the nervus intermedius is in close contact with the pars vestibularis of the vestibulocochlear nerve. Rhoton et al. (1968) called this part the proximal segment of the nerve which according to their findings has a total length of 21 (18–26) mm. This value corresponds to the results obtained in our investigations.

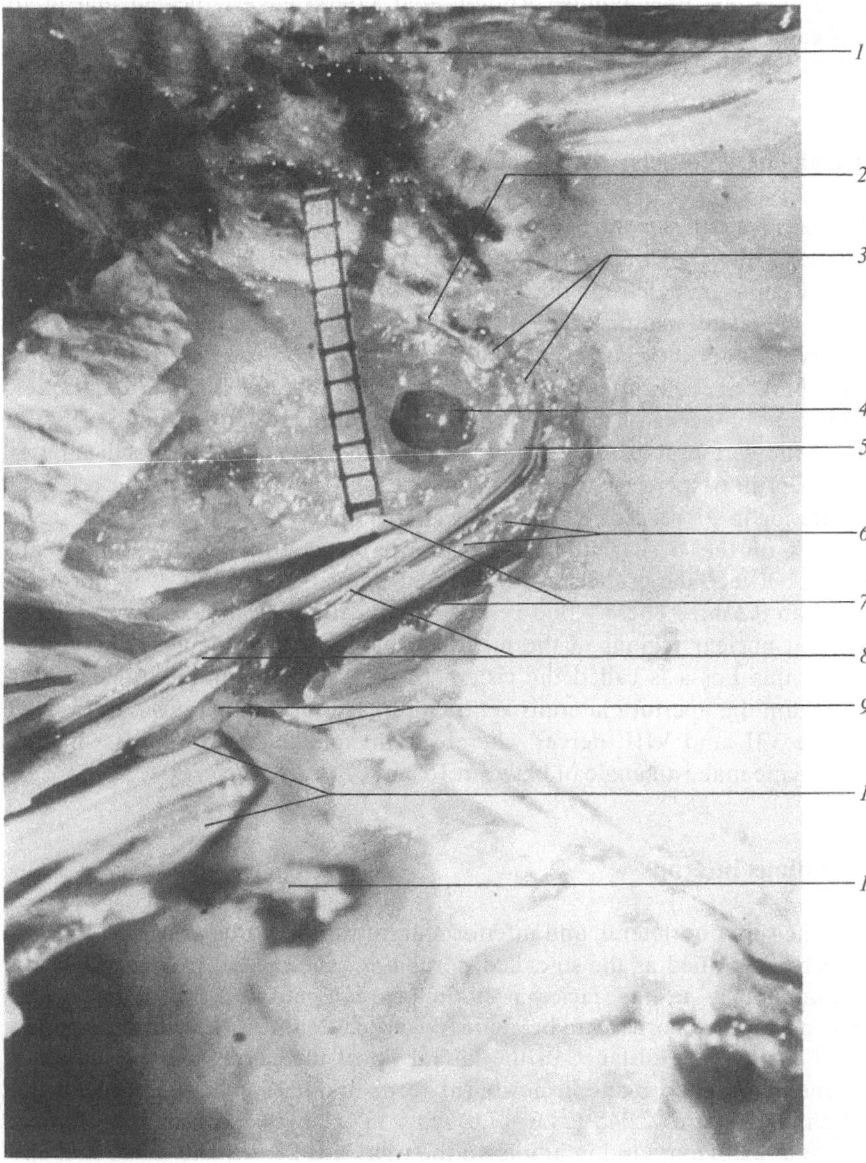

Fig. 1. Meatus acusticus int. Internal acustic meatus, roof removed; *1* = Middle meningeal artery, *2* = Greater petrosal nerve, *3* = Ganglion geniculi, *4* = Cochlea, *5* = N. VII, *6* = Ganglion vestibulare and pars vestib. sup. *7* = Dura mater meatus ac., *8* = N. intermedius, *9* = A. cereb. inf. ant. and A. subarcuata, *10* = Nn. IX to XI, *11* = transcisternal vene

The intermediate segment continues after the proximal segment freely between the VII. and VIII. nerves. The detachment from the pars vestibularis occurs after traversing a distance of about 6 mm. Its length varies mostly between 7 and 12 mm, in 22 percent of the cases it is 13 mm or more. On an average, they calculated a value of 10 (1–18) mm and pointed out that in 30 of the 73 specimen it was made up of more than one fiber bundle. Rhoton et al. (1968) have indicated that in 20 percent of cases the intermediate nerve within the posterior basal cistern cannot be identified, because it sits very tight to the pars vestibularis.

Fossa parolivaris, Vessels, and Cerebellarpontine Angle

The fossa parolivaris lies caudal to the pons and lateral to inferior olive. Laterally, it is bordered with cerebellum. The glossopharyngeal nerve leaves the fossa about 1.79 (1.0–3.0) mm caudal from the pontomedullar sulcus and 3.19 (1.5–5.0) mm lateral from the lateral margin of the olive. Caudal to it are the tenth nerve and the cranial radix fibers of the eleventh cranial nerve. Into the fossa enter the branches of the vertebral, cerebelli inferior posterior, basilar and cerebelli inferior arteries. We called these branches of the arteries the rami parolivares. We could verify the branches of the vertebral artery in 70 percent of the cases, of the cerebelli inferior posterior artery in 61 percent, of the basilar artery 81 percent and of the cerebelli inferior anterior in 91 percent. Considering their total cross section in percentage, the branches of the basilar and vertebral arteries dominate. Often there are anastomoses between the branches of individual source-vessels; however, normally not wider than 0.2 mm. These blood vessels supply, although in very diverse ways, the important nuclear regions of the medulla oblongata and spinalis. The cistern projected in this Fossa is called the cistern of the cerebellopontine angle. To its posterior region the apertura lateralis ventriculi quartii normally opens; in front of this pass the VII. and VIII. nerves whereby right and left nerve cords with the transversal plane make an angle of between 18 and 22 percent.

Porus acusticus internus

Normally, the superior, lateral, and inferior margins of the porus acusticus internus can be clearly identified as the so-called porus lips. The medial margin goes over almost continuously to the facies posterior partes petrosae. Therefore, width measurements of the porus can be defined very differently. Recently, we have determined the average distance of the lateral lip of the porus acusticus internus from the median sagittal plane in newborns to be about 13 (11.5–15) mm; in two year old children about 22.46 (21.0–27.0) mm; in six to seven year old children about 25 (23.0–27.0) mm; and in adults on the right side 28.65 (23.0–33.5) mm and on the left side 28.16 (22.0–34.0) mm (Fig. 2). A significant right-left difference in these distance measurements does not exist. The investigations show a rapid lateral displacement up to the second year followed by slight distance increase which remains until adult age. We have also determined the postnatal distance increase to the lateral wall of the cranium in the region of posterior margin of the meatus acusticus externus and to the posterior wall of cranium (sagittally up to a zone below the sinus transversus sulcus). Important from the medical point of view is also the roof thickness of meatus acusticus internus, which according to Jackson (1938), varies (in various degrees of pneumatisations) between 3.1 and 3.8 mm. The upper porus lip in about 60 percent is made up of stronger bone torus, and in 40

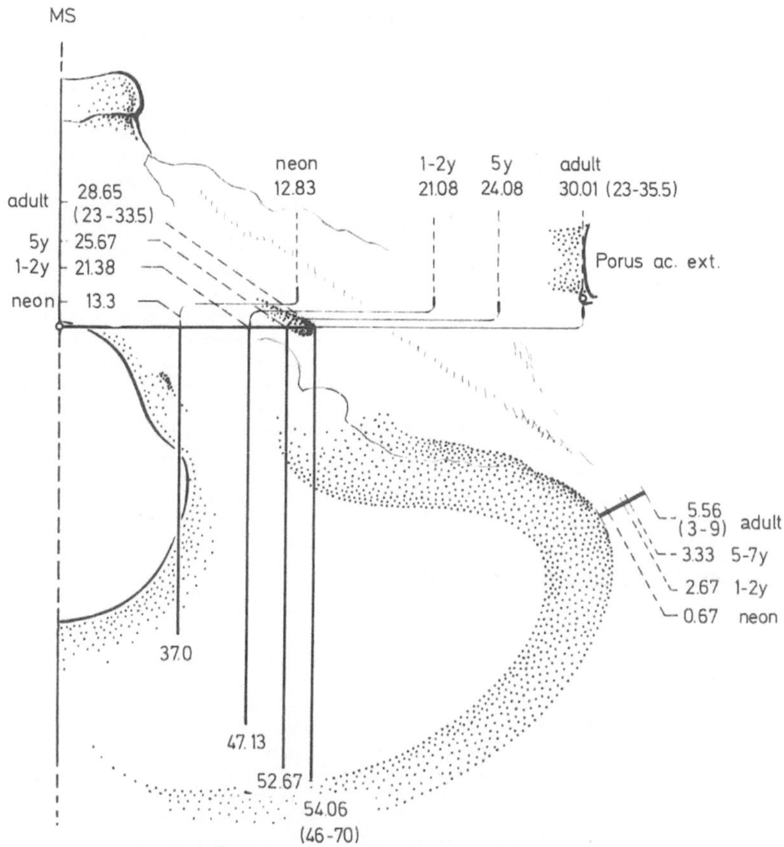

Fig. 2. Porus acusticus internus (lateral lip) distances

percent of smaller bone lip. The porus acusticus internus in newborns is about 3 (2.5–4.5) mm high and in 9 to 11 year old children about 4.7 (4.5–5.0) mm high. In adults the average values of 4.2 ± 1.6 (2.0–11.0) mm were obtained for the height of porus acusticus internus (Fig. 3). It is to be noted that the porus lies, in going over from the medial two-fifths to the lateral three-fifths, on the upper edge of the pars petrosa.

Porus acusticus internus, Nerves, and Blood Vessels

As it is known, the dura mater coat completely surrounds the internal auditory meatus. Inside it is arachnoid which encloses a fluid space of the internal auditory canal, nerves and blood vessels. According to Fisch, the arachnoid accompanies the first segment of the facial nerve canal up to the geniculate ganglion. The nerve-vessel relations in the porus region are of medical importance because of the

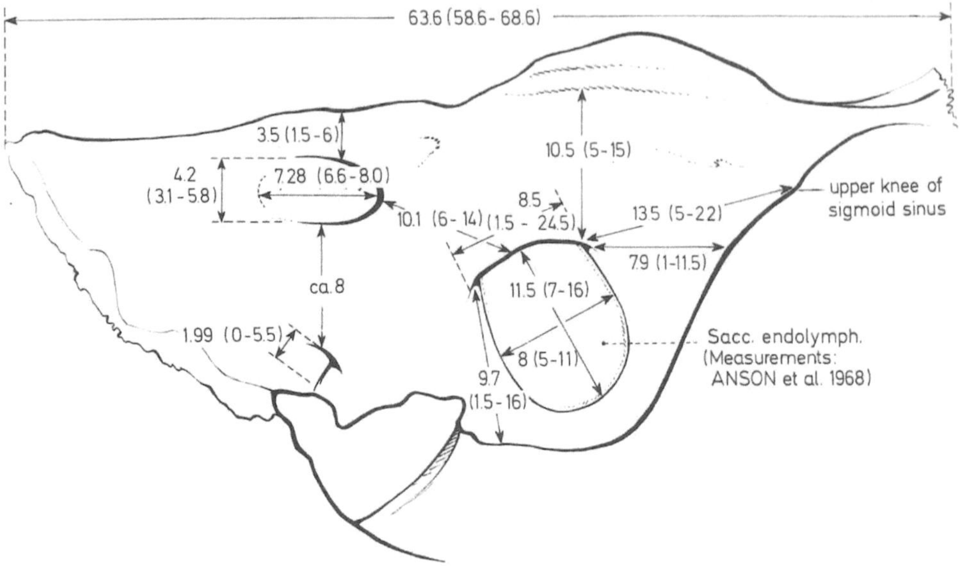

Fig. 3. Facies posterior partis petrosae, measurements

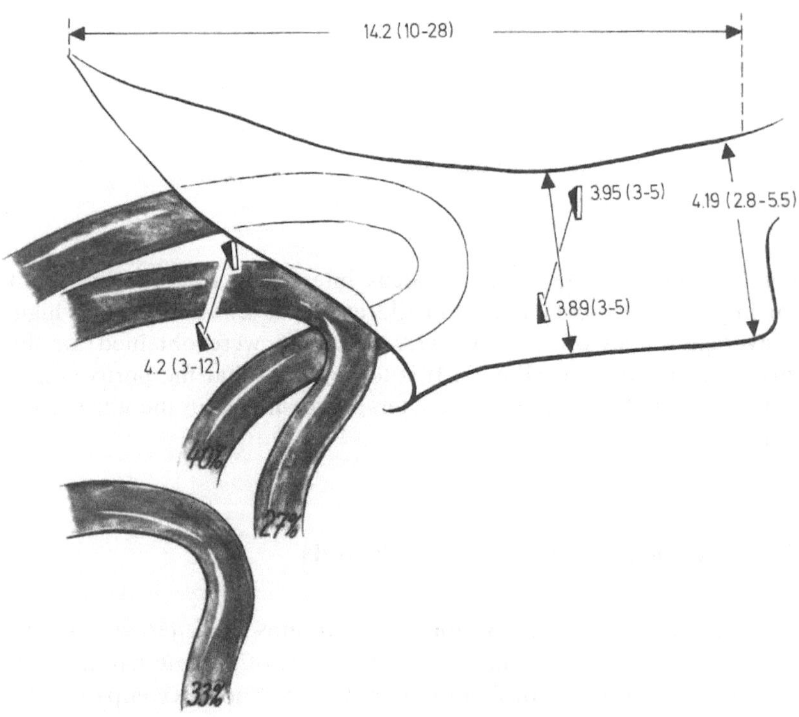

Fig. 4. Internal acoustic meatus, measurements and relation to anterior inferior cerebellar artery

extraordinary variability, especially, in the path of the anterior inferior cerebellar artery. We agree with the results of Mazzoni (1969), over the fixation of the vessels adjacent to the porus through direct embedment of the loop in the dura (6 percent) or through the subarcuata artery (6 percent). As far as the position of the vessels on the porus acusticus internus or inside the internal auditory meatus is considered, our results correspond with the findings of the Stopford, Sunderland, and Mazzoni. According to these authors, the loop in about 40 percent lies inside the meatus (Fig. 4). It enters below the nerves and leaves between the VII. and VIII. nerves (31 percent). In a large percentage of the cases, the loop is situated in the region of the porus acusticus internus and in about 40 percent there is no relation to the entrance of the internal auditory canal. As it is known, the facial nerve runs medial and rostral, the pars vestibularis lateral and more dorsal, and the pars cochlearis medial and below. The nervus intermedius, when it is separated from the vestibular part, lies above it. Prott (1974) has determined the minimum diameter inside the dura-coated meatus to be on the average, 3.3 (1.8–5.0) mm. He found the diameter of the nerves passing through the internal auditory canal as 2.3 (1.0–3.0) mm. According to Pulec and House, the facial nerve occupies only 12 to 19 percent of the cross sectional area.

Meatus acusticus internus, Postnatal Enlargement

The length of the meatus acusticus internus, as measured in the middle region of xanthopren-blue-cast specimens, is in newborns 5.0 (3.0–6.0) mm, in two year olds 7.23 (4.0–9.0) mm. Up to the fourth year, this segment elongates about 1 mm on the average, until eight years of age somewhat more than 1 mm. In 15 to 17 year olds an average value of 11 (9.0–12.0) mm is given for the length of the meatus. It is difficult to determine the medial border region of the medial or anterior wall of the meatus acusticus internus. We have performed some measurements of this type in two year old children and came up with a value of 10 mm and in adults with 14.15 (10–20) mm. The length of the lateral wall, which is easier to define, was in two year old children 5.9 mm, in adults on the right side 8.1 (4–11) mm and on the left 7.6 (4–11) mm.

The postnatal vertical development of the meatus acusticus internus is minimal. In newborns the average values of 3.0 mm on the right and of 3.1 mm on the left have been verified. The values in one year old children have been found as 4.25 and 4.5 mm on the right and left, respectively (Fig. 5).

In cast specimens of our investigations in 1975 it was found out that the meatus acusticus internus in adults is about 3.8 ± 0.6 mm wide and it often expands itself near the fundus meatus acustici to 4.2 ± 0.7 mm. Further, we determined, as Fisch did in 1968 and 1969, the narrowest parts in non-cylindrical canals near the fundus and in the porus region. Papangenlou (1971) found the vertical diameter to be 4.6 (2–7) mm.

The transverse diameter of the meatus acusticus internus in newborns is about 3 mm, in five year olds about 4.5 mm thus reaching the average value of the adults. The limit values in adults vary, after Papangenlou, between 3.0–7.0 mm.

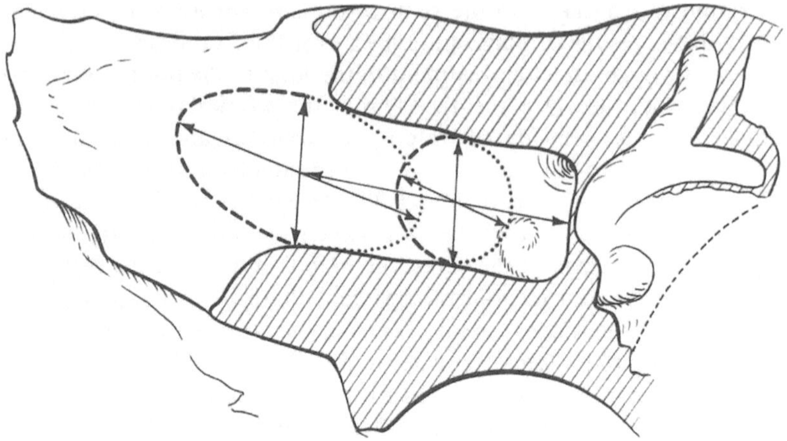

age	Porus-width	Porus-height	Meatus length	Meatus height	Meatus width
adult		3.10-5.80	11.15	3.0-7.0	6.46
15-17y	9.63	4.75	11.10	6.0	5.50
2y	7.04	4.08	7.23	4.6	4.30
neon	5.90	3.06	5.00	3.0	2.88

Fig. 5. Internal acoustic meatus, measurements

Meatus acusticus internus, Topography of the Cranial Nerves

Inside the meatus acusticus internus are placed the VII. intermedial and VIII. nerves respectively from top to bottom. Within the canal the facial nerve traverses forward above, the cochlear nerve (pars cochlearis) forward below, lateral and above runs the pars superior of the pars vestibularis and lateral below its pars inferior. According to Rhoton et al. (1968) the nervus intermedius unites with facial nerve at a point 5 (1–11) mm proximal to the fundus meatus acustici. Rhoton et al. (1966) believe, as Kehr 1962, that the pain fibers of nervus intermedius in dorsal parts of the spinal tract of trigeminal nerve descend to the superior cervical segment. The sensory fibers of taste, as maintained by the authors, reach the principal nucleus of trigeminal nerve in pons.

As Van Buskirk (1945) has identified inside the nervus intermedius as well as in pars vestibularis small bipolar ganglion cells may be found. The vestibular ganglion can be divided into a pars superior and a pars inferior, which are separated from each other by a narrow isthmus (Bergström 1973). It is situated in the lateral base and side-wall region of the meatus acusticus internus, and is rich in vascularisation. The larger pars superior contains the ganglion cells of the anterior and lateral ampullary nerves as well as of the utricular nerve. The pars inferior is comprised of the ganglion cells of saccular and posterior ampullary nerves. After Bergström, the pars vestibularis has, on the average, about 18,000 fibers, which in aged persons may reduce to approximately 11,000 fibers. Of interest is that

Ehrenbrand, in 1972, found a vestibular paraganglion which looks like glomus organ and sits close to the vestibular ganglion. He believes that it receives fibers from nervus intermedius over the communicating rami and has an endocrine neurosecretory function.

Fundus meatus acustici interni

The nearly round fundus is divided by the transverse crest into an upper and a lower part. Above and medial is the region of facial nerve, which preferably is called the internal apertura canalis n. facialis. Above and lateral is the area of superior vestibular which is limited medially by a vertical fold of dura and bone: Bill's bar. Below the transverse crest, medially, is situated the cochlear area. Through its small spiral openings leave the central neurons of the tractus spinalis foraminosus, and enters the retrograde Rasmussen bundle. Lateral and dorsal to the cochlear area, there is the area of inferior vestibular whose openings serve as exit for the centripetal nerves of the saccule. Below, is the foramen singulare for the nerve fibers of the posterior semicircular canal. Krmpotić-Nemanić et al. (1971) emphasize that in the cochlear areas, in persons over 20 years of age, bone depositions take place on the margins of the canals which are quite conspicuous at the openings for nerve fibers of the basilar cochlear convolution; they become compressed and get atrophic.

Hardy, in 1934, determined that between the lower part of the vestibular ganglion, fibers pass to the cochlear ganglion, pierce with it through the cochlear area and run forwards to the anterior part of the saccule: the cochleo-saccular nerve. The saccular ramus (Voit nerve) emerging from the pars superior reaches the anterior and posterior parts of the Macula sacculi. She designated a branch of the inferior part of the pars vestibularis as great saccular nerve; whereas, the superior saccular ramus (Voit) stems from the pars superior of the pars vestibularis. The larger and posterior section of macula is innervated from the great saccular nerve. Even in these small nerves, there are numerous variations. Bergström (1973) indicated that the great saccular nerve passing the transverse crest leads to the superior vestibular area. He further maintained that practically in every case a posterior accessory ampullary nerve exists which sometimes branches off from inside the internal acoustic meatus or directly from ganglion and enters in a bone canal somewhat above the foramen singulare. After a distance of 2 to 3 mm the accessory nerve unites with the posterior ampullary nerve, seldom, however, it runs separately to the ampullar of posterior semicircular canal.

Labyrinthine Artery

Siebenmann (1897) emphasized that as a result of his investigations in 1893 the vascularisation of labyrinthine has been understood thoroughly, a view which no researcher should maintain concerning his own findings. According to his opinion, there exists a main artery (labyrinthine artery) which divides itself into three equally strong main branches. Konaschko (1927) found that often a bi-arterial type was observed, a view also supported by Fisch (1968).

Table 1. A. labryrinthi origin

Origin	%	Authors
a) A. cerebelli inf. ant.	63	Stopford, 1916
	83	Sunderland, 1945
	80	Mazzoni, 1969
b) A. basilaris	70 re 67% li	Cavatorti, 1908
	36	Stopford, 1916
	5	Watt and McKillop, 1935
	17	Sunderland, 1945
	17	Mazzoni, 1969
c) A. cerebelli inf. post. or A. vertebralis	3	Mazzoni, 1969 and Rare Walker, 1965
d) More then one vessel	15	Ferrari-Lelli, 1939
	23	Guerreer and Villaceque, 1949
	45	Mazzoni, 1969
	4 (3 vessels)	Mazzoni, 1969

Table 2. A. cerebelli inf. ant. and Meatus acusticus internus

Origin	%	Authors
1. Loop		
a) in meatus ac. int.	67	Mazzoni, 1969
	64	Sunderland, 1945
b) porus acusticus internus	25	Sunderland, 1945
c) without relation to porus	11	Sunderland, 1945
	33	Mazzoni, 1969
2. Relation to N. VII et VIII second part of the loop		
a) between Nn. VII et VIII meatus	31	Sunderland, 1945
porus	11	Sunderland, 1945
meatus	35	Mazzoni, 1969
b) below Nn. VII et VIII meatus	4.5	Mazzoni, 1969
without relation to meatus	25	Mazzoni, 1969
porus	14	Sunderland, 1945
	18	Mazzoni, 1969
c) above Nn. VII et VIII	1	Mazzoni, 1969
d) anterior Nn. VII et VIII	8	Mazzoni, 1969
e) between Nn. VII et VIII	8	Mazzoni, 1969
f) between Nn. VII et VIII and an posterior wall	5	Mazzoni, 1969

Labyrinthine Artery, Branches

Presently in anatomic nomenclature the vestibular rami and cochlear rami are considered as the branches of labyrinthine artery. Certainly there are also small branches going off the labyrinthine artery such as the anterior inferior cerebellar artery and other vessels which enter the path of the intracisternal nerves and of the internal acoustic meatus and the dura. Very often the labyrinthine artery lies below the nerves. Once two are together, one passes, according to Fisch, between the pars cochlearis and facial nerve. From it then arise the cochlear ramus and vestibular ramus. The lower vessel which is regularly observed crosses the pars cochlearis to its posterior surface and follows mainly the inferior ramus of the pars vestibularis to the inferior vestibular area. From it, several vessels go off to the vestibular ganglion. The arteries inside the internal acoustic meatus are, according to Fisch (1968) and according to our findings, not more than 150 μm thick.

The intra-osseous branches of the internal ear vessels have been studied particularly by Mazzoni who took into account the course and branching areas of the subarcuate artery. I would like to show you a schematic picture of these vessels and the most important findings regarding the blood supply of facial nerve, with which particulary Blunt (1954) was quite engaged. It is to be noticed that the glomeruli of cochlear artery twigs have been already described in the past centuries by the German anatomists. Presently, it is assumed, since pericapillary tissues are particularly rich in enzyms, that here a metabolic process between the modiolus, fluid and blood and other secretory functions may play a role.

Krmpotić-Nemanić et al. (1971) pointed out that the bone portals for the artery branches in aged humans are surrounded by bone cuffs. In his way the arteries can be compressed endangering the blood supply of the internal ear, especially the stria vascularis.

Facial Canal

The first segment of the canal part of the facial nerve is bent forward against the axis of the internal acoustic meatus about 30 to 50 degree (Fig. 6). Usually, it is 1 mm wide and 1 mm long. The fossa for the geniculate ganglion is 2 to 3 mm wide and elliptic in form. Medially, there is a variably long canal leading to the hiatus canalis n. petrosi majoris, which can be absent as well. Then there is the genu of facial canal. Here a deflection of 74 to 80 or 90 degree occurs and pars labyrinthica (tympanica, horizontalis) begins. This segment, according to Banfai (1976) is between 8 and 11 mm long. Baxter (1971) identified their sections:

1. Area geniculi
2. Area cochleariformis
3. Area fenestrae ovalis

The so-called pars horizontalis or labyrinthica seldom traverses in a straight line. Often it is somewhat convex upwards or upwards laterally. It normally casts up a protuberance of facial canal above the vestibular fenestra onto the paries labyrinthicus. In the first part, after Dietzel (1961) in 9.7 percent of cases dehiscences occur so that between the muscle tensor tympani and facial nerve no osteoseptum exists. He supposed that these have occurred due to pneumatisation processes because no such epitympanale dehiscences have been observed up to age four.

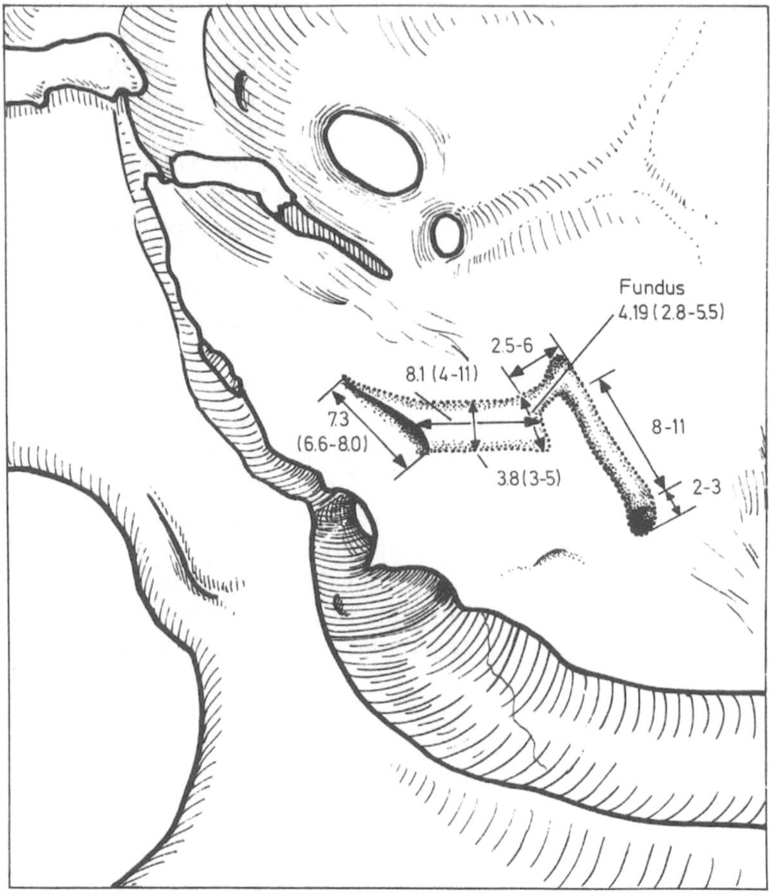

Fig. 6. Internal acoustic meatus and facial nerve canal

In the second portion of the canal of pars tympanica, dehiscences were observed in 57 percent of the well pneumatised partes petrosae. It is to be noticed that the pars labyrinthica (horizontalis) with a paramedian sagittal plane makes an angle of 37 degree which is open backwards. This does not continue horizontally, rather has a slope of about 37 degree towards the back (Cuerrier 1977). Then begins the pars pyramidalis as deflection zone in the third intraosseous segment of the facial nerve which is called also pars pyramidalis because it lies above and behind pyramid eminence. The transitional zone is variably round and seldom has almost a rectangular shape. On the average, it is 2 to 3 or 2.5 to 6 mm in length, depending on the measuring procedure. The distances of this genu segment from the suprameat spine varies between 14 and 20 mm (Banfai).

The third vertical portion of the facial canal is called pars mastoidea which proceeds mostly straight-lined downward and is 9 to 11 mm long. Bollobas (1972) as cited by Banfai, has divided the vertical segment in pars parameatalis and pars mastoidea. This vertical pathway lies on a frontal plane together with tympanomastoid suture or somewhat rostral from it (Batson 1938). Hawley (1922) examining 300 specimens found that in four cases it was 3 to 4 mm in front of the nerve canal. The nerve canal can be bent dorsally. It can be double (very rare). Litton et al. (1969) maintain that the vertical segment is wider than the horizontal. In 50 percent it is formed latero-concave, in 48 percent straight, and in 2 percent latero-convex. According to Wright and Taylor (1972, tomographic techniques), there is a forward or backward bent in 50 percent and a medial or lateral curvature in 29 percent.

The chorda tympani nerve usually arises 5.3 (1.2–10.9) mm proximal to the stylomastoid foramen; in 6 percent less than 1 mm proximal from it (Kullman et al. 1971). It is emphasized that the cavity opposite to the stapedius muscle which lies mostly ventral to the vertical portion of the facial canal is separated from the third canal segment by a connective tissue sheath and bony spur. From this fold (cavum m. stapedii) and a connective tissue septum stem the fibers of about 7 mm long muscle which is assymetrically double pinnated and contain numerous muscle spindles and motor end-plates. The muscle can also be situated medial and lateral to the nerve path. More on this subject will be discussed by Mr. Helms. Plester, Wende, and Nakajama (1978) have illustrated a total of 14 known variations of the course of facial canal.

Basec (1962) who examined about 500 temporal bones twice observed a duplicate pathway of the facial nerve in the third segment, whereby a lateral, thicker branch swept diagonally downward from which the chorda tympani went off. In another case duplication was partial. Streit (1903) first described a flat course of the facial nerve. Decussations have also been observed. Miehlke has noticed a duplication and chorda tympani going off from anterior branch. Even a triple partition has been observed by Jongkees. Medial and lateral curving of the third segment may be seen in 29 percent of cases (Wright et al. 1967). According to Nori (1972) the whole facial canal is, on the average, 30.37 mm long. The first segment makes 13.2 percent, the second 40 percent and the third 46 percent of the total length. No variations on the basis of sex or lateral differences have been observed in 12 Japanese.

Following Hofmann (1924) several researchers examined the position of individual nerve segment inside the facial canal and came up with extremely different and not consistent results. Also there are several opinions regarding fasciculations and cavities.

Summary

The origin, course, and intracisternal length of the VIIth and VIIIth cranial nerves are described with their variations. The postnatal growth displacement of the internal acustic porus and meatus are demonstrated. The nerve-vessel-relationships outside and inside the internal acustic porus are discussed.

References

Banfai P (1976) Die angewandte klinische Anatomie des N. facialis. HNO 24:253–264
Basek M (1962) Anomalies of the facial nerve in normal temporal bones. Ann Otol Rhinol Laryngol 71:382–390
Batson OV (1938) Surgical Anatomy of the Temporal Bone. In: Nelsons Loose-Leaf surgery of the ear. Thos Nelson & Sons, New York
Bergström B (1973) Morphology of the Vestibular Nerve. I. Anatomical Studies of the Vestibular Nerve in Man. Acta Otolaryngol (Stockh) 76:162–172
Bergström B (1973) Morphology of the Vestibular Nerve. II. The Number of Myelinated Vestibular Nerve Fibers in Man at Various Ages. Acta Otolaryngol (Stockh) 76:173–179
Bergström B (1973) Morphology of the Vestibular Nerve. III. Analysis of the Calibers of the Myelinated Vestibular Nerve. Fibers in Man at Various Ages. Acta Otolaryngol (Stockh) 76:331–338
Blunt MJ (1954) The Blood Supply of the Facial Nerve. J Anat 88:520–526
Bollobas B (1972) zit Banfai P (1976)
Buskirk C Van (1945) The seventh nerve complex. J Comp Neurol 82:303–333
Cavatori P (1908) Il tipo normale e le variazioni delle arterie della base dell'encefalo. Monit Zool Ital 19:248
Dietzel K (1961) Über die Dehiszenzen des Facialiskanals. Z Laryngol 40:366–379
Ehrenbrand F (1972) Über ein Paraganglion vestibulare bei der Maus. Z Anat Entw Gesch 137:285–300
Ferrari-Lelli G (1939) Comportamento dell' Arteria Uditiva Interna e dei Suoi Rami Labirintici nell' Uomo. Z Anat Entw Gesch 110:48–80
Fisch U (1968) The surgical anatomy of the so-called internal auditory artery. In: Proceedings of tenth Nobel Symposium on Discerolers of the Skull Base Region. Almquist von Wiksell, Stockholm, p 121–130
Guerrier Y, Villaceque G (1949) Origin et Comportement des Arteres Cerebelleuse Moyenne et Auditive Interne. C R Ass Anat 36:377–382
Hardy M (1934) Observations on the Innervation of the Macula Sacculi in Man. Anat Rec 59:403–418
Hawley CW (1922) IMJ 41:116. Zentralbl. Hals-, Nasen- und Ohrenheilkunde 1:156
Hofmann L (1924) Der Faserverlauf im Nervus facialis. Z Hals-, Nasen- u Ohrenh 10:86–89
Jackson R (1938) Morphologic and Roentgenologic Aspects of the temporal bone. Arch Otolaryngol 28:561–580
Jongkees LBW (1973) Practical Application of Clinical Tests for Facial Paralysis. Arch Otolaryngol 97:220–223
Kerr FWL (1962) Facial, vagal, and glossopharyngeal nerves in the cat. Arch Neurol 6:264–281
Konaschko PI (1927) Die Arteria auditiva interna des Menschen und ihre Labyrinthäste. Z Ges Anat I Abtg 83:241–268
Krmpotić-Nemanić J, Nemanić G, Kostović I (1971) Alterserscheinungen im inneren Gehörgang und am Gehörnerv. Arch Klin Exp Ohren-, Nasen- und Kehlkopfheilk 199:468–473
Kullman GL, Dyck PJ, D TH Cody (1971) Anatomy of the Mastoid Portion of the Facial nerve. Arch Otolaryngol 93:29–33
Litton WB, Krause CJ, Anson BA, Cohen WN (1969) The Relationship of the facial canal to the annular sulcus. Laryngoscope 79:1584–1604
Miehlke A (1958) Über die Topographie des Faserverlaufes im Facialisstamm. Arch Ohren-, Nasen- und Kehlkopfheilk 17:340
Mazzoni A (1969) Internal auditory canal arterial relations at the porus acusticus. Ann Otol 78:797–814
Nori S (1972) Topography of the facial nerve in the temporal bone. Nippon Ika Daigaku Zasshi 39:49–59
Papangelou L (1975) Study of the human internal auditory canal in relation to age and sex. J Laryngol Otol 89/1:79–89

Plester D, Wende S, Nakayama N: Kleinhirnbrückenwinkel-Tumoren. Diagnostik und Therapie. Springer, Berlin Heidelberg New York 1978

Pulec JL, House WF (1964) Facial nerve involvement and testing in acoustic neuromas. Arch Otolaryngol 80:685–692

Rhoton AL Jr, O'Leary JL, Ferguson JP (1966) The trigeminal facial, vagal, and glossopharyngeal nerves in the monkey. Arch Neurol 14:530–540

Rhoton AL, Kobayashi, SH (1968) Nervus intermedius. J Neurosurg 29:609–618

Siebenmann, F (1894) Die Blutgefäße im Labyrinth des menschlichen Ohres. Bergmann, Wiesbaden

Siebenmann F (1897) Mittelohr und Labyrinth. In: Bardelebens K (Ed) Handbuch der Anatomie des Menschen. 5. Bd. Sinnesorgane 2. Abt. Fischer, Jena

Sunderland S (1945) Arterial Relationships of the Internal Auditory Meatus. Brain 68:23–27

Stopford JSB (1916) The arteries of the pons and medulla oblongata. J Anat Physiol 50:131–164

Streit H (1903) Beitrag zum Flachverkauf des Nervus facialis. Arch Ohrenheilk 58:233–235

Vraa-Jensen G (1942) The Motor Nucleus of the facial nerve. Munksgaard, Kopenhagen

Walker EA (1965) The Vertebro-Basilar Arterial Systems and Internal Auditory Angiography. Laryngoscope 75:369–407

Watt JC, McKillop AN (1935) Relation of arteries to roots of nerves in posterior cranial fossa in man. Arch Surg 30:336–345

Wright JW Jr., Taylor CC, McKay DC (1967) Variations in the Course of the Facial Nerve as Illustrated by Tomography. Laryngoscope 77:717

Microsurgical Anatomy of the Arterial Loops in the Ponto-Cerebellar Angle and the Internal Acoustic Meatus

G. E. OUAKNINE *, Quebec/Canada

Introduction

The conflict between an arterial loop and a nervous element of the acoustico-facial bundle (A.F.B.) in the ponto-cerebellar angle (P.C.A.) appears to be responsible for many symptoms of irritative nature, such compression of the VIIth nerve in hemifacial spasm (Jannetta 1970, Neagoy and Dohn 1974, Jannetta et al. 1977), the VIIIth nerve in audio-vestibular disturbances (Jannetta 1975, Gros et al. 1975, Bertrand et al. 1977) and the intermediate nerve in geniculate neuralgia (Ouaknine et al. 1980). On the other hand, many anatomical studies report that a loop of the Anterior Inferior Cerebellar Artery (A.I.C.A.) is normally found in this region in a high percentage of cases.

We are reporting our detailed study of the patterns of relationship between the A.I.C.A. and the acoustico-facial bundle in the P.C.A. and the internal acoustic meatus (I.A.M.). A pathophysiological explanation of the role of the arterial-nerve conflict in the irritative pathology of the P.C.A. nerves will be exposed.

Material and Methods

Sixty-five dissections were performed in thirty-five anatomical blocks of the base of skull of cadavers after fixation in formaldehyde. In some specimens, polymer (Batson's solution) was injected into the vertebral arteries. Dissections were not performed in five specimens because gross disturbances of normal anatomical relationship occurred during the removal of the specimens from the cranial cavity.

The nervous and vascular structures of the P.C.A. and I.A.M. were systematically studied with the use of a surgical microscope and microsurgical techniques. The arterial variations in the course of the A.I.C.A. and the relationship between the loops of that vessel, or one of its branches, and the VIIth and VIIIth nerves, were carefully noted.

After opening of the I.A.M. with microdrill by two classical approaches – suboccipital and trans-tentorial – the microdissection of the different branches of the auditory arteries was performed until their entry in the fundus acousticus with the different nervous structures.

* The author realized this work at the Department of Anatomy and Anthropology, Tel Aviv University Medical School, Israel

Results

We found that in 82 percent of specimens, the A.I.C.A. arises, as a single trunk, from the basilar artery. In 12 percent, two arteries corresponding to the A.I.C.A. arise from the basilar artery and in 6 percent, the A.I.C.A. is a branch of the P.I.C.A. which arise from the basilar artery and not from the vertebral artery. The A.I.C.A. arises at the lowest two-third junction of the basilar artery and passes laterally and slightly downwards across the pons to the P.C.A. Here, the A.I.C.A. crosses the acoustico-facial bundle, makes a loop and after giving several collaterals, turns backwards to reach the cerebellum. When there are two A.I.C.A., both of them make a loop at different distances one from the other.

In nine percent of specimens, when the A.I.C.A. crosses the nerves, it gives off one or two branches, the so-called cerebello-labyrinthine artery, which also makes a loop. Therefore, there are sometimes two or three recurrent cerebellar arteries. There are constant anastomosis between these different branches of the A.I.C.A. and branches originating from the superior cerebellar artery or the P.I.C.A. Loops of the A.I.C.A. or one of its branches, are found in 97 percent of specimens in the P.C.A. In 56 percent the loops remained outside the meatus, in 25 percent they

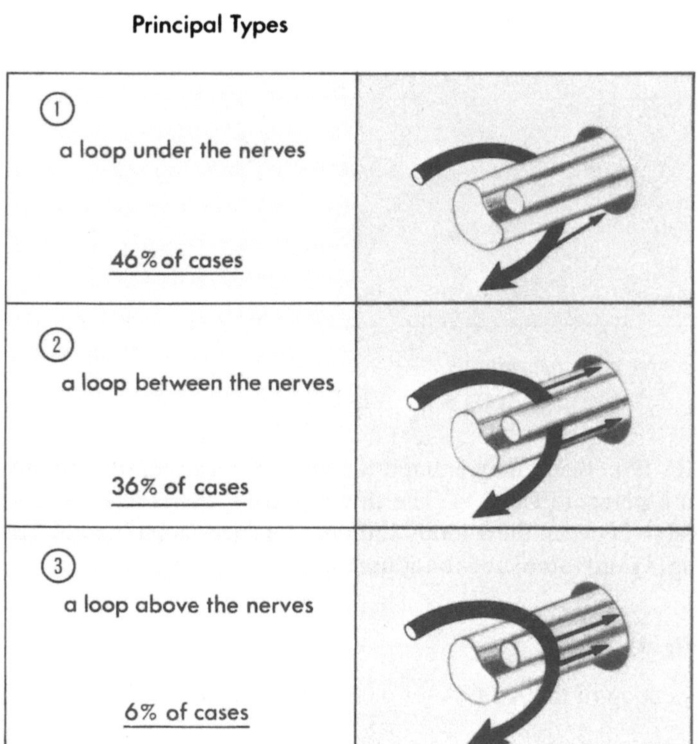

Fig. 1. Patterns of the relationships between the acoustico-facial bundle and the loop of the A.I.C.A. in the ponto-cerebellar angle

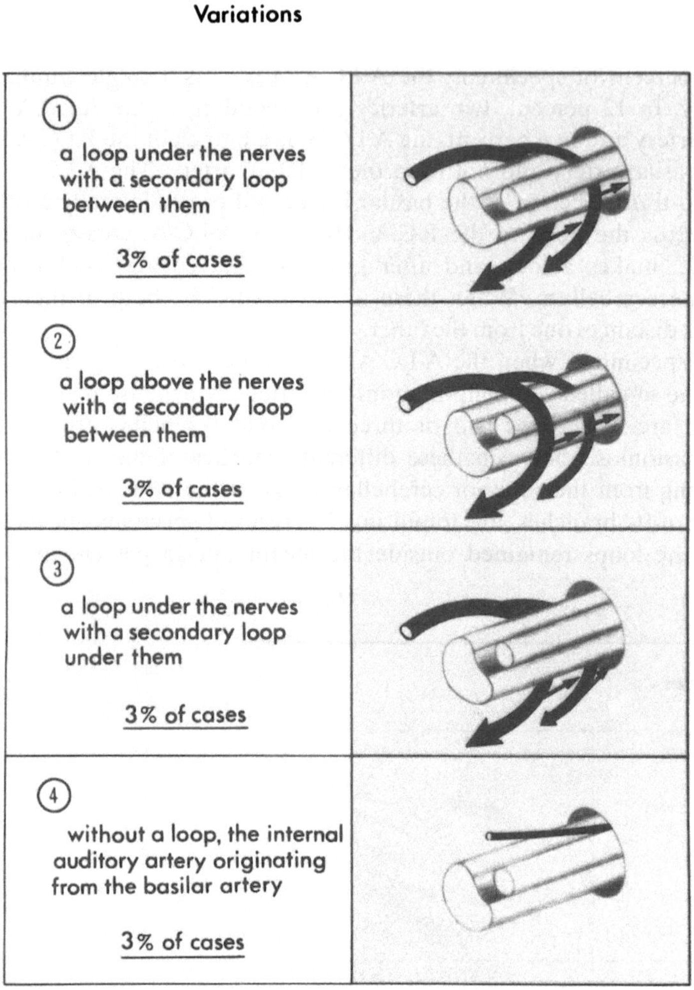

Fig. 2. Subvariations of the three principal patterns

reached the orifice and in 19 percent, they entered the meatus, reaching the middle of the auditory canal in 6 percent (Table 1). The findings are symmetrical in only 23 percent. The relationship between these loops and the acoustico-facial bundle fits into three main types (Fig. 1) and three subvariations (Fig. 2).

Types of Relationship (Fig. 1)

Type 1: (46 percent). The loop of the A.I.C.A. or one of its branches is found under the nerve (Fig. 3).
Type 2: (36 percent). The loop is found between the nerves, generally between the VIIIth nerve complex and the VIIth nerve (Fig. 4).
Type 3: (6 percent). The loop is found above the nerves (Fig. 5).

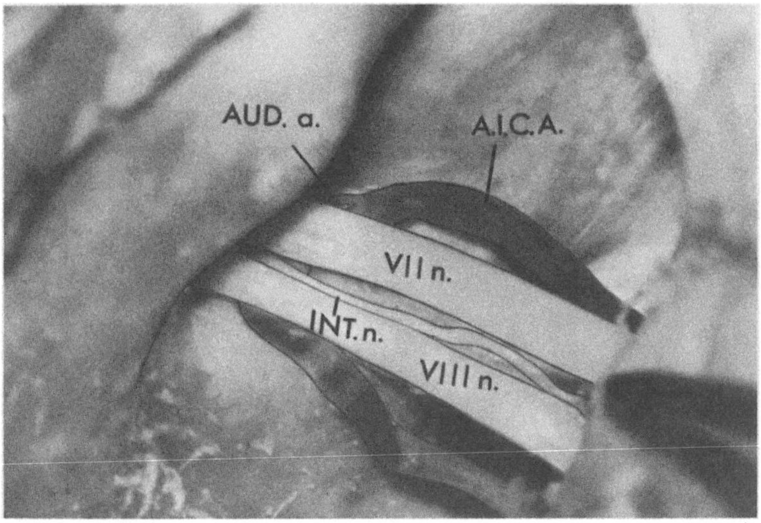

Fig. 3. Left P.C.A. There is a loop of the A.I.C.A. under the nerves and reaching the orifice of the meatus. An auditory artery arises from the apex of the loop; Int. n.: intermediate nerve

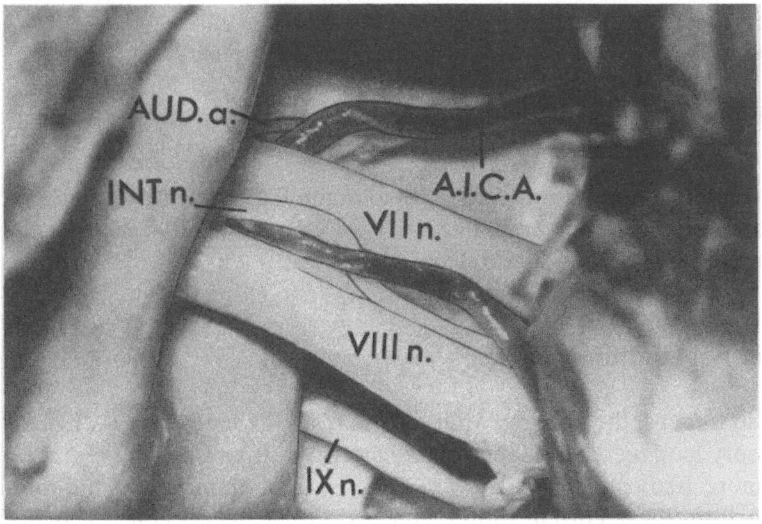

Fig. 4. Left P.C.A. There is a loop of the A.I.C.A. between the nerves. The afferent limb of the loop enters the meatus between the VIIIth nerve and the intermediate nerve, then passes under the VIIth nerve. The auditory artery arises from the recurrent limb of the loop

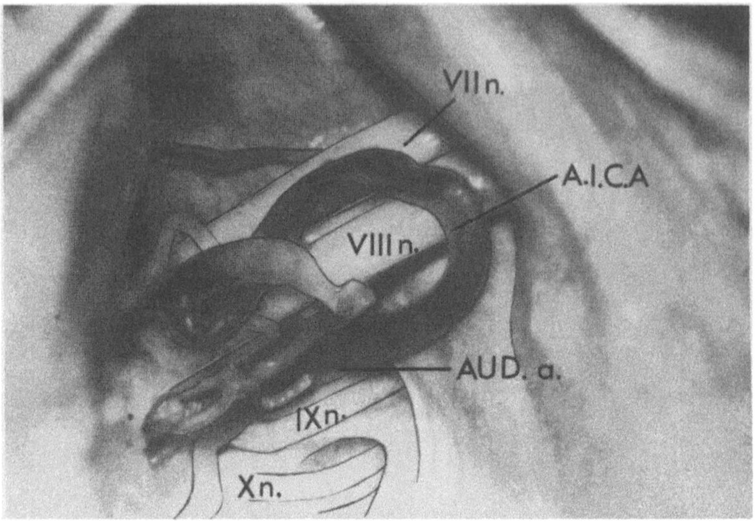

Fig. 5. Right P.C.A. There is a loop of the A.I.C.A. above the nerves and outside the meatus. The auditory artery arises from the recurrent limb of a secondary loop situated also above the nerve and behind the loop of the A.I.C.A. This auditory artery penetrated the meatus between the nerves and the floor of the auditory canal

Subvariations

We found three main subvariations of the basic types:

1. A loop is found under the nerves with a secondary loop, generally the cerebello-labyrinthine artery, between them (three percent) (Fig. 6).
2. A loop is found above the nerves with a secondary loop between them (three percent).
3. A loop is found under the nerves with a secondary loop under them (three percent).

In only three percent of specimens, we find no loop in the P.C.A. In these two cases, the auditory arteries arise from the basilar artery. No loop was found at the root entry zone, between the nerves and the brain stem.

The Auditory (or Labyrinthine) Artery

In 91 percent of specimens, the auditory artery arises from the main loop (A.I.C.A.) or from an accessory loop (cerebello-labyrinthine artery) or from both of them. The auditory arises more frequently from the proximal limb or the apex of the loop (65 percent) than from the recurrent limb of the loop (35 percent) (Fig. 7). In six percent, the auditory arteries arise from the basilar artery (with a loop under the nerves in three percent), and in three percent from the choroid plexus (with also a loop of the A.I.C.A. under the nerves).

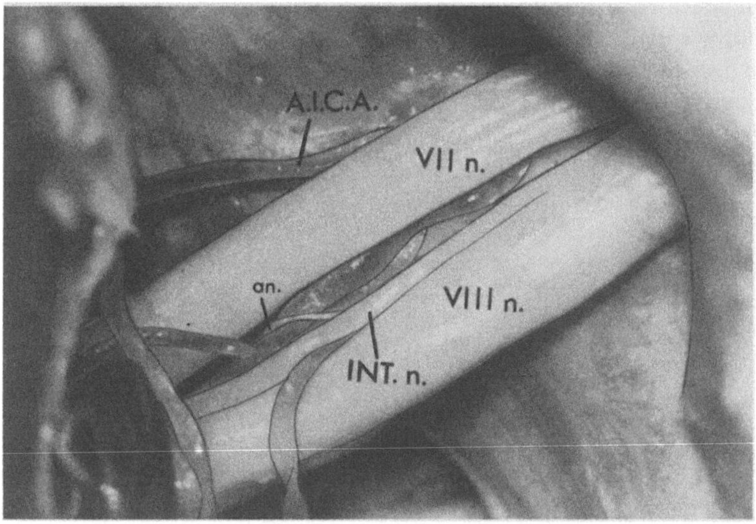

Fig. 6. Right P.C.A. There is a loop of the A.I.C.A. under the VIIth nerve and a secondary loop between the intermediate nerve and the VIIIth nerve. In this case, the auditory artery arises under the VIIth nerve from the apex of the loop which is outside the meatus. an.: anastomose between the facial and the intermediate nerves

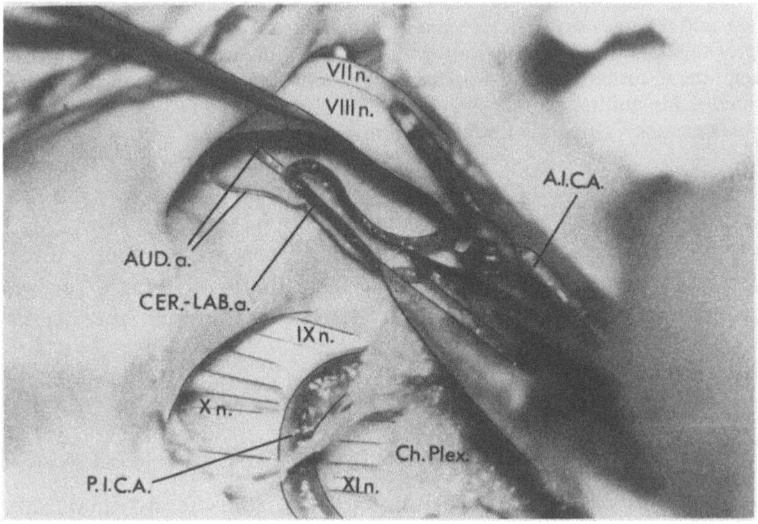

Fig. 7. Left P.C.A. The A.I.C.A. makes a short loop above the origin of the nerves. A cerebello-labyrinthine artery arises from the A.I.C.A. and makes 2 double sharped angulated loops, one above and one under the nerves. From the lower loop arise two auditory arteries, one very thin (0.1 mm) originating from the afferent limb and the second one, originating from the apex of the loop

Recurrent branches of the auditory artery itself are also observed, generally making anastomoses with other branches of the different loops. The auditory arteries were dissected in the P.C.A. and I.A.M. until their entry in the fundus acousticus. Their number was variable (Table 3). In 29 percent, we found only one auditory artery which sometimes bifurcated into the auditory canal. In most of the speci-

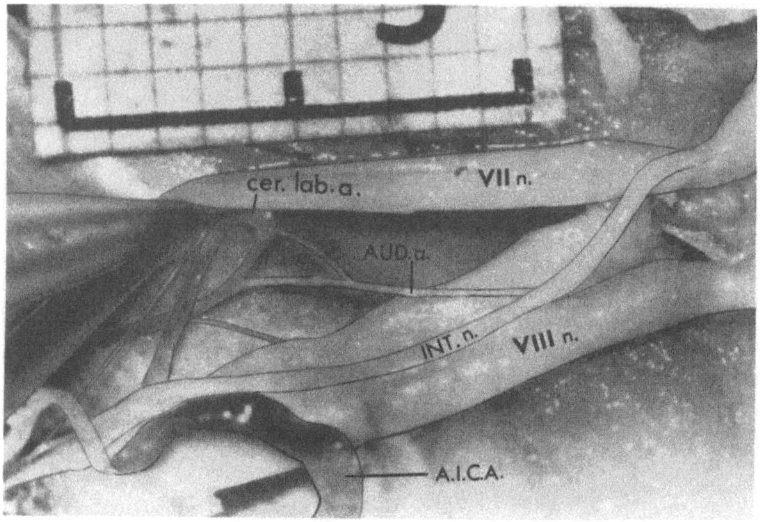

Fig. 8. Left auditory canal. The roof of the internal auditory canal has been removed by microdrill. The nerves and the auditory arteries have been dissected from the porus to the fundus. There is a loop of the A.I.C.A. above the nerve and reaching the meatus. A cerebello-labyrinthine artery (cer. lab. a.) forms a second loop from which arises three auditory arteries and a thin recurrent branch. One auditory artery is under the nerves and the two other merge to form a single artery between the VIIth nerve and the vestibulo-cochlear nerve

mens there were two auditory arteries (44 percent). In 18 percent, we found three auditory arteries, and in 9 percent, four or more arteries with, in a few cases, several anastomoses between them, comprising an arterial network between the nerves (Fig. 8).

The Subarcuate Artery

This important and rarely described artery, arises generally from the proximal limb or the apex of the loop, sometimes from the auditory artery itself outside the I.A.M. It courses laterally and superiorly and enters the temporal bone and the subarcuate fossa which is a small depression situated above and behind the porus. The subarcuate artery passes directly through the dura and the wall of the meatus. Contrary to other publications, we found it in only 55 percent of our specimens.

Discussion

Many anatomical works dealing with the arterial relationship of the acoustico-facial bundle exist. In 97 percent of our 65 specimens, we found a loop of the A.I.C.A. or one of its branches in the P.C.A. Ferrari-Lelli (1940) noted that in 40 specimens, the A.I.C.A. or one of its branches almost always forms a loop either within the I.A.M. or close to its origin. Sunderland (1945) found that in 64 percent of 264 specimens, the A.I.C.A. was intimately related to the VIIth and VIIIth nerves either within (39 percent) or at the mouth (25 percent) of the I.A.M. In 36 percent of specimens, he found no relationship between the A.I.C.A. and the I.A.M. He also found that the A.I.C.A. makes a loop in 67 percent of specimens, under (26 percent), between (49 percent), or above the nerves (two percent) (Table 2). Guerrier and Villaceque (1949) found a loop in 100 percent of their specimens. In 80 percent, the A.I.C.A. makes a single loop which falls into one of three categories: anterior type (60 percent), the A.I.C.A. makes a loop within the I.A.M.; intermediate type (18 percent), the A.I.C.A. stays five mm away from the porus; posterior type (22 percent), the A.I.C.A is close to the cerebellum. In the last two types, cerebello-labyrinthine branches, arising from the A.I.C.A., reach the porus, make a loop and give recurrent cerebellar arteries. In 20 percent of the specimens, two branches arise separately from the basilar artery and each one makes a loop.

Three recent studies performed under microsurgical magnification, give more accurate finding and will be compared to our own work (Table 1).

Mazzoni and Hansen (1970) in 100 cases and Boussens et al. (1972) in 50 specimens, found a loop in the P.C.A. in 100 percent of cases. Salah et al. (1978) found a loop of the A.I.C.A. or one of its branches in 80 percent of 95 specimens. Our findings concerning the relationship of the loops of the A.I.C.A. with the I.A.M. and the VIIth and VIIIth nerves, are very similar to the findings of these last authors (Tables 1 and 2). These loops always arise from the A.I.C.A. or one of its branches, but Mazzoni and Hansen (1970) reported that the loop arises in three percent of specimens from the P.I.C.A.

The knowledge of the varying relation of the A.I.C.A. is of particular importance in operations on the P.C.A. Atkinson (1949) called attention to the fact that clipping the A.I.C.A. where it crosses the acoustic nerve, can lead to infarction of the lateral pons. In fact, branches supplying the middle cerebellar peduncle, pontine and upper medullary portions of the brain stem originated both from the afferent and recurrent limbs of the loops and also from the auditory arteries. Preservation of these branches is paramount in preventing brain stem damage during P.C.A. surgery.

The auditory artery is a very narrow artery 0.15 mm in external diameter (Fish 1968) which generally arises from a loop of the A.I.C.A., lies on the gutter of the VIIIth nerve and gives three terminal branches, the vestibular, the cochlear, and the vestibulo-cochlear arteries.

Nabeya (1923) in more than 200 specimens, stated to have found the auditory artery constantly to be a branch of the A.I.C.A. Adachi (1928) added to this statement that the auditory artery could arise from the P.I.C.A. We found that the auditory artery arises directly from the basilar artery in six percent of specimens, a finding confirmed by Watt and McKillop (1935) in five percent, Sunderland (1945) in 17 percent and Salah et al. (1978) in four percent.

Table 1. Relationship of loops of the A. I. C. A. with the internal auditory meatus

	Mazzoni and Hansen (1970)	Boussens (1972)	Salah et al. (1978)	Ouaknine (1980)
Loop outside the meatus	33%	60%	64%	56%
Loop at the orifice	27%	25%	22%	25%
Loop inside the meatus	40%	15%	14%	19%

Table 2. Relationship between the nerves and the arterial loop in the P. C. A.

	Sunderland (1945)	Mazzoni and Hansen (1970)	Salah et al. (1978)	Ouaknine (1980)		
				Main types	Subvariations	
A loop under the nerves	26%	51%	50.5%	46%	6%	52%
A loop between the nerves	49%	43%	39%			36%
A loop above the nerves	2%	6%	10.5%	6%	3%	9%
Absence of loop	23%	–	–			3%
	100%	100%	100%			100%

Table 3. Number of internal auditory arteries in the internal auditory meatus

No of I. A. A.	Mazzoni and Hansen (1970)	Boussens (1972)	Ouaknine (1980)
1	51%	30%	29%
2	45%	59%	44%
3	4%	10%	18%
4 and more	–	10%	9%

One or two auditory arteries are generally found, rarely three or four. The main anatomical reports on this point can be compared with our results in Table 3.

The subarcuate artery has been well described by otological surgeons such as Nager (1954) and Mazzoni and Hansen (1970). These last authors found that the subarcuate artery is present in 97 percent of specimens and arises from a cerebellar loop in 44 percent, from an auditory artery in 10 percent and from a collateral cerebellar loop in 43 percent. We found it in 55 percent only. Before reaching the subarcuate fossa near the meatus, this artery may have a long course beneath the acoustico-facial bundle where it can be easily injured during neurosurgical manipulations. Thus, some audiovestibular disturbances may be explained despite an apparently atraumatic operation. Portman et al. (1975) have been struck by the fact that this vessel passes through the petromastoid canal to gain the aditus where it anastomoses with the arteries of the middle ear. They stressed that the subarcuate artery is the only communication between the artery supply of the labyrinth and the middle ear.

The acoustico-facial bundle is a complex structure formed by 4 nerves closely bound together by several and complex anastomoses (Ouaknine 1978), whose relations are varying progressively from the brain stem to the fundus acousticus through the ponto-cerebellar angle and internal auditory canal. A small lesion, such as an arterial loop, in one of these regions can affect one or several elements of this bundle. This group of nerves is in close relation with a loop of the A.I.C.A. which normally exists in more than 95 percent of cases.

In practice, the two related questions that arise are whether compression by a normally found structure, as an arterial loop, can explain the occasional irritative disturbances of these nerves and whether removal of this arterial compression can explain the relief of symptoms of the offended nerves. Generally, the offending artery is a branch of the A.I.C.A. (Bertrand et al. 1977, Gros et al. 1975, Jannetta 1970, 1975, 1977), rarely it is a loop of the P.I.C.A. (Ouaknine 1980). If these arterial loops do not normally cause any trouble, they may injure the nerves when elongated (on a congenital basis or not) indurated by an arteriosclerotic process and fixed by arachnoid adhesions. In this perspective, it is interesting to note that children rarely have hemifacial spasm (Ehni and Woltman 1945), 'tic douloureux' or Meniere's disease (Dandy 1934).

The pathophysiology of the artery-nerve conflict is still uncertain. The problem of deficiency symptoms due to tumors compressing cranial nerves must be differentiated from irritative symptoms of cranial nerves like hemifacial spasm of 'tic douloureux'. Gardner (1962) thinks that both are expression of an unstable and reversible pathophysiologic state caused by the mild compression of a cerebello-pontine angle vessel on the nerve root. This compression causing atrophy of the insulated myelin sheath, permits transaxonal short circuit while not interfering with axonal conduction. A reverberating short circuit between the afferent and efferent fibers of the compressed nerve root could explain hemifacial spasm and trigeminal neuralgia.

This theory is supported by the fact that an artificial synapse can be produced between afferent and efferent fibers by gentle ligature of a sciatic nerve, without interruption of the nerve impulse (Granit 1944). This artificial synapse disappears when the pressure by the ligature is released. Jannetta (1970, 1977) stressed that in cases of hemifacial spasm or trigeminal neuralgia, the vascular compression must be cross-compression at right angles to the nerve and must be at the root exit zone of the nerve from the brain stem. He added that the junction zone defects, which exist at the root entry zone, may predispose to disordered conduction when a cross-compression exists at this point. Kumagami (1974) also stressed that the ultrastructural lesions of the peripheral nerve fibers of idiopathic hemifacial spasm and 'tic douloureux' are of the same type.

In fact, as demonstrated by Tarlov (1937) a nerve root consists of a central glial and a peripheral non-glial segment. The transition zone or pial ring is arch shaped and is at a variable distance from the brain stem. The central glial segment increases in length from birth to adult life and is directly related to the body length. The eighth nerve – both cochlear and vestibular parts – present the longest glial segment (8 mm) followed by the Vth (sensory root 2.2 mm; motor root 0.5 mm), the Xth nerve (1.3 mm), the IXth nerve (1.1 mm), the IVth (1.0 mm) and the VIIth nerve (0.8 mm). The other cranial nerves, except the optic and ophthalmic nerves, which represent a fiber tract of the brain, have even a shorter glial segment. The pial ring through which the nerve root passes is reinforced by a plexus of neuroglial and connective tissue fibers. Many of the axons in passing through the pial ring may be seen to undergo constriction. There is a net diminution of myelin at the transition zone. Peripheral to the transition zone, the axones and their myelin sheath are thicker than centrally. Tarlov (1937) also stressed that the cranial nerves, contrary to the peripheral nerves have no peri- or epineurium but only endoneurium. Therefore they are more sensitive to traction or compression.

We then can present the following mechanism to try to explain the irritative syndrom of the ponto-cerebellar angle nerves by a redundant arterial loop:

The compression by an arterial loop at the level of the pial ring may, indeed, cause a transaxonal short circuit, the myelin sheath being thinner at this point. This short circuit could be between efferent fibers in continuous facial spasm, as after facial nerve palsy, or between afferent and efferent fibers in idiopathic hemifacial spasm and trigeminal neuralgia. The fact that the central glial segment is very short in the VIIth nerve explains that the arterial cross-compression must be at the root entry zone near the brain stem, at the level of the pial ring. On the contrary, the central glial segment of the Vth nerve is relatively longer and cross-compression easier to visualize. The arterial cross-compression on the VIIIth nerve should be near the meatus where the pial ring is situated. These anatomical facts explain why Dandy, like many neurosurgeons after him operating without microsurgical techniques, has described compression of the nerves by an offending vessel in trigeminal neuralgia (30 percent) in 215 cases, Dandy 1934) or Meniere's disease (20 percent in 560 cases, Dandy 1934) but has not seen this arterial compression in cases of hemifacial spasm. As stressed by Granit (1944), the artificial synapse may disappear temporarily by manipulating the nerve, or completely by removal of the nerve compression.

Conclusions

This work has not only an academic anatomical interest but is also of importance for the E.N.T. and the neurological surgeons for the precise microsurgical approach of lesions of the ponto-cerebellar angle and the internal acoustic meatus. The loops and the branches of the anterior inferior cerebellar artery have many anatomical variations and different patterns of relationship with the acoustico-facial bundle. The knowledge of these variations and relationships is of importance for the realization of an atraumatic microsurgery during procedures like the removal of the intracranial portion of an acoustic neurinoma or the vascular decompression in an irritative syndrome due to an artery-nerve conflict.

Acknowledgement: The author wishes to express appreciation to the staff of the Department of Medical Illustration at the Notre-Dame Hospital for their technical help and to Mrs. Micheline Lévesque for secretarial assistance.

References

Adachi B (1928) Das Arteriensystem der Japaner. Tome 1: 123

Atkinson WJ (1949) Anterior inferior cerebellar artery. J Neurol Neurosurg Psychiatry 12: 137

Bertrand RA, Molina P, Hardy J (1977) Vestibular syndrome and vascular anomaly in the cerebello-pontine angle. Acta Otolaryngol Stockh 83: 187–194

Boussens J, Caille JM, Koehler R, Boyer M, Piton J, Bisch X, Martin PL (1972) A propos de la vascularisation du conduit auditif interne. Cah ORL (Montpellier) 7: 763–774

Dandy WE (1934) Concerning the cause of trigeminal neuralgia. Am J Surg 24: 447–455

Dandy WE (1934) Treatment of so-called pseudo-Ménière's disease. Johns Hopkins Med J 55: 232

Ehni G, Woltman WH (1945) Hemifacial spasm. Review of one hundred and six cases. Arch Neurol Psychiat 53: 205–211

Ferrari-Lelli G (1940) Comportaments dell' arteria auditiva interna e dei suoi rami labyrintici nell' uomo. Z Anat Entwicklungsgesch 110: 48–80

Fisch U (1968) L'anatomie chirurgicale du système artériel du conduit auditif interne chez l'homme. Rev Laryngol Otol Rhinol (Bord) 89/11–12: 659–671

Gardner WJ (1962) Concerning the mechanism of trigeminal neuralgia and hemifacial spasm. J Neurosurg 19: 947–958

Granit R, Leksell L, Skoglund CR (1944) Fiber interaction in injury or compressed region of nerve. Brain 67: 125–140

Gros G, Ben Rhouma T (1975) Conflit artère-nerf. Atteinte du groupe acoustico-facial. Neurochirurgie 21: 329–336

Guerrier Y, Villaceque G (1949) Origine et comportement des artères cérébelleuses moyennes et auditives internes. CR Assoc Anat 36 Réunion: 377–382

Jannetta PJ (1970) Microsurgical explanation and decompression of the facial nerve in hemifacial spasm. Curr Top Surg Res 2: 217–220

Jannetta PJ (1975) Neurovascular cross-compression in patients with hyperactin dysfunction symptome of the eighth cranial nerve. Surg forum 26: 467–468

Jannetta PJ, Abbasy M, Maroon JC, Ramos FM, Albin MS (1977) Etiology and definitive microsurgical treatment of hemifacial spasm. Operative techniques and results in 47 patients. J Neurosurg 47: 321–328

Kumagami H (1974) Neuropathological findings of hemifacial spasm and trigeminal neuralgia. Arch Otolaryngol 99: 160–164

Mazzoni A, Hansen CC (1970) Surgical anatomy of the arteries of the internal auditory canal. Arch Otolaryngol 91/2: 128–135

Nabeya D (1923) A study in the comparative anatomy of the blood vascular system of the internal ear in mammalia and in homo (Japanese). Acta Sch Med Univ Kioto 6/1: 1–27

Nager GT (1954) Origins and relations of the internal auditory artery and subarcuate artery. Ann Otol Rhinol Laryngol 63: 51–61

Neagoy DR, Dohn DF (1974) Hemifacial spasm secondary to vascular compression of the facial nerve. Cleve Clin Q 41: 205–215

Ouaknine GE (1978) Microsurgical anatomy of the nervous and vascular structures in the ponto-cerebellar angle and the internal acoustic meatus. Proc. for the XXI International Biennial Congre. s, International College of Surgeons, Jerusalem, Israel, p 81

Ouaknine GE, Rehavi G, Nathan H (1978) Microsurgical anatomy of the arterial loops of the anterior cerebellar artery in the ponto-cerebellar angle and the internal acoustic meatus. Isr J Med Sci 14/8: 902

Ouaknine GE, Robert F, Molina-Negro P, Hardy J (1980) Geniculate neuralgia and audio-vestibular disturbances due to compression of the intermediate and eighth nerves by the postero-inferior cerebellar artery. Surg Neurol 13: 147–150

Portman M et al. (1975) The internal auditory meatus. In: Churchill, Livingston (eds)

Salah S, Bock FW, Perneczky A, Koos WT, Tschabitscher M (1978) Vascular anatomy of the cerebello-pontine angle. In: Koos WT, Bock FW and Spetzler RF (eds) Microneurosurgery. Thieme, p 70–71

Sunderland S (1945) The arterial relations of the internal auditory meatus. Brain 68:23–27

Tarlov IM (1937) Structure of the nerve root: 1. Nature of the junction between the central and peripheral nervous system. Arch Neurol Psychiat 37:555

Tarlov IM (1937) Structure of the nerve root: 2. Differentiation of sensory from motor roots; observations on identification of function in roots of mixed cranial nerves. Arch Neurol Psychiat 37:1338–1355

Watt JC, McKillop AN (1935) The relation of arteries to roots of nerves in posterior cranial fossa in man. Arch Surg 30:336–345

Variations of the Course of the Facial Nerve in the Middle Ear and Mastoid

J. HELMS, Mainz/FRG

The variations of the course of the facial nerve in the middle ear and mastoid are shown in Fig. 1.

1. Normal course.
2. Elongation of the pars tympani, so that the lateral knee has a more posterior position [3].
3. Posterior and inferior displacement of the lateral knee [3].
4. Displacement of the lateral knee to the surface of the sigmoid sinus [3].
5. Blunting of the lateral knee and displacement of the pars tympani over the niche of the oval window which is thereby narrowed [3].
6. Vertical course of the nerve through the middle ear from the geniculate ganglion crossing the anterior pars of the middle ear [3].
7. Displacement of the pars tympani medially through the stapes footplate [5].
8. Course of the nerve through the crura of the stapes [6].
9. Protrusion of axon bundles out of a bony dehiscence and a dehiscent epineurium posteriorly and anteriorly of the stapes superstructure [5].
10. Doubling of the pars tympani anteriorly and posteriorly of the stapes (Caparosa a. Fowler after [7].
11. Doubling of the pars mastoidea of the course of the nerve [3].
12. Doubling of the pars mastoidea of the course of the nerve with doubling of the foramina stylomastoidea [3].
13. Another doubling of the pars mastoidea of the nerve with 2 foramina stylomastoidea [7].
14. Development of 3 branches of the facial nerve in the pars mastoidea with 3 stylomastoid foramina [1].
15. Displacement of the labyrinthine part of the facial nerve to a course lateral of the labyrinthine bone. The nerve enters the pyramid lateral of the posterior semicircular canal and runs to the geniculate ganglion underneath the horizontal semicircular canal. The course from the geniculate ganglion to the stylomastoid foramen is normal [2].

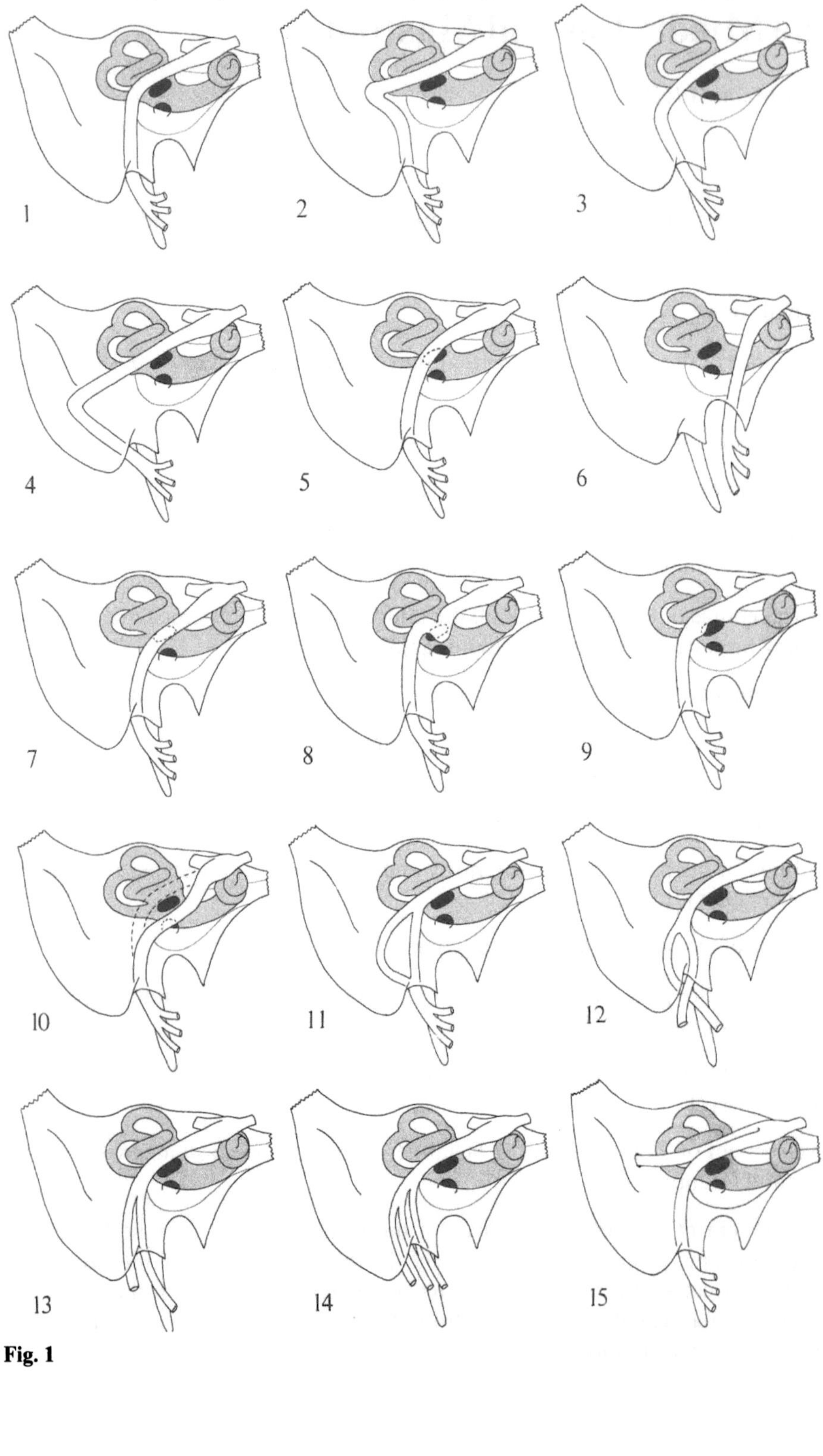

Fig. 1

References

1. Botmann JWM, Jongkees LBW (1955) Endotemporal branching of the facial nerve. Acta Otolaryngol (Stockh) 45:111
2. Feldmann H (1975) Supraganglionärer Verlauf des Nervus facialis durch Warzenfortsatz und Epitympanon; eine bisher nicht beobachtete Anomalie. Arch Ohr- Nas- Kehlk- Heilk 210:346
3. Fowler EP jr (1961) Verlaufsanomalien des N. facialis im Schläfenbein. Z Laryng Rhinol Otol 40:360
4. Hahlbrock KH (1960) Zweiteilung des N. facialis im Warzenfortsatz. Arch Ohr- Nas- Kehlk- Heilk 174:465
5. Helms J (1978) Zur Chirurgischen Anatomie des Felsenbeins. In: D Plester, S Wende, N Nakayama (Ed) Kleinhirnbrückenwinkeltumoren. Springer-Verlag, Berlin Heidelberg New York S 3–23
6. Johnson LG, Kingsley TC (1970) Herniation of the facial nerve in the middle ear. Arch Otorhinolaryng 91:598
7. Miehlke A (1973) Surgery of the facial nerve, 2nd Ed. Urban & Schwarzenberg, München Berlin Wien

Intraneural Topography of the Extracranial Facial Nerve

H. Millesi and G Meissl, Vienna/Austria

Clinical experience and studies of the intracranial topography of the facial nerve in cadavers are confronting us with the distribution of the nerve fibres to different functional areas within the cross-section of the facial nerve at different levels. An attempt should be made to pay attention to the intraneural topography when bridging defects of the facial nerve trunk.

Introduction

The facial nerve has an excellent potential for recovery after repair. However, often nerve regeneration results in mass movement without control of the individual muscles. Thus the ability for individual facial expression is lost, which means a great handicap for the patient.

The reason for the loss of coordinating movements may be found at different levels:

a) Loss of dendritic connections at the neurom, as described by Kreutzberg (1977). It is evident that this development cannot be influenced surgically.
b) Irregular outgrowth of axon sprouts. Such irregular outgrowths may be reduced to some degree by a meticulous technique.
c) The axon sprouts from nerve fibres, supplying a certain muscle, are not able to grow into the correct peripheral pathway to reach the same muscle again. If the nerve fibres, supplying a certain muscle, are distributed diffusely over the cross-section, there is only a random chance that axon sprouts meet the corresponding pathway in a peripheral stump. If certain rules exist regarding the distribution of nerve fibres of the same function over the cross-section, and these rules are obeyed during nerve repair, the chances may be increased significantly.

Miehlke postulated already in 1958 that nerve fibres of certain functions are located in distinct areas of a cross-section. The same view was held by May (1973). Sunderland (1977) focussed the attention to the plexiform arrangement of the fascicles within a nerve trunk and postulated a diffuse distribution.

It was our impression that an attempt to restore the original structure of the facial nerve as good as possible reduces the amount of mass movement and increases the control of the individual muscles. This impression is based on clinical observations with peripheral lesions of facial nerves at the level of branches and rami, and with lesions at trunk levels with one branch, for instance the ramus marginalis mandibulae intact, which permitted an orientation regarding the remaining fascicles of the cross section.

Study of the Intraneural Topography in Cadavers

G. Meissl studied ten facial nerves in human cadavers using serial sections and following the nerve fibres from section to section. The plexiform pattern of the facial nerve was confirmed.

At the stylomastoid foramen the pattern of the facial nerve is polyfascicular. Many fascicles are arranged in three fascicle groups (A).

The fascicle fuse to form one thick fascicle (monofascicular pattern) within the proximal third of the facial nerve trunk (B).

At the level of the middle third there is again a polyfascicular pattern with several individual fascicles which arrange themselves in the distal third to three distinct fascicle groups, a cranial, a middle, and a caudal one (C, D). Towards the end of the distal third a fascicle group in the middle divides, its cranial half joins the cranial group forming the upper branch, its lower part joints the caudal group forming the lower branch of the facial nerve.

As regards the individual fibres, the arrangement is as follows:

A. At the stylomastoid foramen:
   Nerve fibres to the upper face supplying the frontal epicranial muscle, the orbicular muscle of the eye, and parts of the cygomatic muscles (Ramus temporalis and Ramus cygomaticus) are located in the craniomedial sector of the nerve trunk.
   Nerve fibres to the middle face:
   Supplying the muscle of the upper lip and the cheek (Ramii infraorbitales and buccales) are preferably located in the cranio-lateral sector.
   Nerve fibres to the lower face and the neck: (marginal mandibular and cervical branches) are mainly concentrated in the caudal sector. The fibres of a certain function do not form well defined fascicles, but are more concentrated in some areas than in others, with fluid boundaries between them.
B. Proximal third.
   There is a monofascicular pattern. Nerve fibres for the upper face are concentrated in the cranial, nerve fibres for the middle face in the caudal-lateral, and nerve fibres for the lower face and the neck in the caudal-medial sector. Note that there is a anti-clock-wise turn of about 90 degrees.
C. Middle third.
   There is again the polyfascicular pattern. The distribution about the sectors remains the same with the nerve fibres to the upper face in the cranial and the nerve fibres to the middle face in the caudal-lateral sector and the nerve fibres to the lower face and the neck in the caudal-medial sector.
D. Distal third.
   The pattern is polyfascicular, three fascicle groups can be distinguished, a cranial one, containing about half of the fibres for the upper face, a middle one, and a caudal one. In the upper half of the fascicle group of the middle there are also nerve fibres for the upper face, in the caudal half of the middle one, there are nerve fibres for the middle face, which are also to find in the cranial half of the caudal fascicle group. The nerve fibres for the lower face and the neck are concentrated in the caudal half of the caudal fascicle group.

E. Main Trunk before Division.
The fascicle group in the middle is divided into two halves, the cranial half joining the cranial, the caudal half joining the caudal fascicle group. After this division the cranial fascicle group contains all the fibres going to the upper face, it is bound to form the upper branch of the facial nerve. The lower fascicle group contains fibres for the middle face in its cranial half, and fibres for the lower face and the neck in its caudal half. It will form the lower branch of the facial nerve.

Application to Clinical Practice

Based on this knowledge an attempt can be made to offer a better chance for axon sprouts to reach the correct pathway in the periphery.

If one has to deal with a clean cut without a defect, an end-to-end nerve repair is the treatment of choice. An exact fascicular coaptation should be achieved with minimal surgical manipulation. At the proximal third the coaptation will be a trunk-to-trunk coaptation, due to the fact that we basically have to deal with a monofascicular pattern. Towards the periphery a group-to-group coaptation after interfascicular dissection will increase accuracy.

After loss of nerve substance a defect has to be overcome. We prefer to bridge a defect by nerve grafts instead of forcing an end-to-end repair after mobilization.

The best source for a nerve graft is the sural nerve. At its distal end the sural nerve has a polyfascicular pattern and strands of different size and of different fascicular pattern can be provided as necessary.

A : D: If the lesion is located at the stylomastoideum and the peripheral stump is represented by a cross-section somewhere in the proximal third, three sural nerve grafts are used. One of them uniting the cranio-medial fascicle group of the proximal stump with the cranial and cranio-medial sector of the distal stump. The second graft units the cranio-lateral fascicle group of the proximal stump with the caudal-lateral sector of the peripheral stump. A third graft is put between the caudal fascicle group of the proximal stump and the caudo-medial sector of the peripheral stump (Fig. 1).

A : C: If the defect expands between the proximal stump of the stylomastoid foramen and the middle third of the main trunk, again three sural nerve grafts are used to bridge a defect. One is put between the cranio-medial fascicle group in the proximal stump and the cranial fascicle group in the distal stump, the second graft is used to unite the cranio-lateral fascicle group of the proximal stump and the caudo-lateral fascicle group ot the peripheral stump, and the third graft units the caudal fascicle group of the proximal stump and the caudo-medial fascicle group of the peripheral stump (Fig. 2).

A : D: In a defect between the proximal at the stylomastoid foramen and the distal stump in the distal third of the main trunk, three sural nerve grafts can be used, the proximal ends of which are united with the sectors of the proximal stumps, as described above. The first graft attached to the cranio-medial fascicle group in A has a split distal end, one united with the cranial fascicle group, one united with the upper half of the middle fascicle group. A second nerve graft is attached to the cranio-lateral fascicle group A and has also a split end, one part is attached to the lower half of the middle group in the distal stump, the other part to the upper half of the caudal fascicle group. A third graft is used for the caudal fascicle group in the proximal stump and the lower half of the caudal fascicle group in the peripheral stump. Instead of three sural nerve grafts two of which having split ends, one can also take five thin sural nerve grafts (Fig. 3).

A : E: In defects between the proximal stump at the stylomastoid foramen and the peripheral stump proximal to the division of the nerve, four sural nerve grafts are used. Two are united with the cranio-medial fascicle group in A and with the cranial fascicle group in a distal stump, one graft is put between the cranio-lateral fascicle group in A and the cranial half of the lower fascicle group in the distal stump, and the fourth one connects the caudal fascicle group in A with the caudal half of the caudo-fascicle group in the distal stump (Fig. 4).

In a large defect between the proximal stump at the stylomastoid foramen and the peripheral stumps already represented by the individual branches, six thin sural nerve grafts are used, uniting the corresponding fascicle groups of the proximal stump with corresponding individual branches. A connection with the Ramus colli is optional instead of this branch, two grafts can be used to connect a proximal stump with the buccal branches, if several of them are available (Fig. 5).

B : C: In a defect between a proximal stump in a proximal third and the distal stump in the middle third, three nerve grafts are used, uniting the cranial and cranio-medial sector of B with the cranial fascicle group of C, the caudal lateral sector of B with the caudo-lateral fascicle group of C and the caudo-medial sector of B with the caudo-medial fascicle group of C (Fig. 6).

B : D: In case of a defect between the proximal stump and the proximal third and of the distal stump and the distal third, three sural nerve grafts, two of them with split ends, or five thin sural nerve grafts are used similar as in A : D (Fig. 7).

B : E: In a defect between the proximal third and the main trunk before its division, four sural nerve grafts are used similar as in A : E (Fig. 8).

In a defect between the main trunk and the proximal third, and the peripheral rami, the procedure is as depicted in Fig. 9.

C : D: The procedure in a defect between the proximal stump in the middle third and the distal stump in the distal third is suggested in Fig. 10.

C : E: In a defect between the proximal stump in the middle third and the distal stump before the division, again four sural nerve grafts are used, as suggested in Fig. 11.

In a defect between the proximal stump in the distal third and the peripheral rami, six grafts are used, as suggested in Fig. 12.

D : E: In a defect the proximal stump in the distal third and the distal stump, just prior to the division of the nerve, four sural nerve grafts are used, as suggested in Fig. 13.

In a defect between the proximal stump at the distal third of the main trunk and the peripheral rami, six nerve grafts are used, as suggested in Fig. 14.

Figs. 1–14. The sketch gives a schematic view of the fascicular pattern at different levels. The figures indicate the distribution of nerve fibres, supplying different muscle groups over the cross-section

1 to 5: Nerve fibres to the upper face,
6 to 8: Nerve fibres to the upper face,
9 to 10: Nerve fibres to the middle face.

A suggestion is made as to how to prepare the stump (resection or interfascicular dissection) and how many grafts should be used to unite the corresponding sectors of the cross-section, respectively the corresponding fascicle groups

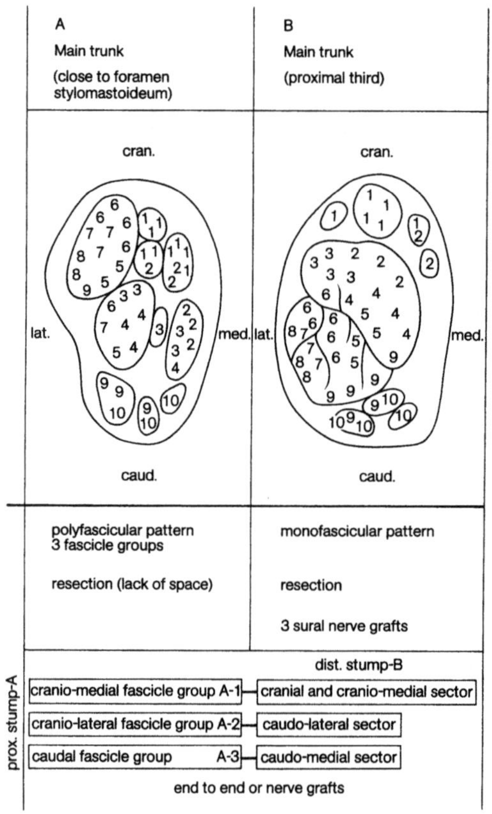

Fig. 1

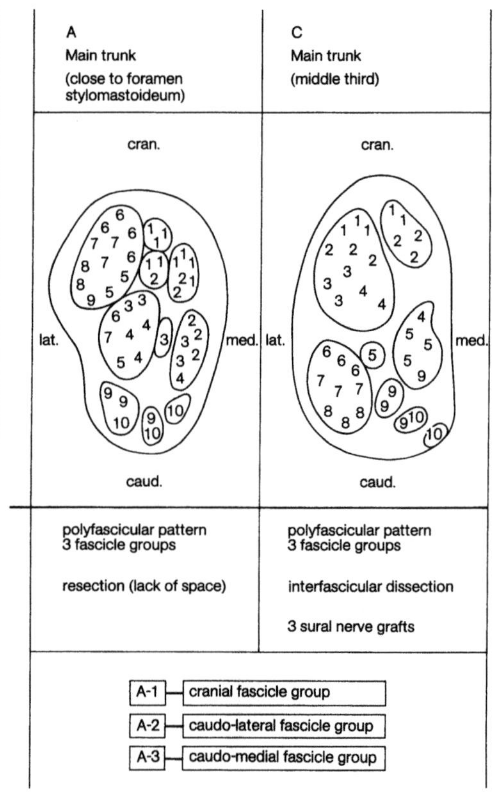

Fig. 2

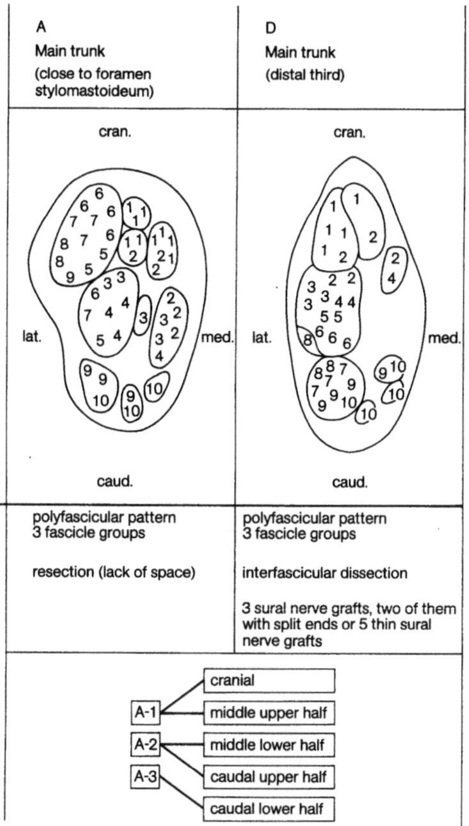
A
Main trunk
(close to foramen stylomastoideum)
D
Main trunk
(distal third)
cran.
lat.
med.
caud.
polyfascicular pattern
3 fascicle groups
resection (lack of space)
polyfascicular pattern
3 fascicle groups
interfascicular dissection
3 sural nerve grafts, two of them with split ends or 5 thin sural nerve grafts
A-1
A-2
A-3
cranial
middle upper half
middle lower half
caudal upper half
caudal lower half

3

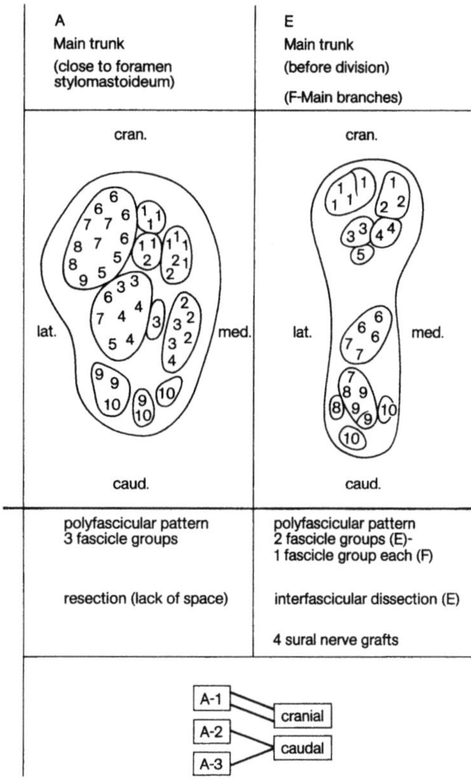
A
Main trunk
(close to foramen stylomastoideum)
E
Main trunk
(before division)
(F-Main branches)
cran.
lat.
med.
caud.
polyfascicular pattern
3 fascicle groups
resection (lack of space)
polyfascicular pattern
2 fascicle groups (E)-
1 fascicle group each (F)
interfascicular dissection (E)
4 sural nerve grafts
A-1
A-2
A-3
cranial
caudal

4

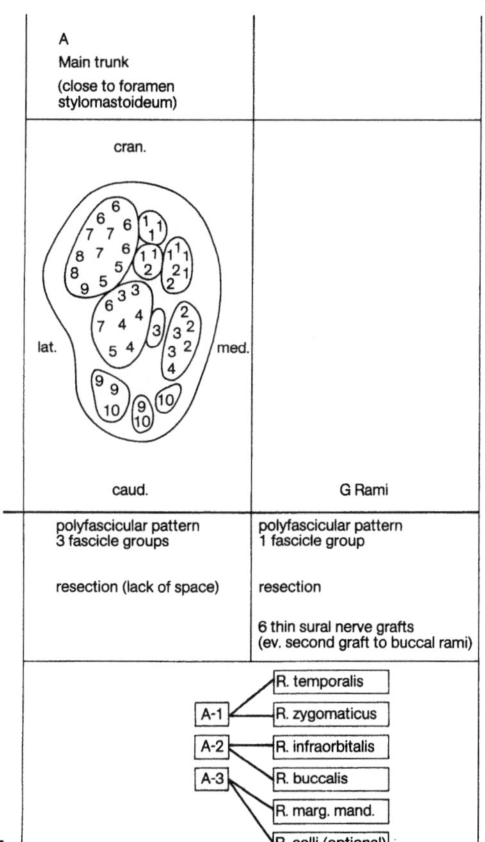
A
Main trunk
(close to foramen stylomastoideum)
cran.
lat.
med.
caud.
G Rami
polyfascicular pattern
3 fascicle groups
resection (lack of space)
polyfascicular pattern
1 fascicle group
resection
6 thin sural nerve grafts
(ev. second graft to buccal rami)
A-1
A-2
A-3
R. temporalis
R. zygomaticus
R. infraorbitalis
R. buccalis
R. marg. mand.
R. colli (optional)

5

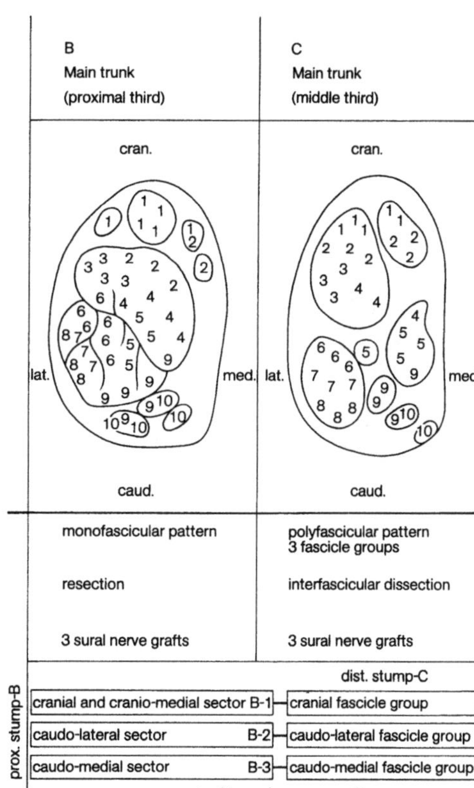
B
Main trunk
(proximal third)
C
Main trunk
(middle third)
cran.
lat.
med.
caud.
monofascicular pattern
resection
3 sural nerve grafts
polyfascicular pattern
3 fascicle groups
interfascicular dissection
3 sural nerve grafts
dist. stump-C
prox. stump-B
cranial and cranio-medial sector B-1
caudo-lateral sector B-2
caudo-medial sector B-3
cranial fascicle group
caudo-lateral fascicle group
caudo-medial fascicle group
end to end or nerve grafts

6

Figs. 3–6

B Main trunk (proximal third)	D Main trunk (distal third)

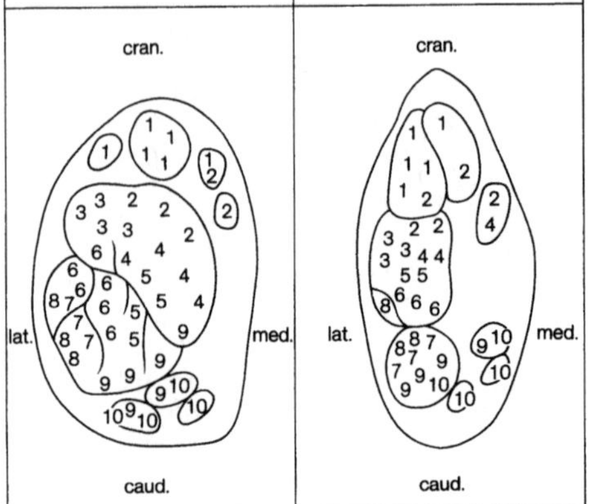

monofascicular pattern	polyfascicular pattern 3 fascicle groups
resection	interfascicular dissection
3 sural nerve grafts	3 sural nerve grafts, two of them with split ends or 5 thin sural nerve grafts

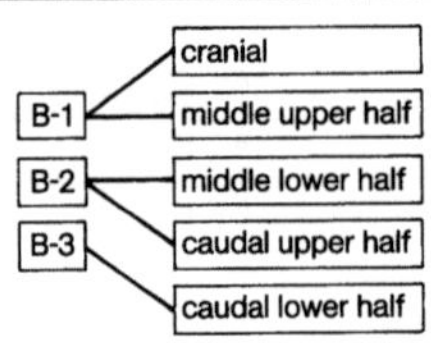

7

B Main trunk (proximal third)	E Main trunk (before division) (F-Main branches)

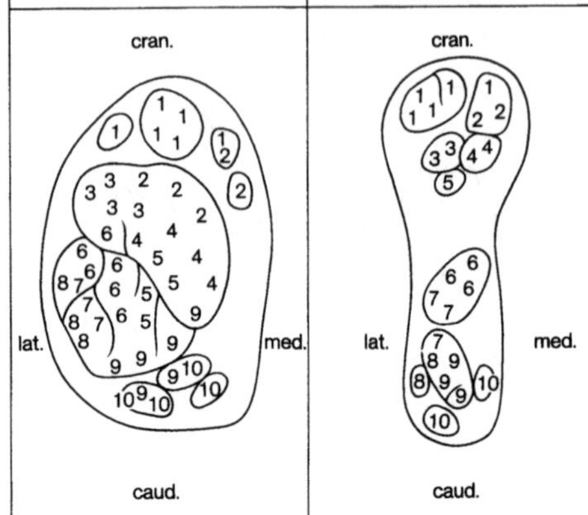

monofascicular pattern	polyfascicular pattern 2 fascicle groups (E)- 1 fascicle group each (F)
resection	interfascicular dissection (E)
3 sural nerve grafts	4 sural nerve grafts

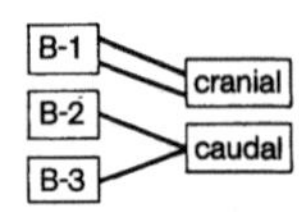

8

B Main trunk (proximal third)	

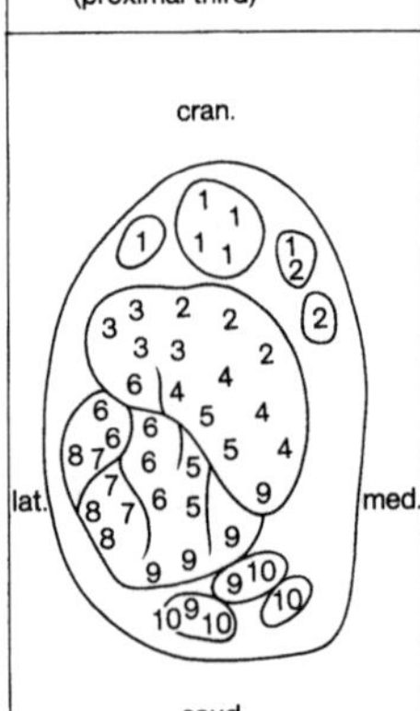

G Rami

monofascicular pattern	polyfascicular pattern 1 fascicle group
resection	resection
3 sural nerve grafts	6 thin sural nerve grafts (ev. second graft to buccal rami)

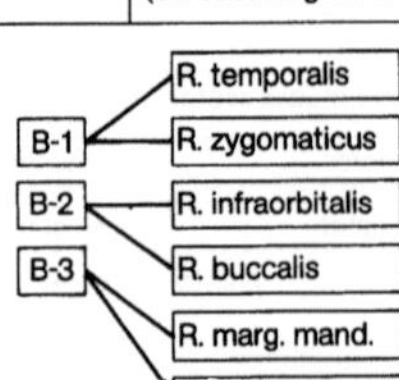

9

Figs. 7–10

C Main trunk (middle third)	D Main trunk (distal third)

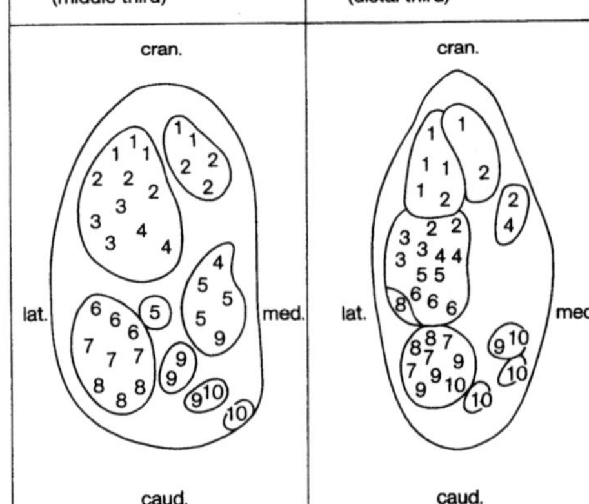

polyfascicular pattern 3 fascicle groups	polyfascicular pattern 3 fascicle groups
interfascicular dissection	interfascicular dissection
3 sural nerve grafts	3 sural nerve grafts, two of them withsplit ends or 5 thin sural nerve grafts

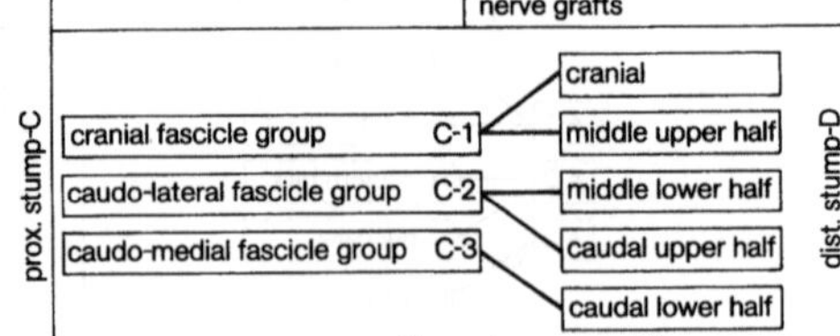

10

11

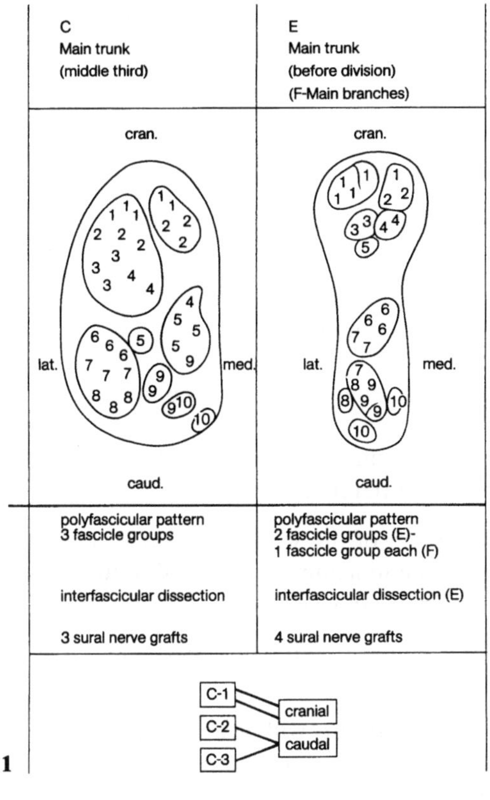

12

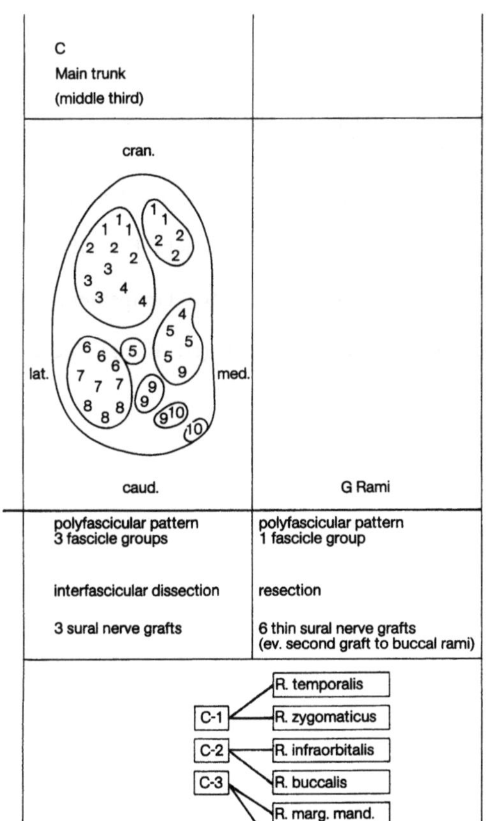

13

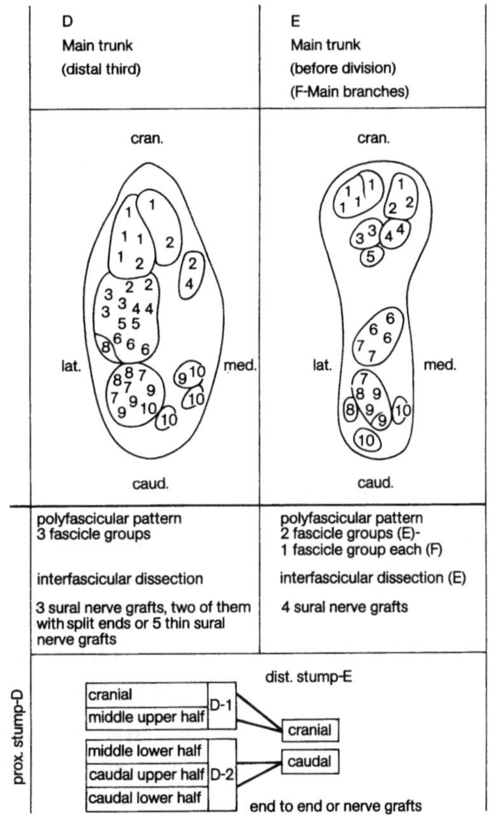

14

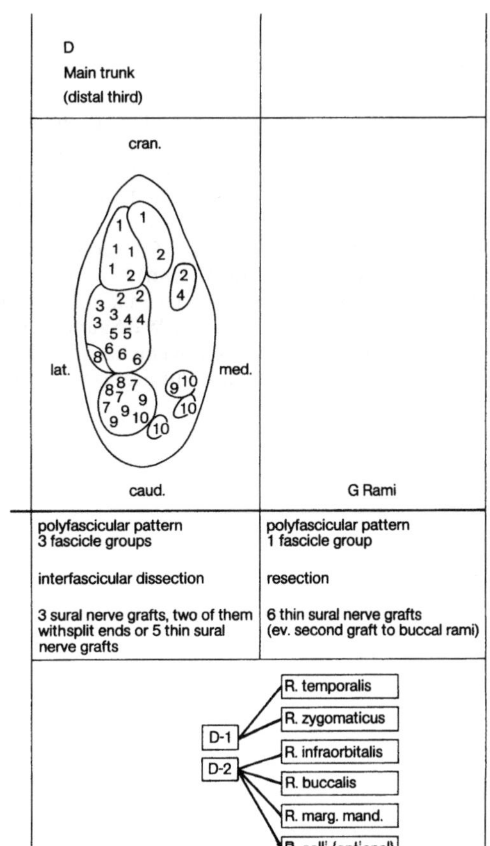

Figs. 11–14

Conclusions

It is evident that by following these suggestions, mass movement will not be avoided completely for the following reasons:

1. The boundaries between areas of prevalence of certain fibres are fluid, and it will not be possible to prevent some fibres going the wrong way.
2. The surgical accuracy has its limits.
3. It will not always be possible to define the individual parts of the fascicular pattern.
4. Anastomosis between the rami in the periphery may contribute to the fact that nerve fibres from the same branch are going to different muscles.

Since the ramus cygomaticus contains forty percent of the whole number of facial nerve fibres (Samii 1979), it may rather be possible to achieve individual motion of the mouth without accompanying motion of the lips, than vice versa.

5. The possibility of mass movements due to irregular outgrowth of axons and loss of dendritic connections has been mentioned already.

In spite of these restrictions a larger portion of axon sprouts will be able to grow into the correct peripheral pathway, and the chances of avoiding mass movement will be increased if an attempt is made to restore the original structure of the facial nerve as good as our present possibilities permit.

References

Kreutzberg GW (1977) Neurobiology of the Regenerating Facial Motor Unit. In: Fisch U (ed) Facial Nerve Surgery. Kugler Medical Publications, Amstelveen

May M (1973) Anatomy of the facial nerve. Laryngoloscope 83, 8: 1311–1329

Meissl G (1979) Die intraneurale Topographie des extrakraniellen Nervus facialis. Acta Chir Austr Suppl 25

Miehlke A (1958) Topography of the course of fibres in the facialis stem. Arch Klin Exp Ohren Nasen Kehlkopfkunde (Berlin) 171: 340–347

Samii M (1979) Nerves of the Head and Neck. In: Omer GE, Spinner M (eds) Management of Peripheral Nerve Problems. WB Saunders Comp, Philadelphia

Sunderland S (1977) Mass movements after facial nerve injury. In: Fisch U (ed) Facial Nerve Surgery. Kugler Medical Publications, Amstelveen p 285–289

Distribution of Nerve Fibres in the Extra-Temporal Branches of the Facial Nerve

I. Søgard, M. Samii, and J. M. Schröder, Aalborg/Denmark, Hannover, Mainz/FRG

Introduction

In 1971, J. W. Smith described a new treatment of facial paralysis. Some of the peripheral branches of the facial nerve from the intact side were connected by means of nerve grafting to the corresponding branches on the affected side (facio-facial anastomosis). The method has since been used in several instances, but there has been disagreement as to the peripheral branches which should preferentially be taken from the donor nerve.

Therefore, the present study was undertaken for estimating the number of nerve fibres in the various peripheral motor branches of the facial nerve. It was thought that the number of nerve fibres might be of major influence on the efficiency of nerve grafting.

Material and Method

The extracranial portion of the facial nerve was obtained on both sides in 11 autopsy cases, selected at random. None of the cases had degenerative neurological disorders. There were 3 women and 8 men, aged 28 to 75 years, with an average of 52 years.

The facial nerve was exposed from the stylomastoid foramen about 2–3 cms in front of the parotid gland.

A number of investigators observed that there is a wide variation in the peripheral course of the facial nerve which can be confirmed by the present study. Frequently, the course differed on the two sides in the same individual.

In all cases, however, it was possible to isolate the main branches. The greatest variation was found in the course of the buccal branch, which could either originate from the temporo-facial or cervico-facial trunks, or elsewhere from an independent branch of the main nerve.

About 1 cm was removed from the main nerve immediately in front of the stylomastoid foramen, from the temporo-frontal, zygomatic and buccal branches, and from the main cervical branch before its division into the marginal and the cervical branches.

The pieces of nerve were fixed in 3.9% glutaldehyde with phosphate buffer for about one hour. The epineurium was partially removed, and the nerve subsequently fixed in 2% buffered osmium tetroxide, and embedded in epoxy resin. Sections, 1–1.5 in thickness, were cut on an ultra-microtom and stained with toluidine blue and paraphenylendiamine. Photographs were obtained of whole sections at a final magnification of 80×. In addition, three representative areas were selected from each branch, and photographs were obtained at a final magnification of 800×.

The main nerve shows usually only one, or a number of very small fascicles. The nerve fibres were counted and measured by using a semi-automatic particle size analyser (TGZ 3 of Zeiss, Oberkochen). The total area of the fascicles was calculated by means of a microweight method. The nerve section was enlarged 100 times in a epidiascope, and the outline of the fascicles was traced on paper. Cut-outs of the total area of the fascicles were then weighed and converted to real areas by means of a known reference weight.

Results

There was an average of 6,948 myelinated fibres (range 5,048 to 10,543) in the main trunk of the nerve (Table 1). The frontotemporal branch contained 1,256 fibres, corresponding to 18% of the fibres in the main stem, the zygomatic branch 2,089, corresponding to 30%, the buccal branch 2,034, corresponding to 29%, and the cervical branch an average of 1,459 fibres, corresponding to 21%. In the main stem there was no difference between the number of fibres on the left and the right side, but it appears that on the right side there is a larger number of fibres in the zygomatic than in the buccal branch, while the opposite is true on the left side.

Table 1. Distribution of fibers in the extracranial part of the facial nerve (mean values in 22 nerves)

	Main stem	Frontal branch	Zygomatic branch	Buccal branch	Cervical branch
Right	7,097 (5,048 – 10,543)	1,187 (461 – 2,055)	2,433 (1,029 – 4,767)	1,807 (845 – 2,780)	1,424 (373 – 2,463)
Left	6,800 (5,077 – 7,323)	1,326 (600 – 2,247)	1,745 (853 – 2,789)	2,262 (1,137 – 3,155)	1,495 (635 – 2,294)
Mean	6,948	18%	30%	29%	21%

Discussion

The present counts of the number of myelinated nerve fibres in the main trunk of the human facial nerve (mean value 6,948 fibres) are well in agreement with the counts of the number of motor nerve cells in the facial nucleus (about 7,000, van Buskirk 1945) and with previous descriptions of the mastoid portion of the facial nerve (Kullman et al. 1971).

In addition, the proportion of fibre numbers in the main branches of the facial nerve have been determined. It is apparent from the fibre counts that the zygomatic and the buccal branches of the facial nerve may be the most suitable ones for surgical reconstructive purposes, whilst the frontal branch, in accordance with common clinical experiences, appears to be the least suitable one.

References

Kullman GL et al. (1971) Anatomy of the Mastoid Portion of the Facial Nerve. Arch Otolaryngol 93:29–33

Samii M (1977) Rehabilitation of the Face by VIIth Nerve Substitution. In: Fisch U (ed) Facial Nerve Surgery, Aesculapius, Birmingham, Ala. p 243–245

Van Buskirk C (1945) The Seventh Nerve Complex. J Comp Neurol 82:303–333

Clinical Aspects of Facial Nerve

Clinical Diagnosis in Bell's Palsy

E. Stennert, Göttingen/FRG

Concerning the different etiologies and also the possible functional and cosmetical disorders, facial paralysis should be regarded as an emergency. It offers excellent chances for optimal healing when treated in its initial stage. This does not only apply to Bell's palsy. Fisch (1976) in his 'Guidelines for the Management of Traumatic Injuries of the Facial Nerve', has recently emphasized the urgency of an early diagnosis (within six days) which permits a therapeutic decision. What diagnostic possibilities do we have, and how are they to be assessed?

Bell's palsy is etiologically the most frequent diagnosis, comprising about 75 percent of all cases. But this high incidence is often responsible for a premature, false diagnosis. These errors lead to the actual diseases being neglected. We have therefore to adhere to the following principle: One can only speak of an actual case of Bell's palsy if all other possibilities have been safely eliminated!

The basic diagnostic technique must consequently and on principle include the following standard investigations:

1. Careful evaluation of the history.
2. Otoscopic investigation in order to exclude inflammatory middle ear processes, purulent cholesteatomas, glomus tumors and malignomas originating from the auditory meatus or the tympanic cavity.
3. A careful palpation of the ear-region, especially of the retromandibular fossa, is very important for the exclusion of malignant tumors of the otobasis and particularly of malignant tumors of the parotid gland.
4. Owing to the close topographical relationship of the facial nerve to the eighth cranial nerve, it is indispensable to perform a pure tone audiogram, a nystagmogram, and the excitability test of Hallpike, in order to exclude tumors of the cerebellopontine angle, acusticus neurinomas, and the like.
5. X-ray examination according to Schüller and Stenvers help to exclude both inflammatory and space-requiring processes in the region of the petrous bone. If a particular suspicion exists, these tests can be supplemented by tomography of the internal auditory meatus or the pyramidal tip.

Only if all these investigations have not resulted in a specific suspicion, the special tests of facial function and localization may be applied. Their discussion should also be preceded by a principal annotation:

The facial nerve is a mixed nerve possessing motory, secretory (parasympathetic) and sensory fibers, besides a small sensible portion innervating Ramsey Hunt's cutaneous zone. These different fiber qualities are reacting to compression as well as to hypoxia with different intensities, so that functional deficiency is often not only graduated but also dissociated. Thus, the functional state of a single group of fibers does not permit to assess the situation of the whole nerve without certain qualifications.

Stapedial Reflex

The limitations just mentioned apply to the stapedial reflex, which is recommended by a number of authors as a suitable procedure for a general assessment of nerve function. Two factors advocate against such an interpretation:

1. The fibers of this reflex arc are not representative enough owing to their small number.
2. As reflex-transmitting neurons, these fibers are particularly myelin-rich and therefore more susceptible to pressure than the other motoneurons, and hence are much sooner liable to undergo neurapraxia.

All this means in effect that the assessment of the stapedial reflex is not suited as a sole procedure for the assessment of nerve function. Its value is confined mainly to topodiagnosis.

The Schirmer Test

This test is especially significant in topodiagnosis because it permits, with a relatively high degree of certainty, to differentiate between injuries of the nerve that have occurred distal to the geniculate ganglion (which makes operative intervention easy and low in risk) and those that are located proximal to the geniculate ganglion (which require a much more sophisticated surgical procedure). The test should be assessed as follows (Fig. 1):

SCHIRMER'S TEST

1. Wipe eyes dry
2. Anasthesia not necessary
3. Testing for at least 5 min.

Test is
a) *evaluable:* ≧ 1,5 cm wetted
b) *positive:* side-difference > $_{30}$‰

Fig. 1. Criteria for the assessment and evaluation of Schirmer's test

Prior to insertion of the litmus paper strip, both eyes ought to be wiped with a swab. This prevents misleading results which could be produced by a lacrimal lake in the lower conjunctival sac created by lagophthalmus on the paretic side.

Anesthesia of the conjunctiva is not necessary. The test strips should remain in place for at least five minutes. The Schirmer test permits evaluation if at least 1.5 cm of the strips have become wet, discounting the portion that had laid inside the conjunctival sac. The test is positive if the side difference amounts to more than 30 percent. This value was obtained by studies of Gontier and Fisch (1976) who found that a difference of up to 30 percent lies within the normal range, so that only differences of more than 30 percent can be regarded as statistically different.

Not rarely, and particulary in older people, a nearly complete lack of tear secretion may be observed on both sides. In these cases stimulation of tear secretion can be achieved by inhalation of a trigeminal stimulant, for instance ammonia vapor.

Examination of Taste

Here, too, some critical remarks should be made first. As it is obvious from Fig. 2, the anterior two thirds of the tongue are innervated by 2 types of afferent nerve fibers: On the one hand by the sensory fibers transmitting taste sensation via the tympanic chord, and on the other hand by the sensory fibers conveying an extremely high surface sensitivity via the lingual nerve as a branch of the trigeminal nerve.

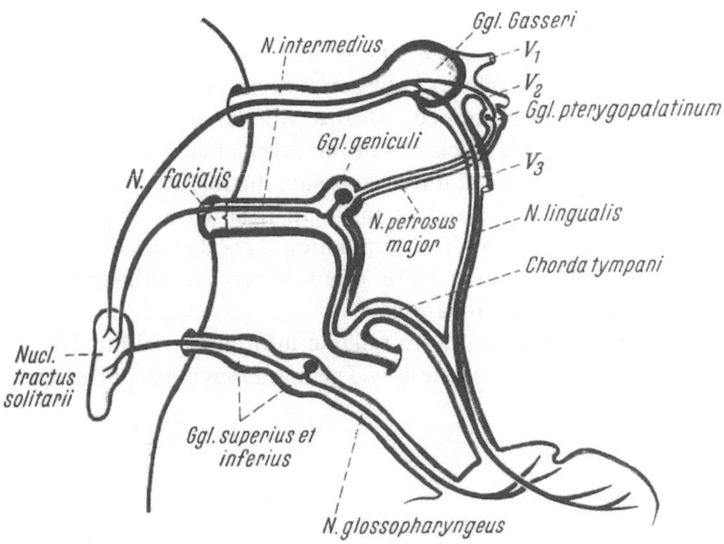

Fig. 2. Pattern of the sensory innervation of the anterior two thirds of tongue by two different types of afferent nerve fibers, transmitting taste sensation via the tympanic nerve and surface sensitivity via the lingual nerve.
From: Miehlke; Surgery of the Facial Nerve, Urban & Schwarzenberg, München 1973 according to Ferner: Anatomie des Nervensystems und der Sinnesorgane, Basel 1952

It is therefore understandable that with electrogustometry these sensitive terminals are also stimulated even at relatively low stimulus intensities, which can result in a false response by the patient. According to Kida and Rollin (1975), such electrical stimuli can be perceived from as low as 50 microamps up. Interpretation of results therefore requires extended experience of the investigator, but also a sufficiently high I.Q. of the patient.

Occasionally the use of a simple flashlight-battery is recommended. But also with this simple test one should consider the same limitation as the intensity of current is normally 2 milliamps and therefore much higher than the critical value.

We have for these reasons returned to the traditional examination criteria for taste sensation. These include the 4 sapid qualities of 'sweet', 'sour', 'salty', and 'bitter' which are applied in varying concentrations to the anterior two thirds of the paretic half of the tongue with a cotton swab. It is in any case advisable to assess very critically the findings especially of any examination of taste perception.

Salivary Flow and pH

To complete the presentation of clinical examination techniques, the investigation of *salivary flow* according to Magielski and Blatt (1958) shall be mentioned. This test, for example, is recommended by Diamant et al. (1972, 1977) as a reliable prognostic test. Moreover, the analysis of *submandibular salivary pH* as a diagnostic aid for prognosis of facial palsy was recently favoured by Saito et al. (1977).

Mimic Function

Although the facial nerve is a mixed one, it is first of all a motor-nerve. A careful investigation of its motor function is therefore of utmost importance.

Resting tone should not be over-estimated, because it is largely dependent on the smoothness of the skin surface, the thickness of the layer of subcutaneous adipose tissue, the mass and firmness of the connective tissue, the turgor of the cells in the cutis, subcutis, and muscular layers, and so forth. In fresh cases of paresis in younger individuals, and especially in children or pyknics, a good resting tone with a high degree of facial symmetry is therefore often observed, although electromyography reveals marked or even total paresis.

Motility on the other hand gives much more reliable information of the degree, the course and sometimes also of the site of a lesion. The main functions, particularly

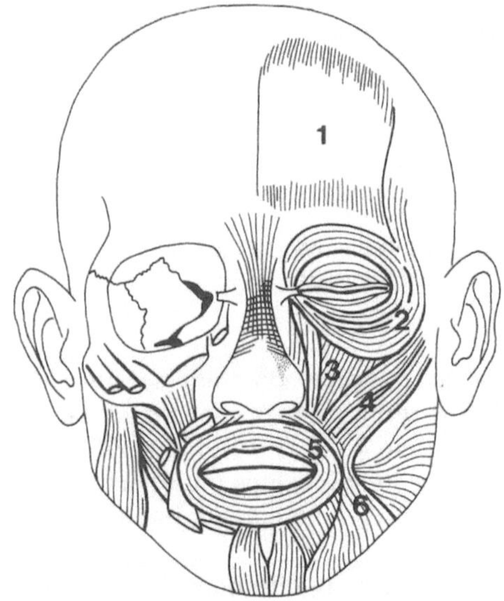

Fig. 3. Diagram of the main muscles responsible for the most important functional and cosmetic disturbances: *1* = frontal muscle (frowning), *2* = orbicularis oculi muscle (closing eyes), *3* = levator labii muscle (wrinkling nose), *4* = zygomaticus muscle (showing teeth), *5* = orbicularis oris muscle (whistling), *6* = risorius and depressor anguli oris muscle (dropping corners of the mouth).
Their function should always be checked first by comparison of both halves of the face and second by observation of the paralyzed side only while pressing the thumb on the midline of the face

involving the muscles demonstrated in Fig. 3, are the following and should therefore always be examined: Frowning (frontalis muscle), closing eyes (orbicularis oculi muscle), wrinkling nose (levator labii muscle), exposure of teeth (zygomaticus and buccinatorius muscle), whistling (orbicularis oris muscle), and, if necessary, dropping the corners of the mouth (risorius and depressor anguli oris muscle plus platysme).

These five or six functions should always be examined first by comparison of both halves of the face, but also subsequently by careful observation of the paralyzed side only. In this examination it is very important to press the thumb on the midline of the forehead, the dorsum of the nose, and the philtrum of the upper and the lower lip, in order to prevent transmission of movements from the healthy to the paretic side.

In this connection attention ought to be directed to a situation which often leads to erroneous interpretation: If a patient is clinically investigated for the function of the orbicularis oris muscle when in a supine position, complete lid closure can often be observed even if there exists a total paralysis of this muscle. This finding is explained by the fact that the upper eyelid is not innervated by the facial nerve and the lower eyelid moves passively following the rotation of the bulbus which is known as Bell's phenomenon. A safe diagnosis can therefore only be made by electromyographic investigation.

A last statement is indicated in connection with this subject: The facial nerve offers several clinical tests whose diagnostic and, moreover, prognostic value is pointed out by different authors. But anyone familiar with the varying picture of facial pareses knows about the uncertainty of all of them. According to own experience and in good agreement with other experienced physicians (see panel discussion No. 3 in Fisch, 1977) it is not worthwhile to use only one test, but it is recommended to assemble as much information as possible. All these clinical tests should be looked upon as pieces in a puzzle game, in which they may be helpful to ascertain a diagnosis concerning etiology, degree and especially topography. However, it is the author's opinion that all these tests do not permit any reliable prognosis regarding the further course of the paralysis.

References

Diamant H, Eckstrand T, Wiberg A (1972) Prognosis of idopathic Bell's palsy. Arch Otolaryngol 95:431–433

Diamant H (1977) Taste Examinations. In: Fisch U, Kugler-Aesculapius (eds) Facial Nerve Surgery. Amstelveen-Birmingham/Alabama, p 154–158

Fisch U (1976) Richtlinie zur Versorgung traumatischer Verletzungen des Nervus facialis. ORL (Suppl. 1) 38:42

Gontier J, Fisch U (1976) Schirmer's Test: Its Normal Values and Clinical Significance. ORL 1:38

Kida A, Rollin H (1975) Wo liegt die Grenze zwischen sensibler und gustatorischer Wahrnehmung in der Elektrogustometrie? HNO 23:72

Magielski JE, Blatt IM (1958) Submaxillary salivary flow: a test of chorda tympani nerve function as an aid in diagnosis and prognosis of facial nerve paralysis. Laryngoscope 68:1770

Saito H, Higashitsuji H, Kishimoto S, Miyamoto K, Kitamura H (1977) Submandibular salivary pH as a diagnostic aid for prognosis of facial palsy. In: Fisch U, Kugler-Aesculapius (eds) Facial Nerve Surgery. Amstelveen-Birmingham/Alabama p 143–153

Functional Testing of the Facial Nerve

L. B. W. JONGKEES, Amsterdam/Netherlands

In cases of facial palsy it is extremely important to start with a thorough examination of the clinical function of the nerve. This may seem an easy task, since the loss of movement of the facial muscles is so clear that it can hardly be missed. It is certainly trickier to find and assess the seriousness of a facial paralysis in cases of trauma to head and face. Swelling, haemorrhage, and general condition of the patient are factors which hamper the perception of a muscular dysfunction. Also in the young child diagnostic difficulties may be present, since the turgor of the facial skin can make it almost impossible to discover the asymmetry, especially seeing that voluntary movements cannot be easily provoked. After operation upon the tem-

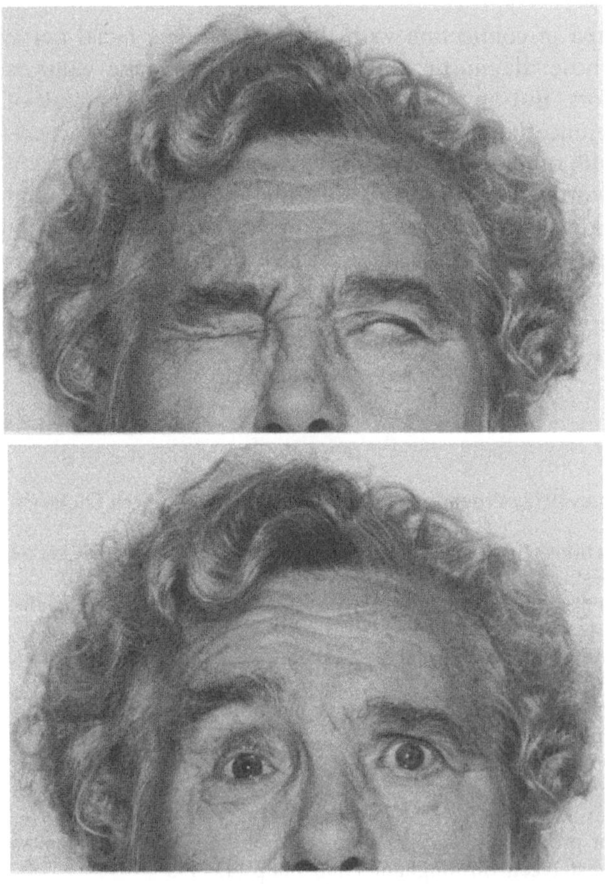

Fig. 1. Complete facial paralysis of the left side of the face. The movements of the forehead on the right side cross the midline

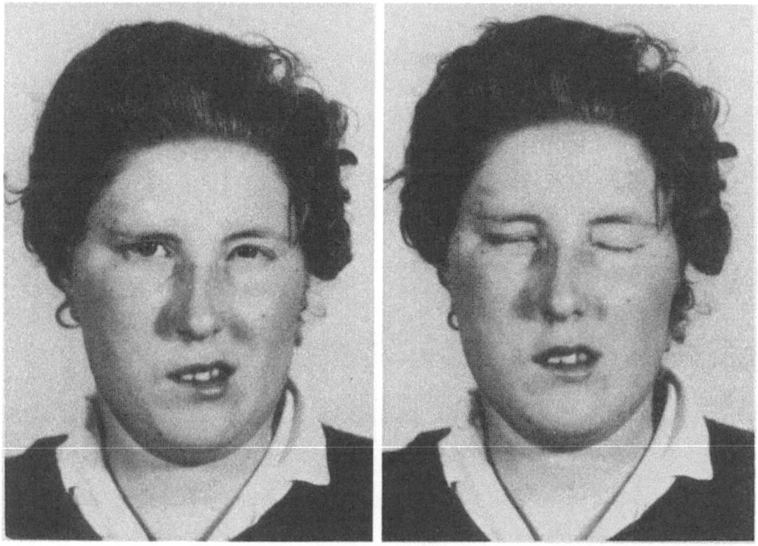

Fig. 2. Complete facial paralysis on the right side. The right eye is closed by the upper eyelid, innervated by the oculomotor nerve

poral bone, it must be deemed impossible to determine the presence of a facial nerve lesion before the patient has awakened from general anaesthesia.

The most important first step is to determine whether the palsy is of peripheral or central origin. If all branches are involved, the cause is peripheral. If the upper branches (forehead and eyes) show no involvement the affection has a central cause, with the exception of a few easily detectable extratemporal lesions caused by trauma or tumor in the region of the parotid gland.

Since the prognosis of the affection is very important, both for therapy and for the patient's psychological condition, the degree of the palsy must be carefully evaluated. It may seem to be an easy task to find out whether the paralysis is either complete or partial. Often it is not! If the function of the forehead is examined, it is not unusual for the paralysed (Fig. 1) side to show some wrinkles that may be provoked by the contraction of the muscles on the healthy side via traction on the skin. In order not to be misled, it is useful for the examiner to fix the patient's skin with one finger in the midline on the underlying bone of forehead or nose.

When looking at the closure of the eyes, the examiner must realize that closing of the eyes with only the lower eyelid indicates (Fig. 2) facial nerve function. The eye can also be closed by active relaxation of the muscles of the upper eyelid, but these muscles are innervated by the oculomotor nerve.

It is very important, both for an experienced and for an unexperienced observer, to be sure about what he is confronted with (Fig. 3). Therefore perfect illumination is of utmost importance. It is also necessary to examine the patient under such conditions that he is relaxed and at ease. The best position for the patient is the supine position on a couch in a well-heated room. In this way all kinds of irrelevant twitchings can be avoided.

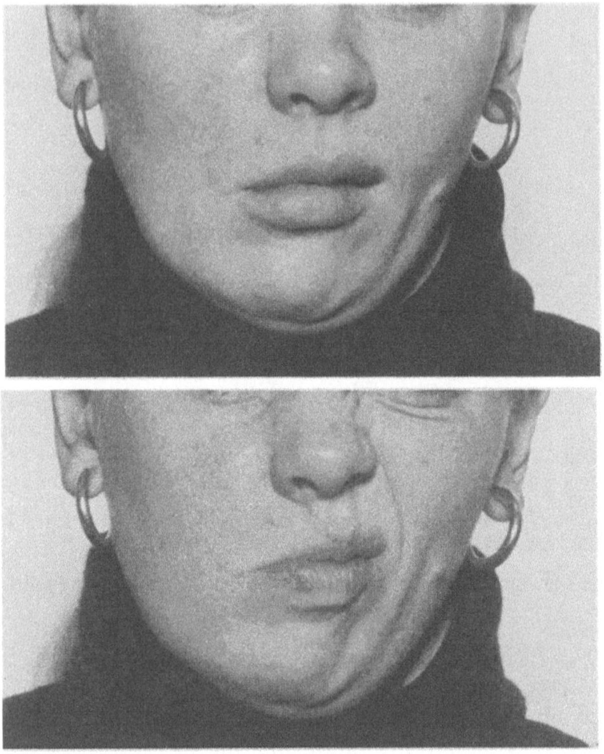

Fig. 3. Facial paralysis on the right side. The angle of the mouth on the paralyzed side moves when the facial muscles on the left side are set in action

Always look at the face at rest and at all the movements in the field of the various branches of the facial nerve. Always use an identical sequence.

Mistakes can be made at first examination of the face at rest or during movements but more often they are even made in the course of affection. It is not uncommon that the patient tells his doctor that his complaints diminish and that the function of the facial muscles improves. He does not loose saliva as much as the day before, he does not bite on the inside of his cheek anymore, eating and speaking are easier, etc. Adaptation is important in patients with unaltered paralysis. This often happens without any real improvement only for the reason that the patient gets used to his affliction, which in the beginning was to him an ominous catastrophe. Finding himself alive after some days makes him see the future, and his ailment, with less pessimism. On the other hand it may be that the turgor of the paralyzed half of his face is increasing but this does not herald a real improvement either. It is, in itself, certainly not the basis for the assumption of more improvement.

For determining the prognosis of a facial paralysis in a patient, the severity of the paralysis, the degree of muscle tone and the presence or absence of a naso-palpebral reflex are important. As long as there is still an evident sign of muscular response in the patient's efforts to move his face, the paralysis is not complete. It is then a paresis where the loss of function of the nerve has not gone so far yet that there is an immediate danger of degeneration.

But a paresis may progress and become a complete paralysis. The muscle tone may diminish. Then we need more information in order to be able to judge the condition of the nerve, and thereby, the prognosis of the palsy.

Electromyography is essential in determining the complete absence of nervous impulses reaching the muscle and making the fibres contract, and for the answering of this question EMG is useful. But it is not a good test for the important questions about the presence or absence of denervation.

Fibrillation potentials indicating denervation are not found within about two weeks, too late for timely decisions in emergency cases and, as I stressed so often, a facial paralysis is an emergency. Therefore, in this respect EMG lets us down.

Under normal conditions muscle fibers contract when they receive the appropriate stimulus via their motor nerve. As long as the conductivity of the nerve is intact, muscle contraction can be produced by stimulation of the nerve trunk in its peripheral course. In cases of peripheral motor nerve lesions, the propagation of the stimulus may be impaired or lacking. In the nerve excitability test the threshold value of excitation is determined by measuring the intensity of the minimal electrical stimulus required to produce muscle contraction.

With an electric stimulator stimuli (square wave impulses) of measurable duration and strength are delivered to the nerve trunk in front of the auricle at gradually increasing intensity until the first muscle contraction is recorded from the well and tangentially lit face, first on the normal, thereafter from the paralyzed side.

Serial examinations are necessary in fresh cases. Denervation is not a static situation but a process.

Absolute values are not important since slight changes in temperature and humidity can alter them greatly. As long as the difference between the thresholds of the normal and the paralyzed sides remain below 3.5 mA, there is no indication of degeneration. Above this till about 20 mA difference few to all fibers must be judged to be degenerated. Above 3.5 mA difference between normal and paralyzed side it is nearly certain that the function of the paralyzed nerve will never be completely normal again.

Fisch and his coworkers have great faith in a test with supraliminal stimuli: electroneurography from which they postulate to be able to find the proportion of still active fibres and blocked ones.

Contrary to many other authors I have never been able to find any connection between the amount of aural pain (usually located behind the ear, radiating to the occipital region, neck, or shoulder, often 'twitching', sometimes tearing) and the final outcome of the paralysis.

Loss of taste can be an important symptom. If the patient mentions it himself, one can be almost certain that electrogustometry will show its presence. The absence of subjective taste disturbances proves nothing. About 50 percent will show hemiageusia or hypogeusia. Though many authors regard taste as important in both the typical diagnosis of facial nerve lesions and in determining the prognosis of the palsy, my experience based on about 600 operations performed upon the facial nerve, has taught me to be very careful, since the point at which the chorda tympani curves away from the nerve shows considerable individual variations (Fig. 4). In Bell's palsy, the site at and the distance over which the nerve is swollen are also subject to considerable variation. In view of the great variability of these two factors,

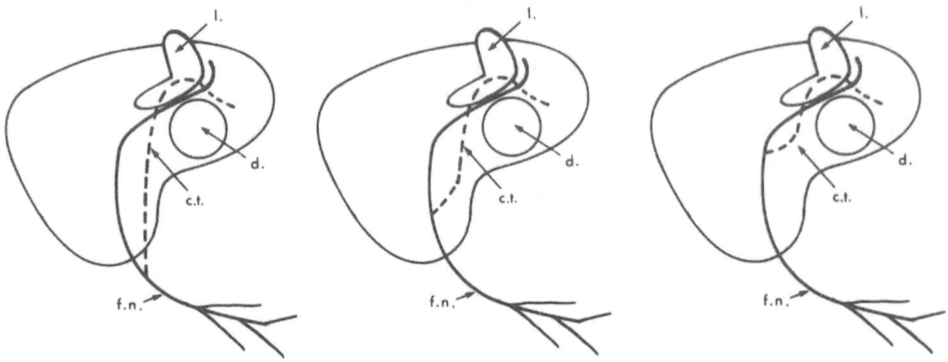

Fig. 4. Various courses of the chorda tympani curving away from the facial nerve. *l* labyrinth, *c.t.* chorda tympani, *d* outer ear canal, *f.n.* facial nerve

the absence of taste disturbances cannot be expected to yield exact topical or prognostic indications in facial paralysis. Their presence, however, can be of importance. Electrogustometry is a very simple test (Fig. 5). A small electric current is used to determine the thresholds of perception of a gustatory sensation on the two sides, which are then compared. As attendant information, it can help us to decide about prognosis and therapy.

The function of the chorda tympani can also be examined by measuring and comparing the flow of saliva on both sides. According to May (1970) 'the salivation test can be done in the office with inexpensive materials: a slice of lemon, a lacrimum punctum dilator, 0–00 lacrimal probe, No. 50 polyethylene tubing, and a fine wire stylet'. Since it is really not so easy to introduce the tubes into the submaxillary duct in order to count and compare the number of drops of saliva on both sides, but on top of that, since the drawbacks of this test are similar to those of the easier electrogustometry, I do not see much advantage in the use of the salivation test.

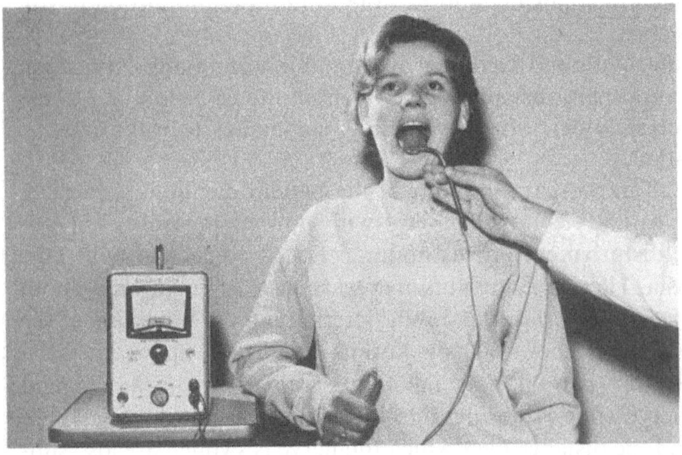

Fig. 5. Electrogustometry

Hyperacusia tests are not very attractive for the clinician either. The determination of acoustic impedance is not simple and the test is of dubious value because of the uncertain origin of the phenomenon. It is a fact that the tensor tympani muscle supplied by the trigeminal nerve can strongly influence the results of dysfunction of the stapedial muscle.

The Schirmer test with which one can measure lacrimal secretion is not a difficult test to perform. By suspending a strip of filter paper bent to form a hook in the conjunctival sac of each eye, the extent and speed of lacrimal fluid absorption can be measured. Any clinician can measure lacrimal secretion, but it is not easy to interpret the results. Whatever the value of the lacrima test may be, it is, in any case exclusively of topical diagnostic interest, and does not contribute a thing in our insight in the prognosis of a given case.

We may get some important information from the above mentioned clinical tests, but they do not answer two fundamental questions: whether the paralysis is transient or degenerative, and if transient, whether it shows any indications of unfavourable development. The clinical data give us a statistical prognosis but do not enable us to prognosticate individual patients early enough to take therapeutic steps. For these answers we need accurate, quantitative methods which are reproducible and comparable. As usual in many medical examinations a variety of tests can be used, and the usefulness does not depend upon the test only, but also upon the experience an investigator has with the test.

Reference

May M (1970) Facial Paralysis: peripheral type Laryngoscope 80:331–390

Neurophysiological Diagnosis of Facial Nerve

A. Struppler and R. Dengler, München/FRG

Introduction

The facial nerve mainly contains motor fibers supplying the mimic musculature and additional secretory and taste fibers running in the associated nervus intermedius. The most frequent disease affecting the nerve is idiopathic facial palsy leading to a more or less complete, usually unilateral paresis of the facial muscles. The major purpose of neurophysiological investigations in this disorder is to provide early information on the natural prognosis and the direction of the process. The tests used in this and other disorders of the facial nerve mainly investigate motor function giving objective and quantitative data. The examination of the taste and secretory function contributes to the topographical diagnosis of facial nerve lesions.

Methods and Results

Table 1 shows the clinical problems and questions which are to be answered by neurophysiological investigations. The largest topic deals with idiopathic facial palsy. Since it is the most frequent facial nerve disorder, the implications of neurophysiological diagnosis on this disease shall be considered first. Consecutively the other topics of Table 1 will be discussed.

1. Idiopathic Facial Palsy

The major purpose of the tests applied in assessing idiopathic facial palsy is to provide early reliable information on the natural direction and prognosis of the disease. Sometimes the question must be answered as to if and when a decompressive operation may be indicated. Principally the motor function serves as indicator of the general condition of the nerve. Of particular importance is to determine as early as possible the relation of reversibly blocked to degenerated nerve fibers and frequent (in the beginning, daily), follow up of the functional loss. Several tests as listed in Table 2 are available to fullfill this task.

a) Strength-Duration-Curve

Current pulses of variable intensity and duration are applied to a facial muscle to achieve a just visible muscle twitch. The results are plotted to give an i/t-curve with the stimulus duration on the abscissa. Since denervated muscles exhibit an increased threshold to electrical stimulation, the obtained curves are shifted to the right and can thus indicate nerve fiber degeneration. The test is positive only after seven or more days have elapsed (Alford, 1967). Since it is not very accurate and rather time-consuming, it is no longer in common use.

b) Chronaximetry

The chronaxy is the stimulus duration at twice the stimulus strength of the rheobase. Except that the test is quicker performed it has no diagnostic advantages as compared to the strength-duration-curve.

c) Excitability Test

The excitability test (Laumans, 1965; Jongkees, 1969) has gained considerable diagnostic importance. The facial nerve is stimulated near the foramen stylomastoideum with a pulse of 0.3 ms and of variable intensity to evoke a just visible muscle twitch. The stimulus intensities required on the normal and the affected side are compared. A more than 3.5 mA higher threshold on the paretic side is agreed to be pathological. The test may become positive after about 72 hours and should be repeated at daily or shorter intervals to assess the direction of the process. It is ap-

Table 1. Neurophysiological diagnosis in facial nerve disorders

Facial palsy
reversible conduction block – degeneration
reinnervation
aberrant regeneration
Restorative operations
facio-facial sutures
spino-facial anastomoses
Lexer-Rosenthal Operation
Spontaneous facial movements
facial hemispasm – psychogenic tic
facial myokymia

Table 2. Neurophysiological tests in idiopathic facial palsy

Strength-duration curve
Chronaximetry
Excitability test
Maximal excitability test
Distal latency determination
Evoked compound muscle action potential
Electromyography
Orbicularis oculi reflex
Stapedius reflex
Electrogustometry

propriate to indicate early degeneration of nerve fibers, although not quantitative. Complete inexcitability does not exclude the demonstration of some volitional activity on EMG-examination. The excitability test is still in common use and is involved in establishing the indication for decompressive operations.

d) Maximal Excitability Test

In the maximal excitability test (May, 1976) the current strength applied to the facial nerve is maximal to stimulate all excitable nerve fibres. The intensity of the evoked muscle twitch is assessed by clinical observation comparing the responses on the healthy and paralytic side. With some experience the test seems to provide information on nerve fiber degeneration somewhat earlier than the excitability test.

e) Distal Latency

The latency of the muscle action potential following the stimulation of the facial nerve near the foramen stylomastoideum was introduced by Taverner (1966) to assess the natural prognosis of facial palsies. In patients, where degeneration of nerve fibres occured, the latency increased over a critical value of 4 ms within the first week of the disease often progressing to absolute nerve inexcitability.

f) Electrically Evoked Compound Muscle Action Potential

The method was developed by Esslen and is extensively described in his monograph (1977). The amplitude of the compound action potential following supramaximal stimulation of the facial nerve is determined by means of standardized surface electrodes placed at the nasolabial fold. It is assumed that at this site a representative record of the facial musculature can be obtained. The amplitude of the paretic side is expressed as percentage of the response on the healthy side. The difference of both sides thus provides a quantitative measure of the degree of nerve fibre degeneration in percent. On the basis of these calculations and the time course determined by repeated testing a scheme has been established containing nine groups of patients from 0 to 100 percent degeneration with the corresponding implications concerning the natural prognosis. The method seems to be very sensitive to detect degeneration early and provides quantitative data. It can easily be combined with the excitability test and distal latency determination.

g) Electromyography

Conventional needle electromyography does not contribute very much to answer the question 'neurapraxia – degeneration' before 10 or more days have elapsed. This is the earliest time when pathologic spontaneous activity (fibrillation-potentials, positive sharp waves) as a sign of denervation can be detected. A reduced interference pattern on maximum volition or an absence of any volitional activity cannot discriminate between reversible conduction block and degeneration. A response to facial nerve stimulation, however, argues for a still reversible block. Otherwise, the preservation of some volitional activity in a clinically complete palsy over a period of seven to eight days indicates that degeneration is incomplete and

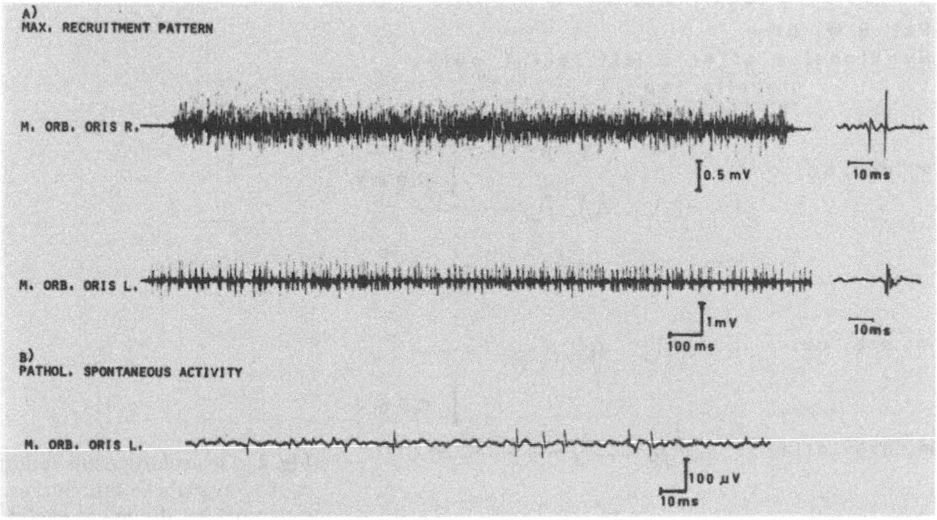

Fig. 1 A, B. EMG recorded in the m. orb. oris on both sides with concentric needle electrodes. In **A** the activity on max. volition is recorded. On the right side a full interference pattern, on the left side a reduced recruitment is observed. At the right margin of either trace motor unit potentials on fast time base are illustrated. The upper trace shows two normal potentials, the lower trace a polyphasic potential of increased duration. In **B** fibrillation potentials recorded in the left m. orb. oris are demonstrated

may predict a favourable outcome. The same is valid for an early return of volitional activity.

In the phase of recovery, prolonged polyphasic motor unit potentials point to a collateral reinnervation by sprouts of surviving motor neurons. Later on small motor unit potentials indicate beginning reinnervation by regenerating nerve fibers. These rather important signs of reinnervation are first to be detected by careful search in the retroauricular muscles.

Figure 1 shows the EMG records of a patient with a facial palsy in recovery. On examination of the left m. orb. oris fibrillation potentials could be demonstrated as well as prolonged polyphasic motor unit potentials and a single unit discharge pattern. The records of the right side were normal.

During recovery from facial palsy with nerve fiber degeneration an aberrant regeneration frequently occurs. The resulting synkinesias can be unequivocally separated from other associated movements by means of polygraphic EMG recordings, i.e. from the m. orb. oculi, m. orb. oris and m. mentalis. Synchronous discharges in these muscles identify muscle fibers which are supplied by the same motoneuron as a result of aberrant regeneration.

h) Orbicularis Oculi Reflex

The anatomical, physiological and methodical rationale of the OOR has been described in the section 'Neuro-physiological Diagnosis of the Trigeminal Nerve'. Since the common efferent path for both, the early and the late response, runs in the

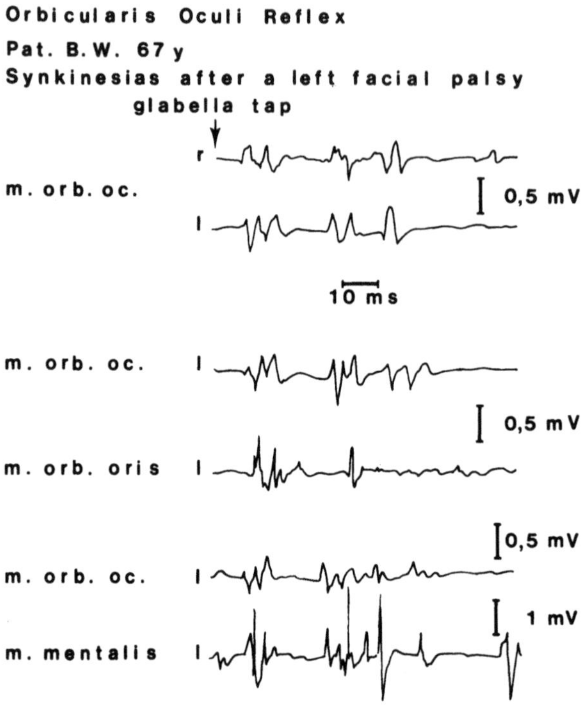

Fig. 2. Orbicularis oculi reflex evoked by glabella tap. Surface electrodes on the lower eyelid, concentric needle electrodes in the m. orb. oris and m. mentalis. A spread of the OOR to the m. orb. oris and m. mentalis can be recognized indicating synkinesias

facial nerve, the OOR has also some importance in testing the function of this nerve. Concerning idiopathic facial palsy, attempts have been made to predict the natural prognosis on the basis of OOR recording combined with determination of the electrically evoked compound action potential of the m. orb. oris (Manz and Schenck, 1975) and of distal latency (Kimura et al., 1976).

Since the OOR in normals can be recorded from the m. orb. oculi, only its demonstration in other facial muscles following facial palsy proves synkinesias (Kimura et al., 1975). In Fig. 2 polygraphic records from the m. orb. oculi, m. orb. oris and m. mentalis in a patient with facial palsy seven years ago show a spread of the OOR to all three muscles as a result of aberrant regeneration.

2. Other Facial Nerve Disorders

It is not the purpose of this article to discuss the applicability of the available neurophysiological tests to any of the numerous facial nerve diseases. Generally can be said that the tests already described in the section concerning idiopathic facial palsy are equally useful in the examination of other facial nerve disorders. Sometimes in lesions due to trauma or to a localized compression by a space occupying process a topographical diagnosis may be desirable. In this context the Schirmer test and the salivation test shall be mentioned which give some clues to the localization of a facial nerve lesion proximal of the branching of the n. petrosus superf. major or the chorda tympani respectively. Additionally two electrodiagnostic tests will be described.

a) Stapedius Reflex

The m. stapedius is the most proximal muscle supplied by the facial nerve. Its contraction results in a change of the impedance of the sound conducting apparatus. This can be measured by means of an appropriate equipment producing acoustic impulses and determining the reactive change of impedance. A loss of the stapedius reflex associated with facial nerve dysfunction points to a lesion site proximal of the branching of the stapedial nerve. Although the value of this test in idiopathic facial palsy seems to be limited (Miehlke, 1973; Chüden, 1978), a preservation in an individual case may predict a good prognosis. In petrosal fractures, however, the test can provide reliable information on the exact site of the lesion (Dieroff, 1964).

b) Electrogustometry

The test has been described by Krarup (1958). Anodal currents of up to 300 mA are applied to the lateral border of the anterior two thirds of the tongue. The threshold currents of the two sides, when a metallic taste is perceived, are compared. A loss of this sensation or a considerable increase of the threshold associated with a facial nerve disorder points to a lesion site proximal of the branching of the chorda tympani. Disorders of the facial nerve involving a decreased conduction velocity can be objectivated by means of the OOR or by determining the distal latency.

Figure 3 shows the OOR of two patients suffering from Charcot-Marie-Tooth disease and a chronic relapsing polyradiculitis respectively. In both cases an extreme delay of the otherwise well preserved early and late components can be recognized. The distal latency was determined in the second patient with 15.5 ms right and 15.0 ms left, by far exceeding the normal range (4 ms).

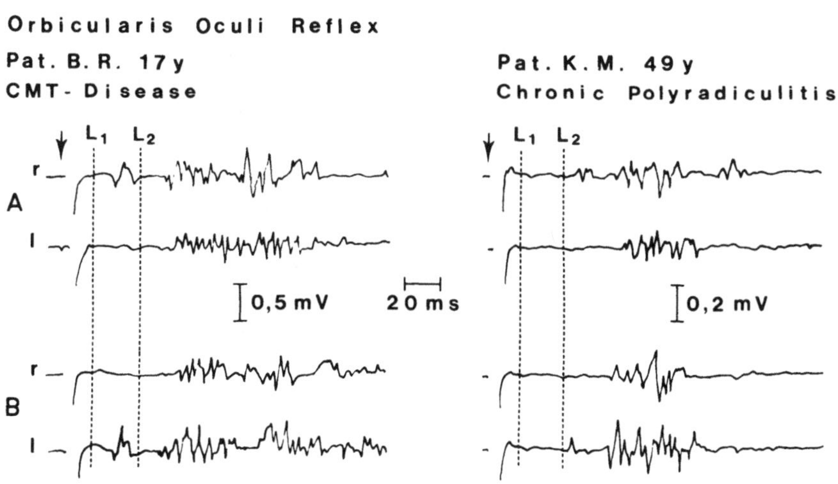

Fig. 3 A, B. Orbicularis oculi reflex evoked by electrical stimulation of the supraorbital nerves. Arrows indicate stimulation on the right **A** and left **B** side. The vertical interrupted lines demonstrate the upper limit of the latencies of the early (*L1*) and the late (*L2*) response. Increased latencies of both responses can easily be recognized in both patients

3. Restorative Operations

Before the indication for a restorative operation can be established the existence of excitable muscle tissue must be assured. This can be performed by direct stimulation of facial muscles in the mode of the strength-duration-curve. More convenient may be the demonstration of insertion- or spontaneous activity in needle electromyography.

Independent of whether facio-facial sutures with or without grafting or spino-facial anastomoses have been carried out, the assessment of reinnervation and of postoperative coordination of the mimic muscles is a domaine of electromyography. Reinnervation potentials, giant motor units, synkinesias and the distribution of these phenomena to the various facial muscles can be easily recognized. Reinnervation by the donor nerve may be proved by polygraphic records involving the tongue in hypoglosso-facial or the m. trapezius in accessory-facial anastomoses demonstrating discharges in facial muscles when the primarily supplied muscle is innervated. In Fig. 4 such simultaneous discharges are demonstrated in a patient having undergone accessory-facial anastomosis.

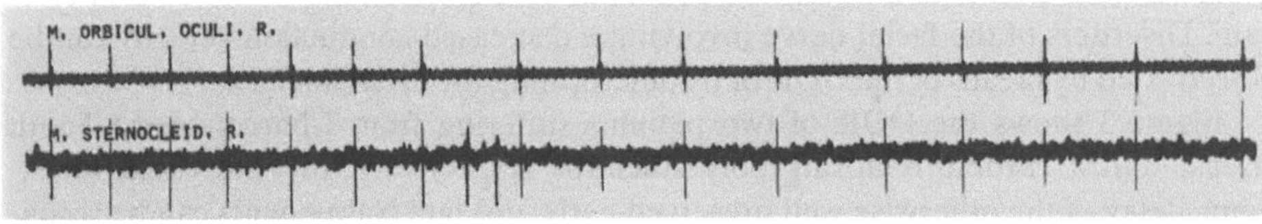

Fig. 4. EMG recorded with concentric needle electrodes in a patient with an accessory-facial anastomosis. Synchronous discharges in the m. orb. oculi and sternocleidomastoideus can be recognized

A very fascinating question is whether after spino-facial anastomosis gross syncinetic movements only or at least partially the former facial muscle function with typical mimic movements may be regained. In addition to careful clinical observation electromyographical analysis of facial muscle functions like spontaneous or reflex blinking can provide conclusive information. Struppler and Dobbelstein (1963) demonstrated an OOR on the operated side in a case of right-sided hypoglosso-facial anastomosis (Fig. 5). This finding was later corroborated by other workers (Kilimov and Linke, 1978; Stennert, 1979). Since the reinnervation of the eyelid muscles by the cut facial nerve was carefully ruled out, a shift of the efferent OOR path from the facial to the hypoglossal nerve must be seriously discussed. Stennert presumes preformed linkages of the afferent trigeminal path and the facial and hypoglossal motoneurons. A controversial question is if peripheral trigemino-facial anastomoses could be involved. A transfer of function, however, seems also to be possible from the facial to the accessory nerve. In Fig. 6 electromyographical evidence of spontaneous blinking on the side of a accessory-facial anastomosis is provided. Note the delay of the EMG activity on the operative right as compared to the left side. Presumably this delay is caused by central factors as the interposition of several interneurons as well as by peripheral factors associated with this type of anastomosis.

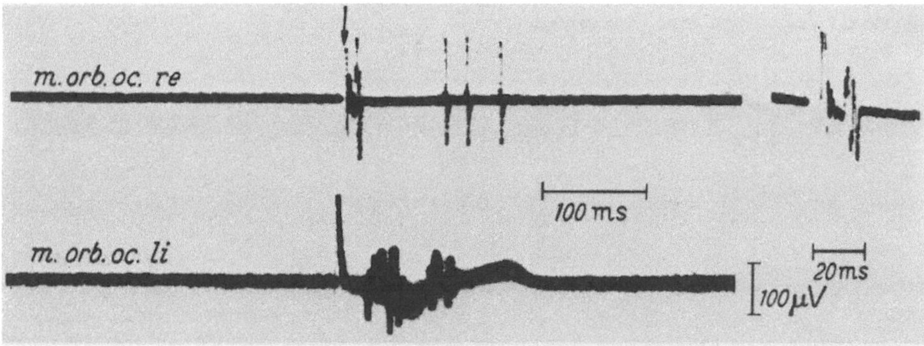

Fig. 5. Right-sided hypoglosso-facial anastomosis. Orbicularis oculi reflex evoked by electrical stimulation of the right supraorbital nerve (arrow). Recording by means of needle electrodes. An early component with a latency of about 16 ms can be recognized in the right m. orb. oculi

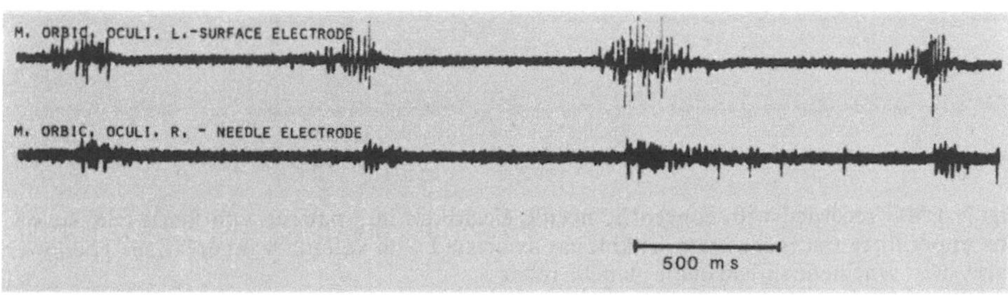

Fig. 6. Right-sided accessory-facial anastomosis. Spontaneous blinking. Recording by means of surface (left) and needle electrodes (right). Note the delayed onset of the EMG activity on the operated side (see text)

In the case of the Lexer-Rosenthal operation the rationale is not only to restore symmetrical face proportions, but also to induce a neurotisation of the facial muscles by trigeminal motoneurons. Struppler and Scheininger (1961) testing exteroceptive reflex inhibition in the masseter and facial muscles, were not able to find evidence in favour of a trigemino-facial neurotisation in the described cases. Clearly this cannot be taken as an argument against reconstructive operations using chewing or free muscle transplants.

4. Spontaneous Facial Movements

Hemispasmus facialis is a disorder with spontaneous burst-like facial movements probably caused by a lesion of the facial nerve after leaving the brain stem (Jacobi et al., 1965; Auger, 1979). By clinical examination alone it can be difficult to distinguish it from conditions like essential blepharospasm, tardive dyskinesia, severe dyskinesias after aberrant nerve regeneration or psychogenic tic. In conventional needle electromyography frequently signs of slight denervation can be detected. On polygraphic EMG examination of several facial muscles, however, synchronous dis-

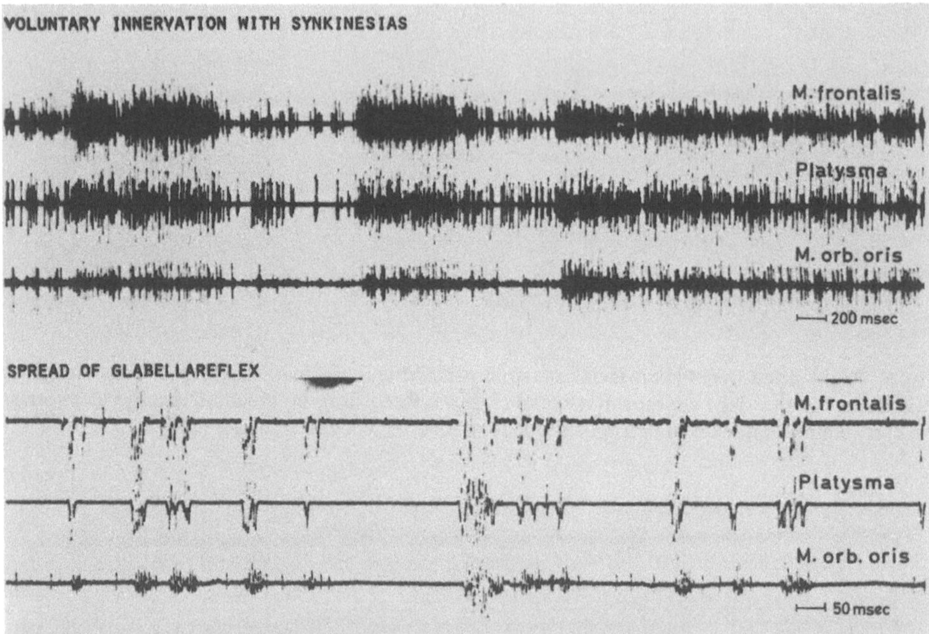

Fig. 7. EMG recorded with concentric needle electrodes in a patient with facial hemispasm. The upper three traces illustrate synkinesias associated with voluntary innervation. The lower traces show syncinetic spread of the glabella reflex

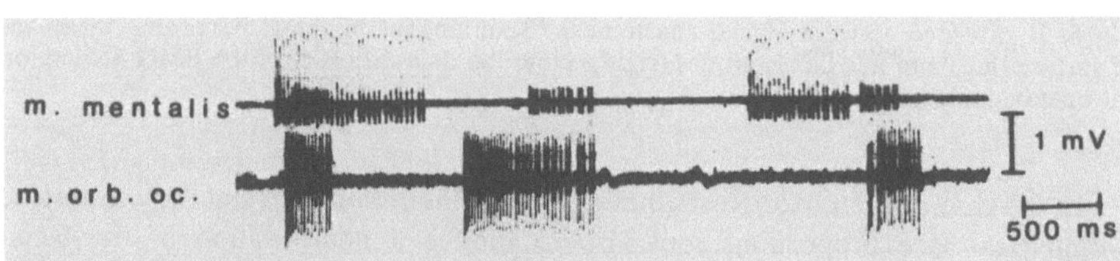

Fig. 8. EMG recorded with concentric needle electrodes in a patient with left-sided facial myokymia. Incoordinated bursts of motor unit discharges with a frequency of up to 50/s can be seen

charges during the spontaneous bursts can be recorded corresponding with typical synkinesias. The same can be seen in testing the OOR during the bursts, whereas in the free interval no synkinesias are present (Auger, 1979). Figure 7 shows a polygraphic EMG record of a patient with facial hemispasm objectivating characteristic synkinesias.

Facial myokymia presents clinically with fine, undulating spontaneous movements of facial muscles, usually affecting one side only. It occurs mainly in multiple sclerosis, rarely in tumors growing near to the facial nucleus and in polyradiculoneuropathy, suggesting an origin of spontaneous discharges in facial motor neurons within the nucleus or in the peripheral course of the nerve (Andermann et al., 1961; Daube et al., 1979).

Figure 8 shows a polygraphic record from the m. orb. oculi and the m. orb. oris in a patient presenting with facial myokymia on the basis of multiple sclerosis. As can be seen, motor units in both muscles spontaneously discharge in short bursts, obviously without any coordination. A firing frequency of about 50/s is achieved.

Discussion

Neurophysiologic investigation of the facial nerve is difficult due to the fact that direct access is limited to the short extracranial course. Within the last two decades various efforts have been made to overcome this difficulty and to substitute the older methods, such as plotting a strenght-duration curve. The aim of all methods is to allow a statement to the natural prognosis of an acute facial palsy as early as possible. For this purpose it is necessary to distinguish between reversible conduction block and nerve fiber degeneration. The basic considerations in the case of idiopathic facial palsy were that an early decompressive operation might prevent further damage from the nerve and should result in a more favourable outcome. Thus, it becomes clear that the development as well as the application of these methods is closely correlated with the evolution and the tendencies in facial nerve surgery.

Generally can be said that it is still not possible to assess the degree of degeneration and the further direction of the process before four to five days have elapsed. In fact, degeneration may be complete only by the tenth or eleventh day (Esslen, 1977). Before this time frequently repeated investigations using the excitability test and the method described by Esslen as well as the clinical experience of the physician may allow to draw conclusions on the further development of the disease and help to decide whether an early decompressive operation may be indicated or not. If the matter is only to assess the natural prognosis the results of additional tests can give valuable clues. Thus, preservation of some volitional activity in the EMG, of the taste sense or the stapedius reflex in an otherwise complete facial palsy as well as an early return of the OOR allow a fair prognosis.

Topographical diagnosis is not very meaningful in idiopathic facial palsy, but has its particular value in intratemporal lesions. Electrodiagnostic measures like the stapedius reflex or electrogustometry can contribute to topographical questions.

Recovery from facial nerve lesions or from restorative operations is best assessed and followed by electromyography. In particular, early signs of reinnervation can be detected at a time when the clinical impression is still that of a complete palsy. Aberrant regeneration leading to synkinesias can be separated from other associated movements by polygraphic EMG records and by a spread of the OOR to muscles other than the orb. oculi.

In the same way spontaneous facial movements like hemispasm or myokymia can be reliably identified by their typical discharge pattern and distinguished from supranuclear disorders or tic-like movements.

Conclusions

Associated with the evolution of new trends in facial nerve surgery, neurophysiologic tests have been developed which shall as early as possible provide information on the natural prognosis and the direction of facial palsies. But to present it is not possible to reliably assess the degree of nerve fibre degeneration before four or more days have elapsed. The described tests are equally useful in the diagnosis of other facial nerve diseases and in the follow-up of decompressive and restorative operations. In conditions with synkinesias and spontaneous facial movements they allow a separation from supranuclear disorders or psychogenic tics.

References

Alford BR (1967) Electrodiagnostic studies in facial paralysis. Arch Otolaryngol 85:259–264
Andermann F, Cosgrove JBR, Lloyd-Smith DL (1961) Facial myokymia in multiple sclerosis. Brain 84:31–44
Auger RG (1979) Hemifacial spasm: clinical and electrophysiologic observations. Neurology (Minneap) 29:1261–1272
Chüden H (1978) Impedanz-Hörprüfung. Urban u. Schwarzenberg, München Wien Baltimore
Daube JR, Kelly JJ, Martin RA (1979) Facial myokymia with polyradiculoneuropathy. Neurology (Minneap) 29:662–669
Dieroff HG (1964) Zur Impedanzprüfung bei intratemporalen Facialisparesen. Z Laryngol Rhinol 43:428
Esslen E (1977) The acute facial palsies. Springer, Berlin Heidelberg New York
Jacobi HA, Jusic A, Struppler A (1965) Hemispasmus facialis – peripher oder zentral bedingt. Proc. 8th Internat. Congress of Neurology. Vienna IV:351–352
Jongkees LBW (1969) Tests for Facial Nerve Function. Arch Otolaryngol 89:127–130
Kilimov N, Linke D (1978) Blink Reflex in Facial-Hypoglossal Anastomosis. Arch Psychiatr Nervenkr 225:307–313
Kimura J, Rodnitzky RL, Okawava S-H (1975) Electrophysiologic analysis of aberrant regeneration after facial nerve paralysis. Neurology (Minneap) 25:989–993
Kimura J, Giron LT, Young SM (1976) Electrophysiological study of bell palsy. Arch Otolaryngol 102:140–143
Laumans EPJ (1965) Nerve Excitability Tests in Facial Paralysis. Arch Otolaryngol 81:478–488
Manz F, Schenk E (1975) Orbicularis Oculi Reflexe und Summenpotentiale des Orbicularis oris bei idiopathischer Facialislähmung. J Neurol 210:271–281
May M (1977) Maximal Excitability Test. In: Fisch U (ed) Facial Nerve Surgery. Kugler, Amstelveen, p 87–92
Miehlke A (1973) Surgery of the Facial Nerve. Urban und Schwarzenberg, München Berlin Wien. WB Saunders, Philadelphia London Toronto
Stennert E (1979) I. Hypoglossal Facial Anastomosis: Its Significance for Modern Facial Surgery. II. Combined Approach in Extratemporal Facial Nerve Reconstruction. Clin Plast Surg 6:471–485
Struppler A, Scheininger R (1961) Elektromyographische Untersuchungen zur Frage der Innervationsübernahme im Bereich motorischer Hirnnerven beim Menschen. Pfluegers Arch 274:48
Taverner D (1965) Electrodiagnosis in Facial Palsy. Arch Otolaryngol 81:470–477

Indications and Operative Technique for Endoscopy of the Cerebellopontine Angle

F. OPPEL, G. MULCH, M. BROCK, and D. ZÜHLKE, Berlin/FRG

Introduction

Considerable progress in the field of early recognition of processes of the cerebellopontine angle and the internal auditory meatus has been made in recent years thanks to the development of new audiological methods, improved vestibular function tests and cisternography (Fisch and Wegmüller, 1974; Mulch, 1978; Zöllner et al., 1978). At present the surgical technique aims at preserving the facial and, if possible, the cochlear nerve (House, 1961; Samii, 1979; Yaşargil, 1978). Depending on tumor size, optimal tumor removal is achieved either by transtemporal, translabyrinthine or by lateral suboccipital approach.

A prerequisite for the choice of the surgical access is precise knowledge of the location and extent of the tumor. In this respect, diagnostic uncertainty is still frequent in the presence of small tumors of the internal auditory meatus or of the cerebellopontine angle. In addition to neuro-otological findings, the most reliable diagnostic information is provided by plain roentgenograms and cisternography. However, these studies do not always give exact information about the size, extent and type of tumor. Computerized tomography (CT), with and without parenteral or intrathecal application of contrast medium, angiography and pneumencephalography, frequently yields no findings in the presence of small tumors.

Based on post mortem studies, Prott (1974) demonstrated the possibility of examining the cerebellopontine angle by endoscopy. He used a transpyramidal, retrolabyrinthine approach through Trautmann's triangle, as already described in the nineteen forties and fifties for draining of the basal cisterns in cases of otogenic meningitis (Link, 1950; Moser, 1952; Mündnich, 1950; Zöllner, 1944). Endoscopy offers the advantage of permitting detailed visualization of the cerebellopontine angle: the entire posterior surface of the pyramid, including its apex and the porus acusticus internus, a part of the floor of the posterior fossa including the jugular foramen as well as the cranial nerves V to XI. First clinical experiences confirmed the diagnostic value of the method (Ehrenberger et al., 1976 and 1978; Mulch and Oppel, 1979; Oppel et al., 1978). Further experience was gained when the indication for cisternoscopy was extended to therapeutic interventions for neurotomy of the nerves V, IX and X (Oppel et al., 1979 and 1980). The diagnostic value of this method is illustrated and discussed in the present paper.

Indications

Diagnostic endoscopy of the cerebellopontine angle is indicated in cases in which there is suspicion of small space-occupying processes in the cerebellopontine angle and the internal auditory meatus, not satisfactorily demonstrable by neuroradiological methods. Typical examples are: 1. when there is only a minor CT-finding which does not permit a precise determination of the tumor size and, thus, optimal choice of surgical procedure; 2. when there is an isolated dysfunction of the cranial nerves located in the cerebellopontine angle; 3. when a tumor of the petrous bone growing into the cerebellopontine angle is suspected in cases with cranial nerve involvement only.

Material

Commercially available arthroscopes are used for endoscopy; they have an 18 cm long shaft and a diameter of 2.7 or 3.8 mm. They are equipped with 0°, 30° and 70° angular optics. Photo and film facilities are available for documentation. The instruments consist of maleable microdissectors, scissors, forceps and an insulated electrode.

Surgical Procedure

The mastoid is exposed with the patient supine having the head turned to the side opposite to exposure. Prior to this, lumbar cerebrospinal fluid (CSF)-drainage is performed. The sigmoid sinus, the posterior vertical semicircular canal, and the su-

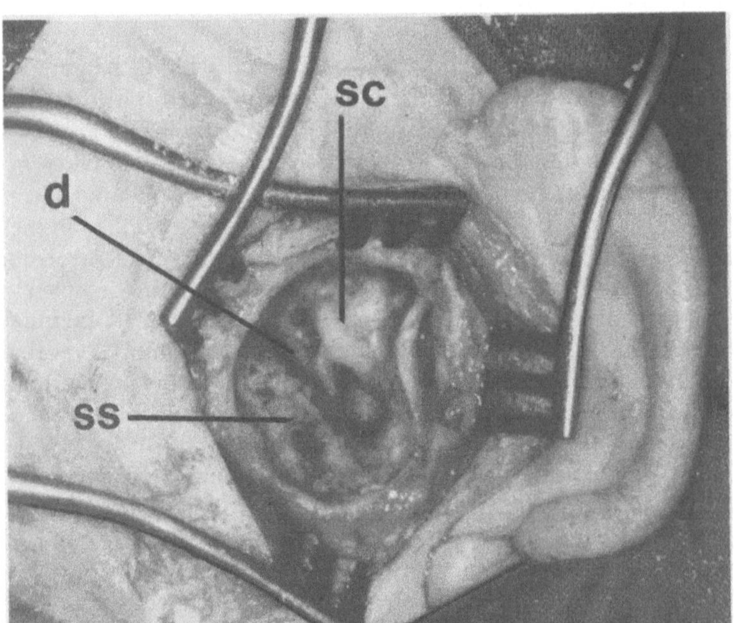

Fig. 1. Surgical approach through a retroauricular skin incision (approximately 4 cm). Trautmann's triangle is exposed. The outer diameter of the bone defect is approximately two cm; the exposed surface of the dura of the posterior cranial fossa is of approximately ten by six mm (*d:* dura; *sc:* posterior semicircular canals; *ss:* sigmoid sinus)

perior petrosal sinus are visualized by an antrotomy. The dura of the posterior fossa is exposed in the area of the Trautmann's triangle (Fig. 1). The short incudal limb is used for orientation. The bony shell above the sigmoid sinus must be completely removed. An angular dural incision follows while preserving the endolymphatic sac. The endoscope, freely moved by hand, is now inserted extra-arachnoidally towards the apex of the pyramid (Fig. 2). Small dural adhesions are detached by blunt dis-

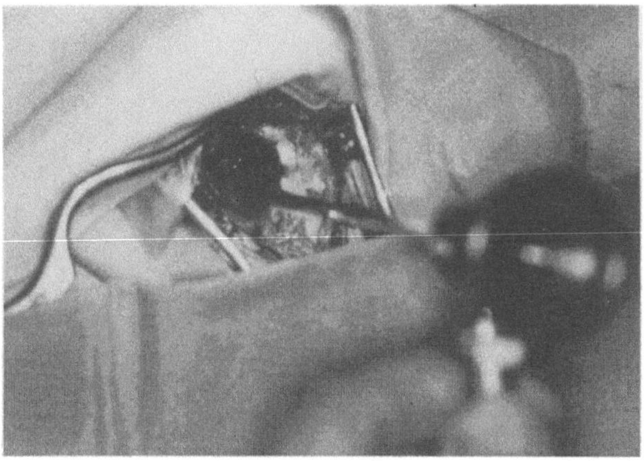

Fig. 2. Operative site, the endoscope being directed towards the apex of the pyramid

section. Arachnoid vessels can be coagulated and sectioned. The instruments are inserted side by side to the endoscope. For assessment of the cranial nerves V, VI and IX to XI, the lateral pontine cistern must be opened. Tumor tissue can be obtained by biopsy. Best visibility is achieved with the 30° angular optic. At the end of the endoscopy, CSF is replaced by saline, and the dura is sutured watertight. Additional gluing has proven effective in the prevention of CSF-leakage. The short incudal limb should be protected by insertion of a silicon strip. The bone defect is covered by a pediculated temporal muscle flap.

Results

We have to present performed seven diagnostic endoscopies. A suspected tumor was confirmed in all patients; in five there was an acoustic neurinoma, part of the tumor protruding into the posterior fossa for 2 to 25 mm, and a meningioma growing en plaques. In one patient, there was a cholesteatoma of the petrous bone, which, however, had not infiltrated or perforated the dura. Tables 1 and 2 provide a summary, and Figures 3 to 7 show the findings in these cases.

No complications occured in the seven endoscopic examinations with diagnostic purpose. However, it must be pointed out that of the 27 endoscopies performed so far, a CSF-fistula had to be corrected in two patients, and a slight conductive deafness remained in three, due to adhesions of the short incudal limb. More recently it has become possible to avoid these complications.

Table 1. Pre-endoscopic findings in the seven patients studied. With the exception of patient 4, the main finding was vestibular hypoexcitability on the side of the tumor. There was unequivocal deafness of retrocochlear type only in the patients with an acoustic neurinoma larger than 10 mm in the posterior fossa (patients 2 and 7) (see Tab. 2), and in the patient with the extradural tumor of the petrous bone (case Nr. 3). The findings were variable (–/+) in patients with a tumor of less than 10 mm. There was a widening of the internal auditory meatus in all patients with an acoustic neurinoma. Emphasis should be placed on the CT-findings, which may be dubious (+) in the presence of larger tumors, and indicate a rather small tumor. Vertebral angiography is of secondary importance for diagnosis of small tumors. (ϕ = not examined)

Patients age/sex	(1) R. H. 56/(f)	(2) W. U. 57/(f)	(3) B. R. 31/(m)	(4) L. R. 41/(m)	(5) M. M. 39/(f)	(6) K. E. 67/(f)	(7) T. J. 57/(f)
Pre-endoscopic findings							
Disturbances of the cranial nerves	V, VII, VIII	VIII	VII, VIII	VIII	VIII	VIII	VIII
Retrocochlear type of deafness	ϕ	+	+	–/+	–/+	–/+	+
Significant reduced vestibular excitability	+	+	+	–	+	+	+
X-ray-findings:							
Widening of the internal acoustic meatus	–	+	–	+	+	+	+
Cisternography	–	+	ϕ	+	+	+	+
CT	–	(+)	–	–	–	–	(+)
Angiography	–	–	–	–	–	–	–

Table 2. Endoscopic and histological findings in the seven patients examined, as well as specification of the surgical procedure chosen on the basis of the endoscopic finding. The histological findings relate to material obtained at biopsy in three cases. Noteworthy is the surprising extent of the finding in patients 1, 2, and 7, which was unexpected in view of the preliminary examinations. (ϕ = not studied)

Patients age/sex	(1) R. H. 56/(f)	(2) W. U. 57/(f)	(3) B. R. 31/(m)	(4) L. R. 41/(m)	(5) M. M. 39/(f)	(6) K. E. 67/(f)	(7) T. J. 57/(f)
Endoscopic findings	en plaque growing meningeoma	acoustic neurinoma	bulging of the dura	acoustic neurinoma	acoustic neurinoma	acoustic neurinoma	acoustic neurinoma
Biopsy	+	+	–	+	–	–	–
Histological findings	meningeoma	neurinoma	ϕ	neurinoma	ϕ	ϕ	ϕ
Location of the tumor	apex of the pyramid	int. acoustic porus	pyramid	int. acoustic porus	int. acoustic porus	int. acoustic porus	int. acoustic porus
Extent of the tumor	whole post. surface of the pyramid	25 mm	extradural	8 mm	2 mm	3 mm	15 mm
Subsequent surgical intervention	lat. suboccipital	lat. suboccipital	temporal extradural	translabyrinthine (same session)	transtemporal	translabyrinthine (same session)	lat. suboccipital

Discussion

The present experience with 27 endoscopies of the cerebellopontine angle for various indications shows that this procedure is highly effective and involves few complications. Only diagnostic endoscopy is discussed here. All the patients examined had long-term history of a hearing loss with varying audiological and neuro-otological findings. Table 1 contains only the findings immediately prior to the endoscopic intervention. Especially in the presence of very small tumors (cases 4, 5, 6; Figs. 3, 4, 5; Table 2), the audiological findings did not yield any clear indication or a retrocochlear lesion. The suspicion of an acoustic neurinoma arose supplementary to the positive radiological findings, which, however, did not permit an exact statement about the size of the tumor (CT: neg.). Only patients 2 and 7 (Fig. 6) showed uniform findings. Endoscopy was performed in these cases due to the dubious CT-findings, which indicated a rather small tumor. Patient 1, who showed the most extensive endoscopic finding, had the least clinical symptoms and a 5 year history. In one case (patient 3; Fig. 7) with a primary cholesteatoma of the petrous bone, the diagnosis seemed clear, but an infiltration of the tumor into the posterior fossa could not be ruled out except by endoscopy.

Endoscopy not only allows confirmation of the diagnosis, but also permits complete translabyrinthine removal of the tumor in the same session, if the patient is

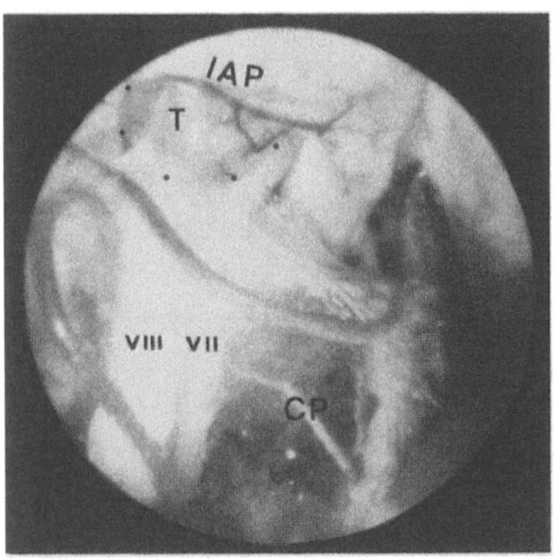

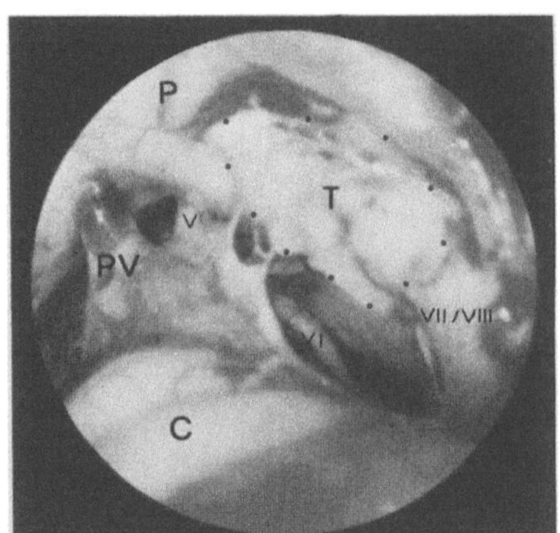

Fig. 3 **Fig. 4**

Fig. 3. Intrameatal acoustic neurinoma (*T*) (left side) extending only two mm beyond the porus acusticus internus (*IAP*). The cranial nerves VII and VIII can be well differentiated. The lateral pontine cistern (*CP*) has not been opened

Fig. 4. Intrameatal acoustic neurinoma (*T*) (right side) growing in a medial direction on the dorsal surface of the pyramid and extending three mm beyond the porus acusticus internus. The tumor adhered the cerebellum (*C*) by way of vascular bridges, which were endoscopically detached. The cranial nerves V, VI, VII and VIII are clearly recognizable. (*P*=pyramid; *PV*=petrosal vein)

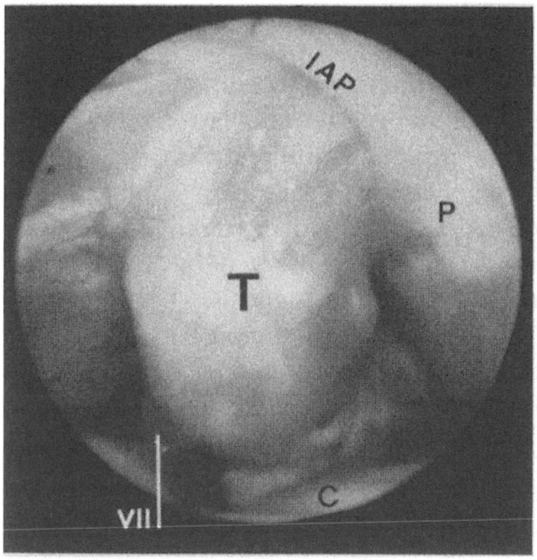

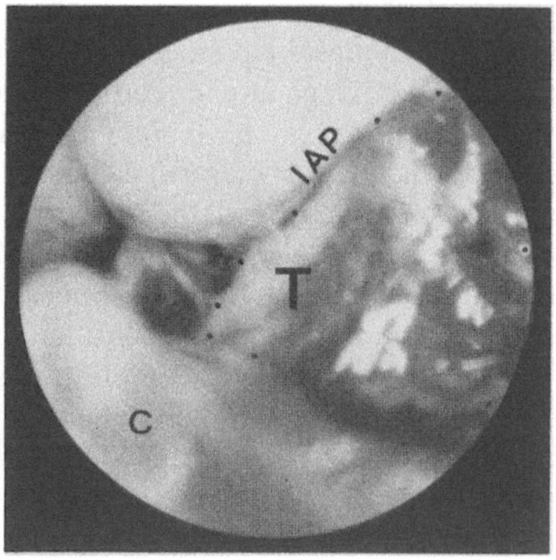

Fig. 5 **Fig. 6**

Fig. 5. An acoustic neurinoma (*T*) (left side) already dissected, projecting eight mm into the cerebellopontine angle. The porus acusticus internus (*IAP*) is considerably widened. The facial nerve (*VII*) can still be clearly differentiated. (*P* = pyramid; *C* = cerebellum)

Fig. 6. Acoustic neurinoma (*T*) (right side) which had grown into the cerebellopontine angle for an extension of 15 mm, as demonstrated by subsequent suboccipital exposure. It had been impossible, in this case, to dissect the tumor by endoscopic route. (*IAP* = porus acusticus internus; *C* = cerebellum)

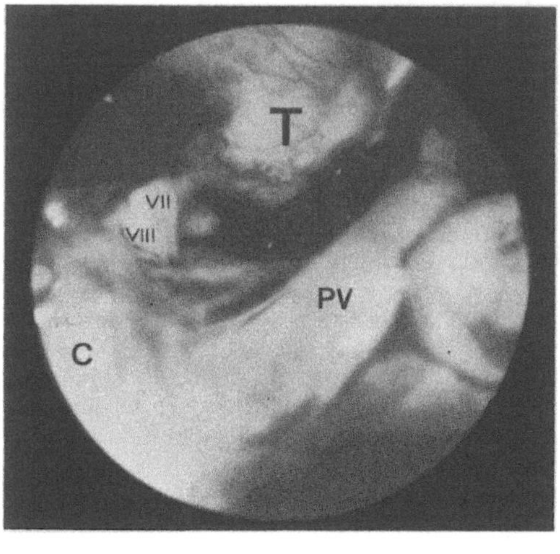

Fig. 7. Endoscopic view in patient three (left side). The dura of the posterior surface of the pyramid protrudes rostrally to the porus (*T*), which is concealed by a drop of blood, but is intact. The branched petrous vein (*PV*) is visible in front and to the right. (*C* = cerebellum; *VII* and *VIII* = cranial nerves)

already deaf. Previous endoscopic freeing of the tumor substantially facilitates this procedure. It must be pointed out that sufficient space and visibility are obtained by controlled drainage of CSF and preoperative treatment with dexamethasone alone. Vascular damage can be avoided by coagulation of even the smallest vessels. Smaller hemorrhages (a few drops) can occur following contact of the endoscope with the retropetrous dura or with the surface of the cerebellum, but they stop spontaneously in a very short time. Suction can easily be performed with a small silicon tube. Hearing loss caused by arachnitic adhesions such as observed by Ehrenberger et al., 1976 and 1978, must be considered in the differential diagnosis.

The above mentioned complications can be avoided by the measures discussed here. It should be stated that patients with slight residual conductive deafness caused by adhesions of the short incudal limb regained normal hearing power after local revision under local anesthesia.

Conclusions

Diagnostic endoscopy of the cerebellopontine angle should be restricted to those cases in which, according to the specified indications, a tumor of the internal auditory meatus or of the cerebellopontine angle is suspected, but cannot be clearly demonstrated by other methods. Our experience, based on 27 endoscopies, seven of them for diagnostic purpose, have shown that this very small procedure, causing a bone defect of maximal 2 cm diameter, can be performed without risk in co-operation with the otosurgeon. In seven patients with a long-term history of hearing loss, the diagnosis of a tumor could be confirmed and its size determined. This allowed the choice of the optimal surgical technique for each patient.

References

Ehrenberger K, Innitzer J, Koos W (1976) Erfolgreiche Akustikusdekompression bei postarachnitischen Hörschäden. Laryngol Rhinol Otol (Stuttg) 55:561–566

Ehrenberger K (1978) Endoscopy of the cerebellopontine angle. Endoscopy 10:260–264

Fisch U, Wegmüller A (1974) Early diagnosis of acoustic neuromas. ORL 36:129

House WF (1961) Surgical exposure of the internal auditory canal and its contents through the middle cranial fossa. Laryngoscope 11:1363–1385

Link R (1950) Die herdnahe Behandlung der otogenen Meningitis durch Basalzisternendrainage. Arch Otorhinolaryngol (NY) 158:453–458

Moser F (1952) Über örtliche cysternale Penicillinanwendung bei otorhinogener Meningitis. HNO 3:250

Mündnich K (1950) Zur Zisternendrainage der Meningitis. Ohrenheilk. 84:297–298

Mulch G (1978) Zur Frühdiagnose der Tumoren des Kleinhirnbrückenwinkels. HNO 26:258–264

Mulch G, Oppel F (1979) Erfahrungen mit der Endoskopie des Kleinhirnbrückenwinkels. Arch Otorhinolaryngol (NY) 223:460–463

Oppel F, Zeytountchian CH, Mulch G, Kunft HD (1978) Endoscopy of the cerebellopontine angle: Its diagnostic and therapeutic possibilities. In: Frowein RA, Wilcke O, Karimi-Nejad A, Brock M, Klinger M (eds) Advances in neurosurgery, vol 5. Springer, Berlin Heidelberg New York, p 269–275

Oppel F, Mulch G (1979) Selective trigeminal root section via an endoscopic transpyramidal retrolabyrinthine approach. Acta Neurochir Suppl 28:565–571

Oppel F, Mulch G, Brock M (1980) Endoscopic section of the trigeminal root, the glossopharyngeal nerve and the cranial part of the vagus for intractable facial pain caused by upper jaw carcinoma. Surgical Neurology (in press)
Prott W (1974) Möglichkeiten einer Endoskopie des Kleinhirnbrückenwinkels auf transpyramidalem-retrolabyrinthärem Zugangsweg – Cisternoscopie. HNO 22:337–341
Samii M (1979) Operative treatment of cerebellopontine angle tumors with special consideration of the facial and the acoustic nerve. In: Marguth F, Brock M, Kazner E, Klinger M, Schmiedek P (eds) Advances in neurosurgery, vol 7. Springer, Berlin Heidelberg New York, p 138–145
Yaşargil MG (1978) Mikrochirurgie der Kleinhirnbrückenwinkeltumoren. In: Plester D, Wende S, Nakayama N (eds) Kleinhirnbrückenwinkeltumoren. Springer, Berlin Heidelberg New York, p 215–257
Zöllner F (1944) Verfahren zum Aufsuchen und Entleeren tiefer subduraler Eiterherde an der Schädelbasis. Z Hals-Nas-Ohr-Heilk 49: 183–189
Zöllner CH, Karnahl TH, Weigel K (1978) Elektrische Reaktionsaudiometrie (Hirnstammpotentiale und späte Potentialkomponente N_1) bei Patienten mit Akustikusneurinom oder raumforderndem Prozeß im Bereich des Hirnstammes. Neurochirurgia (Stuttg) 21: 191–208

Preservation and Reconstruction of the Facial Nerve in the Cerebellopontine Angle

M. Samii, Hannover/FRG

The portion of the facial nerve in the cerebellopontine angle, with a length of 23 to 24 mm, is endangered by space occupying processes. About 71 percent of all tumors of the cerebellopontine angle are acoustic neurinomas. During the growth of a cerebellopontine angle tumor, facial nerve function remains intact for a long time. Primary intrameatal tumors with extension into the cerebellopontine angle sometimes result in early paralysis, especially when arising from the facial nerve itself. In the cerebellopontine angle, the position and course of the facial nerve may be displaced in different directions by space occupying processes. The identification of the facial nerve may prove to be extremely difficult during tumor surgery. Accurate exposure and preservation or reconstruction of the continuity of the facial nerve through microsurgical technique during removal of the cerebellopontine angle tumors should be part of the modern surgical concept.

As a neurosurgeon, I would like to underline the fact that, due to the delicate location of the tumor next to the brain stem, our first aim in the removal of an acoustic neurinoma is to save the life of the patient.

The second aim is to remove the tumor totally in order to avoid a recurrence. Our final aim is the preservation of the facial nerve or its reconstruction when traumatized.

The neurosurgical lateral suboccipital approach of the cerebellopontine angle permits either dorsolateral of dorsocaudal exposure of the tumor. After retracting the cerebellum craniomedially, the caudal cranial nerves often slightly compressed by the tumor must be identified and freed from the tumor capsule.

Immediate identification of the facial nerve in the cerebellopontine angle will be possible only in those patients in whom the tumor is relatively small (Fig. 1a and Fig. 2a). The condition after total removal of the tumor is seen in Fig. 1b. The posterior wall of the internal auditory canal is removed and the tumor dissected from all fascicles of the seventh and eighth cranial nerves. In this case the tumor, two centimeter in diameter, has not reached the brain stem.

Next is demonstrated a small acoustic neurinoma with enlargement of the internal auditory canal and extension into the cerebellopontine angle up to the brain stem (Fig. 2a). After partial removal, the tumor can be isolated from the brain stem as well as the anterior inferior cerebellar artery (Fig. 2b). The tumor originates from some fascicle of the vestibular nerve (Fig. 2c) so that the continuity of the facial and cochlear nerve may be preserved. The facial nerve in such a case can be traumatized just in front of the internal auditory canal. Removal of the posterior wall of the internal auditory canal guarantees total tumor removal and the preservation of the facial nerve (Fig. 2d).

When there is a large tumor (Fig. 3a), the facial nerve is not visible at the brain stem or in the internal auditory meatus. Starting from a five to ten mm opening of

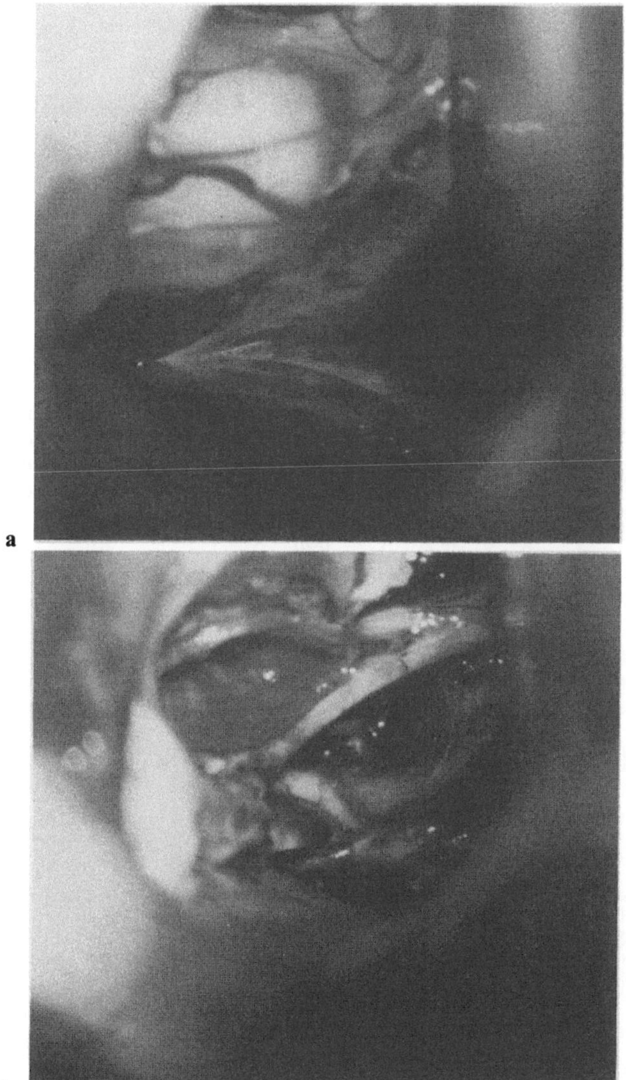

Fig. 1 a, b. Small intrameatal neurinoma with extension into the cerebellopontine angle without compression of the brain stem. The two cm size tumor is located between the fascicles of the seventh and eighth cranial nerves (**a**). The posterior wall of the internal auditory canal is removed and the tumor which was arising only from one small fascicle of the vestibular nerve is dissected from all fascicles of the seventh and eighth cranial nerves and totally removed. The preoperative function of both nerves was completely preserved (**b**)

the tumor capsule, reduction of tumor size is performed using the operating microscope. Thus the tumor capsule loses its primary tension. By gradual resection of the tumor capsule the facial nerve can be identified at the brain stem (Fig. 3 b).

Any direct manipulation of the facial nerve in the cerebellopontine angle may lead to postoperative loss of function. The continuity of the nerve must be preserved. The facial nerve, therefore, must be followed from the brain stem to the internal auditory meatus under highest magnification and with extreme patience and caution.

The nerve may not be detached from the tumor capsule, but the tumor capsule itself must be dissected carefully from the nerve using microsurgical instruments.

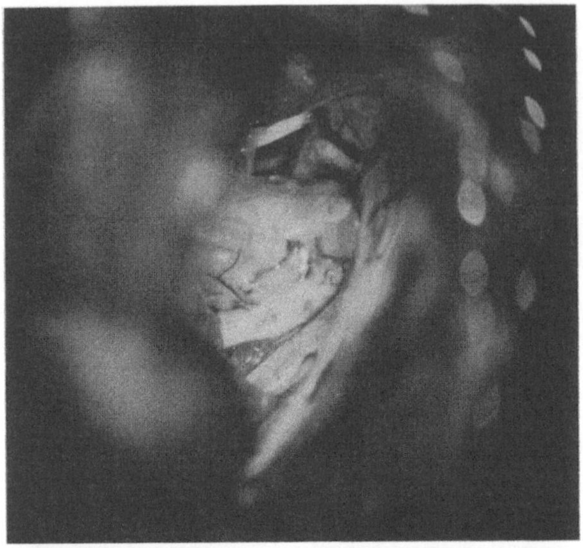

Fig. 2a. Exposure of the right cerebellopontine angle. The tumor reaches the brain stem and is compressing the seventh and eighth in dorso-caudal direction

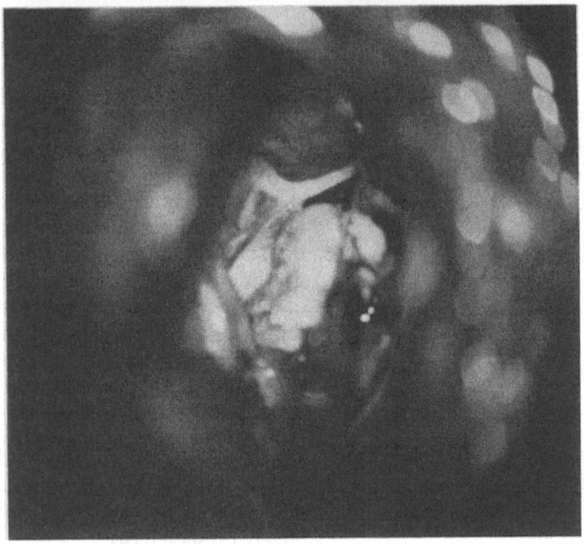

Fig. 2b. After partial removal the tumor is isolated from the brain stem as well as the anterior inferior cerebellar artery

Stretching of the nerve, with its adhesion to the tumor capsule, must be strictly avoided. The tumor capsule may be slightly stretched with one hand while with a microsurgical scissors in the other hand the membrane between the tumor capsule and the nerve is precisely transected. Not infrequently the nerve, owing to an expansive compression, is stretched around the tumor capsule as a thin surface of approximately two to three cm. The preservation of the continuity and function of the facial nerve in such a case is quite difficult. However, it is technically possible (Fig. 3c).

The facial nerve may be preserved in its continuity in two thirds of all cerebellopontine angle tumors by using microsurgical technique and observing the

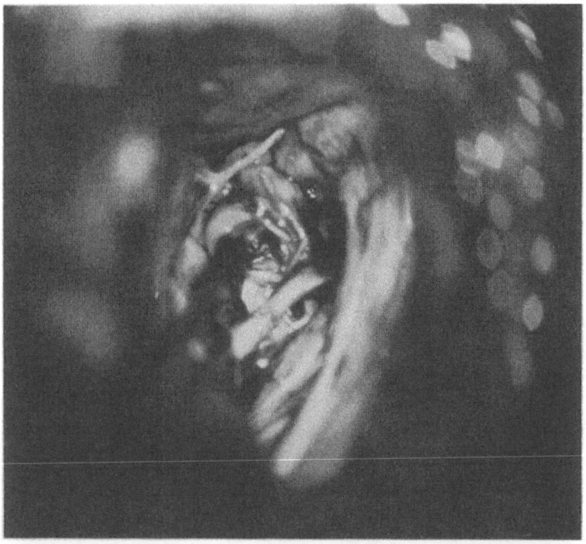

Fig. 2c. At the internal acoustic porus one can see that the rest of the tumor originates from some fascicles of the vestibular nerve

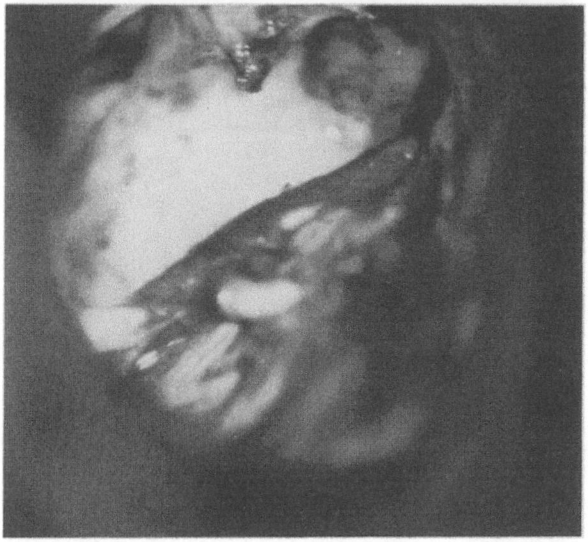

Fig. 2d. Total extirpation of the tumor after removal of the posterior lip of the internal auditory canal. The facial and cochlear nerves are preserved in continuity

above mentioned principles (Drake, 1973; Yaşargil, 1973, 1977; Hitselberger and House, 1973; Koos et al., 1973). If the facial nerve is injured in one area the surgeon should still continue the preparation of the nerve. Because of the tumor growth in the region of the cerebellopontine angle, the nerve becomes stretched in length so that in the event of interruption of continuitiy and loss of substance of about one and a half centimeter during tumor extirpation, one is still able to perform an end-to-end suture without any tension (Fig. 4a and b). Because the results of suture of the facial nerve in the cerebellopontine angle are satisfactory and are superior to any other intervention, the effort towards reconstruction of the continuity of the facial nerve through nerve suture at the cerebellopontine angle is a rewarding task.

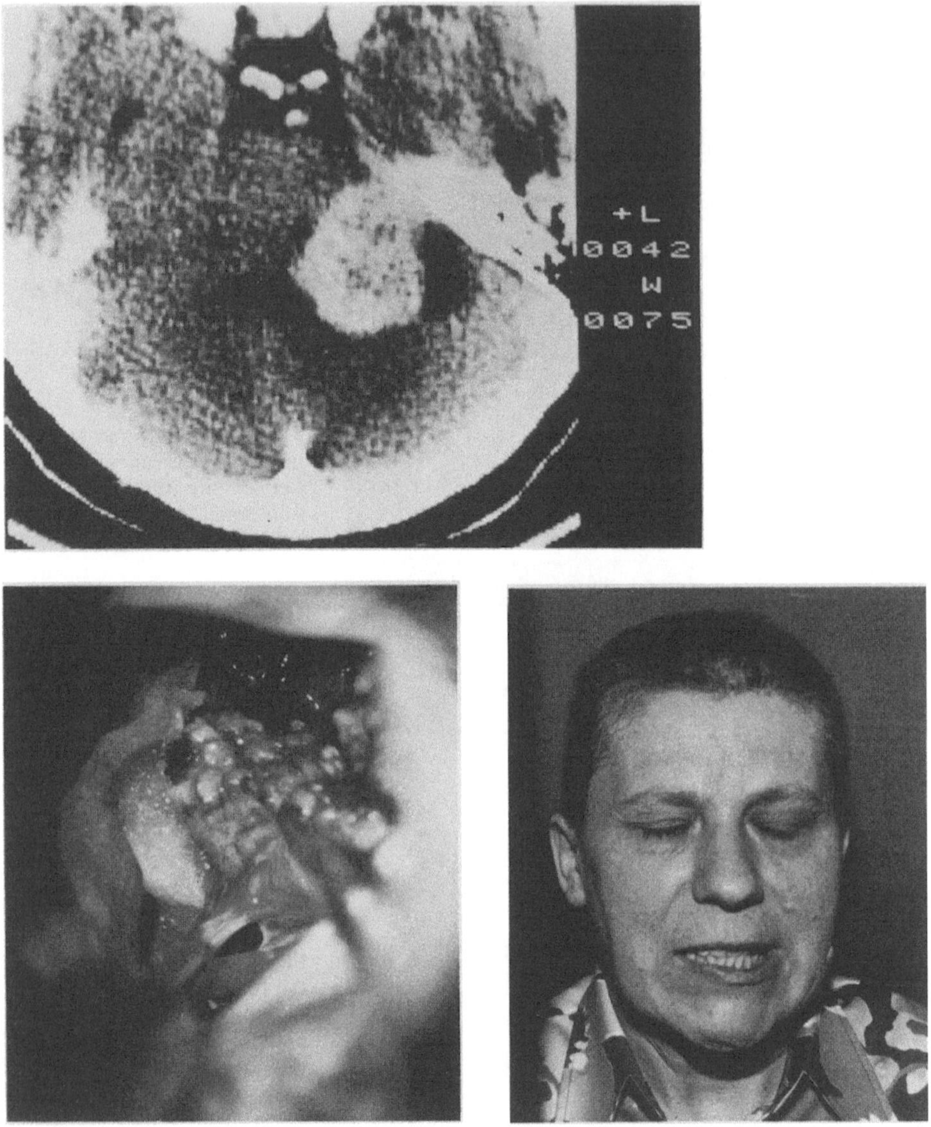

a b c

Fig. 3a. CT scan of a right-sided neurinoma of the cerebellopontine angle

Fig. 3b. By gradual resection of the large neurinoma in the right cerebellopontine angle the facial nerve is identified at the brain stem

Fig. 3c. Postoperative facial nerve function of the same patient as Fig. 3b

In cases of large defects of the facial nerve end-to-end-suture is impossible and a nerve graft has to be performed. Identification of the distal nerve stump at the internal auditory meatus is hardly possible when the tumor grows in cone-shaped fashion into the auditory canal. Even electrostimulation cannot help to distinguish

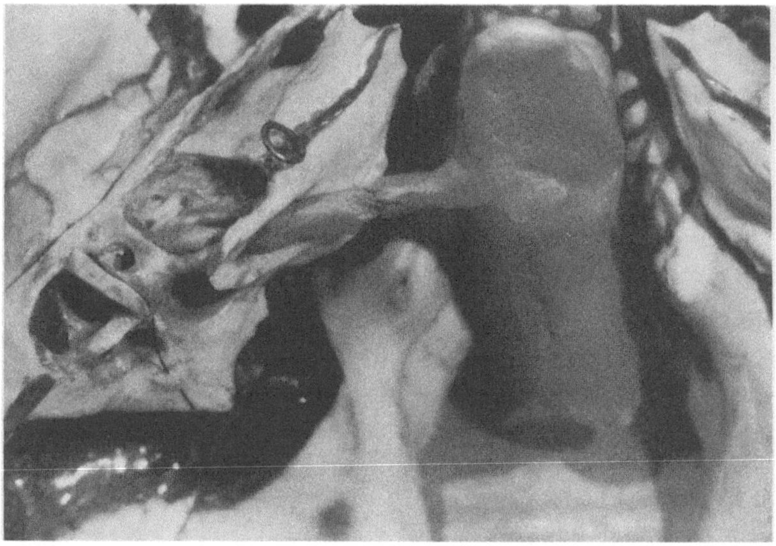

Fig. 4a. Model of the facial nerve in the cerebellopontine angle after interruption of continuity and end-to-end suture

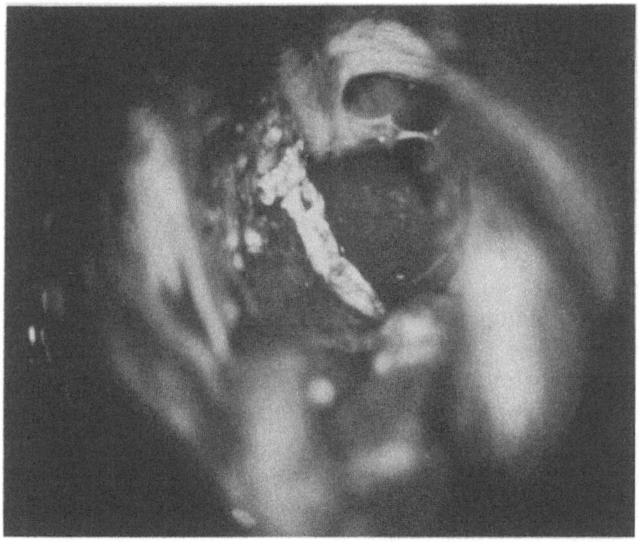

Fig. 4b. After removal of a very large left-sided acoustic neurinoma with interruption of continuity of the facial nerve, an end-to-end suture in the cerebellopontine angle is accomplished

the distal stump of the facial nerve from the vestibulo-cochlear nerve. Stimulation of each distal stump of the facial nerve causes a contraction of the face muscles. Dott (1958), therefore, recommended the intracranial-extratemporal repair of the facial nerve grafts of 15 to 20 cm in length (Fig. 5). The method of Dott is performed in

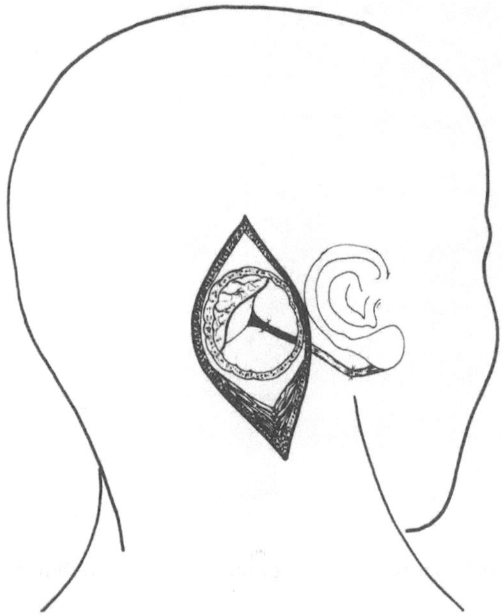

Fig. 5. Intracranial-extratemporal repair of the facial nerve using nerve graft according to the method of Dott

two stages. The first stage is the suture of the graft to the central stump of the facial nerve. The nerve graft is led out of the skull through the craniotomy. The graft is then passed through a tunnel below the mastoid between the sternocleidomastoid and the splenius capitis muscles. The distal end of the graft is marked with a silver clip and fixed in the retromandibular fossa. In a second stage, three months later, the distal end is found and anastomosed to the peripheral end of the facial nerve in front of the stylomastoid foramen.

We have used this method in a 46 year old man with a large left acoustic neurinoma. He previously had undergone an enucleation of the left eye because of angiomatosis retinae. Here we achieved a good result 18 months after the operation.

In 1958, Dott reported his results in four patients. He had achieved satisfactory results in two, and in the other two the results were excellent. After performing the operation in five patients, Drake (1960) was able to achieve good results in four. In 1962, Loew published one case he had operated upon with Miehlke where the result was good. In 1967, Miehlke and Bushe also achieved a good result with this technique in one case.

It seems somewhat surprising after Dott's publication in 1958 that despite the good results achieved with this method, we have found only seven registered cases over the last twenty years. This is probably due to the fact that the exposure of the facial nerve at the brain stem in very large acoustic neurinomas, without the use of an operating microscope and microsurgical technique, is too difficult. Now, that microsurgical operations have become somewhat routine, one can expect that, in the future, the operative treatment of cerebellopontine angle lesions will include reconstruction of the facial nerve.

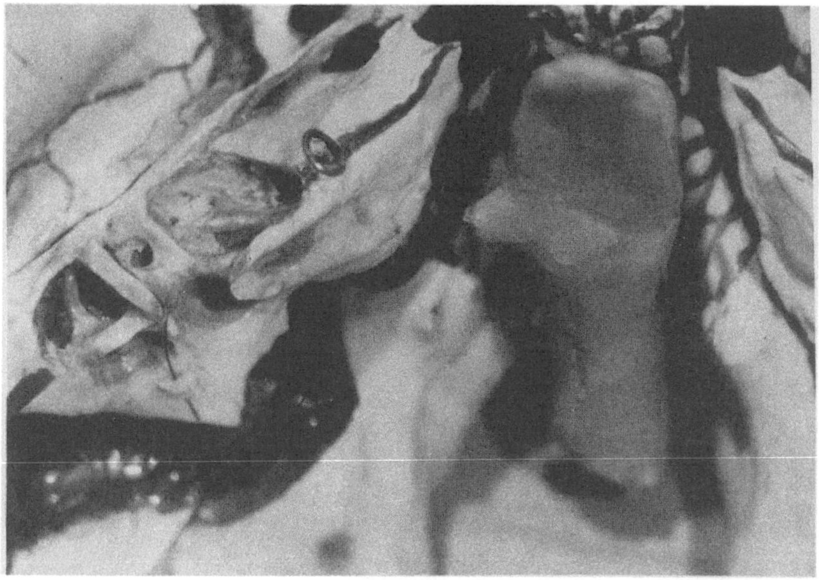

Fig. 6a. Model of a nerve defect of the facial nerve in the cerebellopontine angle and internal auditory canal

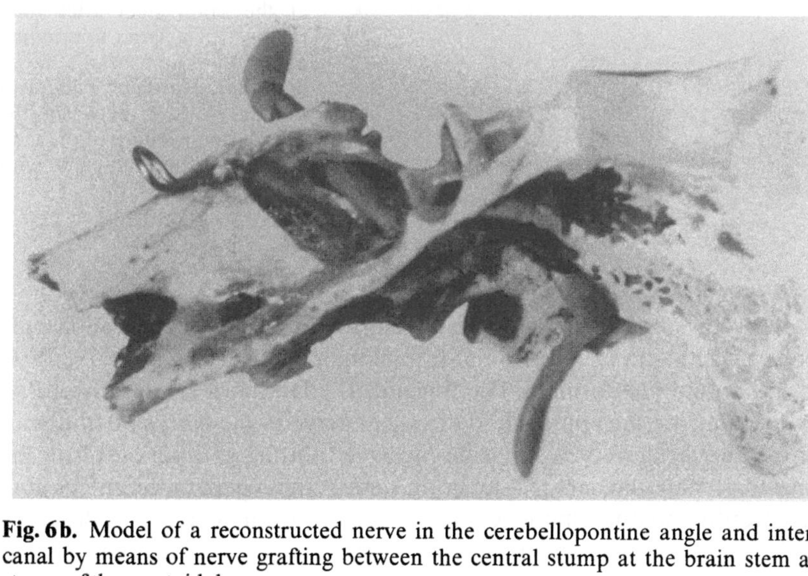

Fig. 6b. Model of a reconstructed nerve in the cerebellopontine angle and internal auditory canal by means of nerve grafting between the central stump at the brain stem and the distal stump of the mastoidal course

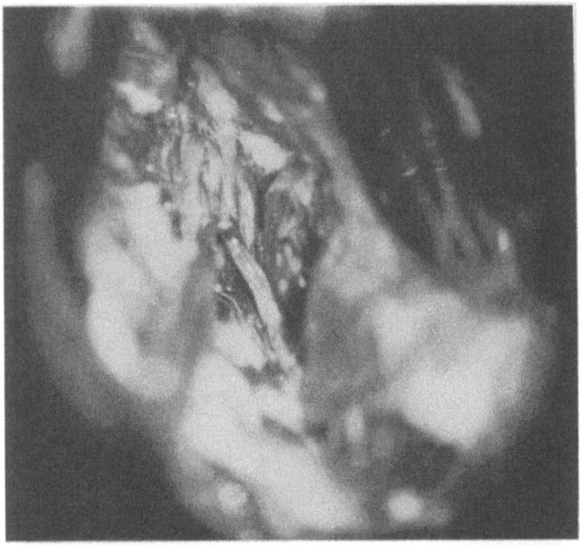

a

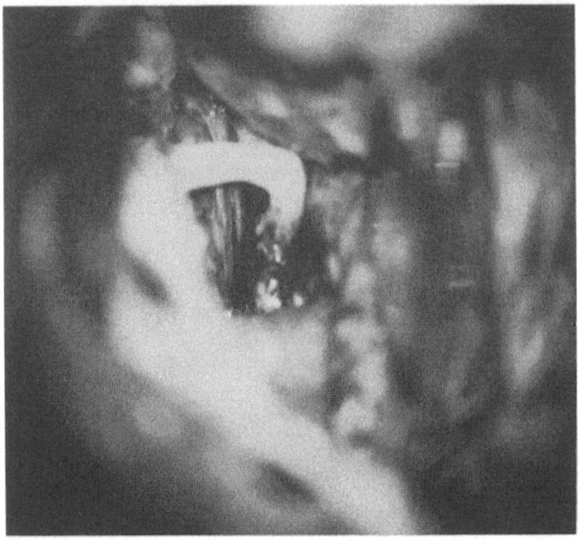

b

Fig. 7a, b. Exposure of the central stump of the facial nerve at the brain stem after total removal of a large neurinoma along with part of the facial nerve (**a**). The same patient as Fig. 7a. Suture between the central nerve stump of the facial nerve at the brain stem with a sural nerve graft (**b**)

Instead of Dott's surgical method, we developed in 1975 in cooperation with ENT surgeons a technique of intracranial-intratemporal repair (Samii 1979, 1980) Fig. 6a and b. I would like to thank Dr. Wigand, Dr. Draf and Dr. Osterwald for their help in teaching me the approach to the facial nerve in the tympanal and mastoidal course. If the facial nerve cannot be preserved during extirpation of the tumor, we strive to prepare the nerve at the brain stem in the region of the sulcus ponto bulbaris. According to our experiences it is possible to gain a stump of the facial nerve of at least one to one and a half centimeter long, even in huge tumors (Fig. 7a). Subsequently, an autologous nerve graft about 5 cm in length is taken

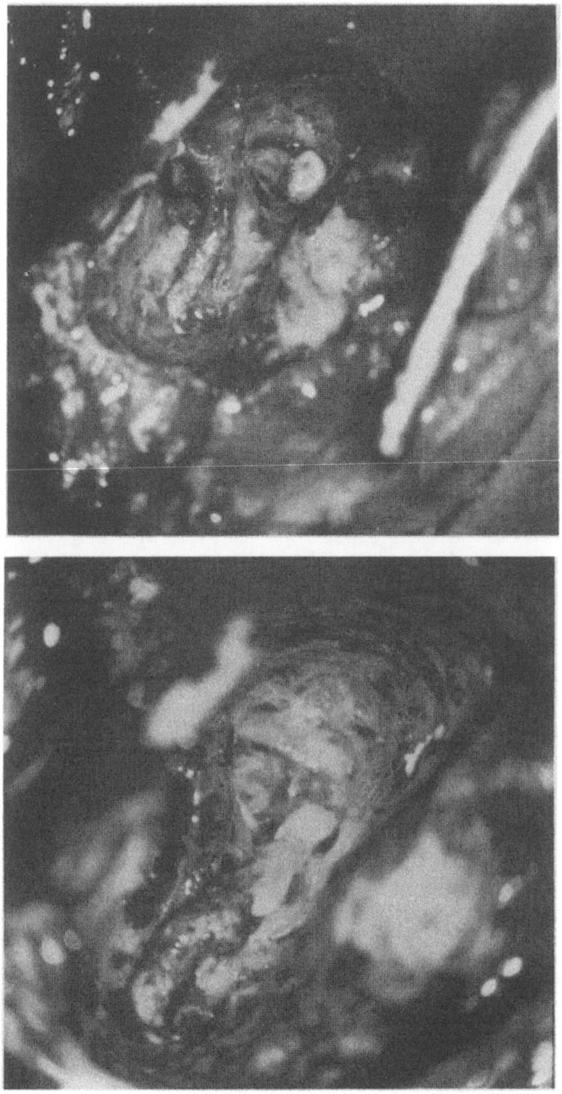

c

d

Fig. 7 c, d. The same patient as Fig. 7 a and b. Exposure of the facial nerve in the mastoidal and tympanal course (**c**). The same patient as Fig. 7 a, b, and c. The facial nerve is transected below the geniculate ganglion. The distal stump is mobilized dorsally and sutured with the nerve graft (**d**)

from the sural nerve and sutured to the central stump of the facial nerve at the brain stem (Fig. 7 b). The distal end of the graft is placed dorsal to the internal auditory meatus between the labyrinth and the sigmoid sinus. The facial nerve is exposed in its mastoidal and tympanal course through a mastoid approach (Fig. 7 c). Now the distal end of the graft can be transferred to the mastoid through a small incision in the dura, between the sigmoid sinus and the labyrinth. After transection of the facial nerve distal to the geniculate ganglion, the nerve stump is mobilized and anastomosed with the distal end of the graft (Fig. 7 d). In this manner an intracranial-intratemporal reconstruction of the facial nerve is performed with a graft 5 cm in length.

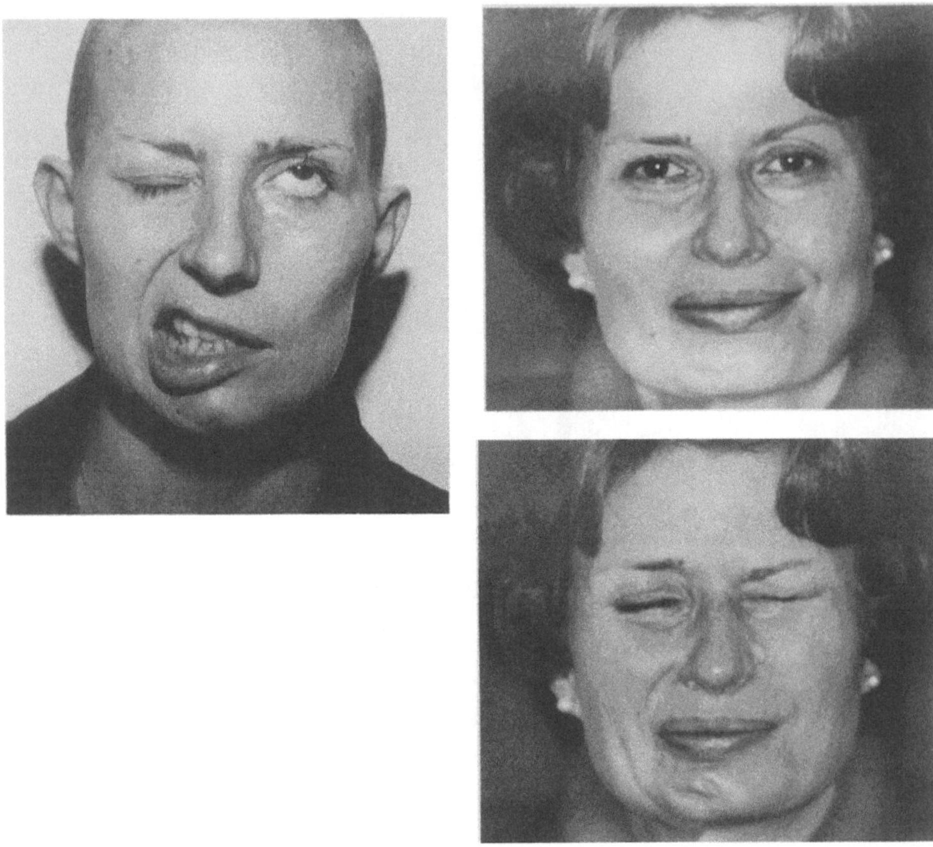

a b c

Fig. 8a. Ten days after removal of a large acoustic neurinoma on the left side with reconstruction of the facial nerve by means of a five cm long graft between the proximal stump at the brain stem and the mastoidal segment in the petrous bone. Total paralysis of the facial nerve on the left side

Fig. 8b, c. The same patient as Fig. 8a. Functional return 13 months after nerve grafting between the intracranial and the intratemporal part of the facial nerve

Fig. 9a. Postoperative paralysis of the left facial nerve. Another example of intracranial-intratemporal facial nerve repair

Fig. 9b. The same patient as Fig. 9a. Satisfactory function nine months after the operation

Fig. 9c, d. The same patient as Fig. 9a and b. An excellent functional result 15 months after nerve grafting

Fig. 8 a shows complete paralysis of the facial nerve on the left side following removal of a large acoustic neurinoma, and performing intracranial-intratemporal grafting of the facial nerve. Postoperative results thirteen months later are demonstrated in Fig. 8 b and c.

Another example of intracranial-intratemporal facial nerve repair is shown in Fig. 9 a. Postoperative paralysis of the facial nerve is seen. Fig. 9 b shows satisfactory nerve function nine months after the operation. The result 15 months later is excellent (Fig. 9 c and d).

The satisfactory results in all eight patients operated upon with a follow up between eleven months and five years justify the future application of this technique (Table 1). The one and a half hours necessary for the operation means minimal additional strain to the patient.

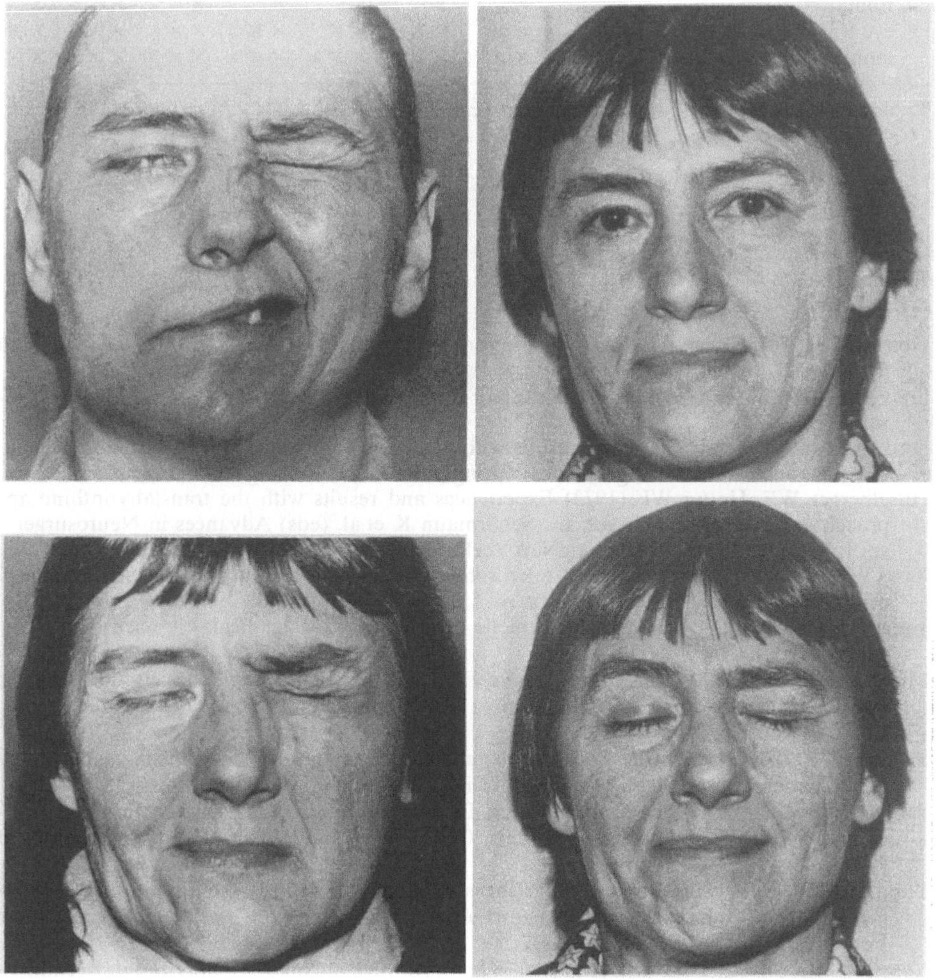

a c b d

Figs. 9 a–d (Caption see opposite Page)

Table 1. Results of intracranial-intratemporal grafting of the facial nerve in eight patients with acoustic neurinoma

Case	1	2	3	4	5	6	7	8
Age	17	24	39	46	55	41	46	27
Year of operation	1975	1976	1976	1977	1979	1979	1979	1979
First active muscle movement (months)	10	9	10	8	7	8	8	7
Follow up in months	60	45	42	40	15	12	12	11
Results in May, 1980:								
Symmetric state of repose	yes	yes	yes	yes	yes	yes	yes	yes
active muscle movement:								
frontal	×	×	×	×	×	×	×	×
eye	××	××	××	××	××	××	××	××
mouth	××	××	×××	×××	×××	×××	×××	××

Explanation of symbols: – = negativ / × = weak / ×× = good / ××× = very good

References

Dott NM (1958) Facial paralysis. Restitution by extrapetrous nerve graft. Proc Soc Med 51:900–902

Drake CG (1960) Acoustic neurinoma. Repair of facial nerve with autogenous graft. J Neurosurg 17:836–842

Drake CG (1973) Experiences and results with posterior approaches. In: Schürmann K et al. (eds) Advances in neurosurgery, vol 1. Springer, Berlin Heidelberg New York, p 251

Hitselberger WE, House WF (1973) Experiences and results with the translabyrinthine approach and related techniques. In: Schürmann K et al. (eds) Advances in Neurosurgery, vol 1, Springer, Berlin Heidelberg New York, p 289

Koos WT et al. (1973) Experiences in microsurgery of acoustic neurinomas. In: Schürmann K et al. (eds) Advances in Neurosurgery, vol 1, Springer, Berlin Heidelberg New York, p 251

Loew F (1962) Die kombinierte intrakranielle extratemporale Fazialisplastik nach Dott. Langenbecks Arch Chir 298:934–935

Miehlke A, Bushe KA (1967) Die operative Freilegung der mittleren Schädelgrube und des Porus acusticus internus zur Behandlung interlabyrinthärer Läsionen des Nervus facialis. Chir Plas Reconstr 3:37–46

Samii M (1979) Neurochirurgische Gesichtspunkte der Behandlung der Akustikusneurinome mit besonderer Berücksichtigung des N. facialis. Laryngol Rhinol Otol (Stuttg) 58:97–106

Samii M (1980) Nerves of the head and neck. In: Omer-Spinner (eds) Management of peripheral nerve problems, W. B. Saunders Company, Philadelphia, London, Toronto, p 507–547

Yaşargil MG (1973) Microsurgical experiences in surgery of acoustic neurinomas. In: Schürmann K et al. (eds) Advances in neurosurgery, vol 1. Springer, Berlin Heidelberg New York, p 250

Yaşargil MG (1978) Mikrochirurgie der Kleinhirnbrückenwinkel-Tumoren. In: Kleinhirnbrückenwinkel-Tumoren – Diagnostik und Therapie. Springer, Berlin Heidelberg New York, p 215–257

Facial Nerve Preservation in Acoustic Neuroma Surgery

Comparison Between Trans-Temporal and Retro-Sigmoid Approaches

J. M. STERKERS, Paris/France

Introduction

'The Facial nerve is the key that opens the door to earlier surgical removal of acoustic neuromas' (W. F. House, 1968). Since 1965, I have operated upon 190 acoustic tumors with a rate of 67.4 percent of immediate postoperative preservation of the Facial nerve function. This series is remarkable by the limited size of the tumor at the time of removal, and the possibility of comparing the results obtained by the same surgeon who has used the trans-labyrinthine or the middle fossa approach as well as the retro-sigmoid approach in the acoustic neuroma surgery.

Material and Approach

One hundred and ninetynine acoustic neuromas were operated upon, 181 unilateral, 9 bilateral tumors. The size of the tumor was in 28 patients less than 10 mm (intra- canalar tumors), in 122 between 10 and 25 mm (middle size tumors) and in 40 more than 25 mm, reaching 50 mm at maximum (large size tumors).

The removal was total in 170 and partial in 20 patients; two of these had a planned decompression on the second ear.

Three approaches were used: the middle fossa approach in 21 patients, the trans-labyrinthine approach in 89, and the retro-sigmoid approach in 80.

The techniques of the trans-temporal approaches were identical to the descriptions of W. F. House (1968) with only some modifications to locate the Facial nerve; I identify the Facial nerve directly in the internal auditory canal with an electrical stimulator using the Hilger apparatus. I do not think that it is necessary to open the Fallopian aqueduct. Another modification is the preservation of the Cochlear nerve to sustain the Facial nerve.

The third route to the internal auditory meatus is the retro-sigmoid approach, which is a variant of the posterior approach. I have used it since the early nineteen seventies (Sterkers J. M., Billet R., 1972).

Some details of my technique are original. The patient is in a supine position; the incision is vertical behind the mastoid; the craniotomy is located behind the sigmoid sinus, between the linea nuchalis superior and inferior; the diameter of the craniotomy is not more than three cm; the cerebellum is retracted by the effect of an intravenous infusion of Mannitol (500 ml, 25 percent) and also by the issue of the cerebrospinal fluid when the arachnoid of the lateral cisterna is opened; the cerebellum is protected by sheets of lyophilised dura-mater. I do not use a retractor.

The method of preservation of the Facial nerve in the retro-sigmoid approach depends upon the size of the tumor. The Facial nerve is identified in the angle if the tumor is small; the nerve is situated in front of the cochlear and vestibular nerve. If the size of the tumor is so large that the nerves are completely hidden by the tumor, the Facial nerve is first identified in the internal auditory canal. The posterior wall of the meatus is drilled away to two thirds of its length; the tumor is removed by careful dissection of the arachnoid sheet between the capsule of the tumor and the nerve. Its identification is done under high optic magnification and with the help of the electrical stimulator. It is of great importance to know that there is no contraction of the muscles if the anesthesia is too deep. During removal of the part of the tumor which is situated in the angle, identification of the Facial nerve is done after the intra-capsular removal of the tumor. The nerve lies in 99 percent of patients in front of or underneath the tumor. Electrical stimulation is absolutely necessary to detect the location of the nerve throughout its entire length. As in the other approaches, it is essential to avoid any suction and traction on the nerve and its vascular supply if function is to be preserved.

Results

The pre-operative state of Facial nerve function was clinically normal in 163 of the 190 patients. A complete facial palsy preceded the operation in four. Some facial weakness was observed before the operation in 23. All these patients are included in the following results. The post-operative results in 190 cases are classified into three groups. Normal post-operatory function, which means no facial weakness one month after surgery, was obtained in 128 patients (68 percent). Residual facial weakness, synkinesis and contracture in 50 (26 percent) and a permanent facial palsy in 12 (six percent).

The comparison of the preservation of Facial nerve function with each approach is summarized in Table 1.

Normal facial function was preserved in 77.5 percent by the retro-sigmoid approach, in 62 percent by the middle fossa approach, and in 60 percent by the translabyrinthine approach.

Facial function related to the size of the tumor in each approach are summarized in Tables 2, 3, 4. After the removal of the intra-canalar tumors, the function of the Facial nerve always remained normal when the approach was trans-labyrinthine. In the two other approaches, normal function was preserved in more than 85 percent. After the removal of the middle size tumors, normal facial function was ob-

Table 1. Results of facial nerve function in 190 acoustic neuromas comparison between middle fossa (MFa), translabyrinthine (TLa) and retrosigmoid (RSa) approach

	MFa		TLa		RSa	
	n	%	*n*	%	*n*	%
Normal facial function at one month	13	62	53	60	62	77,5
Residual facial weakness	6	29	28	31	16	20
Permanent facial palsy	2	9	8	9	2	2.5

Table 2. Comparison between middle fossa (MFa), translabyrinthine (TLa) and retrosigmoid approach, in intra-canalar acoustic neuroma (28 cases)

	MFa	TLa	RSa
Normal facial function	11	6	8
Residual facial weakness	2		1 [a]
Permanent facial palsy			

[a] In this exceptional case, the facial nerve was located behind the tumor, and not as usual in front.

Table 3. Comparison between middle fossa (MFa), translabyrinthine (TLa) and retrosigmoid approach (RSa) in 122 middle-size acoustic neuromas

	MFa		TLa		RSa	
	n	%	*n*	%	*n*	%
Normal facial function	2	29	36	61	45	80
Residual facial weakness	4	57	19	32	11	20
Permanent facial palsy	1	14	4	7		

Table 4. Comparison between middle fossa (MFa), translabyrinthine (TLa) and retrosigmoid approach (RSa) in 40 large size acoustic neuromas

	MFa		TLa		RSa	
	n	%	*n*	%	*n*	%
Normal facial function	–	–	11	46	9	60
Residual facial weakness	–	–	9	37	4	27
Permanent facial palsy	1	–	4	17	2	13

tained in 80 percent of the patients operated upon by a retro-sigmoid approach, in 61 percent operated by a trans-labyrinthine approach, and in 29 percent operated by a middle fossa approach. After removal of the large tumors, normal function was preserved in 60 percent by a retro-sigmoid approach, and in 46 percent by a trans-labyrinthine approach. Facial function was completely lost in less than 20 percent, in one or other approach. These last results include postoperative deaths (three patients, 1.6 percent).

Discussion

The preservation of Facial nerve function is related to the size of the tumor and to the surgical technique. The rate of Facial nerve preservation is excellent after re-

Table 5. Results of preservation of hearing in 94 acoustic neuromas. Comparison between middle-fossa (MFa) and retro-sigmoid approach (RSa). No hearing preservation was possible after removal of large size tumors, neither by MFa (1 case) nor by RSa (17 cases)

	Hearing preservation		Intracanalar acoustic neuroma		Middle size acoustic neuroma	
	n	%	*n*	%	*n*	%
MFa	8/20	40	7/13	54	1/6	17
RSa	23/74	32	6/9	67	17/48	35

moval of intracanalar tumors. The risk of damage to the Facial nerve is smaller by the trans-labyrinthine route and the retro-sigmoid route than by the middle fossa approach, if the tumor fills completely the canal and expands a few millimeters into the angle. In our experience, the best result was obtained by the trans-labyrinthine approach, although the only case of Facial weakness that occurred with the retro-sigmoid approch could be explained by an abnormal situation of the nerve which was posterior to the tumor.

The rate of facial preservation in middle size tumors has been the best with the retro-sigmoid approach. The rate was good with the translabyrinthine approach and the worst in the few cases, where a middle fossa approach was used. It is perhaps surprising that the results have been so good by the retrosigmoid approach as the Facial nerve is not as directly exposed to view as in the trans-labyrinthine approach. The experience I have acquired in locating the Facial nerve in the meatus when doing trans-temporal approaches might be an explanation.

Another explanation proceeds from the technique used to remove the tumor via the retro-sigmoid approach: the nerve is dissected at the end of the removal of the tumor, and as it is not necessary to make a close dissection of the nerve, it is easier hereby to preserve its arachnoid sheet and its vascular network than by the other approaches. Electrical stimulation is essential to locate the nerve through its arachnoid sheet. Briefly, by the trans-temporal approaches the Facial nerve is dissected from the tumor and, conversely, by the retro-sigmoid approach the tumor is dissected from the nerves.

The choice of the approach must not only be decided with the aim of Facial nerve preservation, but also to preserve the hearing function (Pertuiset et al., 1966; Sterkers et Billet, 1972; Bremont et al., 1974). This can be obtained by both a retro-sigmoid approach or a middle fossa approach (Table 5). We have noticed that post-operative facial function was always in a normal state when the hearing function was preserved.

Conclusions

To improve the functional preservation in Acoustic Neuroma surgery, an earlier diagnosis and the knowledge of every approach is recommended. It is actually possible to preserve the Facial function in more than 75 percent of patients after removal of intra-canalar and middle size tumors.

References

Bremond G, Garcin M, Magnan J, Bonnaud G (1974) L'abord à minima de l'espace ponto-cérébelleux. Cah d'ORL 9:443–460

House WF (1968) Monograph II – Acoustic neuroma. Arch Otolaryngol 88:575–715

Pertuiset B, Maspetiol R, Semette D, Pecheyre G (1966) La conservation des fonctions auditive et faciale au cours de l'exérèse totale des neurinomes de l'acoustique par voie sous-occipitale (d'après 4 observations). Presse Médicale 74:2327–2330

Pertuiset B et al. (1970) Les neurinomes de l'acoustique développés dans l'angle pontocérébelleux. Neurochirugie 16, Suppl. 1, Masson, Paris

Sterkers JM, Billet R (1972) Petites tumeurs de l'acoustique. Diagnostic et cure précoces. Ann. Otolaryngol (Paris), 89:323–339

Sterkers JM (1979) Neurinome de l'acoustique et autres tumeurs de l'angle et du conduit auditif interne (126 cas). Ann Otolaryngol chir Cervicofac 96:373–386

Microsurgery of the Extratemporal Portion of the Facial Nerve

A. Miehlke, Göttingen/FRG

Let me state at the beginning that, as often occurs in operative techniques, there are many ways to skin a cat. Every surgeon has his own special experience, and one or the other method is expecially suited to his abilities. I shall therefore present for each facial nerve segment only the particular approach I personally am using and, due to the limited time, refrain from demonstrating different operative methods which may be suited equally well for the same purposes. In discussing problems of extratemporal facial nerve surgery we are involved in anatomically very dissimilar structures which have followed completely different paths of surgical development. However, the combination of the operative methods of parotid surgery with those of neurosurgery has produced the present state of extratemporal facial nerve surgery.

Exposure of the facial nerve in its extratemporal course means nothing else but resection of the outer lobe of the parotid gland. The postauricular incision is carried to the mastoid periosteum. The anterior margin of the sternocleidomastoid muscle is next freed from the posterior surface of the gland. Although many landmarks have been employed in finding the nerve, we utilize the tympanomastoid fissure in locating the nerve, as described by Hogg and Kratz. Spezifically, the facial nerve lies 6 to 8 mm medial to the endpoint of the tympanomastoid fissure.

The tympanomastoid fissure is traced to its terminus. Two Freer elevators (one in each of the surgeon's hands) are then employed for careful blunt dissection within the depths of the retromandibular fossa, and are used to reflect the capsule of the posterior portion of the parotid gland anteriorly. As the gland is mobilized it can be carefully retracted anteriorly. The facial nerve can be defined as a glistening silver-white cable, which is approximately of knitting-needle thickness and can be found passing diagonally through the retromandibular fossa.

Once the main trunk of the facial nerve has been clearly identified, the Freer elevators can be used for further blunt anterior mobilization of the lateral portion of the parotid gland. The dissection is thus brought to the level of the bifurcation of the facial nerve.

We utilize a 'tunnel' technique. This principle is based on a division of the gland into sectors that overlie the branches of the facial nerve. A Freer elevator is directed peripherally beneath the substance of the gland but directly over the exposed branches of the facial nerve. Thus, the nerve is kept under direct view and is protected from injury by the elevators. Scissors can be used to cut the gland within this 'tunnel'. By continuing blunt dissection of the gland and advancing the elevators above the branches of the facial nerve, the glandular parenchyma can be safely excised. The dissection is complete when all the gland has been removed.

It is important that the procedure is so performed that the tumor-bearing sector of the gland is removed without damaging the capsule, when present, or the normal

Table 1. Surgical concept of Göttingen University ENT Department for parotid tumors. The use of surgery in parotid tumors

Group 1	Group 2	Group 3	Group 4
Lateral or total parotidectomy with preservation of the facial nerve	Lateral and total parotidectomy with preservation of the facial nerve or partial resection with reconstruction by direct or indirect anastomosis (Conley's 'big-little' operation)	Total parotidectomy with preservation of the facial nerve or total parotidectomy with neck dissection, resection, and reconstruction of the facial nerve by autogenous nerve grafting or by combination nerve grafting	Total parotidectomy and neck dissection, where necessary, together with resection of the lower jaw and mastoid and sacrifice of the facial nerve without nerve reconstruction (Conley's 'big-big' operation)
No irradiation	No irradiation	With irradiation	With irradiation
Monomorphic adenoma (oncocytoma, basal cell adenoma)	Acinic cell tumor (benign form)	Acinic cell tumor (malignant form or tumor recurrences)	Adenoid-cystic carcinoma (previously known as cylindroma)
Pleomorphic adenoma (mixed cell tumor)	Mucoepidermoid tumor ('low grade' type)	Carcinoma in a pleomorphic adenoma (previously known as secondary malignant mixed cell tumor)	Carcinoma in a pleomorphic adenoma at an advanced stage
Papillary cystadenoma lymphomatosum (Warthin's tumor)		Mucoepidermoid tumor ('high grade' type) when locally confined	Mucoepidermoid tumor ('high grade' type) at an advanced stage Squamous cell carcinoma and undifferentiated carcinoma
Lymphangioma		Adenocarcinoma (locally confined)	Infiltrating adenocarcinoma
Neurinoma of the facial nerve (to gain access to the tumor; in only a few cases, however, is it possible to preserve the facial nerve or to reconstruct it when necessary)		Carcinoma of the parotid duct	All tumors, basically, which are associated with facial paresis prior to operation and extensive, infiltrating tumor recurrences

In the not rare cases, when tumor metastases are present in the intra- and paraglandular lymph nodes – possibly with a defined primary tumor – the surgeon must be flexible as regards the preservation or resection of the facial nerve. This also applies to the eventual reconstruction of the nerve (using group 3 or group 4 operations or a combination of both groups).

adjacent glandular parenchyma. Should the tumor prove to be malignant, a most radical approach to parotidectomy is required.

When a significant cosmetic defect is made in the retromandibular fossa by the parotidectomy, we utilize a superiorly based transposition muscle-flap from the sternocleidomastoid muscle in order to minimize and improve the defect. The flap is placed over the primary branches of the facial nerve and is then sutured into place.

Total parotidectomy with preservation of the facial nerve is indicated if a benign tumor is located within the isthmus or deep portion of the parotid gland as well as for definitive treatment for recurrent parotid tumors. In order to allow complete removal of the deep portion of the gland, the branches of the facial nerve must be carefully elevated and retracted. This can be readily accomplished by placing small rubber slings around the individual branches of the facial nerve for retraction, and then mobilizing each branch from the underlying gland by sharp dissection with fine-tipped scissors.

During removal of the so-called 'iceberg tumors' there may be danger of damaging the facial nerve by overstretching. In this case it would be best to open the Fallopian canal in order to mobilize the intratemporal segment of the nerve. Once the nerve has been mobilized, it is relatively easy to retract it so that tumor removal can be effected without injury to the facial nerve.

It was realized during the last decade that radical removal of parotid tumors is indispensable in the interest of the patient. This awareness requires operative measures that have to take into account the grade of malignancy to be reckoned with in any given case. The arsenal of adequate surgical procedures contains operations of various degrees of radicality, from parotidectomy with preservation of the facial nerve, on the one hand, extending to total parotidectomy with sacrifice of the facial nerve en bloc together with radical neck dissection and, if necessary, resection of the mandible, on the other. Between these two cornerstones for our surgical concept there exist operations including reconstruction of trunk and branches of the facial nerve, if these had to be previously removed together with the tumor, for safety reasons.

We will now present the different techniques available for the reconstruction of the previously sacrificed facial nerve. There are four possibilities for the reconstruction of the facial nerve, depending on the size and location of the defect:

1. Direct anastomosis
2. Indirect anastomosis
3. Autogenous nerve transplantation
4. Combined transplantation – diversification method.

When anastomosis of the nerve endings is still possible after the excision of a relatively small tumor, we use the Millesi technique involving perineurial or epineurial microsurgical suturing after preparative epineurial resection. We protect the suture line with a collagen cylinder or cover it with an artificial nerve sheath made of amniotic tissue.

It is conceivable that a wide resection of one of the important nerve branches must be undertaken in connection with the removal of the tumor whilst another less important branch is resected to a limited extent, or not at all. The longer por-

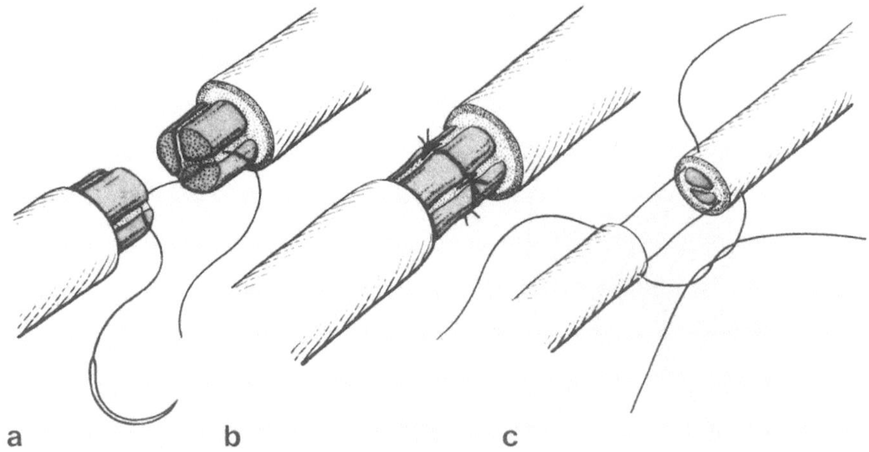

Fig. 1 a, b. Perineural suture (schematic representation). **c.** Epineural suture

tion of nerve left in the latter case allows anastomosis with the considerably more important branch. This is the so-called indirect anastomosis.

However, when the facial nerve must be sacrificed at the level of the trunk or when several branches must be resected at the periphery, then neither of the methods just described can be used, but only the free grafting of an autogenous nerve. I prefer to use the great auricular nerve or other branches of the cervical plexus as donors because these are approximately equal to the facial nerve in the width of their trunk and in the sequence of their branches. For very extensive grafting we use the sural nerve.

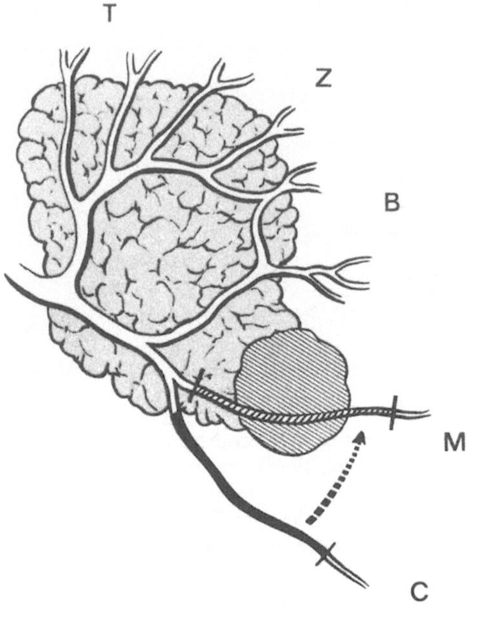

Fig. 2. Indirect anastomosis. *T* = temporofrontal branches, *Z* = zygomatic branches, = buccal branches, *M* = marginal mandibular branch, *C* = colli branch. (After Miehlke, Dtsch. Med. Wschr. 85 (1960), 506)

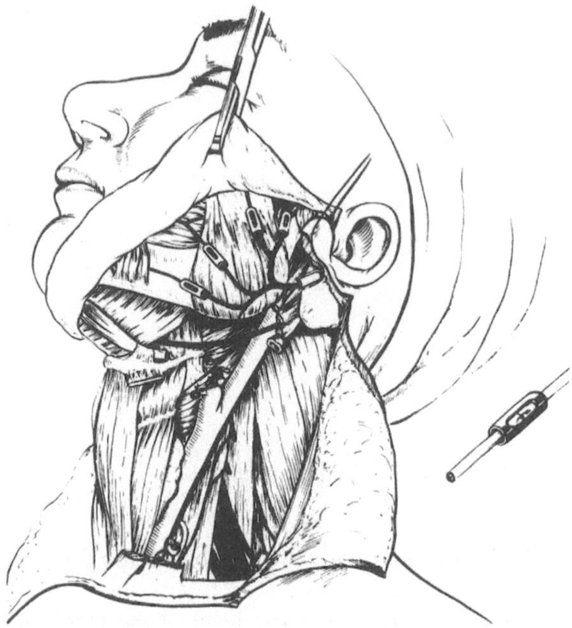

Fig. 3. Situation after reconstruction of the trunk and branches of the facial nerve. (From Conley, J, 'Concepts in Head and Neck Surgery' Thieme, Stuttgart 1970)

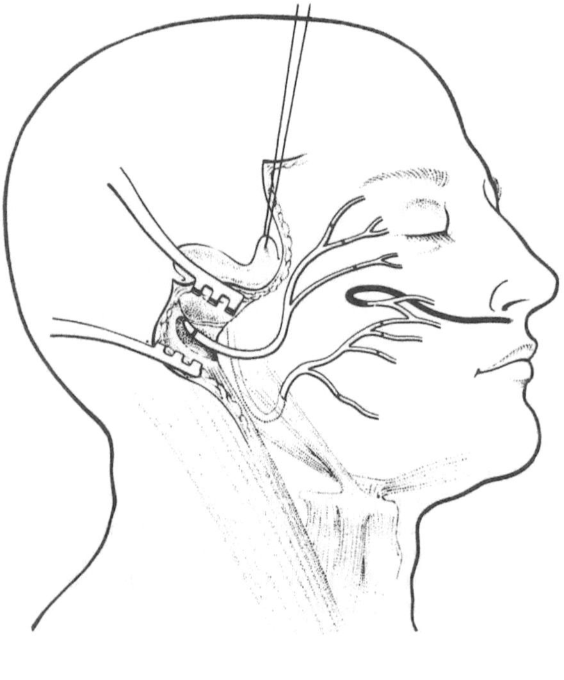

Fig. 4. Reconstruction of the Parotid. Plexus by means of the Diversification technique (for details see text) (From Miehlke A, Seifert G, Haubrich J, and Becker W, „Entzündungen der Speicheldrüsen", Thieme, Stuttgart, im Druck)

The most recent development in our grafting techniques can be described by the term 'diversification'. We have found that a further, significant improvement in our results can be achieved by a combined graft where anastomosis between the original facial nerve stem and simultaneous graft in the hypoglossal nerve are linked, if necessary, with a cross-face anastomosis. Diversification thus prevents the development of disturbing involuntary movements whilst, on the other hand, it allows individual nerves to contribute their full motor capacity at preferred sites of action.

In the meantime, the technique of morphological restoration of the peripheral facial nerve by one of the methods discussed has justified itself completely. Lost facial expression has been restored to many patients and, with it, a not inconsiderable part of their enjoyment of life.

Any kind of tumor surgery in this region may involve extremely difficult and time-consuming surgical procedures. Operations lasting for six to eight hours are not uncommon. If such is to be expected, there are no contraindications. The reconstruction of the facial nerve and hence the direct microsurgical technique has to be performed in a second operation following the first after an interval of a few days. The surgeon is then relaxed and can use his good condition to achieve a good result employing the sophisticated and difficult reconstruction technique in these extremely thin peripheral nerves.

We come now to the second and equally important point, the question of precautionary measures to be taken, resorting to immediate or two-stage grafts in these categories. In order to present the whole scope of the surgery employed here, let us now turn from tumor surgery to accident surgery in this region. We can take as an instance an accident involving deep rupture of the parotid gland and other defects of the facial nerve. A condition of this kind demands special consideration. At this point I would like to emphasize that every practicing doctor, and especially otologists and maxillo facial surgeons, should know that in such injuries the treatment given initially will determine whether or not an injured facial nerve will recover its function.

The best procedure is without doubt one which combines primary care of the wound with attempted restoration of the facial nerve. A primary facial suture or nerve graft offers an excellent prospect of success. However, we are all aware that occasionally, for various reasons such as severe shock, lack of instruments at the scene of the accident etc., it is simply impossible to give the necessary primary attention to the nerve. In such cases one should realize that reactive and even local inflammatory processes in the injured area will later make detection of the facial nerve very difficult. The first doctor to treat the patient should therefore appreciate our urgent request that the nerve stumps should be marked by provisional suture, if possible using coloured silk, which at the same time prevents their retraction. These small but very important measures are most important for subsequent success.

If the positions of the facial nerve stumps are safely marked, the so-called secondary early suture can be done in the third week after the acute shock has settled. Many neurologists and surgeons consider that with this procedure the chance of success are as good as those with a primary suture. This opinion is borne out by the fact that proliferation of Schwann's cells is most pronounced in the third week after the nerve lesion has occurred and that suturing is greatly facilitated by thickening of the nerve stumps.

Even if neither primary nor early secondary suturing is done and no exact report on the condition of the wound is available, there is no cause for resignation or an attitude of 'waiting hopefully', as such an attitude only tends to make the situation even more hopeless. Here I should like to mention a chronological schedule: If only contusion of the nerve has occurred, the first signs of returning function appear after two to three weeks. If the damage to the axon cylinder is so severe that functional rehabilitation is only possible by anatomical regeneration, the first signs of functional recovery can be expected after approximately three months while the affected muscles are open to reneurotization for roughly one year. This suggests that exploration of the nerve should take place if the first signs of expected functional recovery are still absent after three to five months. In such important decisions, electrical examination methods, particularly electromyography, are clinically extremely valuable.

Now, coming to the end, let us discuss very briefly, how we should handle cases in which nerve reconstruction, along the lines I have already described, has failed. Experience has taught us that regeneration generally takes place over a period of six to eighteen months, depending upon the extent of the defect and the operation undertaken. It appears that maximum recovery of function is generally achieved within two years.

Therefore, when there is no functional recovery after about one and a half years, one should not hesitate to reoperate, resect the scar, freshen up the nerve endings and perform a reanastomosis. The regenerative powers of the facial nerve are considerable and perhaps greater than those of other peripheral nerves. It is our task to carry out truly functional surgery using the extensive capacity for regeneration and directing the re-growing nerve bundles towards the paralysed muscles as long as these are still capable of neurotisation. For only thus can we recapture the emotional expressiveness of the face which in its immensely delicate gradations acts as a kind of mirror of the human soul.

Neurosynthesis of the Facial Nerve; Electrical vs. Clinical Results

M. E. WIGAND and W. THUMFART, Erlangen/FRG

Introduction

As was pointed out by some foregoing contributions (Samii, Pulec, Miehlke) there is full agreement about the necessity of surgical interventions for different kinds of facial nerve lesions of other than Bell's origin (Table 1). The indications for the individual case, however, that are the questions 'whether to operate' and 'when to operate', seem to vary with both the personal experience of the author and with his technique of preoperative examination.

Table 1. Indications for facial nerve synthesis

Petrous bone fractures
Iatrogenic nerve lesions
Infratemporal facial trauma
Neuroma, glomus-tumor, benignoma
Malignancies

I would like to summarize our attitude toward surgery in this respect:

Reluctance to operation	after delayed onset of the paralysis
Reluctance to operation	if residual movements are visible
Reluctance to operation	if residual voluntary activity is present in the EMG
Indications for surgery	are based on the electromyographical proof of denervation
Emergency operation	is advised, if the palsy occurred immediately with the trauma, and a tendency to degeneration is observed.

It should be emphasized that the functional state of a facial palsy is described most exactly and most sensitively by the electromyogram (EMG), better than by other electrical tests, and that our surgical indications were based predominantly on the EMG since 1965 (Wigand 1967). The beginning degeneration may be traced earlier by the stimulated EMG.

Material

The figures of our material, that is the number of facial nerve sutures, of neurosynthesis by fibrinogen tissue adhesive, and of nerve grafts are given by Table 2.

Table 2. Facial nerve synthesis

	Graft sutured	Graft glued	Nerve suture	Other	Total
Supralabyrinthine	6	4	–	–	10
Tympano-mastoidal	2	1	–	1	4
Infratemporal	20	5	12	–	37
Total	28	10	12	1	51

Technique

According to the different structural properties of the facial nerve in its different portions during its course from the brain stem down to the facial muscles the techniques of neurosynthesis have to be adapted to the site of the lesion.

While in the *infratemporal portion* fascicular sutures (Millesi) were the method of choice, this technique was not appropriate in the upper temporal portions because of the more diffuse arrangement of the facial nerve fibres. Only very thin fascicles are to be identified in the tympanal area, while at the geniculate ganglion and in the internal auditory canal it is almost impossible to suture separate fascicles without further destruction of preserved fibres.

We, therefore, have confined the *intratemporal* nerve synthesis to readaptation of the nerve stumps or grafts after dissection of their epineurium, and have fixed their position with blod clot and gelfoam. During the last two years fibrin tissue adhesive was used for nerve synthesis, according to Matras et al. (1972) and Kuderna (1979).

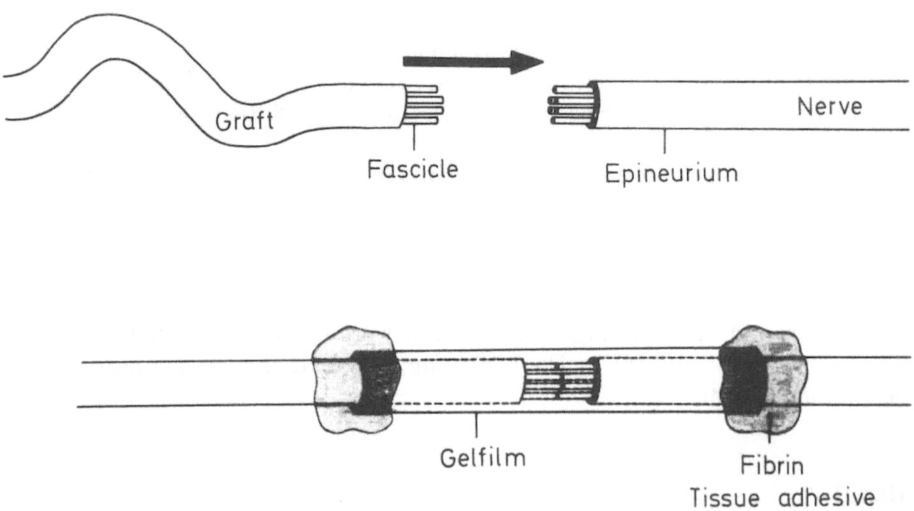

Fig. 1. Fixation of a free nerve graft to the proximal stump of the facial nerve in the intrapetrosal region with fibrinogen tissue adhesive (schematic drawing). Care is taken, not to cover the nerve fascicles with the glue

This new tool in ear surgery helps much to facilitate nerve grafting within the *internal auditory canal*. The floating proximal stump can be united with the graft by mere adaptation of the nerve endings. A piece of gelfilm is used for manteling the nerve junction, and is then covered with fibrin glue (Fig. 1), what keeps the graft in an adequate position. The prevention of csf pulsation by sealing off the porus with a fibrin glued muscle graft helps to immobilize the nerve stumps.

In all cases of nerve synthesis at or above the geniculate ganglion the major petrosal nerve was identified in its channel and resected over more than two millimeters, according to Fisch (1974), in order to avoid unwanted outspreading of axons into this nerve.

Results

Surgical nerve repair in the *internal auditory canal* and at the cerebello-pontine angle is technically difficult. Nerve sutures are possible in this region, and three of my patients were grafted by Prof. Samii in a combined oto-neurosurgical operation with the grafts extending from the brain stem to the mastoid portion of the facial nerve. All of them had excellent reinnervation of their facial muscles, correlating with the voluntary activity in the EMG.

Also a fourth own case with a free sural nerve graft of 7 cm length, interposed between the internal auditory canal and the mastoidal portion of the facial nerve achieved a beautiful functional and cosmetic result (Fig. 2).

Three other cases with supralabyrinthine nerve synthesis, using fibrin glue, also had good reappearance of voluntary action potentials in the EMG, but the clinical results are up to now, that is about one year after the operation, only partly satisfactory. We have got the impression that more time is required for more regenerating nerve fibres. The time interval between the first electrical response in the EMG and the final stage of clinical rehabilitation may range from 6 months to one year and to even more. We don't know why this is so, but we have to take it into account, and must not label the end results too early.

Our series of *tympano-mastoidal* facial nerve lesions is too small to allow particular conclusions. Miehlke has demonstrated his excellent technique and results. We don't hesitate to follow his rules, but have used fibrinogen tissue adhesive recently as a very effective fixative.

After large ablative surgery for malignomas of the parotid region the immediate *infratemporal* nerve grafting showed only very limited rehabilitation. Inspite of electrical signs of restored voluntary activity only improved muscular tonus and restricted coordination of facial movements became visible. Excellent results were achieved at the same anatomical site and with the same techniques after minor interventions with only partial nerve repair. In my opinion this is due to the very bad preconditions of graft immobilization in the great wound after parotidectomy with neck dissection.

The evaluation of functional results after facial nerve repair is complicated by the fact that regeneration of nerve fibres always induces mass movements and aesthetic dysharmony. For the patient himself, however, automatic functions of eye closure and lip mobility for speech and food intake have absolute priority. In our

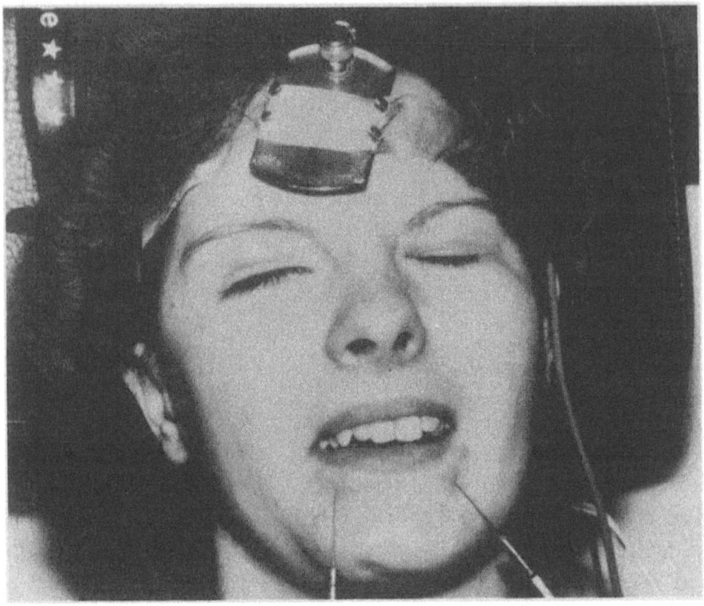

a

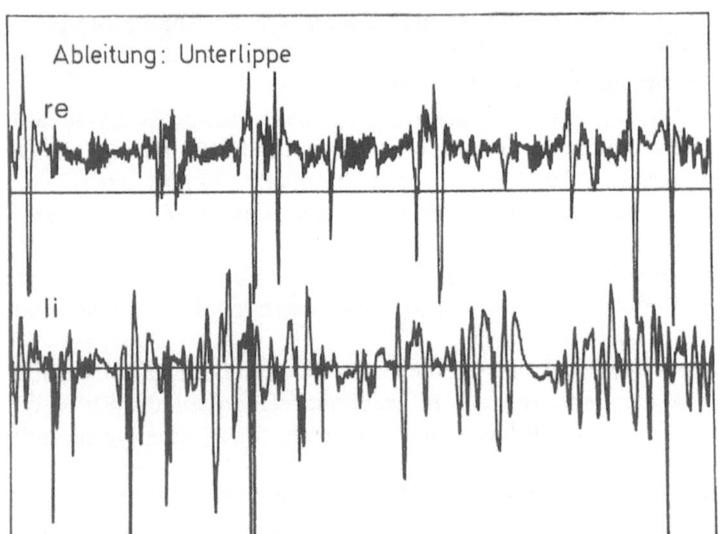

b

Fig. 2a, b. Functional result after facial nerve synthesis because of neurotmesis at the supralabyrinthine portion by cholesteatoma operation. **a** A free sural nerve graft was interposed between the right internal auditory canal and the mastoid portion of the nerve. **b** EMG examination 2 years after the nerve repair

Table 3a. Functional state after supralabyrinthine nerve repair ($n=12$)

Facial movements		Electromyogram	
Satisfactory	5	Normal pattern	4
Slightly reduced	1	Reduced activity	3
Weak	3	Mixed pattern	4
Complete palsy	3	Electrical silence	1
Massive synkinesia	3	Massive synchronisation	4

Table 3b. Functional state after infratemporal nerve repair ($n=21$)

Facial movements		Electromyogram	
Satisfactory	8	Normal pattern	11
Slightly reduced	6	Reduced activity	3
Weak	2	Mixed pattern	2
Complete palsy	5	Spontaneous activity	5
Little synkinesia	2	Some synchronisation	2
Massive synkinesia	5	Massive synchronisation	5

aim to compare results and to find out the best technique of neurosynthesis we, therefore, have to weigh functionality against practicability of the procedure more than the aesthetic outcome. On the other hand, the viability of regenerated nerve fibres should be objectified by the recording of action potentials in the EMG. We have tried to plot the clinical versus the electrical results in a series of 33 controlled patients (Table 3).

While the EMG is most sensitive in the preoperative diagnostic it does not correlate always with the visible movements nor with the aesthetic outcome. We know this fact from the larynx, where the reinnervation of both agonists and antagonists may paralyse the function of the vocal cords, but we cannot give an explanation for similar phenomena of the facial muscles.

Conclusions

All efforts should be done in degenerative lesions of the facial nerve to provide maximal regeneration of nerve fibres to reinnervate the facial musculature, but one has to be aware that the better the reinnervation is (low index of paresis), the worse will be sequelae like synkinesis and disproportion of facial movements. Fibrinogen tissue adhesive has excellent properties to serve as a fixative for nerve synthesis, but has, up to now, not yet proven equal results as those of fascicular nerve sutures. It may enable nerve junction, however, where nerve sutures are not feasible.

References

Fisch U (1974) Facial paralysis in fractures of the petrous bone. Laryngoscope 84:439–451

Kuderna H (1979) Ergebnisse und Erfahrungen in der klinischen Anwendung des Fibrin-Klebers bei der Wiederherstellung durchtrennter peripherer Nerven. 17. Jahrestagung Deutsch. Gesellsch. Plast. Wiederherstellungschirurgie, Heidelberg

Matras H, Dinges HP, Lassmann H, Mamoli B (1972) Zur nahtlosen interfaszikulären Nerventransplantation im Tierexperiment. Wien Med Wochenschr 122:517

Wigand ME (1967) Die Prognose der idiopathischen (Bellschen) Fazialisparese bei elektromyografischer Indikationsstellung zur Dekompressionsoperation. Z Laryngol Rhinol 46:439–451

Documentation and Evaluation of the Results

E. STENNERT, Göttingen/FRG

Facial pareses and their course, diagnosis, and treatment have so far been the subject of a very extensive literature, which demonstrates the striking interest in the disease of this cranial nerve.

All the more surprising is the fact that no consensus has so far been achieved about valid criteria of assessment. There can be no consensus as long as a degree of paresis is merely indicated as 'slight', 'moderate' or 'severe', and healing after facial paresis is characterized as 'good', 'fair' or 'poor', without giving any exactly defined criteria for these assessments. Results are consequently largely dependent on the subjective feeling of the evaluator, and reports on results are therefore of little value because they cannot be verified by comparison with other reports.

Since the facial nerve is mainly a motor nerve governing the muscles of facial expression, the success of any therapy is primarily measured by the degree of restoration of normal facial motor activity. Facial symmetry in repose and in action is therefore a parameter of paramount importance. A basic general evaluation should therefore be based on those clinical characteristics that are relevant to the cosmetic result and to functional defects which inconvenience the patient.

In the literature you will find about one dozen proposals concerning evaluation and documentation of facial paralysis.

To give an idea about the concepts of these evaluation procedures and how they work, I would like to present a short review of the best established systems:

Botman and Jongkees, 1955 (Fig. 1): The oldest and still most famous one was introduced by Botman and Jongkees in 1955 to whom the credit is due that they were the first physicians at all to develop a scoring system for facial palsy. This system is characterized as follows:

1. The degree of paresis is divided into 5 stages, namely from 0 to IV.
2. The single stages describe multiple functions of different muscle groups, even though they might act as antagonists.
3. The different degrees of functional impairment are described verbally (for example: stage I is characterized 'by a certain asymmetry when laughing and whistling', stage II by 'asymmetry in talking and laughing', stage III by 'dysfunction in movements'.
4. Different late sequelae are not especially mentioned or scored.

Janssen, 1963 (Fig. 2): He introduced, for the first time, a point scheme, in which:

1. Symmetry at rest scores 30 points, function of the frontal branch is rated by 10 points and of the ocular branch as well as of the oral branch by 30 points.
2. Late defects are not taken into consideration.

0 = normal mobility of mimic muscles;

1 = slight paresis: shown by a certain asymmetry when laughing or whistling, but normal at rest and when talking. The eyes can be closed;

2 = medium paresis: shown by asymmetry when talking or laughing. The eyes cannot be closed; but normal at rest;

3 = severe paralysis: asymmetry at rest, dysfunction of movement;

4 = total paralysis: loss of muscle tone, complete loss of nerve function. Muscular contractures may give the impression of some improvement, but muscular atrophy may produce worsening of the picture.

Groups 3 and 4 may represent end-results after total loss of function.

Fig. 1. Evaluation scheme for facial nerve paralysis proposed by: Botman and Jongkees (1955)

	Normal points	Case 1		Case 2	
		% of normal	points	% of normal	points
Symmetry function	30	100	30	100	30
Frontal branch	10	40	4	0	0
Ocular branch	30	90	27	70	21
Oral branch	30	90	27	70	21
Total	100		88		72

Fig. 2. Evaluation scheme for facial nerve paralysis proposed by: Janssen (1963)

Granger, 1967 (Fig. 3):

1. Muscle strength is graduated in a very sophisticated way, which leads to 10 stages.
2. The stages are also indicated by percentages.
3. The stages are again characterized by verbal descriptions.
4. Also in this scheme late defects are not taken into consideration.

May, 1970 (Fig. 4):

1. Facial innervation is divided into 10 different functions – including resting tone which equals 10 percent of the whole score.
2. Although these 10 items describe the different mimic function in a well differentiated way, again every function is estimated by a percentage from 0 to 10, so it is up to the investigator what he supposes the degree of paresis might be.

Adour and Swanson, 1972 (Fig. 5): This scoring system reveals the following characteristics:

1. Resting tone is neglected.
2. The face is divided into 3 levels: forehead, eye, and mouth.

Muscle strength		Description of muscle strength
Grade	%	
		Supine
0	0	No contraction
1	10	Faint contraction without gross motion
2	25	Definite motion
		Erect
2+	30	Completes less than half range of motion
3−	40	Completes more than half range of motion
3	50	Full range of motion
3+	65	Full range of motion plus slight resistance
4	75	Full range of motion plus moderate resistance
4+	90	Full range of motion but less than normal resistance
5	100	Full range of motion against normal resistance

Fig. 3. Evaluation scheme for facial nerve paralysis proposed by: Granger (1967)

	Normal	Weak	Absent
1. Tone	10	5	0
2. Wrinkle forehead	10	5	0
3. Close eyes tightly	10	5	0
4. Blink	10	5	0
5. Wrinkle nose	10	5	0
6. Grin	10	5	0
7. Whistle	10	5	0
8. Blow out cheeks	10	5	0
9. Depress lower lip	10	5	0
10. Tense neck	10	5	0
	100%	50%	0%

Fig. 4. Evaluation scheme for facial nerve paralysis proposed by: May (1970)

3. Return of facial function is 'measured' in units of 25 percent.
4. These estimations are indicated by numbers, respectively points, so that in a case of 75 to 100 percent recovery the patient will receive 10 points.
   The total number of points indicate the *'Facial Paralysis Recovery Profile'*.
5. From those plus-points the negative (minus) points, due to any late complication, are subtracted.
6. All these late complications (which are of different clinical significance) are valued as being equal.
   Thus the whole scoring procedure results in the definite *'Facial Paralysis Recovery Index'*.

In our opinion, however, these evaluation schemes do not adequately fulfill the requirements which, we believe, should be fulfilled:

The investigations required for the evaluation should not be prolonged, so that they can be made during normal office hours. The evaluation should be technically

Site	No. of points assigned to each unit of recovery *				
	0	0% – 25%	25% – 50%	50% – 75%	75% – 100%
Forehead	0	+1	+1	+2	+2
Eye	0	+1	+2	+3	+4
Mouth	0	+1	+2	+3	+4

Complication	No. of points
Early:	
Pain	–1
Epiphora	–1
Ageusia	–1
Decreased lacrimation	–1
Hyperacusis	–1
Late:	
Contracture	–1
Synkinesis (mass facial motion)	–1
Crocodile (gustatory) tears	–1
Facial spasm	–1
Ptosis of eyebrow	–1

Fig. 5. Evaluation scheme for facial nerve paralysis proposed by: Adour and Swanson (1972)

simple, and should not require special experience but be practicable for all otologists and neurologists.

Despite the necessary simplification, the method should be as objective as possible. The evaluator should be required only to make yes or no decisions on the basis of as many unequivocal characteristics as possible. Verbal description of functional conditions is unsuitable for comparative studies. With the aid of a rating system, a score should be determined as a yardstick for an overall evaluation.

The scheme of evaluation should be so designed that it quickly provides comprehensive information on the status of the individual patient, and permits comparison of whole groups, both as to overall result and as to separate functions. An obvious choice for such a procedure is a check-list of the sort long used successfully in technical work but also in medicine, for example the non optimal score in premature births or the Apgar index in neonates.

We, therefore, felt justified in introducing a further scoring system which, in our opinion, approximately fulfills the above mentioned criteria.

Paralysis Score

Figure 6 shows a diagnostic card by means of which a paresis index is determined in accordance with the above discussion. Every single question in the order of sequence given should be checked of. The sum of negative points gives the paralysis score.

Score sheet for evaluation of clinical degree of paresis following facial nerve injury

Resting tone	Difference between palpebral fissures		less than 3 mm		3 mm and more	
	Ectropion		no		yes	
	Loss of nasolabial sulcus (if present on normal side)		no		yes	
	Drop of angulus oris		less than 3 mm		3 mm and more	
Motility	Frowning (at least 50% of normal side)		possible		not possible	
	Incomplete lid closure	slight innervation (as in sleep)	no		yes	
		maximal innervation	no		yes	
	Exposure of teeth	canine teeth: upper and lower	visible		not visible	
		2nd upper incisor (full width)	visible		not visible	
	Whistling (decrease in distance between filtrum and angulus oris compared with normal side)		50% and more		less than 50%	
			Paralysis-score			

Fig. 6. Check-list for the assessment of the clinical degree of paresis after facial nerve injury. The list comprises 10 criteria for evaluation, demanding simple yes or no decisions. Every question must be answered positively or negatively by checking the appropriate field. The sum of the number of checks for each negative finding equals the paralysis score.

In an attempt to fulfill the requirement of routine clinical work for succinct but comprehensive information, we have for some time given the paralysis score as a double score. This double score immediately shows the relative importance of loss of tone on the one hand, and disturbed motility on the other. For example paralysis score 6 can mean normal resting tone without conspicuous difference between paretic and intact side, but total paresis with no voluntary innervation. This is the typical finding in fresh cases of paresis in younger patients and should therefore be indicated as 0/6 (Fig. 7).

But the same paralysis score can also mean a poor resting tone combined with imperfectly restored motility, indicated by 3/3. This is often observed in the case of deficient functional restoration (Fig. 8).

As it is shown in Figure 9, the scheme of investigation evaluates the functional condition of the muscles of facial expression in two separate stages: the stage of repose (resting tone) is assigned 40 percent, and the stage of active movement (motility) 60 percent. For evaluation of the resting tone as well as for that of motility, the face is divided into three areas, corresponding with the muscular structures: forehead, periocular region and perioral region. In the overall evaluation, the following percentage values are assigned to these areas: forehead 10 percent, periocular re-

Resting tone	Difference between palpebral fissures		less than 3 mm	×	3 mm and more		
	Ectropion		no	×	yes		
	Loss of nasolabial sulcus (if present on normal side)		no	×	yes		
	Drop of angulus oris		less than 3 mm	×	3 mm and more		
Motility	Frowning (at least 50% of normal side)		possible		not possible	×	
	Incomplete lid closure	slight innervation (as in sleep)	no		yes	×	
		maximal innervation	no		yes	×	
	Exposure of teeth	canine teeth: upper and lower	visible		not visible	×	
		2nd upper incisor (full width)	visible		not visible	×	
	Whistling (decrease in distance between filtrum and angulus oris compared with normal side)		50% and more		less than 50%	×	
			Paralysis-score			6	0/6

Fig. 7. A typical distribution of checks for fresh complete paralysis in younger patients

gion 40 percent and perioral region 50 percent. In our view these percentages correspond with the various important cosmetic and functional degrees.

The limited time at my disposal does not allow presentation of all the arguments that have been the basis for establishing the different scoring items in this specific way and how their evaluation should be performed. These considerations have been already described elsewhere in detail (Stennert et al. 1979).

Today I only wish to point out the fact that every check point of this scoring system is *measurable* in a simple way and permits only clear-cut yes or no decisions.

Secondary Defect Score

Apart from the functional condition of the musculature, healing of the defect is important in assessing conditions after facial nerve lesions. Figure 10 lists the parameters of importance in this respect. We are convinced, however, that these findings should be assessed separately from the clinical degree of paresis. This conviction is based on the following considerations:

In all cases of severe lesions of nerves with partial or total destruction of neural architecture (particularly the connective tissue structure), functional restoration can only be achieved via extrafascicular heteromorphous reneurotization, that is, mis-

Resting tone	Difference between palpebral fissures		less than 3 mm	×	3 mm and more		
	Ectropion		no	×	yes		
	Loss of nasolabial sulcus (if present on normal side)		no	×	yes		
	Drop of angulus oris		less than 3 mm	×	3 mm and more		
Motility	Frowning (at least 50% of normal side)		possible		not possible	×	
	Incomplete lid closure	slight innervation (as in sleep)	no		yes	×	
		maximal innervation	no		yes	×	
	Exposure of teeth	canine teeth: upper and lower	visible		not visible	×	
		2nd upper incisor (full width)	visible		not visible	×	
	Whistling (decrease in distance between filtrum and angulus oris compared with normal side)		50% and more		less than 50%	×	
			Paralysis-score			6	3/3

Fig. 8. A typical distribution for patients with deficient functional restoration, or fresh incomplete paresis in older patients.

Resting tone			Motility		
Forehead			Frowning	1	10%
Eye	Difference between palpebral fissures	1	Incomplete lid closure (slight innervation)	1	40%
	Ectropion	1	Incomplete lid closure (maximal innervation)	1	
	Loss of nasolabial sulcus	1	Exposure of teeth: canine teeth	1	
Mouth	Drop of angulus oris	1	Exposure of teeth: 2nd upper incisor	1	50%
			Whistling	1	
		40%		60%	100%

Fig. 9. Proportion (in percent) of assessment criteria: resting tone is assigned 40 percent, and motility 60 percent of the total score. Facial portions at the levels of forehead, eyes, and mouth are assigned percentages of value according to their cosmetic and functional significance.

Hyperacusis	no ☐ yes ☐		
Gustation impaired	no ☐ yes ☐		
Synkinesia between:	☐ forehead ☐ eye ☐ nasolabial sulcus ☐ corner of the mouth ☐ chin	no	yes
	More than 3 areas		
Blinkreflex generalized ('secondary spasm', 'twitching')			
Contractures			
Lacrimation	less than 70%		
	less than 70% plus incomplete lid closure		
	0%		
Crocodile tears			
	Secondary defect-score		

Fig. 10. Score sheet for evaluation of secondary defects following facial nerve injury. Five individual parameters are differently weighted depending on their functional and cosmetic significance. The secondary defect score is composed of 8 evaluation criteria permitting only yes or no answers. All of them must be checked separately in systematic order from top to bottom. The hyperacusis and impaired gustation scores are included only for purposes of documentation and are not counted in the evaluation.

direction. This means that secondary defects such as synkinesis, twitching as a consequence of generalized blinkreflex, crocodile tears, and contractures can only develop when a sufficient number of axons again grow out into the periphery. Although there is no linear correlation, there is some justification for the postulate that the better the reinnervation, the more pronounced are the secondary defects. In a uniform assessment of innervation and defect healing therefore, the positive point of good reneurotization is cancelled out by the negative points of accompanying synkinesis and other secondary defects. In our opinion, the assessment of a patient with good reinnervation and many defects should differ from that of a patient with poor reinnervation and correspondingly few defects.

Finally, a few remarks about the selection of criteria which permit only yes or no decisions. This ensures a clearly defined classification in the functional categories 'satisfactory' and 'unsatisfactory', which reflect the authors' personal estimate on the basis of their clinical experience.

Restriction to yes or no decisions may seem to be less differentiated than a percentage evaluation of individual functions, but the many possible combinations of 18 individual decisions nevertheless lead to a well-differentiated overall assessment. Moreover, these clearly defined yes or no decisions ensure greater interscorer reliability. Precisely this should be demanded of a scheme of evaluation by which assessments are supplied for comparison. The selection of the criteria of evaluation proposed here is based on experience gained in over 1,000 individual examinations. Their validity was tested in a follow up on 50 patients after facial nerve reconstruction, carried out by three investigators. Their evaluation showed 93 percent agreement, an interscorer reliability of 0.93.

References

Adour KK, Swanson PJ (1971) Facial paralysis in 403 consecutive patients. Trans Am Acad Ophthalmol Otolaryngol 75: 1284–1301

Botmann JW, Jongkees LBW (1955) The result of intratemporal treatment of facial palsy. Pract Otorhinolaryngol (Basel) 17: 80–100

Granger CV (1967) Toward an earlier forecast of recovery in Bell's palsy. Arch Phys Med Rehabil 48: 273–278

Janssen FP (1963) Proefschrift Univers. Jacob van Campen, Amsterdam

May M (1971) Facial paralysis peripheral type: A proposed method of reporting. Laryngoscope 80: 331–390

Stennert E, Limberg CH, Frentrup KP (1979) Paralysis and Secondary Defect Score. In: Miehlke et al. (eds) New Aspects in Facial Nerve Surgery. Clinics in Plastic Surgery, vol 6, No. 3, pp 458–465

Management of Hemi-Facial Spasm

A. MIEHLKE, Göttingen/FRG

We will now discuss a clinical picture, so-called idiopathic hemi-facial spasm, whose etiology and pathogenesis are not yet sufficiently elucidated.

In the pathogenesis of this syndrome, 3 types of lesions of the facial nerve system are discussed: *first*, a supranuclear, *second*, a nuclear, and *third*, an infranuclear lesion.

1. Following the severe encephalitis epidemic in Europe in the twenties one tended to interpret facial spasm as a manifestation of a disorder of the extrapyramidal system. This interpretation has been rejected (Scheller, 1953).
2. I wish to point your attention to observations by Kirchhoff (1944) who found among his patients a conspicuous coincidence of hemi-facial spasm and rheumatic disease. Chronic tonsillitis, dental granuloma, and sinus inflammations were also in the background.
3. Results of electromyographic studies by Esslen could support the hypothesis that the facial-spasm inducing disorder has to be looked for in the secondary neuron. Esslen described an innervation pattern typical for facial spasm which can only be produced by a 'parabiotically' alterated section on the region of the peripheral neuron. Esslen tends to hold the view that the site of disorder has to be searched for in the mastoidal segment of the course of the facial nerve.

When we try to summarize what we have heard so far, we find indeed that we have no safe and final knowledge about the etiology and pathogenesis of primary facial spasm. Whatever really causes the development of the spasm, it seems clear that they induce damage of the peripheral neuron.

The existing etiological and pathogenetical situation is as unsatisfactory as is the therapy so far. Conservative treatment has no convincing effect and at best is of alleviating value. Injections of alcohol into or around the nerve may cause permanent paralysis. Neurolysis of the facial nerve within the Fallopian canal removes the spasm only if trauma with resulting paralysis was caused during operation. After regeneration and restitution of facial nerve function the spasm also returned.

Lathrop (1952) and Martin (1952) have shown that careful atraumatic neurolysis does not lead to removal of the spasm. Cawthorne performed, after atraumatic neurolysis, a controlled contusion of the facial nerve which resulted in paralysis lasting for several weeks. But also here the spasm returned after facial nerve function had been regained.

After that Cawthorne completely transected the nerve stump in its mastoidal course and left the two stumps apposed in the groove of the Falloppian canal thus permitting regeneration of nerve fibers. But also in this case recurrences nearly always occurred after return of facial nerve function so that Cawthorne relinquished this method.

Hemi-facial spasm is in most cases much more pronounced in the upper facial half in contrast to the region of the mouth which is affected mostly very little or not at all. This fact made me eliminate selectively the predominantly affected nerve fibers. Difficulties arise in the mastoidal segment of the facial nerve for such a selective elimination of the frontal and ocular branches. These difficulties result from the topographic course taken by the fibers.

Extratemporal methods, however, could offer a possibility, some of which try to achieve selective elimination: Scoville (1955) performed a two-thirds transection of the facial trunk with partial resection already before it divides into the two main branches. But in doing so he sacrifices the advantage of a selective spasmolysis of the most affected facial regions. Lathrop (1952) recommends the complete transection of single branches far peripherally. German (1942) proposes partial transection with partial resection of those branches at the anterior margin of the parotid that are predominantly affected by the spasm. In 1960 I tried to find a compromise between German's and Lathrop's procedures and Scoville's technique, by exposing the most severely affected nerve branches along their course through the parotid gland and performing here partial resections of about five mm length.

We avoid inclusion of the cervico-facial branch into the schedule of partial resection in order to involve the region of the mouth not too much in the paralysis.

The patients whom I operated in this way at first experienced disappearance of their hemi-spasm. But the majority of them suffered recurrence after about one year. A second operation became necessary which was not always successful.

Fisch even went further by cutting through, similar to Lathrop, about 90 percent of the facial nerve branches at the anterior margin of the parotid, after first removing the parotid outer lobe, and performing an exheresis. I used this even more radical procedure in my own program, but also here I saw recurrences after about one to two years. Paulsen then has tried to limit impulse conduction by the facial nerve fibers by exposing the nerve in its mastoidal course and treating it with very fine electrocoagulation. Also here recurrences are found after one to two years. Very recently Dr. Jannetta pointed out that, in the cerebello-pontine angle, a loop of the anterior superior artery exerts pressure from below towards the facial nerve trunk which in his opinion causes hemi-facial spasm to occur. On the basis of this concept an operation was devised by which a plastic cushion was introduced between this artery loop and the facial trunk, by that to remove the effect of pressure. Dr. Jannetta will very soon tell us about the success of this operative technic.

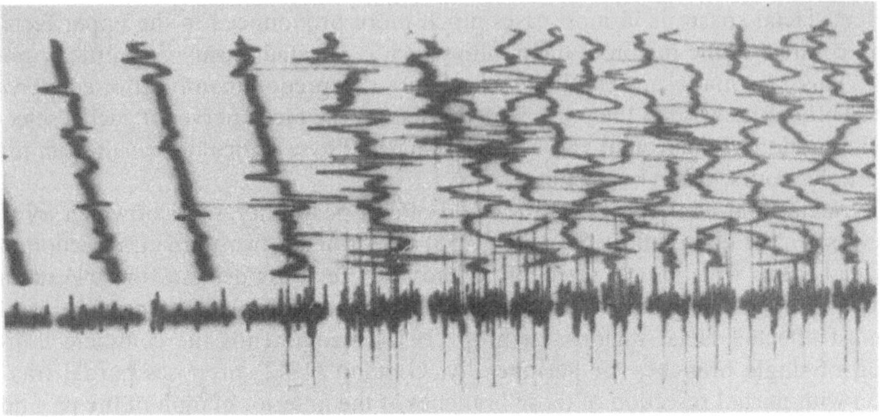

Fig. 1. Electromyogram in primary hemifacial spasm

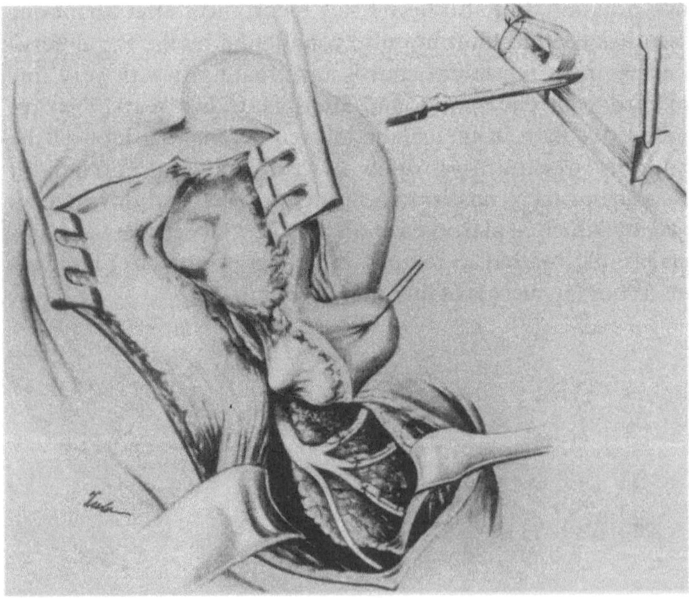

Fig. 2. Exposure of the facial nerve in its course between the superficial and the deep lobes of the parotid gland. Partial excision of individual branches of the facial nerve for primary facial spasm. (Miehlke-Technique)

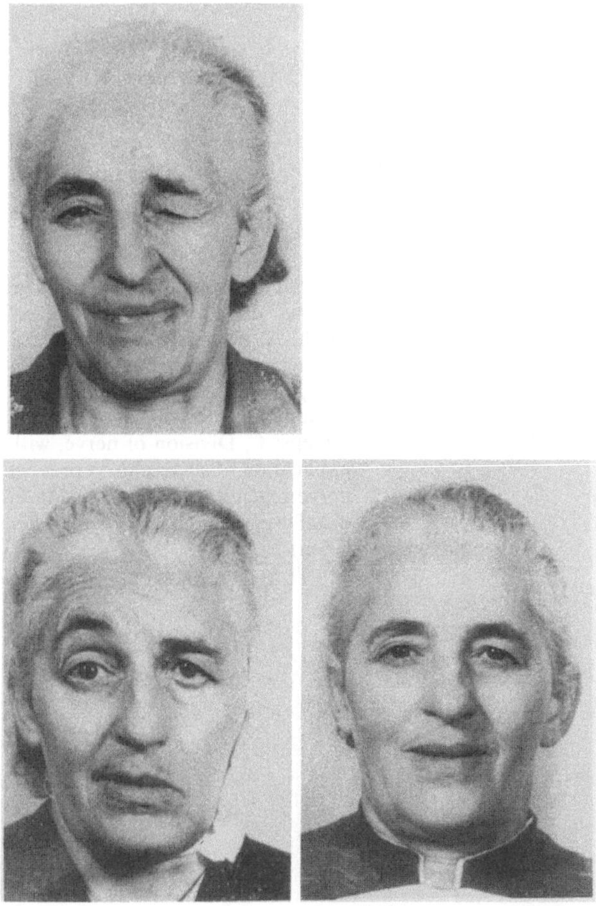

Fig. 3 Hemifacial spasm: Extratemporal operation according to Miehlke-technique

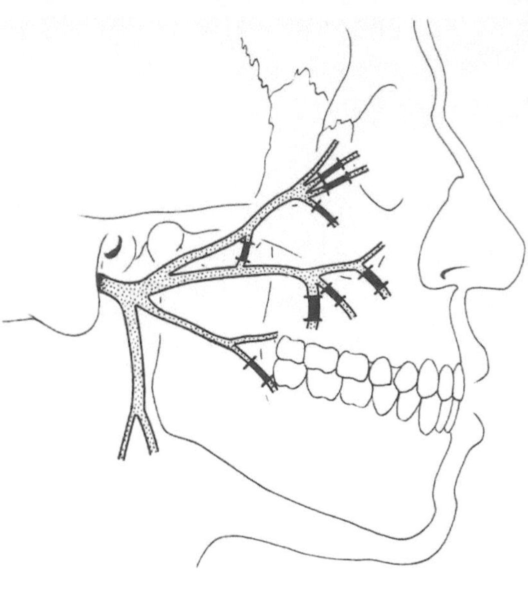

Fig. 4. Operation for hemifacial spasm, using the Fisch-technique

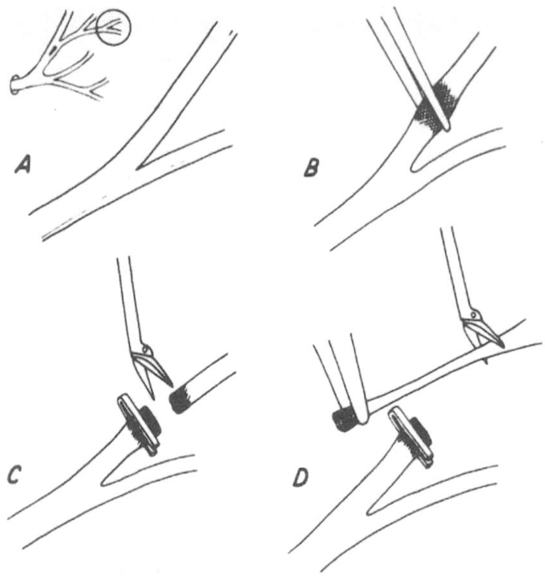

Fig. 5. Operation for hemifacial spasm, using the technique of Fisch. A, Peripheral branch of facial nerve to be sectioned; B, Crushing proximal site of nerve to be sectioned by bipolar coagulation forceps; C, Division of nerve, with application of silver clip to prevent nerve regeneration; D, Division of distal segment of nerve. (After Fisch)

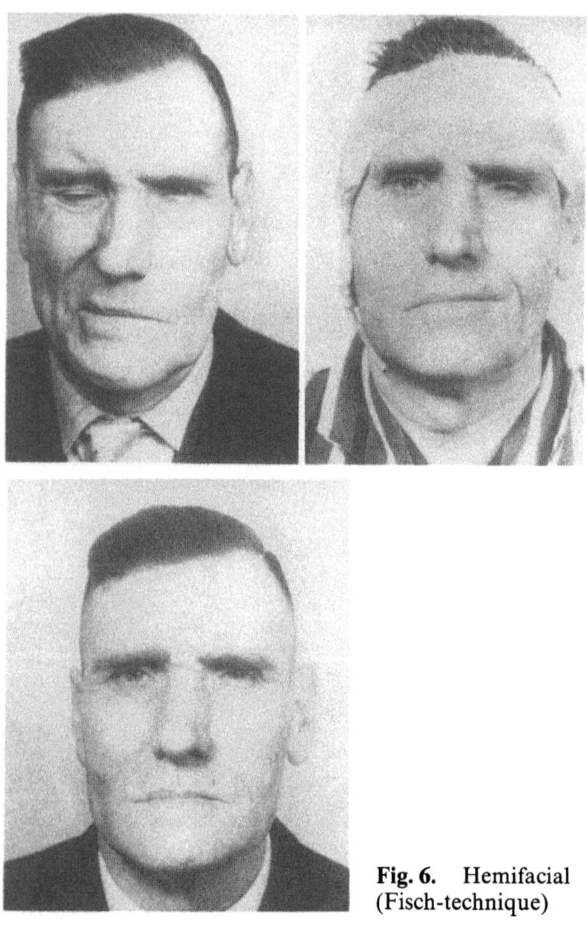

Fig. 6. Hemifacial spasm extratemporal operation (Fisch-technique)

References

Cawthorne T (1956) Br Med J 11: 1197
Esslen E (1957) Dtsch Z Nervenheilk 176: 149
Fisch U (1972) In: Miehlke A (ed) Surgery of the Facial Nerve, Urban & Schwarzenberg, München
German WJ (1942) Surgery 11:912
Jannetta PJM (1980) Management of hemi facial spasm. Symposium of Cranial Nerve, Hannover
Jannetta PJM, Abbary JC, Maroon FM, Ramos MS, Albin (1947) Etiology and definitive micro surgical treatment of hemi facial spasm J Neurosurg 47:321
Kirchhof J (1944) Zentralbl Neurologie, 177:363
Lathrop FD (1952) Bull. New York, Akad Med 28:796
Lathrop FD (1953) J Am Med Assoc 152: 19
Martin H (1952) Surgery 5:670
Miehlke A (1959) Archiv Ohr Heilk. u. Z. Hals 175:464
Paulsen K, Neveling R (1975) HNO 23:47
Scoville WG (1955) Surg Gynecol Obstet 101:495
Scheller H (1953) Handbuch der inneren Medizin, Bd. V/2 Springer Berlin Göttingen Heidelberg

Hemifacial Spasm

P. J. JANNETTA, Pittsburgh, PA/USA

Hemifacial spasm (HFS) is a symptom complex of hyperactive dysfunction of the facial nerve caused by an abnormality at the root entry zone (REZ) of the nerve [13]. This abnormality, almost always vascular cross-compression, most commonly occurs as a result of the aging process just as in the other cranial nerves which are subject to hyperactive dysfunction. In this chapter, we will discuss the clinical findings in a series of 229 patients who have undergone retromastoid craniectomy (RMC) and microvascular decompression (MVD) in treatment of intractable HFS, the operative findings and results, plus an analysis of both the early work upon which provides the basis for the current experience and of the experience of several other current investigators.

The History and Physical Examination

Hemifacial spasm classically begins with slight intermittent twitching of an orbicularis oculi muscle. The onset can usually be localized precisely to the inferior orbicularis oculi. Gradually and relentlessly, the twitching becomes more severe and more persistent as it spreads down over all the muscles of facial expression and in time, ultimately involves the platysma muscle. Involvement of the frontalis muscle occurs in only about 15 percent of patients with classical HFS. The progression is usually slow but spasms may occasionally become very severe in a few months. In time, mild peripheral weakness of the facial muscles develops. The earliest sign is usually decreased ability to bury the eyelashes on the affected side. This is eventually accompanied by the so-called 'tonus phenomen', prolonged severe contractions of all the involved muscles causing severe and ugly grimacing with partial closure of the eye and drawing up of the corner of the mouth. Early on the patient is frequently told he has a nervous tic or habit spasm. A multitude of tranquilizers and mood elevators are given with no relief. A history of worsening or easing of the spasm by changes in head and body position can be extracted in over half the patients. The spasm is painless except for occasional dull ache in the buccal region with severe prolonged tonus. The spasm is exacerbated by using the muscles of facial expression and in some patients by tension and fatigue. It frequently occurs during sleep (spouses will verify this) and may awaken the patient from sleep. Clicking noises in the ipsilateral ear may be noted with severe spasm in some patients (tensor tympani spasm). The weakness gradually worsens. The patient cannot kiss or whistle. Patients are frequently referred for psychiatric help. Of the first 12 patients the author saw with HFS, 11 were sent to psychiatrists. The twelfth, who told me he knew that he had problems but that the HFS was unrelated, was a psychiatrist himself. The symptoms become psychologically, socially, and economically disabling.

Patients become reclusive if they can. Those who must appear in public adopt numerous tricks in the hope that they can improve their appearance. These include wearing oversize darkly shaded sunglasses, wearing their hair over their face, wearing large high collars and hats with floppy brims, keeping their hand pressed to their face, and looking down or away from other people. These techniques work only variably. The patient becomes worried because he looks so suspicious. He may have trouble reading, watching television, or driving because the tonus of the orbicularis oculi interferes with binocular vision.

A subgroup of HFS exists which we have termed 'atypical' HFS. The onset and progression in this group are different from the classical group in that the spasm begins in the buccal muscles and progresses upward over the face. At later stages, this is indistinguishable from classical HFS except that frontalis muscle involvement is very common and platysma involvement less common. It is important to attempt to differentiate these two groups when analyzing the patient's case as significant clinical-pathological correlations exist which influence treatment.

Forced prolonged closure of the eyes ('pretend there is soap in your eyes') will usually precipitate the tonus phenomenon. The presence of weakness may be difficult to evaluate with total confidence, especially in the lower face, because the examiner may not be sure exactly how much limitation of the corner of the mouth is attributable to muscular weakness and how much to contraction of antagonists. This uncertainty is clarified only postoperatively when the spasm is gone, leaving the residual degree of true preoperative weakness unopposed for a time before the return of strength to normal supervenes.

Clinical-Pathological Correlations

Two major points may be made regarding clinical findings with the pathological abnormality. First, the site of vascular cross-compression is at the REZ (the Obersteiner-Redlich Zone) of the nerve. At this point, the myelin of the central nervous system provided by oligodendroglia is replaced by peripheral myelin provided by Schwann cells. By ultrastructural techniques, defects in the myelin are noted to be present here. Second, classical HFS is caused by a blood vessel on the anterior-caudal aspect of the nerve REZ (Fig. 1). Atypical HFS is almost always caused by a blood vessel on the posterior-rostral aspect of the REZ (Fig. 2). This compression may be venous rather than arterial and may be quite caudal on the medullary side of the ponto-medullary junction.

Patient Population, Operative Findings, Results

Two hundred and twenty nine patients have undergone RMC and MVD in this series. Table 1 summarizes some of the pertinent characteristics of this patient population. Note that HFS is more common in women than men, and more common on the left than the right. The population is middle aged and older in general, but the age distribution is the usual Gaussian curve.

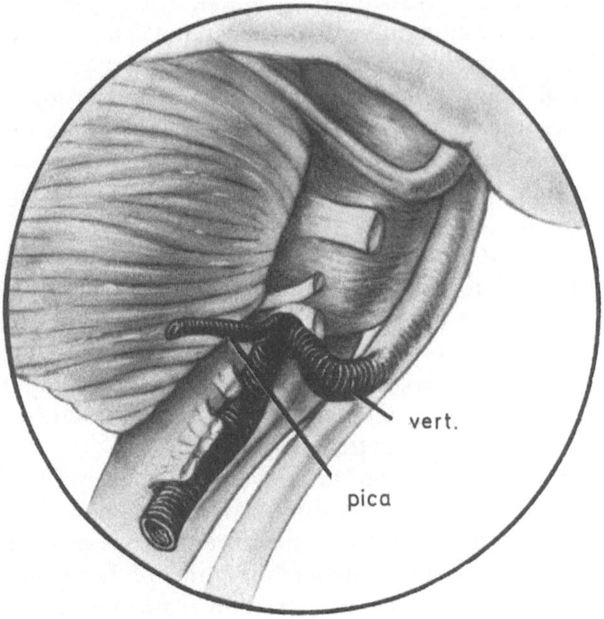

Fig. 1. Classical hemifacial spasm (Drawing of right side of brainstem). Vessel causes cross-compression of anterior-caudal aspect of root entry zone of facial nerve. This may be quite anterior and caudal on brainstem. (*vert.* = Vertebral artery, *pica* = posterior inferior cerebellar artery)

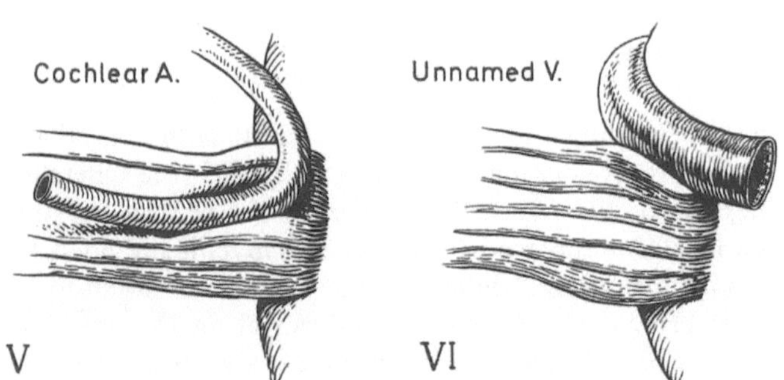

Fig. 2. Atypical hemifacial spasm. Drawing of left facial nerve at brainstem. Vessel causing compression is on rostral-caudal aspect of root entry zone

Table 1. Hemifacial spasm

Patient population:	
229 patients:	150 females, 79 males
Involved side:	91 right, 137 left, 1 bilateral
Syndrome:	205 classical, 24 atypical
Median decade:	50 – 60 years of age
Median duration of symptoms:	5 years

Operative findings are collated in Table 2. Note that the abnormality was overwhelmingly arterial. The Table does not point out that multiple vessels, often lying parallel and with one pushing another into the REZ, are common. The posterior inferior cerebellar artery is the most common vessel by far. If the surgeon finds a vertebral artery as the apparent cause, he must look beyond it to be certain that another smaller vessel is not the true abnormality. Veins, tumors, aneurysms, and arteriovenous malformations are rare cause of HFS although the first described pathology of HFS was an aneurysm [16] and the first patient operated upon by the author had a vein as the cause which was almost missed.

Results of operation are collated in Table 3. It can be noted that 212 patients (93 percent) have had an excellent result, although 12 patients needed a second operation before the vascular compression was relieved, usually because a blood vessel had been missed (see above). The majority of those who are fair results (partially symptomatic < 25 percent of preop level) had prior destructive procedures consisting of nerve crush, a partial section or alcohol injection. Only five patients (2.2 percent) are failures of therapy. Complications are collated in Table 4. It should be noted that hearing loss in the ipsilateral ear is the major risk of this procedure and the patient must have full understanding of this risk before operation is performed. Our incidence of hearing loss is much lower than it was early on. The author has had significant hearing loss in only two of his last 100 HFS patients.

Table 2. Hemifacial spasm (229 patients)

Operative findings:			
Arterial	210	Tumor	3
Mixed	10	Aneurysm	1
Venous	4	AVM	1

Table 3. Hemifacial spasm (229 patients)

Operative Results	No.	(%)
No spasm after one operation	201	87.8
No spasm, second procedure necessary	12	5.2
Partially symptomatic (25% of preop. level)	11	4.8
Failure of therapy	5	2.2

Table 4. Hemifacial spasm (229 patients)

Complications			
Cranial nerve deficit	23	UGI bleed	2
Serous otitis media	18	Pulmonary embolism	1
Aseptic meningitis	13	Pneumonia	4
Bacterial meningitis	1	Tension pneumocephalus	1
CSF rhinorrhea	8		

Operative Technique

The patient is prepared 12 hours preoperatively with 10 mg dexamethasone, and continued on a dose of 4 mg every 6 hours for 48 to 72 hours following operation. The patient is anesthetized and intubated. He is placed in the contralateral lateral decubitus position. The Doppler ultrasound instrument[1] for detection of air embolism is placed over the precordium. The neck is stretched a bit and flexed, and the head rotated to the ipsilateral side about 15 to 20 degrees. Figure 1 in the article 'Vascular Decompression in Trigeminal Neuralgia' shows the contralateral lateral decubitus position for retromastoid craniectomy and microvascular decompression of cranial nerves. Excessive flexion of lateral turning of the head is unnecessary. The ipsilateral hair is shaved posteriorly. An axillary roll is put into place to protect the brachial plexus. The patient must be securely fastened onto the table so that the table may be tilted laterally. The advantages of this position include less postoperative headache from cerebrospinal fluid loss and decreased incidence of air emboli. The disadvantages include increased risk of venous bleeding during soft-tissue dissection, the need for a suction in the cerebellopontine angle, and altered relationships between the facial nerve and vessels. The arterial loop may be 1 mm or more distant from the nerve in this position.

A vertical incision 6 to 8 cm long is made about 2 cm medial to the mastoid eminence roughly parallel to the hairline (Fig. 3). The incision is carried down to the occiput with the electrocautery, and the soft tissues are separated from the bone by means of a large periosteal elevator and electrocautery, and the soft tissues are separated from the bone by means of a large periosteal elevator and electrocautery where necessary. The medial and posterior aspects of the mastoid eminence must be cleared of soft tissue. The nuchal muscles are separated with electrocautery. The transverse occipital artery is identified, ligated, and divided. An inferolateral emissary vein is usually found which must be coagulated and divided. A self-retaining angulated Weitlaner retractor with four posts for the microsurgical retractor[2] is then put into place (Fig. 4). A retromastoid craniectomy, approximately 4 cm in diameter, is made low and laterally. It may be necessary to remove medial mastoid air cells and expose the sigmoid sinus in a dolichocephalic patient to provide an appropriate angle for easy exposure of the facial nerve at the brain stem. Mastoid air cells, if entered, are filled with bone wax. A curvilinear incision is made in the dura mater. The inferolateral flap is incised back to the sigmoid sinus and held out of the way with stay sutures.

The microsurgical self-retaining pillar-and-post retractor is then put into place by a long proximal rod and long narrow blade on a long rod. The blade is bent proximally about 20 to 30 degrees (variable) and placed under the cerebellum inferolaterally over a piece of rubber dam (fashioned from a rubber glove). The surgical binocular microscope with 250 mm objective and a set of angulated micro-dissecting instruments are used for the remainder of the intracranial procedure.

---

[1] Doppler ultrasound instrument manufactured by Roche Medical Electronics, Cranberry, New Jersey.

[2] Weitlaner retractor and microsurgical retractor available from V. Mueller Co, 6600 Touhy Avenue, Chicago, Illinois.

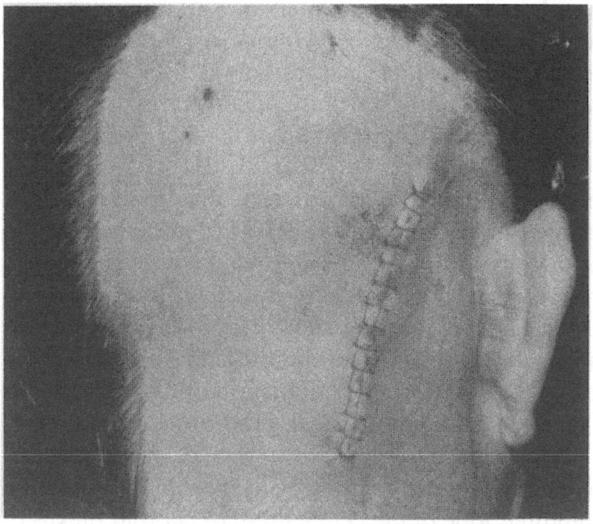

Fig. 3. Incision for retromastoid craniectomy. The incision is placed one fingerbreadth medial to the mastoid eminence and generally parallels the hairline

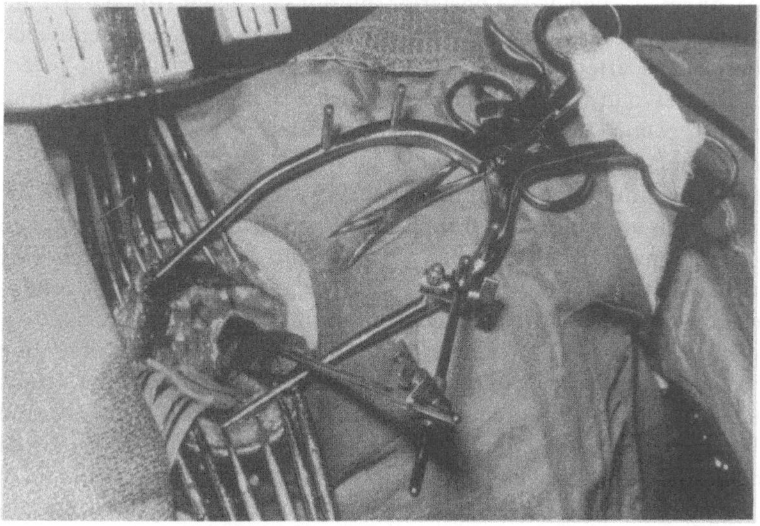

Fig. 4. Retractor arrangement for lower cranial nerve root entry zone exposure. Note that angulated Weitlaner retractor is clamped to the drapes using a sponge through the handles and that retractor blade is connected with one connecting rod to the post of the Weitlaner. We now use a narrower blade than is shown. The blade is bent proximally and not curved at all. Cerebellum is protected with a piece of rubber dam and a small cottonoid

The initial approach for proper exposure of the facial nerve at the brain stem is to elevate the cerebellum from the ninth, tenth, and eleventh cranial nerve. Sharp dissection is used to incise the arachnoid, with progressive medial placement of the retractor blade and elevation of the cerebellum until the choroid plexus of the lateral recess of the fourth ventricle is exposed. This tissue will then be directly in the way of the surgeon in his attempt to follow the facial nerve to the brain stem. Attention is now turned to the seventh and eighth cranial nerves. The arachnoidal incision is opened as necessary to expose these nerves. Arteries are frequently seen compressing, or coursing around or through these nerves between the brain stem and porus acusticus. These have not been found to cause hemifacial spasm in this series. The same vessels may be causing cross-compression of the facial nerve more proximally.

At this point begins a time of coordinated effort between the anesthesiologist and the surgeon. Progressive changes in angulation and height of placement of the microscope by the surgeon and the lateral tilt of the Table by the anesthesiologist may be necessary as dissection is carried more medially under the eighth cranial nerve to see the more anteriorly arising and coursing facial nerve. The retractor tip is usually readjusted medially under the cerebellum several times during this period. The author prefers the precision and safety (no potential 'spring') of a pillar-and-post retractor over the other types in all microsurgical procedures in the cerebellopontine angle.

The facial nerve may not be clearly visualized medially at this time because the offending arterial loop, flocculonodular lobe of the cerebellum, or choroid plexus of the lateral recess may be in the way. The artery may be large, such as the vertebral or basilar arteries, or small, such as the posterior inferior cerebellar (PICA), the anterior inferior cerebellar (AICA), or the cochlear arteries. In classical hemifacial spasm the position of the artery in relation to the nerve is consistent. The artery cross-compresses the nerve at the root exit zone and the nerve is compressed from the anterior caudal direction. Veins were noted in the same precise relationships in some patients, in combination with an artery or alone.

The principle of treatment is to decompress the facial nerve root exit zone by changing the axis of the arterial loop through interposition of a small implant of non-resorbable spongy material between the proximal and distal limbs of the loop and the brain stem. The dissection of the vessel may be easy or difficult. A combination of gentle leverage with sharp and blunt dissection of arachnoidal bands is necessary to mobilize the vessel. After mobilization, a piece of muscle or Ivalon sponge or Teflon felt is shaped to fit that area, grooved to fit and hold the artery, and deeply notched to protect the facial and statoacoustic nerves. The size and shape are variable, depending upon the particular anatomical relationships in each patient. Better methods to hold the new position of the vessel should be available in the future with other materials. More than one piece of material may be necessary to hold the position, prevent arterial kinking, protect the nerves. The implant should be interposed between artery and brain stem and not between artery and cranial nerves.

Tissue adhesive, applied in small amounts to the arachnoid, may be used to hold the implant in place. The facial nerve is deliberately not stroked or manipulated.

The Valsalva maneuver is performed several times in an attempt to ensure that the relationship between implant, artery, nerves, and brain stem will persist. The retractor and rubber dam are removed slowly, with visualization of the neurovascular-prosthesis relationship, as the retraction is released. The arachnoidal opening may be covered with a thin piece of gelatin foam. The dura mater is closed in a watertight fashion. The wound is closed in the usual way. The postoperative care is as for any intracranial procedure. Fluid intake is not restricted. The patient will have variable headache and usually spends 24 hours in the neurosurgical continuous care unit. Codeine sulfate in small doses is given as needed for incisional pain and/or headache.

Special Technical Problems

Three unexpected tumors were found and removed. Small veins were seen in four patients. They were simply coagulated and divided. The patients with atypical onset and progression of hemifacial spasm solely into the upper facial and frontalis muscles had cross-compression of the facial nerve on the posterior aspect of the root entry zone between the facial and statoacoustic nerves by a looping cochlear artery. In this situation, our techniques were unsuccessful in safely decompressing the nerve without threat to eighth nerve function in the early part of this series.

Operative Results

Results of operation in 229 patients with classical hemifacial spasm have been excellent in 201 (87.8 percent) but 12 patients (5.2 percent) required a second procedure for relief. Eleven patients (4.8 percent) are partly symptomatic (less than 25 percent of preoperative level) and five patients (2.2 percent) are failures. Ten patients developed delayed temporary facial weakness with return to fully normal function in all but one. Eighteen patients awoke with ipsilateral hearing loss or developed it later. Temporary stance and gait ataxia was seen in several patients early in the series due to cerebellar retraction, but has not been a problem with the refinements of technique noted in this article.

Postoperative electromyography has shown progressive loss of spasm and loss of pre-existent denervation. Only two late recurrences have been noted out of a 100 percent follow-up survey for up to 14 years. One was in a women whose spasm recurred after an automobile accident, and the second in a man who had 45 years of HFS before he was operated upon. These data support the thesis that the cross-compression at the brain stem is truly etiologic, that decompression is definitive, and that operative trauma is not the cause of the improvement.

Discussion

Theories as to the etiology of hemifacial spasm have been diverse in the past [1–10, 22]. Campbell and Keedy [2] found ectatic vessels in two patients with tic douloureux and hemifacial spasm but did not treat the hemifacial spasm. Gardner [5–8] elegantly correlated the similarities in trigeminal neuralgia and hemifacial spasm, but did not inspect the root exit zone of the facial nerve in his hemifacial spasm patients. Treatment of hemifacial spasm has usually consisted of application of mild to severe trauma to the peripheral facial nerve or to the nerve in the cerebellopontine angle. Scoville successfully treated hemifacial spasm in one patient by moving a rather peripheral artery from the facial nerve in the cerebellopontine angle [21]. He did not use the microscope, nor did he examine the nerve root entry zone in this case, but may have inadvertently decompressed the nerve proximally by moving a more peripheral part of the same looping artery, a situation we have seen a number of times. Recent investigators have shown that vascular cross-compression is the overwhelming common cause of HFS and that it can be treated definitively by microvascular decompression [12–14, 16–20].

In addition to the present series, which includes one case of aneurysm causing HFS reported independently by Maroon [17], Petty and Southby [18], Hankinson and Wilson [11], and Rhoton [19] have published reports of small to large series where vascular compression was identified and treated using microsurgical techniques.

The postoperative sequence in the current series is striking in that if the facial nerve is not touched during the operation, the patient awakens from anesthesia with some hemifacial spasm, which then gradually disappears. If the nerve is touched during dissection, the patient awakens free of spasm; he may develop mild temporary spasm which gradually disappears. If the nerve is gently stroked or manipulated during the procedure, the patient usually awakens from anesthesia free of spasm. Vascular compression-distortion of the root entry zone causes morphological changes in the nerve as has been described elsewhere [20]. With relief of the vascular compression, and without trauma, it may take some time for the abnormal conduction to revert to normal, presumably as the myelin regenerates.

It must be emphasized that the vascular compression must be cross-compressed at right angles to the nerve and must be at the root exit zone of the nerve from the brain stem. Peripheral vessels crossing the facial nerve, and vessels running parallel to and distorting the nerve, have not been shown to cause hemifacial spasm in this series. These latter vessels are left undisturbed. It is known that defects exist in the root entry zone in the cranial nerves at the point where the central myelin is replaced by peripheral myelin. Why the vascular cross-compression must be located precisely at this point we do not know. We can only conjecture that the junction zone defects may predispose to disordered conduction when this part of the nerve is cross-compressed by a blood vessel.

Mild facial weakness is common in hemifacial spasm of long duration, especially if the tonus phenomenon is present. Strength improves gradually after vascular decompression, and is frequently improved in the recovery room. Experience with the surgical binocular microscope and a thorough knowledge of the normal anatomy of the cerebellopontine angle are vital if observations are to be valid and the procedure safe.

References

1. Battle RJV (1963) Facial spasm. Br J Plast Surg 16:257–263
2. Campbell E, Keedy C (1947) Hemifacial spasm: a note on the etiology in two cases. J Neurosurg 4:342–347
3. Diamant H, Enfors B, Wiberg A (1967) Facial spasm. With special reference to the chorda tympani functional and operative treatment. Laryngoscope 77:350–358
4. Ehni G, Woltman HW (1947) Hemifacial spasm. Review of one hundred and six cases. Arch Neurol Psychiatry 53:205–211

5. Gardner WJ (1962) Concerning the mechanism of trigeminal neuralgia and hemifacial spasm. J Neurosurg 19: 947–957
6. Gardner WJ (1960) Five year cure of hemifacial spasm. Report of a case. Cleve Clin Q 27: 219–221
7. Gardner WJ, Sava GA (1962) Hemifacial spasm: a reversible pathophysiologic state. J Neurosurg 19: 240–247
8. Gardner WJ (1971) Personal communication
9. German WJ (1942) Surgical treatment of spasmodic facial tic. Surgery 11: 912–914
10. Greenwood J Jr (1946) The surgical treatment of hemifacial spasm. J Neurosurg 3: 506–510
11. Hankinson HF, Wilson CB (1976) Microsurgical treatment of hemifacial spasm. West J Med 124: 191
12. Jannetta PJ (1970) Microsurgical exploration and decompression of the facial nerve in hemifacial spasm. Curr Top Surg Res 2: 217–220
13. Jannetta PJ (1974) Neurovascular compression of the facial nerve in hemifacial spasm: relief by microsurgical technique. In: Merei FT (ed) Reconstructive Surgery of Brain Arteries. Publishing House of the Hungarian Academy of Sciences, Budapest pp 193–199
14. Jannetta PJ, Abbasy M, Maroon JC, Ramos FM, Albin MS (1977) Etiology and definitive microsurgical treatment of hemifacial spasm. J Neurosurg 47: 321–328
15. Kerber CW, Margolis MT, Newton TH (1972) Tortuous vertebrobasilar system: a cause of cranial nerve signs. Neuroradiology 4: 74–77
16. Maroon JC (1978) Hemifacial spasm. A vascular cause. Arch Neurol 35: 481
17. Maroon JC, Albins MS (1974) Air embolism diagnosed by Doppler ultrasound. Anesth Analg (Paris) 53: 399–402
18. Petty PG, Southby R (1977) Vascular compression of lower cranial nerves: observations using microsurgery with particular reference to trigeminal neuralgia. Aust NZ J Surg 47: 3: 314
19. Rhoton AL (1978) Microsurgical neurovascular decompression for trigeminal neuralgia and hemifacial spasm. J Fla Med Assoc 65: 425
20. Ruby JR, Jannetta PJ (1975) Hemifacial spasm. Ultrastructural changes in the facial nerve induced by neurovascular compression. Surg Neurol 4: 369–370
21. Scoville WB (1969) Hearing loss following exploration of cerebellopontine angle in treatment of hemifacial spasm. J Neurosurg 31: 47–49
22. Wartenberg R (1952) Hemifacial spasm: A clinical and pathophysiological study. Oxford University Press, New York

The Pathogenesis of Hemifacial Spasm: Characteristic Changes of Vasculatures in Vertebro-Basilar Artery System

A. KONDO, J.-I. ISHIKAWA, and T. KONISHI, Tsukimi, Fukui, Fukui/Japan

Introduction

Hemifacial spasm is a very distressing disorder characterized by a subacute, intermittent and involuntary occurrence, and occasionally makes the patients depressive. Treatments for this hyperactive dysfunction of the facial nerve has usually consisted of application of mild to severe trauma to the nerve, either extracranially or intracranially. Posterior cranial fossa approach to this region for decompression of the cranial nerve was enhanced by Jannetta et al. (1977). From experiences of surgery, they emphasized that the facial nerve is, in all cases, cross-compressed by a right- angled artery near the root exit zone from the brain-stem. There have been, however, many controversial opinions concerning the mechanism of the facial spasm and also questions why a special artery is able to make such a 'cross-compression' of the nerve or why the facial spasm invariably develops on one side of the face. The authors treated 61 patients of hemifacial spasm and studied preoperative vertebral arteriograms in 50 patients among them. In this paper, they mentioned the pathogenesis or mechanism causing this clinical symptom-complex of hyperactive dysfunction of the facial nerve from the findings of surgical procedures and preoperative arteriograms.

Cases Operated

Sixty-one patients were operated upon ranging in age from 22 to 68 years and females outnumbering males 46, 60, 15. Neither side of the face was affected more frequently. Thirty-two patients among them had previously undergone other traumatizing procedures to the peripheral part of the facial nerve, resulting in either no relief or recurrence of symptoms. Ten patients complained of tinnitus on the affected side simultaneously with an attack of hemifacial spasm. Fifty patients out of 61 with hemifacial spasm underwent preoperative vertebral arteriography and the findings of arteriograms, namely the vasculatures of vertebro-basilar artery system were closely investigated.

Angiographic Studies

Antero-posterior, lateral, and Stenvers projections of vertebral arteriograms were taken preoperatively and characteristic vasculatures of vertebro-basilar arteries and their branches were verified. The size of the vertebral artery is definitely asymmetric, being larger on the affected side of the face and showing peculiar anatomical change at its third segment. The details of this vascular change will be discussed below. With close observations of these unique vasculature changes on vertebral arteriograms, the responsible compressing artery of the facial nerve is able to be conjectured with and approximately 80 percent accuracy before surgery.

Operative Method

Retromastoid craniectomy with the patient on semiprone position was made to reach the facial nerve. The most important point of this surgery is to identify the artery which is really cross-compressing the cranial nerve, since there are, in some

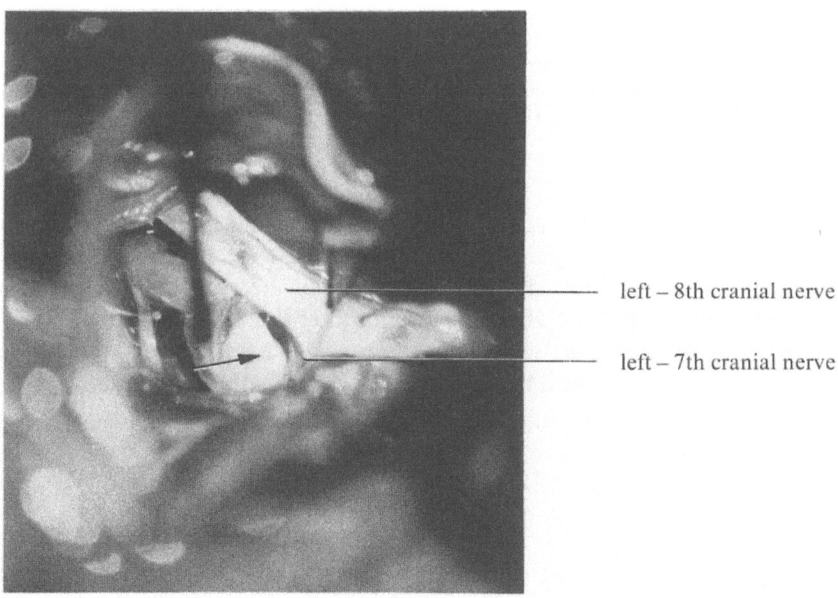

Fig. 1. Operative photograph of a patient with the left hemifacial spasm. A compressing artery (*arrow*) cross-compresses at right-angles to the nerve and also reveals 'arteriosclerotic change of the wall' at the compressing site

instances, several elongated and tortuous arteries found running close to or touching the cranial nerve. The most characteristic findings of the compressing artery is invariably nearly right-angled at its compressing site as mentioned by Jannetta (1970) and furthermore, according to our observations, the wall of the vessels is whitish in appearance and hardened when touched by a microvascular forceps. A small piece of prosthesis is inserted between the artery and the brainstem after freeing the compressing artery from the nerve.

Operative Results

Surgical results were evaluated according to Jannetta's classification (1977) combined with considering postoperative reduction in hearing acuity. Postoperative hearing disturbance continuing more than one year is considered to be a result in placement of the patient to the next less favorable grade; for example, from 'excellent' to 'good'. According to author's classification, the results were: excellent – 25, good – 11, fair – 7, and poor – 1. No recurrence of symptoms occurred in these 44 patients

Table 1. *Surgical results* evaluated according to Jannetta's classification combined with considering postoperative change in hearing acuity

Excellent	25	Fair	7
Good	11	Poor	1

Total 44 cases (out of 60) who have been followed up more than 1 year [a] after the surgery.

[a] Postoperative hearing disturbance continuing more than 1 year is considered to be a result in placement of the patient to the next less favorable grade.

followed up more than one year postoperatively. The average follow up period is two years; the longest, three years. Six patients out of 20 with preoperative facial motor weakness elicited by prior destructive surgery to the peripheral part of the facial nerve well recovered within about six months after the decompressive surgery, whereas eight patients out of 10 with facial motor weakness without undergoing prior destructive surgery recovered better and more rapidly after the operative intervention.

Discussion

In 1960, Bragdon first mentioned a method of intracranial crushing of the facial nerve by a hemostat as a treatment of hemifacial spasm and in 1962, Gardner and Sava first applied a piece of Gelfoam prosthesis between the compressing vessel and the facial nerve for decompression. In 1970, Jannetta, a pioneer of modern microvascular decompressive surgery of cranial nerves first elegantly decompressed the facial nerve with the aid of new microsurgical adjuvants and excellent microsurgical techniques without traumatizing the facial nerve. There are, however, some controversial opinions concerning the mechanism of hemifacial spasm and questions, why a special vessel can be causative of neurovascular compressions despite several arteries are existing around the facial nerve, and why the vast majority of facial spasm occurs on one side of the face, which still remained unsolved. There have been many reports describing that various organic lesions can be causative of hemifacial spasm (1875 Schultze, 1917 Cushing, 1945 Ehni and Woltman, 1947 Campbell and Keedy, 1948 Laine, 1952 McKenzie, 1962 Gardner and Sava). Maroon (1978) described 16 communications reporting a total of 107 cases of hemifacial spasm, probably caused by vascular compression of the facial nerve. Confirmation in these cases was made by surgery (92 cases), angiography (12 cases), and autopsy (3 cases). There is, therefore, extensive evidence pointing to the recognition that fairly consistent pathologic process or organic lesions which exist between the facial nerve nucleus and internal auditory meatus are definitely causative factors of this syndrome. In 1958, Greenfield suggested that myelin seemed to be more vulnerable both to mechanical pressure and to minor degrees of anoxia than nerve cells and axon. In 1944, Granit et al. experimentally created an 'artificial synapse' on the sciatic nerve to verify the 'short circuit' of action current at this synapse by insulating myelin sheaths. In 1962, Gardner proposed the term 'junction zone' at the exit zone of the facial nerve from the brain-stem where the oligodendroglial covering of the myelin sheath was replaced by the tougher neurilemma. Jannetta et al. (1977) pointed out that the 'junction zone' is the place where irritable lesions are most likely to produce disordered nerve function and they hypothesized that at this anatomically discernible junction zone, the physiological threshold to mechanical deformations and pressure might be existing and the stimuli could easily interfere with axonal metabolites and transport.

The 'peripheral hypothesis' for the explanation of pathogenesis of hemifacial spasm is based on the phenomenon of 'fiber interaction' at the site of compression or injured part, several millimeters lateral to the exit zone of the facial nerve from the brain-stem and this 'junction zone' is thought to act as a 'false synapse' and to give rise to potentials which cause spontaneous movements on the face. On the contrary, Hunt (1909) and Wartenberg (1952) conceived that hemifacial spasm might be caused by a lesion in the facial nerve nucleus and furthermore, Ferguson (1978) described his theory opposing the 'peripheral hypothesis'. He was against the hypothesis of Granit et al. (1944) by citing a report of electromyographic study by Wigand et al. (1972) in which differing latencies between the periocular, chin and lip motor units during 'synchronous' spasm were noted and he concluded from this constant difference between latencies that this fact is evidence against impulse initiation from a common point as required by an 'ethapse' hypothesis. For the explanation of the mechanism of hemifacial spasm, Ferguson (1978) proposed that 'the unique central organization of the facial motor system' was the basis not only for a wide range of voluntary movements, but for involuntary or automatic movements of the face as well, and partial and selective differentiation would occur on motor neurons in the nucleus following injury to the facial motor nerve. We partly agree with the opinion of Ferguson (1978) since we realized that 'peripheral hypothesis' does not thoroughly explain the emotional or reflexive effects on eliciting severe hyperkinetic movements of facial muscles. On the other hand, Habel (1898) and Ehni and Woltman (1945) described that the hemifacial spasm was not affected by an ipsilateral hemiplegia caused by a stroke, and also we noticed not infrequently the persistence of facial spasm during surgery even after induction of anesthesia to the patients. These facts might oppose the opinion of Ferguson (1978) who mentioned 'unique central organization' being able to unmask and augument automatic movements of facial muscles, including corticobulbar fibers and motor neurons in the facial nerve nucleus.

The key point of this microvascular decompression surgery is the confirmation of a compressing vessel. Due to Sunderland (1945), anterior inferior cerebellar arteries were running close to the 7th and 8th cranial nerves, and also we realized during surgery that many arteries or veins were running to or touching the cranial nerve. Jannetta et al. (1977) emphasized that vascular compression must be a 'cross-compression' of the nerve at right angles and the compression site must be the root exit zone of the facial nerve from the brain-stem. During surgery, we additionally observed peculiar findings of the compressing artery i.e. the wall of the compressing artery is focally whitish discolored and hardened when touched by a vascular forceps as well. This unique arterial wall changes at the compressing site are very characteristic and noted unrelatedly to the age of the patients and are also noticed merely at the right-angled compressing site, not at other part of the artery.

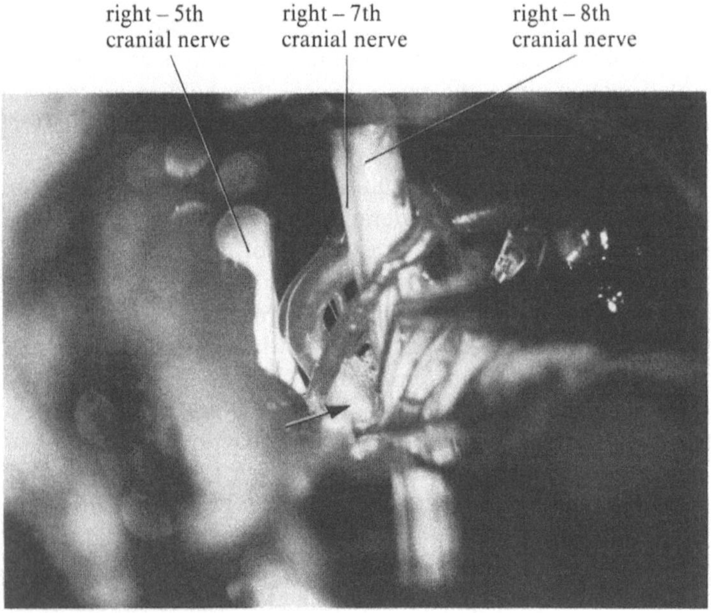

Fig. 2. Another operative photograph of a patient with the right hemifacial spasm shows several arteries which are running closely to the facial nerve. Note only that the compressing site of the artery (*arrow*) shows a specific pathoanatomical process

We have performed vertebral arteriography in 50 out of 61 patients with hemifacial spasm. The most characteristic findings of the arteriogram are that the size of vertebral arteries is found frequently larger on the affected side of the face and the artery makes a sharp, hair-pin like angulation at the beginning of the third segment and from this angulated part, a posterior inferior cerebellar artery which is commonly more ectatic, elongated, and redundant than the contralateral side gives off and directs toward the internal auditory meatus. The other type of peculiar vascular change is that a basilar artery makes an unusual S-shaped curve accompanying an above mentioned specific anatomical change of vertebral artery and also elongated, and tortuous anterior inferior cerebellar artery originated from this basilar artery toward the internal auditory meatus with an aplastic or hypoplastic posterior inferior cerebellar artery on the same side.

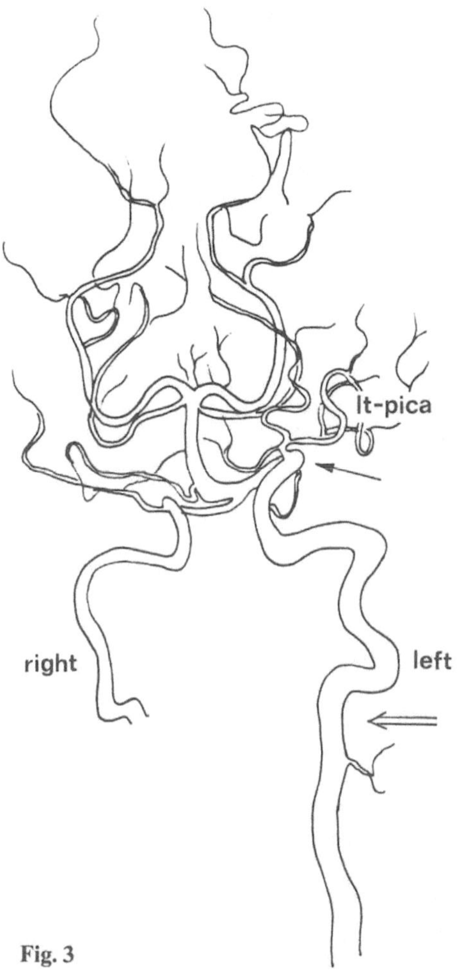

Fig. 3

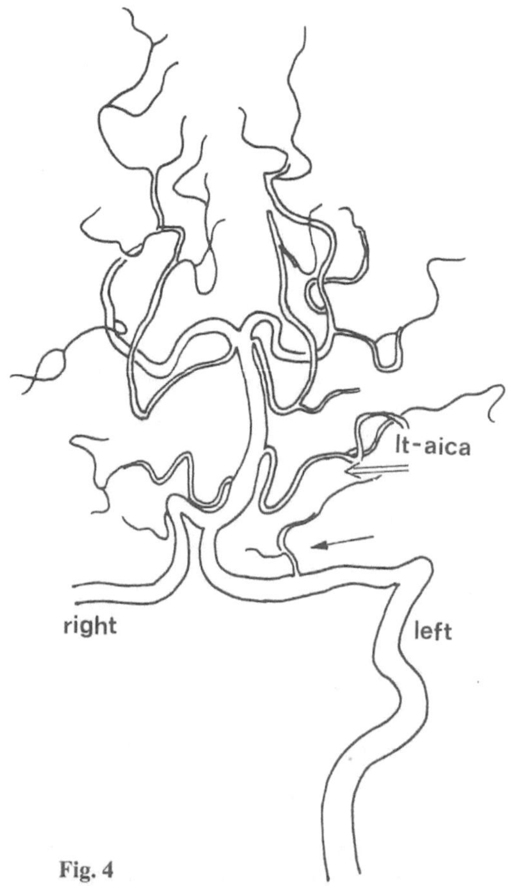

Fig. 4

Fig. 3. Drawing of vertebral arteriogram of a patient with left hemifacial spasm. Note characteristic vasculature changes. The ipsilateral vertebral artery with larger diameter (*large arrow*) makes a hair-pin like angulation at the third segment (*small arrow*) and gives off redundant and dilated posterior inferior cerebellar artery from this angulated site toward the left internal auditory meatus

Fig. 4. Drawing of another vertebral arteriogram with left hemifacial spasm. Note typical vasculature change. Vertebral artery is asymmetric. S-shaped basilar artery originates ectated and tortuous anterior inferior cerebellar artery (*large arrow*) toward the left internal acoustic meatus with (aplastic) or hypoplastic posterior inferior cerebellar artery on the ipsilateral side (*small arrow*)

Although Newton and Mani (1974) reported that the size of the vertebral arteries varied, the left being more often larger than the right, the size of the vertebral artery in our studies is very commonly larger on the involved side of the face despite the fact that neither side of the face was affected more frequently. This vasculature change is, therefore, thought to be definitely characteristic for the patients with hemifacial spasm. There are a number of hemodynamic theories explaining the mechanism of arterial wall thickening which is usually found in the neighborhood of bifurcation, junctions, and curved segment of vessels (Matsuda et al. 1978). We suppose that these unique changes of vasculature of vertebral artery in the patient with hemifacial spasm may be congenital and is influenced by developmental hemodynamic factors as well i.e. the asymmetric size of the diameter and a hair-pin like angulation of the vertebral artery at its third segment may be congenitally present and intraluminal blood stream of the larger sized vertebral artery is likely to give

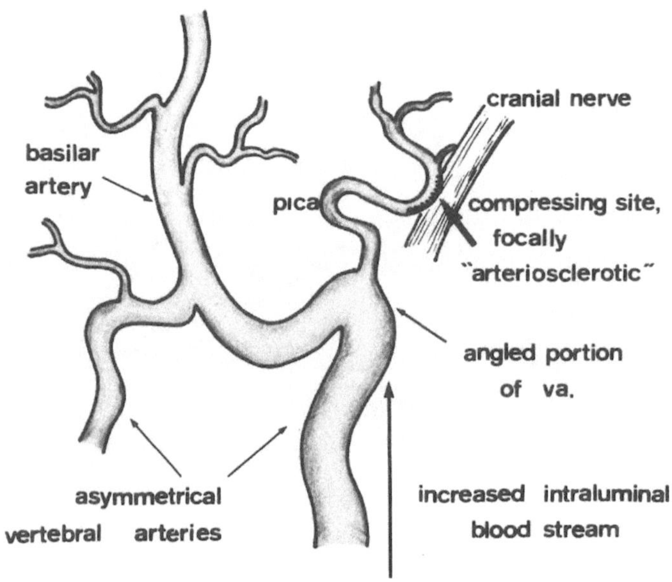

Fig. 5. This figure explains the mechanism of vascular compression of the facial nerve. The vertebral artery shows an asymmetry and characteristic angulation at the third segment. Increased intraluminal hemodynamic forces of this artery are exaggerated to the branching artery, resulting in ectasia, redundancy and wall thickening of these branches at the nerve compression site

stronger forces to the wall of the curved segment afterwards, and that this exaggerated intraluminal blood pressure is exerted to the peripheral part of the branches originating from this angulated part, resulting in ectasia, elongation and wall thickening of the posterior inferior cerebellar artery. For example, after continuous hemodynamic stimulation and provided that the peripheral part of this branch is lying just close enough to be able to make cross-compression of root entry zone of the facial nerve to the brain-stem, the pathological process of the nerve compression might accordingly ensue. These vasculature change of vertebro-basilar artery and their branches might give us a key to clarify the pathogenesis of hemifacial spasm, and to solve the questions why a special artery can be responsible for microvascular compression of the facial nerve and also why this hyperdysfunction of the nerve is invariably elicited on one side of the face.

Conclusions

Vertebral arteriograms and surgical findings of the patients with hemifacial spasm revealed characteristic vasculature changes of vertebro-basilar arteries and their branches as a cause of neurovascular compression of the facial nerve. This peculiar pathoanatomical change of the vessels should be a pathogenesis of hemifacial spasm and invariably unilateral occurrence of this peculiar vascular architecture is a reason why the vast majority of hemifacial spasm develops on one side of the face.

References

Bragdon FH (1960) Intracranial crushing of facial nerve for hemifacial spasm. Presented at the 46th Annual clinical congress of the American college of surgeons. San Francisco, Oct. 10–14

Campbell E, Keedy C (1947) Hemifacial spasm: A note on the etiology in two cases. J Neurosurg 4:342–347

Cushing H (1917) Tumors of the nervus acusticus and the syndrome of the cerebellopontine angle. W. B. Sanders, Philadelphia & London, p 296

Ehni G, Woltman HW (1945) Hemifacial spasm. Review of one hundred and six cases. Arch Neurol Psychiat 53:205–211

Ferguson JH (1978) Hemifacial spasm and the facial nerve. Ann Neurol 4 (2):97–102

Gardner WJ, Sava GA (1962) Hemifacial spasm – a reversible pathophysiologic state. J Neurosurg 19:240–247

Gardner WJ (1962) Concerning the mechanism of trigeminal neuralgia and hemifacial spasm. J Neurosurg 19:947–958

Granit R, Leksell L, Skoglund CR (1944) Fibre interaction in injured or compressed region of nerve. Brain 67:125–140

Greenfield JG (1958) Neuropathology. E Arnold, London, p 640

Habel A (1898) Über Fortbestehen von Tic convulsif bei gleichseitiger Hemiplegie. Dtsch Med Wschr 24:189

Hunt JR (1909) The sensory system of the facial nerve and its symptomatology. J Nerv Ment Dis 36:321–350

Jannetta PJ (1970) Microsurgical explorations and decompression of the facial nerve in hemifacial spasm. Curr Top Surg Res 2:217–220

Jannetta PJ, Abbasy M, Maroon JC, Ramos FM, Albin MS (1977) Etiology and definitive microsurgical treatment of hemifacial spasm. Operative techniques and results in 47 patients. J Neurosurg 47:321–328

Laine E (1948) Hémispasme facial queri par intervention sur la fossa postérieure. Rev Neurol (Paris) 80:38–40

Maroon JC (1978) Hemifacial spasm. A vascular cause. Arch Neurol 35:481–483

Matsuda I, Niimi H, Moritake K, Okumura A, Handa H (1978) The role of hemodynamic factors in arterial wall thickening in the rat. Atherosclerosis 29:363–371

McKenzie KG (1952) The residual hearing following partial resection of the 8th nerve. Laryngoscope 62:562–565

Newton TH, Mani RL (1974) The vertebral artery. In Radiology of the skull and brain. Angiography. In: Newton TH, Potts DG (eds) The C.V. Mosbym St Louis p 1659–1709

Schultze F (1875) Linksseitiger Facialis-Krampf in Folge eines Aneurysma der Arteria vertebralis sinistra. Virchows Arch 65:385–391

Sunderland S (1945) The arterial relations of the internal auditory meatus. Brain 68:23–27

Wartenberg R (1952) Hemifacial spasm. A clinical and pathophysiological study. Oxford Univ Press, New York, p 86

Wigand ME, Spreng M, Bumm P (1972) Electronic evaluation of electromyograms in facial nerve paralysis. Arch Otolaryngol 95:324–330

Surgical Treatment of Hemifacial Spasm

M. Samii, Hannover/FRG

During the last ten years we have operated upon 19 patients with hemifacial spasm (Table 1).

In eight patients we performed selective partial resection of the peripheral branches of the facial nerve using electrostimulation in local anaesthesia (Fig. 1). Peripheral to the parotid gland we exposed the facial nerve at different levels. Selective transection and resection of the individual branches could be done under local anaesthesia in order to prove the functional result. Using this technique we could transect approximately 50 percent of all branches. This procedure did not lead to a

Table 1. Surgical treatment of hemifacial spasm

Operative method	Number of cases	Results
Partial resection of peripheral branches	8	Recurrence in all 8 cases 3 – 18 months
Vascular decompression of VII. nerve (sponge)	6	3 slight improvement 3 no improvement
Vascular decompression of VII. nerve and brain stem (muscle pieces)	5	Excellent, no recurrence

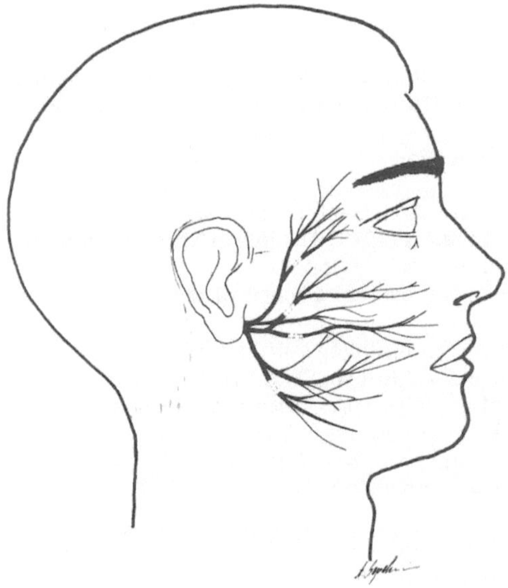

Fig. 1. Scheme of selective partial resection of the peripheral branches of the facial nerve in patients with hemifacial spasm

severe loss of facial nerve function and thus facial muscle movement remained unimpaired. In severe cases of hemifacial spasm, it was necessary to resect more than 50 percent of the nerve fibres in order to achieve satisfactory results. Only in these cases a slight temporary postoperative weakness of the facial nerve function occured. In all these eight cases the patients left the hospital with full satisfaction, but unfortunately permanent healing was not achieved. Symptoms recurred months later. The longest symptom-free interval was 18 months.

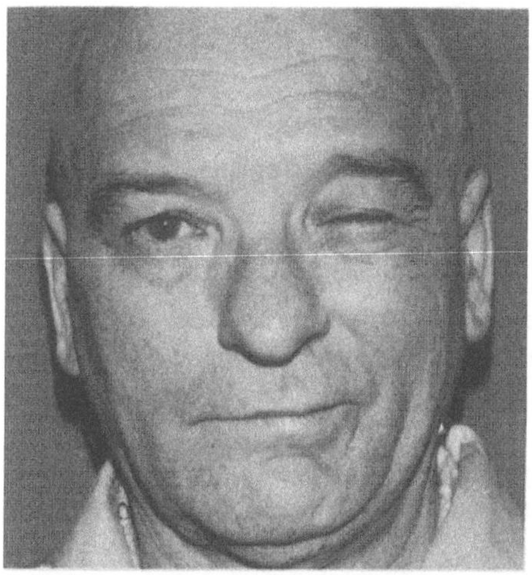

a

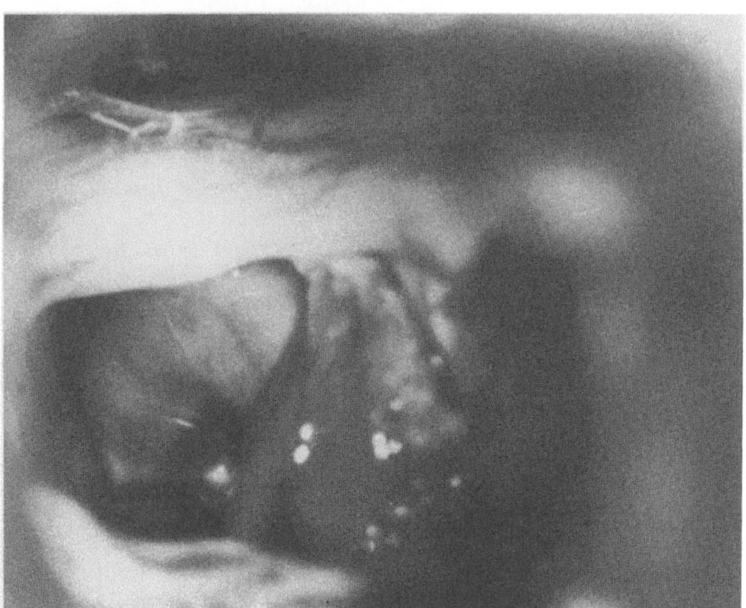

b

Fig. 2a, b. Severe left sided hemifacial spasm (**a**). Vascular decompression of the facial nerve in the left cerebellopontine angle at the brain stem. A muscle implant is placed between the arterial loop and the facial nerve at the brain stem (**b**)

These poor results from one side and the excellent results of operated cases by Jannetta with vascular decompression in the cerebellopontine angle encouraged us to try this technique. In the first six patients who underwent vascular decompression of the VIIth nerve in the cerebellopontine angle we achieved in three cases permanent slight improvement, but in the other three cases the follow up showed no change compared to the preoperative findings. At that time I was not very satisfied with the results and therefore discussed things again with Doctor Jannetta. He explained to me the importance of decompression of the facial nerve at the brain stem and not in the peripheral part at the internal auditory meatus. The next failure was the use of fibrin sponges, which are eventually reabsorbed and disappeared.

In five patients, in which the vascular decompression was carried out at the central part of the facial nerve with exposure of the exit area of the facial nerve at the brain stem, we achieved an excellent result in all five without any complication (Fig. 2a and b). Jannetta's technique seems to be the operative treatment of choice of facial spasm. According to our experience the location of the implant between the arterial loop and the facial nerve at the brain stem is of utmost importance for the result. The risk of inducing deafness must be discussed with the patient. In two patients we had a decrease of hearing function, but in the last patient operated upon six months ago, the patient had preoperatively a severe hemifacial spasm combined with tinnitus and considerable hearing loss. Postoperatively the hemifacial spasm and tinnitus had disappeared and the hearing was reported to be improved, the latter could be proved by an increase of the tone threshold.

Bells Palsy

K. J. Zülch, Köln/FRG

I am somewhat puzzled at the end of these discussions on facial nerve lesions. I think the concept of hemifacial spasm is convincing. However, in Bell's palsy or the so-called 'lesion e frigore' the concept of an intracranial pressure lesion by a normal vessel does not correspond with my clinical experience and I would be reluctant to accept this mechanism particularly in the light of the data and concepts of Esslen (1960, 1977), who found a circumscribed functional block in the intraosseous course of the nerve. Therefore, I still favour the intraosseous mechanism.

With regard to the associated movements after 'regeneration' I still believe that misregeneration theory of Lipschitz (1906) has the highest degree of likelihood. I, in order to overcome the false regeneration and the aberration of the sprouting fibers, have advised patients to make, in the third month, electrical gymnastics of single muscles with galvanic current supported simultaneously by the patients' passive movement of the same muscle by his finger. This is the time when the regenerating axons arrive at the muscles. My concept was that one could perhaps enhance the sprouting of the overshooting axons into the 'right' muscle, possibly even by the aid of the electric current and thus in the long run letting atrophy the unnecessary supernumerous axons (for details see Zülch 1955, 1956, 1961, Fig. 3).

However, there was no different result, and the patients who had performed these combined gymnastics for more than a year just had the usual associated movements (see Zülch 1970, Figs. 17, 20, 24).

References

Esslen E (1960) Electromyographic findings on two types of misdirection of regenerating axons. J Electroenceph Clin Neurophysiol 12:738–741

Esslen E (1977) The acute facial palsies. Neurology Series No. 18. Springer-Verlag, Berlin Heidelberg New York

Lipschitz R (1906) Über aberrierende Bündel bei Facialislähmung. Neurol Zbl 26:380–381

Zülch KJ (1955) Kann die Nachbehandlung während der Regeneration die Wiederherstellung der Leitungssysteme beeinflussen? Zbl Ges Neurol 133, 145–153

Zülch KJ (1956) Der Wert der konservativen Behandlung für die Restitution der gestörten Facialisfunktion. Fortschr Kiefer-Gesichts-Chir 2, 132–135

Zülch KJ (1961) Gedanken eines Neurologen zur konservativen und chirurgischen Behandlung der Facialislähmungen, insbesondere der sogenannten „rheumatischen" Pathogenese. Z Laryngol Rhinol 40:305–318

Zülch KJ (1970) 'Idiopathic' facial paresis. In: Vinken PJ, Bruyn GW (eds) Handbook of Clinical Neurology, Vol 8, North-Holland Publ. Comp., Amsterdam pp 241–302

Infusion Therapy – A New Concept in Treatment of Bell's Palsy

E. STENNERT, Göttingen/FRG

This paper is a short presentation of a new therapeutic concept in the treatment of Bell's palsy, the results of which will be soon published in detail.

Therapy of idiopathic facial paralysis is a matter of controversy since Ballance and Duel in 1932 recommended decompression of the facial nerve by opening the Fallopian canal. This procedure has up to the present day found its supporters as well as critics. Moreover, its discussion has been newly initiated since the exposure especially of the labyrinthine and meatal segment of the facial nerve was regarded as indispensable. On the other hand, either the use of corticosteroides or even complete therapeutic inactivity was recommended as the treatment of choice.

The justification of any surgical decompression is based on the concept of the etiological mechanism of Bell's palsy as it was postulated by Kettel (1947). Although this theory of a primary vascular insufficiency has been widely accepted, the conviction seems to grow that, as far as etiology is concerned, Bell's palsy is not a uniform clinical picture, but that multiple factors may be responsible for this type of pareses. But, as far as this can be judged today, their damaging action always involves a combined inflammatory-vascular component.

Therefore, it is of secondary importance for the fate of the nerve, whether the vicious circle (Fig. 1) starts with ischemia, eventually resulting in edema due to exudation, or whether edema occurs first, leading in a second step to ischemia – by compression first of the lymphatic and the venous drain and later also by compression of the arterial branch. In any case, a combined damage of the neurons develops as a consequence of compression on the one hand and hypoxia on the other. An effective therapy therefore must counteract both components of this vicious circle, the parenchymatous as well as the vascular. This means: Treatment of the edema and at the same time improvement of microcirculation (rheology).

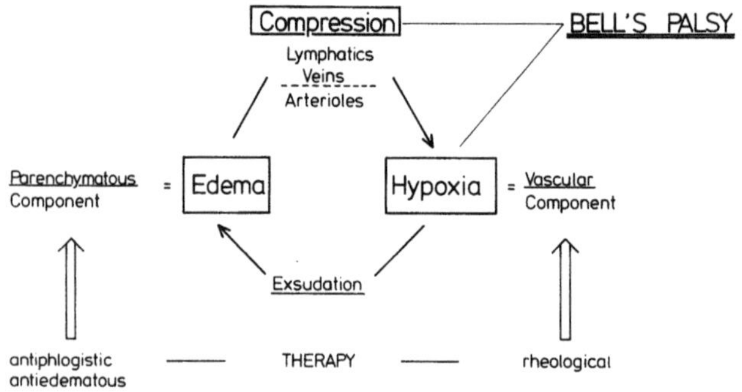

Fig. 1. Estimated pathophysiological mechanism of the 'vicious circle', probably responsible for the development of Bell's palsy

Days of treatment		Dextrane 40 [a] with Sorbitol or Mannitol 5 – 10% (ml/day)	Pentoxifylline [b] (ml/day)	Cortisone [c] (Prednisolone-equivalent dose [mg/day])	< 70 kg	> 70 kg	Substitution
in-	1	2×500/16 h	10		200	250	
patient	2	2×500/16 h	10	per	200	250	1. Potassium [e]
	3	2×500/16 h	15	infusion	150		
	4	500/ 8 h	15		150		
	5	500/ 8 h	15		100		2. Fluid
	6	500/ 8 h	15		100		oral or i.v [f]
	7	500/ 8 h	15		75		(ca. 1000 ml/day,
	8	500/ 8 h	15		50		control of
	9	500/ 8 h	15	oral [d]	40		hematocrit)
	10	500/ 8 h	15	circadian	20		
out-	11			(6 – 8 a.m.)	15		
patient	12				12.5		
	13				10		
	14				7.5		
	15				5		
	16				2.5		
	17				2.5		
	18				2.5		

[a] Onkovertin N with Sorbitol 5%
[b] Trental
[c] Solu-Decortin H
[d] Ultralan
[e] Kalinor Brause-Tbl.
[f] Sterofundin

Fig. 2. Treatment protocol for Bell's palsy (Stennert, E). Therapy with infusions twice per day should last for 3×24 hrs. Cortisone – as well as Pentoxifylline – dose devided into both infusions

On the basis of this pathophysiological concept we have developed an infusion therapy which has been used in our clinic with considerable success for about two years. The details of this therapeutic procedure are given in Fig. 2. As it is seen from this table, we are also using Cortisone in the antiedematous and antiphlogistic therapy, but we differ considerably from all previous therapeutic managements by initially applying very much higher dosages.

For the improvement of microcirculation with the aim of increased perfusion of the peripheral nerve with oxygen, we have used low molecular Dextrane in combination with Pentoxifylline. The selection and combination of these drugs is based on the knowledge of their pharmakokinetics concerning the above mentioned pathophysiological mechanism of Bell's palsy:

1. Cortisone: The strong antiphlogistic and antiedematous effect of Cortisone is clinically and experimentally verified. It is based on its involvement in all phases of the inflammatory tissue reaction. Three main actions cooperate in this effect: an antiexudative, an antitoxic, and an antiproliferative.

There is no contraindication to this infusion therapy in cases of manifest Diabetes mellitus, because: 1. the Steroid-induced Diabetes can be well compensated by Insulin, 2. the Diabetes is not changed in its severity, so that after discontinuation of the Corticosteroids the patient has the same glucose tolerance as before. Despite the high doses, an atrophy of the adrenal cortex is not to be expected, due to the short-term therapy, especially if one switches in time to a circadian application.

2. Dextran: The strong rheological effect of the low molecular Dextrans, especially in the terminal blood vessels, has been demonstrated in many studies. This effect is mainly due to an extensive haemodilution. Moreover, some other characteristics of low molecular Dextran are responsible for their capacity to influence microcirculation. They are: The decrease of the local concentration of hematocrit, of blood viscosity and of blood flow resistance, but the increase of the microcirculatory pressure gradient; furthermore, the decrease of sludge-phenomenon of the erythrocytes as well as of the thrombocytes with an antithrombotic effect and improvement of oxygen-perfusion.

Although the total volume of circulating plasma is, on account of renal clearance, only insignificantly greater than the volume of the infusion itself (Köhler et al. 1947), insufficiency especially of left heart as well as renal insufficiency should be regarded as contraindications. According to Ring and Messmer (1977), the percentage of manifestation of an anaphylactoid reaction is 0.007 percent. Since application of Cortisone is the main therapeutic management of this complication, the risk of an anaphylactoid reaction may even be lower when using our treatment protocol.

3. Pentoxifylline: Investigation on microvascular diseases in recent years gave increasing evidence that vascular disorders with consecutive ischemia are not only due to anatomical or functional changes of the vessels themselves. On the contrary, present knowledge indicates, that these changes are rather influenced by pathophysiological mechanisms concerning the different corpuscular components of blood and their interaction, also causing a vicious circle. Among other pathological changes, aggregation and rigidity of the erythrocyte-membrane in the hyperosmolar and acidic plasma of ischemic areas determinate blood viscosity and passage through terminal vessels, i.e. microcirculation. As a consequence, blood flow is considerably reduced or even blocked distal to the stenosis. In those post-stenotic areas, oxygen perfusion of the tissue, which means in our case: nutrition of the nerve, is no longer sufficiently maintained. Numerous experimental and clinical studies during recent years have demonstrated that Pentoxifylline normalizes those disturbing processes of the blood cells and their membranes, especially by an increase in ATP-level and inhibition of cyclic AMP-formation.

Our treatment protocol (Fig. 2), based upon these clinical and experimental findings, is used as follows: Patients with the tentative diagnosis of Bell's palsy are at once admitted as in-patients, and after taking 10 ml of blood for the initial determination of laboratory values, infusion therapy is started immediately. If there are no contraindications for fluid load, 1,000 ml Dextrane within 16 hours are given during the first three days. Dextran solution should also contain a supplement of 5 to 10 percent Sorbitol or Mannitol. Thus, the glomerular-filtration-rate can be considerably increased and thereby possible damage to the kidneys by crystalline deposits in the tubuli can be avoided. We are using Onkovertin N with five percent Sorbitol, which is commercially available. Since the hyperosmolarity of Dextran leads to intravasal infusion of interstitial fluid and particularly to elimination of potassium during diuresis, one should ensure a sufficient substitution of fluid and potassium.

Only after Cortisone has been decreased to 40 mg per day the remaining treatment is performed orally and in a circadian fashion, which means that application follows the adrenal rhythm. Thus, the risk of irreversible atrophy of the adrenalcortex is considerably reduced. Cortisone, up to an amount of 50 mg Prednisolone-equivalent, as well as Pentoxifylline are added directly into the Dextran solution, so that application is very simple.

The following factors should be regarded as contraindications: 1. Left heart insufficiency, 2. renal insufficiency, 3. recent history of peptic ulcer, 4. pregnancy, 5. florid (bacterial) infections, 6. coagulation defects. During the course of infusion, patients should be monitored as to blood pressure and heart rate, blood glucose, electrolytes, creatinine, and hematocrit.

Results

Of 128 consecutive patients, the first to be treated in this way, 110 patients were available for follow up. Fifty six of them were male and 54 female, so that sex distribution was quite equal. The average age was 39.8 years with range from 17 to 75 years. The mean duration of paresis, i.e. time elapsed between onset of paresis and beginning of treatment, was 5.2 days with range from one to 20 days.

A careful and extensive follow-up examination, including clinical as well as neurophysiological criteria, was performed. Thus, the following main results were obtained:

1. According to clinical evaluation, 96 percent had a complete functional recovery. In other words: From those 110 patients treated by our infusion-therapy, any residual signs of the former palsy could still be detected in only four patients.
   But even the outcome of these four remaining patients has to be regarded as 'good', according to different scoring systems.
2. Furthermore, it could be demonstrated that the development of Bell's palsy is remarkably influenced in its early phase: On their hospital admission, 60 patients (55 percent) had a clinically complete paralysis and, moreover, 29 patients (26 percent) showed a completely silent EMG. During the 10 day infusion-therapy 60 percent of the patients had converted from clinically complete to incomplete paresis, and 86 percent had changed from electromyographically complete to incomplete paresis.

Discussion

We must realize that up to now all our efforts towards the development of any diagnostic procedure, which allows a reliable prognosis of the course of Bell's palsy, have been without success.

NET as well as MST and ENG yield in the first three to four days no information at all and will even take another two or three days before definite data are

Degree	Morphological criteria	Characteristics of repair
1. Neurodyspraxia (Metabolic dysfunction)	? (Disturbance of membranes with inability for polarisation)	?
2. Neurapraxia	Demyelination	Remyelination
3. Axonotmesis	Wallerian Degeneration	
	a) with preservation of perineurium plus endoneural tubes	intrafasciculare 'isomorphic' (Hiller 1949) neurotisation
	b) with preservation of perineurium but with damage of endoneural tubes	intrafasciculare 'heteromorphic' (Hiller 1949) neurotisation
4. Neurotmesis	Partial or complete deterioration of different numbers of fascicles with continuity of epineurium	extrafasciculare neurotisation (always 'heteromorphic' EVEN 'neuromatous' (Hiller 1951)
	Complete section	

Fig 3. Scheme of nerve impairment according to morphological criteria

available. So these tests condemn us to an expectant attitude within a time-range, which seems to be exactly that peroid during which Bell's palsy requires active management.

Furthermore, it is important to stress that all our so-called therapeutic procedures are not curative in the real sense of word. Both, surgical and conservative treatment, can only interrupt the above mentioned vicious circle and thereby stop the progressing disease-process. Thus, we cannot cure but only prevent further nerve damage! All therapeutic procedures can have only one ultimate goal: They can, at least, ensure the normal biological spontaneous recovery process – with the important restriction, that the possibilities for recovery of morphological nerve defects are limited.

If this assumption is correct, how do we explain the fact that 60 percent of our patients changed from clinically complete to incomplete paresis under the medical treatment? To explain this phenomenon, the classification of nerve injury according to Seddon (1943) may be helpful, which distinguishes between the three degrees: neurapraxia, axonotmesis and neurotmesis. Figure 3 shows these stages of nerve impairment according to their morphological criteria. However, it is my personal opinion, that we have to add a fourth degree of nerve injury, for which I would propose the term: 'Neurodyspraxia' and which may be mainly characterized by functional disturbances especially of the membranes with inability for de- and repolarisation.

So, if we can stop the disorders of the nerve fibers during stage I, functional recovery will occur within a few days. And second: As long as we can stop the progressive damage of nerve fibers within stage I to III a – which means that, the regrowth of nerve fibers will occur within their original endoneural tubes and is, according to Hiller (1949, 1951), an isomorphic reneurotisation – no residuals will be detectable even by intensive neurophysiological investigations. The progression of nervous tissues damage in the course of Bell's palsy must therefore be stopped as soon as possible. The empirical data of our study with extraordinarily good results seem to indicate that with our treatment protocol substantial nerve tissue damage and therefore disturbing residuals can be avoided, if at least all patients with clinically complete or progressively incomplete paresis are treated at once. In the meantime, one can perform all investigations to ascertain the diagnosis of Bell's palsy, which of course is important. But this can be done without time pressure while clinical treatment is under way.

References

Ballance C, Duel A (1932) The operative treatment of facial palsy. Arch Otolaryngol 15:1–70

Hiller F (1949) Die Bedeutung des mesodermalen Gewebes bei der Nervenregeneration. Experimentelle Untersuchungen an Nervenverletzungen und Transplantaten. Dtsch Z Nervenheilk 160:176–195

Hiller F (1951) Nerve regeneration in grafts. J Neuropathol Exp Neurol 1:5–25

Kettel K (1943) Facial Palsy of Otitic Origin. Arch Otolaryngol 37:303–348

Ring J, Messmer K (1977) Infusionstherapie mit kolloidalen Volumenersatzmitteln. Anaesthesist 26:279

Seddon HJ (1943) Three types of Nerve Injury. Brain 66:237–288

Anastomosis of the Facial Nerve with Accessory or Hypoglossal Nerves

S. Mingrino and M. Zuccarello, Padova/Italy

Introduction

Microsurgical removal of acoustic neuromas can be accomplished with preservation of the facial nerve in most patients. In large acoustic neuroma successful removal of the tumor may be followed by intracranial nerve interruption. In such an event the treatment of choice is restoration of facial nerve continuity by direct anastomosis or by nerve grafts after completion of the neurosurgical procedure in the cerebello pontine angle.

When repair of the facial nerve is impossible, different types of extracranial anastomosis have been adopted with the following nerves: accessory spinal, hypoglossal, phrenic, controlateral facial.

Some authors (Lodge, 1955; Pool, Pava, 1957; Pertuiset, 1970) have preferred the hypoglossal-facial anastomosis. Some others preferred spino-facial anastomosis (Love, Cannon, 1951; Cecotto, 1957; Migliavacca, 1967).

Another technique performed by Raaf (1967), Schwartz (1968), Perret (1967) is phrenic-facial anastomosis. This technique is most useful when the eleventh and twelfth nerves have been injured intracranially but is contraindicated, if reduced pulmonary function is present, because of the subsequent paralysis of one hemidiaphragm.

We report our experiences with accessory-facial and hypoglossal-facial anastomosis.

Material and Methods

In the Neurosurgical Institute of Padua 45 facial anastomosis were performed in twenty seven years. The facial nerve palsy was the result of large acoustic tumor removal.

Fourty patients were treated by anastomosis between the facial nerve and the spinal accessory nerve; in five patients the anastomosis was between the hypoglossal nerve and the facial nerve. Seventeen patients were men and thirty one women. Their ages ranged from 14 to 60 years, with an average of 41 years. The interval between the onset of the facial palsy and the neural anastomosis extended from one to six months. The follow up extended from one to 13 years.

When performing an accessory spinal anastomosis we prefer to use the entire nerve, instead of the isolated segment to sternocleidomastoid, as suggested by some authors. As a matter of fact this segment is of small size, and in the few cases we adopted it the results were poor, although shoulder motility was spared.

In our cases sectioning of the hypoglossal nerve was never followed by anastomosis of the 'discendens hypoglossi' to the distal stump of the twelfth nerve. Nevertheless, we have observed only a moderate lingual atrophy.

Results

The results were classified on the basis of the following criteria: a good result was when the patient gained facial symmetry at rest, complete voluntary eye closure, voluntary movements of the corner of the mouth and no significant inconveniences from the hypoglossal or accessory nerves palsy. A fair result consisted of incomplete facial symmetry and incomplete eye closure with poor voluntary movements. A poor result consisted of gross facial asymmetry, insufficient eye closure to protect the cornea, no voluntary movements, significant disability from loss of the hypoglossal or spinal accessory nerve.

Among the patients who underwent spinal-facial anastomosis, 13 are classified as good results, 16 as fair and 11 as poor.

The results of the five patients operated on by hypoglossal-facial anastomosis are good in three cases and fair in two cases (Table 1).

Table 1. Facial anastomosis

Result	XI – VII	XII – VII
Good	13 (33%)	3 (60%)
Fair	16 (39%)	2 (40%)
Poor	11 (28%)	–
Total	40	5

Discussion

We have observed a higher percentage of recovery of facial function in women compared to men. It is well known that to achieve maximum benefit from a crossed nerve anastomosis, the patient must exercise the face and develop the habit of voluntarily activating the paretic side of the face. This requires much practise in front of the mirror.

Our results confirm the impression that the hypoglossal-facial anastomosis is more satisfactory than spino-facial anastomosis. Perhaps the hypoglossal-facial anastomosis is better because the cortical representations of the tongue and face are closer than those of the shoulder and face, as suggested by Ballance (1903).

But the selection which nerve to sacrifice for anastomosis to the facial nerve should be made individually for each patient. When speech is crucial to the patient's occupation, the accessory nerve should be employed for the anastomosis, because the hypoglossal facial anastomosis lead to facial syncinesia when talking, which may be socially embarassing and may also provoke disturbances of pronounciation. If normal painless shoulder function is of greater importance than speech for the patient's activity, then a hypoglossal-facial anastomosis is preferred.

References

Ballance CA, Ballance HA, Stewart P (1903) Operative treatment of chronic facial palsy of peripheral origin. Lancet 1:1009–1013

Cecotto C (1957) Trattamento chirurgico della parelisi periferica del nervo facciale con particolare riguardo a quella consequente all'asportazione dei tumori del nervo acustico. Chir Ital 9:555–575

Lodge WO, Gueukdjian SA (1955) De la paralysie faciale. Modifications des opérations d'anastomose facio-hypoglosse et de plastie faciale. Press Med 63:1025–1026

Love JG, Cannon BW (1951) Nerve anastomosis in the treatment of spinofacial paralysis. Special consideration of the etiologic role of tumors of the acoustic nerve. Arch Surg 62:379–390

Migliavacca F (1967) Facial nerve anastomosis for facial paralysis following acoustic neurinoma surgery. Acta Neurochir (Wien) 17:274–279

Pertuiset B (1970) Les neurinomes de l'acoustique développés dans l'angle ponto-cérébelleux. Neurochirugie 16, suppl 1:1–147

Pool JL, Pava AA, Greenfield EC (1970) Acoustic nerve tumors. Ch Thomas, Springfield, Ill.

Raaf F (1967) cited by Pool JL et al.

Schwartz (1968) cited by Pool JL et al.

Facio-Facial Anastomosis

M. Samii, Hannover/FRG

A further development of anastomosis of the facial nerve to other cranial nerves is the facio-facial anastomosis.

The advantage of this technique is that reinnervation of the paralysed muscles can be partially achieved without sacrifying another cranial nerve and without loss of function. This technique was reported for the first time by Smith in 1971 and in the same year by Scaramella. The method was improved by Anderl (1973) and Samii (1975).

The technical principle of facio-facial anastomosis is based on the anatomical fact that the branches of the facial nerve within the face region build a kind of plexus, the pes anserinus, and that parts of these branches may be cut without the risk of visible functional deficit. The central stumps of the transected branches in the healthy side of the face are sutured to nerve grafts crossing the face subcutaneously in the upper lip region to the damaged side. Here they have to be sutured with the analogous branches (Fig. 1).

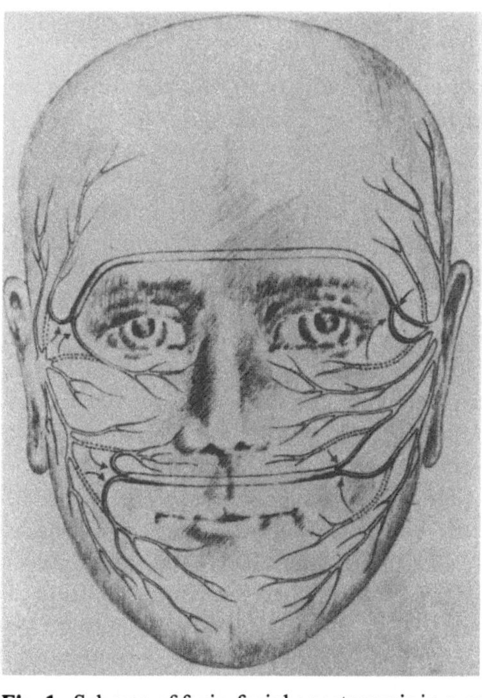

Fig. 1. Scheme of facio-facial anastomosis in a case of a right sided facial paralysis. The central stumps of the left peripheral facial nerve branches are connected to the peripheral stumps of the analogous branches on the right side by means of different nerve grafts

However, it must be taken into consideration that the course of the peripheral branches of the facial nerve is different in each individual. Fujita (1934) found irregularities in this pattern even when comparing the two sides of the face in one person. McCormack and co-workers (1945) established eight different types of facial nerve branch distribution in the face. According to their investigations an anastomosis among the different groups of branches is lacking in only 13 percent of all people. In general a more or less well developed parotid plexus is to be found. Whereas the mandibular branch is very seldom connected through anastomosis with other branch groups, the cervicalis colli branch never is. According to Davis and co-workers (1956) this percentage varies. Intraoperative electro-diagnostic stimulation of the individual branches of the facial nerve confirms these anatomical variations. With this technique, the innervation patterns of the facial nerve of each patient can be accurately evaluated.

It is our impression that the zygomatic branch is the most important of all the facial nerve branches, as electrical stimulation of it produces contraction of both, the orbicularis oculi and orbicularis oris muscles. Because of the overlapping supply by the ocular and mandibular branches of the facial nerve, a complete transection of the zygomatic branch rarely produces a visible paralysis.

Studies of 22 patients with facio-facial anastomosis, in whom each branch was anastomosed with the analogus branch of the opposite side revealed failure of reinnervation of the frontal branch. For this reason we have simplified the technique in later cases, and have abandoned the method of complete exposure of all peripheral branches of the facial nerve. Instead we merely expose both zygomatic branches through two centimeter long incisions. These two branches are identified, transected and sutured, using a sural nerve graft.

Depending on the caliber of the sural nerve, we usually need one and sometimes two sural grafts to anastomose the zygomatic branch (Fig. 2 a and b).

The results in 41 patients with a follow up between two to seven years showed electromyographically proved reinnervation of muscles in 90 percent. In 50 percent of the patients we could ascertain symmetry of the face in state of repose. In the other 40 percent, despite contraction of the reinnervated muscles, we could still recognize the paralysis in state of repose. Only in a few cases could we achieve an optimal symmetrical function in connection with active contraction of the face muscles.

Although reinnervation of the paralysed muscles could be achieved by facio-facial anastomosis, the functional result remained far behind the result of direct grafting of the facial nerve in its entire course. We, therefore, tried during recent years to improve the results of facio-facial anastomosis by additional surgical measures at the same stage described already by Lexer and Rosenthal. We tried to build two muscles strips from the temporal muscles in such a way as to fix one strip with three stitches subcutaneously in a broad region of the orbicularis oris muscle and lead the second strip subcutaneously to the inner corner of the eye, where it has to be fixed with two stitches at the palpebral media ligament. Herewith, the lifting of the lower eyelid and an immediate closing of the eye postoperatively is possible. We performed subsequently the facio-facial anastomosis. Fig. 3 a and b demonstrate the technique of facio-facial anastomosis combined with skin excision of the nasolabial fold and temporal muscleplasty in a 65 year old patient with a left sided facial nerve paralysis.

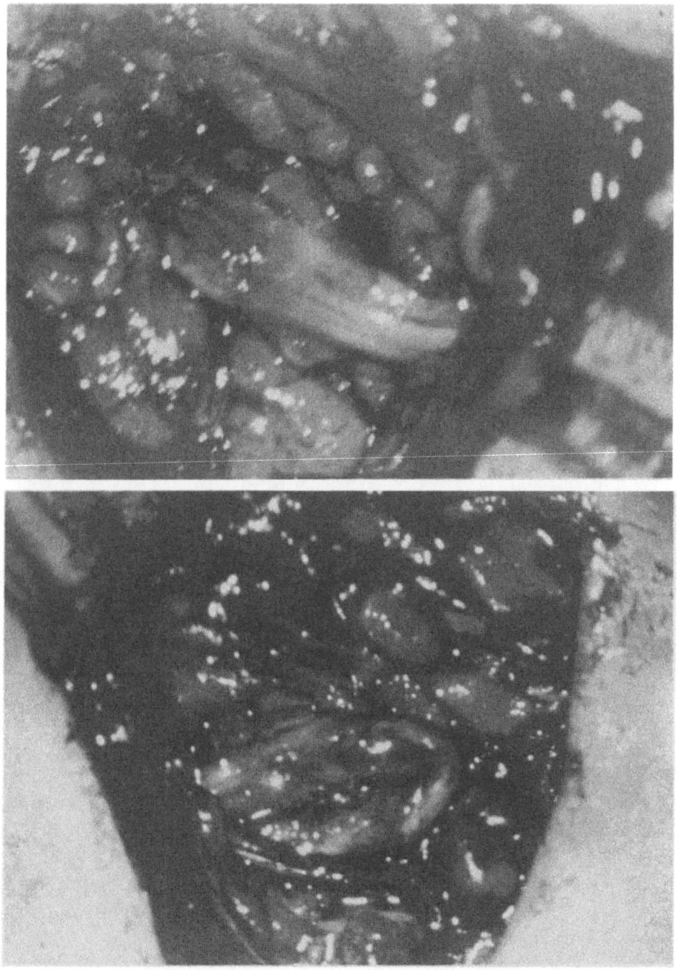

a

b

Fig. 2a and b. Facio-facial anastomosis between both zygomatic branches by means of one sural nerve graft. The zygomatic branch is exposed and transected, the central stump of the intact side is sutured with the sural graft nerve (**a**). The distal end of the graft is sutured to the distal stump of the zygomatic branch of the facial nerve on the damaged side (**b**)

Fig. 3a and d shows the preoperative condition and the immediate result 10 days after the operation. Symmetric position of the face is achieved and eye closure is nearly possible. The voluntary movement of the paralysed muscle as a result of the facio-facial anastomosis is observed 12 months after the operation (Fig. 3e and f). An additional example of this combined technique is demonstrated in Fig. 4a–d.

From 1977 to 1980, we had the opportunity to perform a combined intervention in 21 patients. Postoperatively the symmetry of the face in the relaxed position and closure of the eye was evident. With increasing reinnervation of the muscles, approximately one year after the operation, the result could further be improved. Symmetric voluntary movement could almost be reached in those patients, in whom the postoperative follow up was longer than one year.

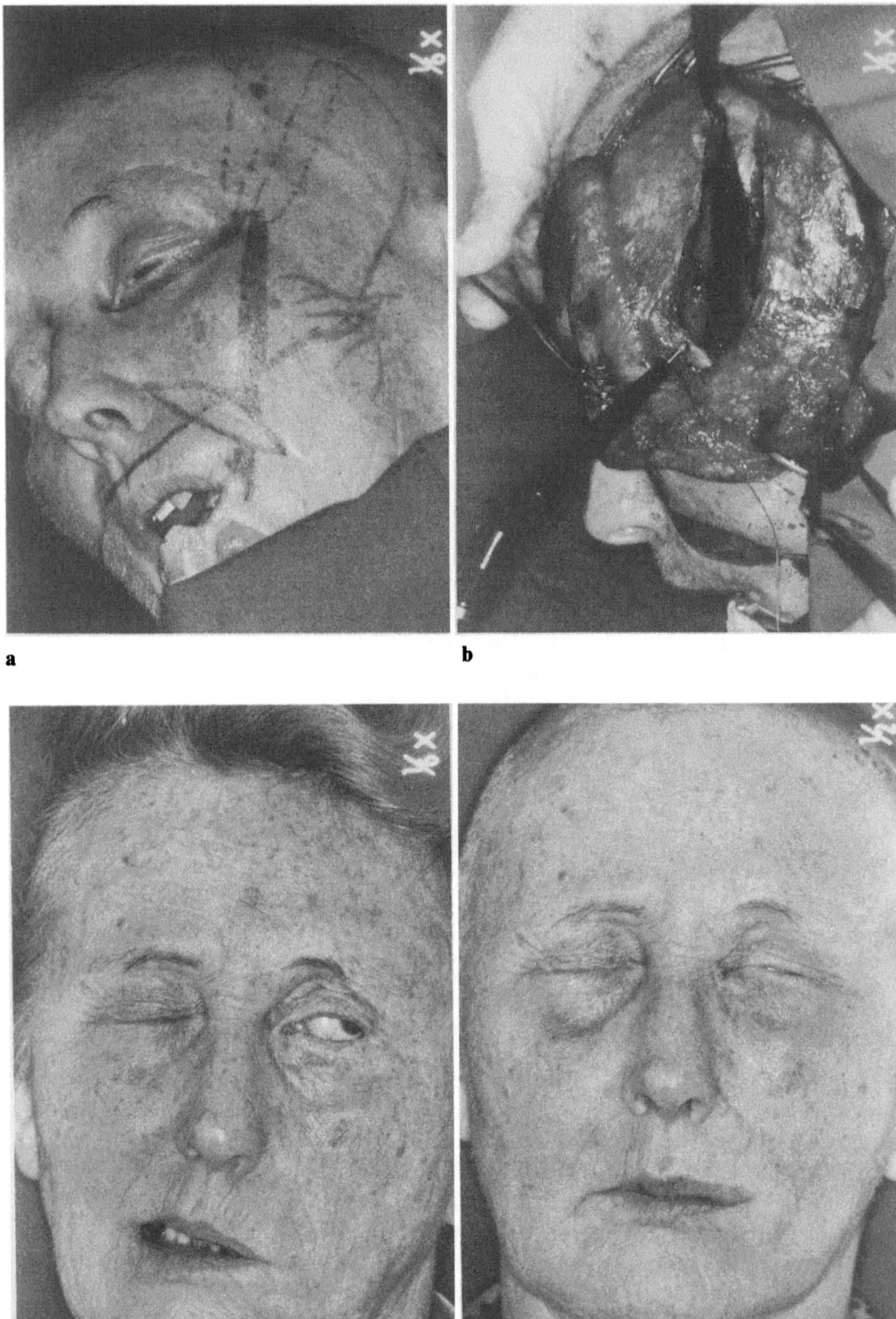

a b c d

Fig. 3a–d (caption see opposite page)

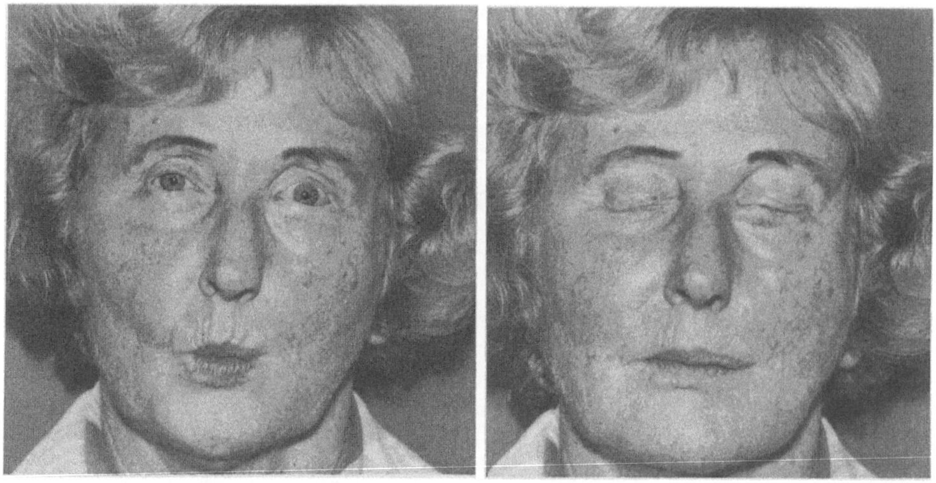

e f

Fig. 3e and f. The same patient as Fig. 3a, b, c, and d. Postoperative result after 12 months. The voluntary movement of the paralysed muscle as a result of the facio-facial anastomosis is observed

In conclusion we can prove in the case of 62 patients that facio-facial anastomosis with and without skin and muscle-plasty is a real development in facial nerve surgery. Due to the fact that not all nerve fibres of the healthy side of the facial nerve are available, the results for facio-facial anastomosis remain far behind the ones of direct nerve grafting in case of facial nerve lesion.

Therefore, facio-facial anastomosis is indicated in those patients in whom direct treatment of the facial nerve is technically impossible or the primarily performed intervention in the region of the lesion did not lead to the desired improvement, and also, where facio-facial anastomosis had to be performed as an additional intervention.

According to our experiences, the combined techniques of facio-facial anastomosis and the skin excision in the region of the nasolabial fold as well as the temporal- and masseter muscle-plasty show the following advantages compared with the facial nerve anastomosis to the other cranial nerves:

1. No sacrifice of other cranial nerves.
2. Symmetric position in state of repose after operation.
3. Emotional movement of the paralysed muscles to a certain degree.

Fig. 3a–d. Operative technique of facio-facial anastomosis combined with skin excision in the nasolabial fold and temporal muscle-plasty. **c and d.** The same patient as Fig. 3a and b. A 35 year old patient with a left facial nerve paralysis (**c**). Postoperative results 10 days after the operation (**d**). Symmetric position of the face is achieved. Closure of the eye is possible

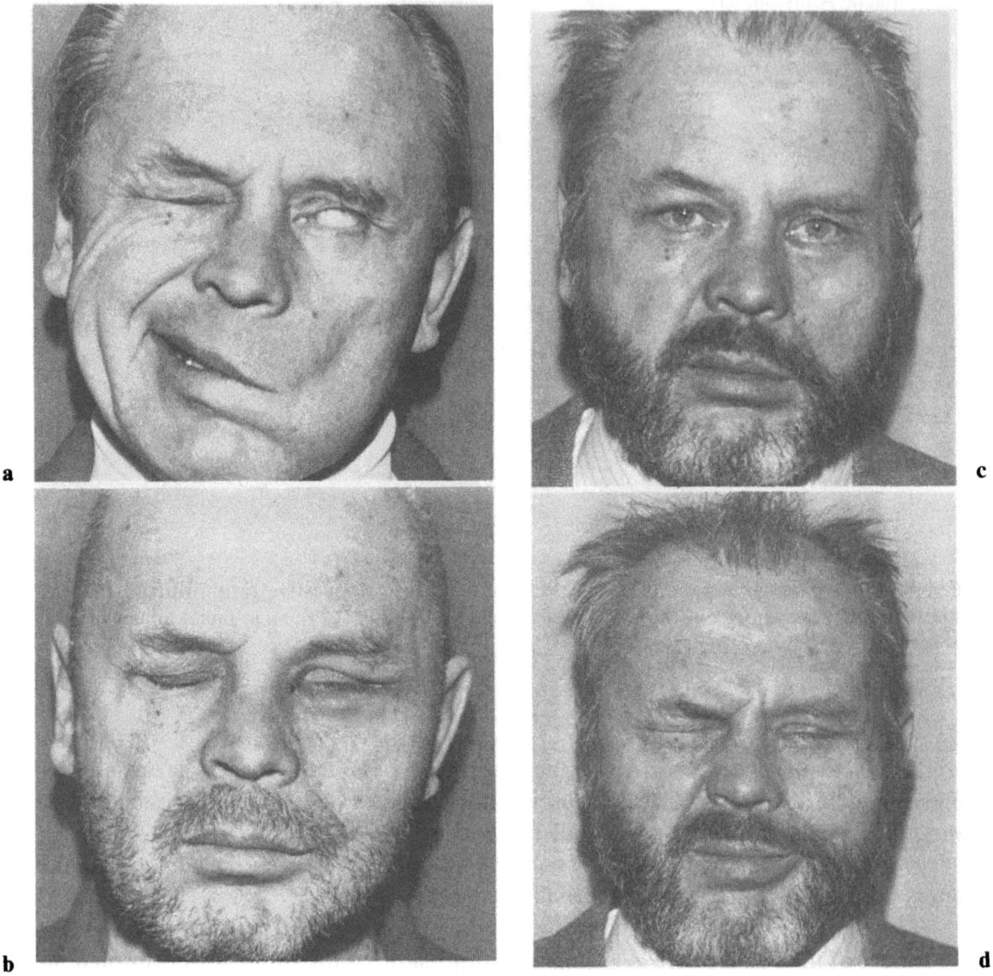

Fig. 4a–d. Preoperative and 10 day postoperative condition of a left sided facial nerve paralysis. The combined technique of facio-facial anastomosis and skin as well as temporal muscleplasty has been accomplished. **c** and **d.** The same patient as Fig. 4a and b. Functional result 12 month postoperatively

References

Anderl H (1973) Reconstruction of the face through cross-face-nerve transplantation in facial paralysis. Chir Plastica (Berlin) 2:17–46

Davis RA, Anson BJ et al. (1956) Surgical Anatomy of the facial nerve and parotid gland based upon a study of 850 cernicofacial halves. Surg Gynecol Obstet 102:385–412

Fujita T (1934) Über die periphere Ausbreitung des Nervus facialis beim Menschen. Gegenbaurs Morphol Jahrb 73:578–614

McCormack LJ, Couldwell EW et al. (1945) The surgical anatomy of the facial nerve with special reference to the parotid gland. Surg Gynecol Obstet 80:620–630

Samii M (1975) Modern aspects of peripheral and cranial nerves surgery. In: Advances and Technical Standards in Neurosurgery, Vol 2. Springer, Berlin Heidelberg New York, p 33–85

Scaramella L (1971) L'anastomosi trai due nervi facialli. Arch Ital Otol 82:207–215

Smith JW (1971) A new technique of facial animation. Transaction Fifth International Congress Plastic and Reconstructive Surgery. Butterworth, Melbourne p 83–84

Cochleo-Vestibular Nerve

Audiological Findings in Retrocochlear Lesions

D. PLESTER and J. POPPENDIECK, Tübingen/FRG

By far the most frequent cause of a retrocochlear lesion of the eighth nerve is acoustic neuroma. Despite the fact that acoustic neuromas almost always originate from the neurilemma of the vestibular ganglion, symptoms of the pars vestibularis of the eighth cranial nerve are rare at the beginning of the disease. However, the first subjective complaints are unilateral hearing impairment with or without tinnitus or tinnitus only.

Many audiometric tests have been developed for the quantification and differential diagnosis of sensori-neural hearing loss and tinnitus. The pure-tone air and bone conduction tests give information concerning the degree and frequency-pattern of the hearing loss and exclude a conductive hearing loss. However, neither the pure-tone loss pattern nor the duration of the hearing impairment are specific in the diagnosis of the existence or size of acoustic neuromas or any other retrocochlear lesion (Cambon et al., 1958; Johnson, 1977; Lehnhardt, 1978; Lundborg, 1952; Plester, 1978; Schuknecht, 1963).

Audiometric tests which have been developed to distinguish between a cochlear and a retrocochlear lesion are based on the recruitment phenomenon and tone decay. These tests require sufficient residual hearing. In 1937, Fowler found an abnormally rapid rise in loudness sensation in diseased inner ears compared to healthy ones. He called this important phenomenon recruitment. The performance of the Alternate Binaural Loudness Balance test (ABLB, Fowler's test) requires a threshold difference of at least 30 dB in one frequency in an individual's ears. The sound pressure level of this frequency is increased in 20 dB steps in the healthy ear, the intensity necessary for the same sensation level in the diseased ear is determined and compared to that of the healthy ear. Tones of half a second duration are presented alternately to both ears.

The patho-physiologic mechanism of recruitment has not been fully established. The isolated damage of the outer hair-cells which usually exists in cochlear diseases is assumed to play a part. The outer hair-cells are said to be sensitive to acoustic stimuli near the hearing threshold, while the inner hair-cells are more sensitive to acoustic stimuli of intensities in the range above 40 dB. Therefore recruitment should be present as long as the inner hair-cells are intact and the hearing loss does not exceed 60 dB (Feldmann 1979, Lehnhardt 1978). The abnormal growth in the sensation of loudness in the diseased ear compared to the healthy ear also means that the diseased ear has the ability to recognize smaller increases in intensity.

Jerger's SISI-test (Short Increment Sensitivity Index) is based on this phenomenon (Jerger et al. 1959). Increments of 1 dB, lasting 200–250 msec, are presented at 20 dB above the hearing threshold, i.e. at 20 dB sensation level. When a patient recognizes 20 percent or less of the 20 presented increments, the test is negative and the patient therefore does not have recruitment. A score of 80 percent or higher represents a positive test and indicates recruitment. The exposure of a normal ear to noise with a high sound pressure level (80 dB or more) for longer periods of time leads to a temporary threshold shift. If this happens at threshold intensities there is a pathological tone decay. This seems to be pathognomonic for lesions of the fibers of the cochlear nerve, for example in patients with acoustic neuromas with pressure on the cochlear nerve (Carhart, 1957; Schubert, 1944). To test this we use Rosenberg's modification of the tone decay test (Rosenberg, 1972). The pure tone is presented at threshold to one ear at a time and the intensity is increased in 5 dB steps when the patient does not hear the tone any longer. A decay of 30 dB or more in one minute strongly supports the diagnosis of a retrocochlear lesion.

The recruitment and tone decay phenomena can also be demonstrated with Békésy audiometry (Békésy, 1947). A tone increasing in frequency from 100 up to 10,000 Hz over 400 seconds is presented to the patient, firstly as an interrupted and then as a continuous tone. The patient regulates the intensity himself by pressing a button when he does not hear the tone any more and releases the button when he just hears it. In this way his thresholds for interrupted and continuous tones are recorded. Normally both tracings nearly overlap. Whereas the interrupted tone tracing corresponds with the hearing threshold measured with the usual pure-tone audiometer, the continuous tone tracing can deviate from it. No separation or a limited separation is a sign of a cochlear lesion. A marked separation of both lines indicates tone decay and therefore a retrocochlear lesion. In the continuous tone tracing large amplitude indicates tone decay as well as a very small one recruitment.

The acoustic resistance or impedance of the ear drum depends on changes in the middle ear, for instance contraction of the stapedius muscle (Metz, 1946; Tröger, 1930). If there are not pathological changes in the middle ear the threshold of the acoustically evoked stapedius reflex, evaluated by measuring impedance alterations of the ear drum, is of value in the differential diagnosis of sensori-neural deafness. In persons with normal hearing the stapedius reflex, which has to be regarded as a protective reflex, can be evoked by intensities of 80 dB or more. Metz found a decreased threshold of the stapedius reflex in patients with unilateral cochlear lesions who have recruitment (Metz, 1952; Spillmann et al., 1974; Anderson, 1970). A stapedius reflex decay, on the other hand corresponding to a tone decay is a sign of a retrocochlear lesion.

Speech audiometry plays an important role in the differential diagnosis of sensori-neural deafness. In speech discrimination tests the individual's ability to correctly repeat a standardized list of phonetically balanced monosyllabic words presented at comfortable loudness levels is determined. In addition we use lists with tetrasyllabic numbers. In cochlear nerve lesions a common manifestation is a loss of speech discrimination out of proportion to the pure-tone threshold loss. This implies that only a few nerve fibers are needed to transmit pure-tone stimuli at threshold whereas many fibers are necessary to carry the complex neural patterns of speech. A rather flat curve or discrepancies in the discrimination of the mono- and tetrasyllabic words are also highly suggestive of a retrocochlear disease (Feldmann, 1979; Lehnhardt, 1978).

Since 1977, our audiometric evaluation has included brainstem electric response audiometry (BERA). The acoustic stimuli are broad-band clicks of 160 microseconds duration. The evoked brainstem potentials are recorded by surface electrodes.

Potentials within the first 10 milliseconds following the stimuli are added up by an averaging computer and the summated end result can be seen on the screen of an summated end result can be seen on the screen of an oscilloscope. By the statistical elimination of the basic interference patterns a five peak tracing is usually seen. Peak one corresponds with the excitation of the spiral ganglion, peak two with that of the cochlear nuclei, peak three with the upper olive, peak four with the lateral lemniscus, and peak five with that of the inferior colliculus (Brackmann, 1977). In 1975, Chinn and Miller demonstrated that compression of the eighth nerve caused an increased latency of the evoked potentials. According to Wang and Dallos (1972), this is not found in hair-cell lesions. A difference of more than 0,2 milliseconds in the latency of the fifth peaks which usually are the largest peaks and therefore clearly visible is pathologic and supports the assumption of compression of the cochlear nerve by a tumor (House et al., 1979). However, demyelinization of the auditory pathways, e.g. in encephalitis disseminata, also leads to a prolonged latency.

At the ENT-Clinic of the University of Tübingen we found the following results in 83 confirmed acoustic neuromas:

Pure-tone audiometry (n = 83)		
Normal hearing	1	(1%)
High tone loss	25	(30%)
Mild hearing impairment	2	(2%)
Moderate hearing impairment	11	(13%)
Severe hearing impairment	12	(14%)
Total or near total deafness	32	(39%)
ABLB test (n = 41)		
Positive	25	(61%)
Negative	16	(39%)
SISI test (n = 40)		
Positive	23	(57%)
Negative	17	(43%)
Tone decay test (n = 41)		
Less than 30 dB/60 sec	39	(95%)
30 dB/60 sec and more	2	(5%)
Impedance audiometry (n = 60)		
Metz recruitment	19	(32%)
No recruitment	13	(22%)
No reflex	28	(47%)
Speech audiometry (n = 43)		
Discrimination loss proportional	26	(60%)
Discrimination loss more than proportional	17	(40%)

BERA (n = 12)

Normal	0 (0%)
Pathologic	12 (100%)

It is evident that audiometric tests in favour of a chochlear lesion cannot exclude a tumor. In 1977, Johnson evaluated the audiometric test of 500 patients with acoustic tumors and reached the same conclusion. The inconsistancies of the audiometric tests can be explained by secondary tumor effects such as compression of the labyrinthine artery or perhaps changes in the CSF circulation. We have not found a normal BERA in any patient with an acoustic neuroma. However, this has been described in the literature in cases where at surgery the tumor was found not to exert pressure on the cochlear nerve (Clemis et al., 1979; Glasscock et al., 1979; Selters et al., 1977).

As is well known, a tumor in the cerebello-pontine angle can only be proved by contrast cisternography or computertomography. These invasive and relatively expensive examinations are only indicated when one has a high index of suspicion. As to this, we believe that regarding audiometry, BERA is the single most valuable test in the work up of patients with unilateral sensori-neural hearing loss.

Summary

To diagnose a retrocochlear lesion by audiologic testing the lack of recruitment, pathological tone decay and poor speech discrimination provide a high index of suspicion. Audiometric signs of chochlear disease do not exclude an acoustic neuroma and were present in more than 50 percent of our patients with confirmed cerebellopontine angle lesions. To date the most reliable single audiometric test for retrocochlear pathology seems to be the brainstem electric response audiometry.

References

Anderson H, Barr B, Wedenberg E (1970) Early diagnosis of VIIIth nerve tumors by acoustic reflex tests. Acta Otolaryngol (Stockh) 263:232

Békésy G (1947) A new audiometer. Acta Otolaryngol (Stockh) 35:411

Brackmann DE (1977) Electric Response Audiometry in a Clinical Practice. Laryngoscope (Suppl) 87:5

Cambon K, Guilford FR (1958) Acoustic neurilemmoma. Arch Otolaryngol 67:302

Carhart R (1957) Clinical determination of abnormal auditory adaptation. Arch Otolaryngol 65:32

Chinn J, Miller J (1975) Animal model of acoustic neuroma. Arch Otolaryngol 101:222

Clemis JD, McGee Th (1979) Brainstem electric response audiometry in the differential diagnosis of acoustic tumors. Laryngoscope 89:31

Feldmann H (1979) Audiometrie bei Erwachsenen. In: Hals Nasen Ohrenheilkunde. In: Berendes J, Link R, Zöllner F (eds) Bd. 5, 11 Georg Thieme, Stuttgart

Fowler EP (1963) Loudness recruitment: definition and clarification. Arch Otolaryngol 78:748

Glasscock ME, Jackson CY, Josey AF, Dickins JRE, Wiet RJ (1979) Brainstem evoked response audiometry in a clinical practice. Laryngoscope 89:1021

Graf K (1955) Die Kleinhirnbrückenwinkelgeschwülste. Fortschritte der Hals Nasen Ohrenheilkunde. Karger, Basel New York

House JW, Brackmann DE (1979) Brainstem Audiometry in Neuro-otologic Diseases. Arch Otolaryngol 105:305

Jerger J, Shedd JL, Hartford E (1959) On detection of extremely small changes in sound intensity. Arch Otolaryngol 69:200

Jerger JF (1960) Békésy audiometry in analysis of auditory disorders. J Speech Hear Res 3:275

Jewett D, Romano M, Williston J (1970) Human auditory evoked potentials: possible brainstem components detected on the scalp. Science 167:1517

Johnson EW (1977) Auditory Test Results in 500 Cases of Acoustic Neuroma. Arch Otolaryngol 103:152

Lehnhardt E (1978) Praktische Audiometrie. 5. Aufl. Stuttgart, Georg Thieme

Lundborg T (1952) Diagnostic problems concerning acoustic tumors. A study of 300 verified cases and the Békésy audiogram in the differential diagnosis. Acta Otolaryngol (Stockh) Suppl 99:1–110

Metz O (1946) The acoustic impedance measured on normal and pathological ears. Acta Otolaryngol (Stockh) Suppl 63:1

Metz O (1952) Threshold of reflex contractions of muscles of middle ear and recruitment of loudness. Arch Otolaryngol 55:536

Plester D (1978) Otologische Diagnose der Kleinhirnbrückenwinkel-Tumoren. In: Plester D, Wende S, Nakayama N (eds) Kleinhirnbrückenwinkel-Tumoren. Springer, Berlin Heidelberg New York

Rosenberg PE (1972) cited in Green DS: Pure tone airconduction thresholds. In: Katz J (ed) Handbook of Clinical Audiology. Williams and Wilkins, Baltimore, p 67

Schubert K (1944) Hörermüdung und Hördauer. Z Hals Nasen Ohrenheilkunde 51:19

Schuknecht HF (1963) Menière's disease: Correlation of symptomatology and pathology. Laryngoscope 73:651

Selters WA, Brackmann DE (1977) Acoustic Tumor Detection with Brainstem Electric Response Audiometry. Arch Otolaryngol 103:181

Spillmann T, Hof E (1974) Das objektive Recruitment bei Innenohrstörungen. Z Laryngol Rhinol 53:59–66

Tröger J (1930) Die Schallaufnahme durch das äußere Ohr. Physik Z 32:26

Wang CY, Dallos P (1972) Latency of whole-nerve action potentials: Influence of hair-cell normalcy. J Acoust Soc Am 52:1678

Functional Testing of the Vestibular Nerve

L. B. W. JONGKEES, Amsterdam/The Netherlands

There are very many persons in this world who, at some moment or the other, are troubled by some sensation of instability, or movement or incertainty. The intensity of this sensation is no indicator for the seriousness of its cause, neither is the exactitude of its description by the patient. The examination of the equilibrium system is certainly possible but it is a time-consuming procedure. It will hardly be feasible to examine, thoroughly and completely, all those patients who come to their doctor with the story that they are or have been giddy, but the doctor should know that dysfunction of nearly any organ or organ system in the body can disturb the fine interaction of all the organs and systems which together lead to that intricate equilibrium which we call health. If anything goes wrong, the patient may translate this disequilibrium into terms of vertigo, dizziness, giddiness or loss of balance, depending upon what he feels, what he knows, and where he comes from. It is easy to understand why patients may have difficulty in explaining their feelings and why their complaints are often so vague as to be meaningful only to a specialist. As those feelings are not clear to the patient either, well-directed question will be necessary to dig up hidden information. Good knowledge of both, the morbid anatomy and physiology of the entire equilibrium system; of the various clinical pictures of disequilibrium; of the background of the methods of examination that can be used; of the information those examinations can give and what they cannot give; how one can make the correct diagnosis, what this diagnosis really means and how it can lead to an appropriate therapy, i.e. treatment of the cause of the ailment.

Though vertigo in the literal sense implies a sensation of rotation, one is never certain that a patient uses the word in this sense. He may also use giddy or dizzy to indicate subjective movements. I agree completely with Williams (1962) when he states that there is no basic difference in the words giddy, dizzy, and vertiginous. All three may be used for the message: "I feel unbalanced or disequilibrated, or even unsure." These sensations are certainly not always caused by vestibular disorders (i.e. originating inside the peripheral labyrinth, the VIII th nerve of their central connections). Even the true rotary sensation of pure vertigo can be provoked by visual, cervical or auditory stimuli.

It must be accepted that the complaints of the dizzy, the giddy, and the vertiginous patient cannot be so easily explained by one malefactor, but originate from lack of coordination of the information from various sense organs, above all optic, vestibular, tactile, and proprioceptive. This clash of information usually leads to reactions originating in the autonomic nervous system: nausea, anguish, vomiting, sweating, etc. There is nothing about the clinical description of vertigo as such which will help the examiner to locate its course, but only if the words 'as such' are strongly emphasized. As a matter of fact, important information is almost always present in the clinical description of the way in which the vertigo presents itself: paroxysmal vertigo, chronic vertigo, acute onset slowly decreasing vertigo with changing intensity, positional or positioning vertigo, vertigo with eyes open, but not with eyes closed, form not a bad basis for specification. Associated phenomena like running ears, tinnitus, deafness, loss of consciousness, visual hallucinations, and the very typical description of phobias are easily found by the doctor who is eager to get a good anamnesis. In many cases the case history suggests the necessary examination which can help to unravel diagnostic puzzles. The combination of deafness and vertigo points to peripheral vestibular disorders. In case of headache, paralysis of cranial nerves other than the eighth, loss of consciousness, etc., central disturbances are more probable.

Not infrequently the case history will give enough information for a tentative diagnosis (Ménière's disease, benign paroxysmal positional nystagmus, orthostatic or epileptic vertigo). In most cases the case history suggests the necessary observation and examination. Never forget that a slight feeling of dizziness can be due to some very serious disease and strong vertigo can be caused by a benign disorder (alcohol, some influenza epidemics like the Bornholm type).

A patient has the right to have his complaints about giddiness taken seriously. This means that the doctor does not stop his investigation before he knows the origin of the complaints. If the history has been intelligently taken, the number of tests necessary to reach a diagnosis may sometimes be small.

The same is true if the vestibular tests provoke perverse reactions, such as a vertical nystagmus in response to routine caloric stimulation. A vestibular examination is of little value if it remains isolated. Only within the entire framework of medical, neurological, ophthalmological, radiological, and even psychiatric data, can the vestibular examination properly show its optimal value. Modern, sophisticated tests are not always necessary for a good diagnosis. In nine out of ten cases a physician in his office can make the correct diagnoses without electronystagmographs, torsion swings, and intricate instruments delivering water of stabilized temperatures.

There are, however, some drawbacks. A clinician who wants to examine a 'vestibular case' will need time because vestibular examination is time-consuming, and he will need knowledge about the function of this tricky organ system. He will sometimes not be able to reach a definite diagnosis, or he may want it substantiated by findings from a vestibular laboratory. But in the majority of cases he himself should be able to find out whether the cause of the complaints is central or peripheral. Very important data can be found by the investigation of deviations in both, the vestibulo-spinal and in the vestibulo-ocular reflexes: Romberg's test (Fig. 1), walking (Fig. 2), and past-pointing (Fig. 3) in the one case, and ocular nystagmus (Figs. 4, 5) in the other. Spontaneous nystagmus not of the combined horizontal-rotatory (horizontal-frontal) type is not provoked by disease of the peripheral labyrinth of the eighth nerve. Vertical, diagonal, rotatory or purely horizontal varieties of spontaneous nystagmus are caused by central nervous system (CNS) disease. Positional nystagmus showing a change in direction in different positions, a disharmony between the direction of the vestibulo-spinal reflexes and the slow phases of a spontaneous nystagmus, as well as a strong spontaneous nystagmus in a patient not suffering from severe vertigo are not indicative of peripheral disease of the vestibular system.

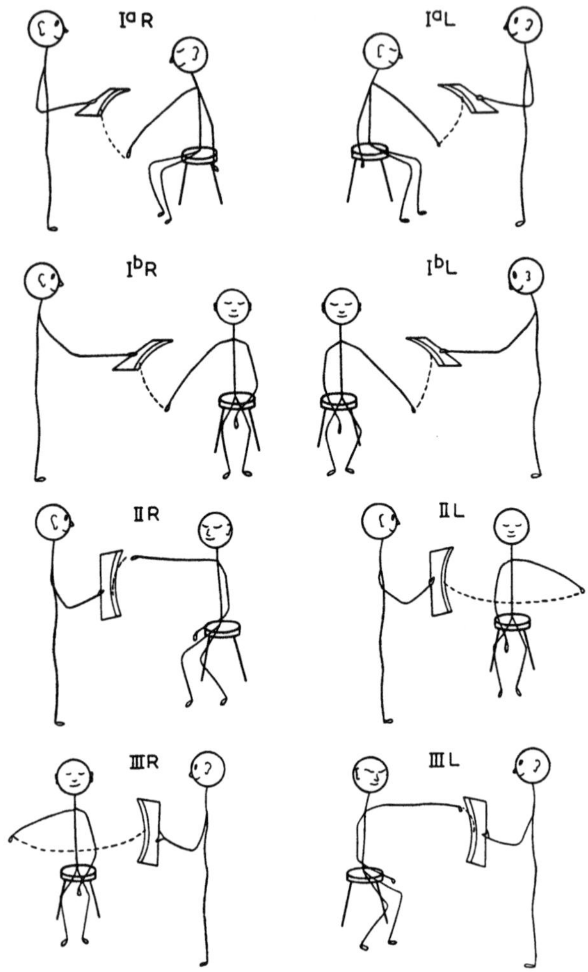

Fig. 1. Past pointing test

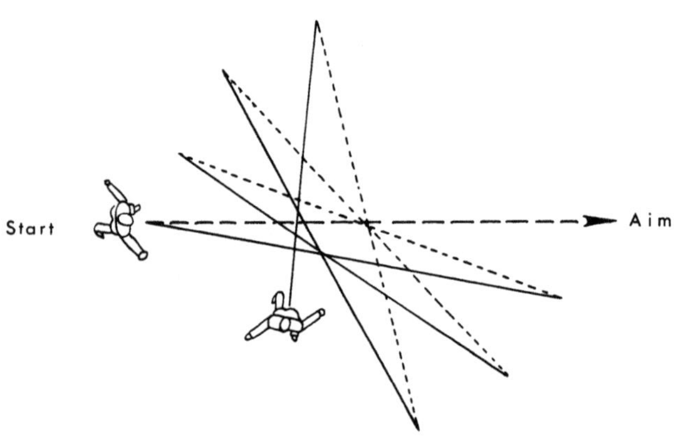

Fig. 2. Walking test

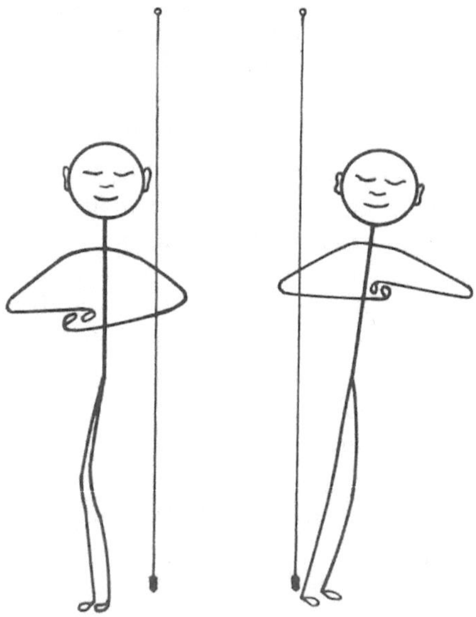

Fig. 3. Romberg test

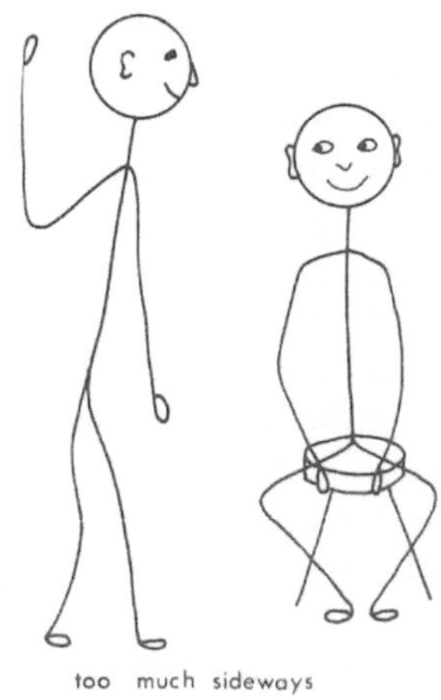

Fig. 5. Frenzel's spectacles

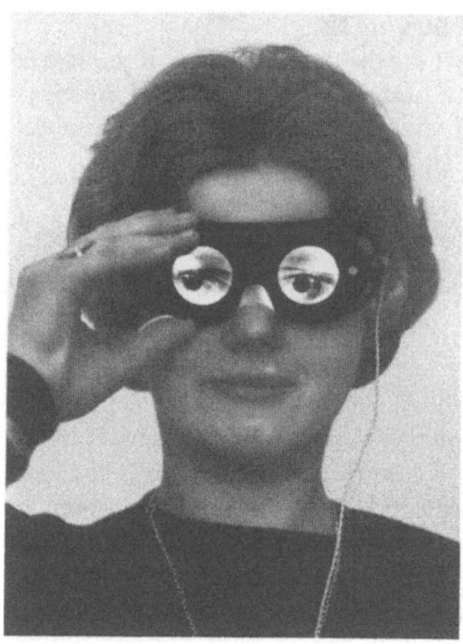

Fig. 4. Testing of spontaneous nystagmus

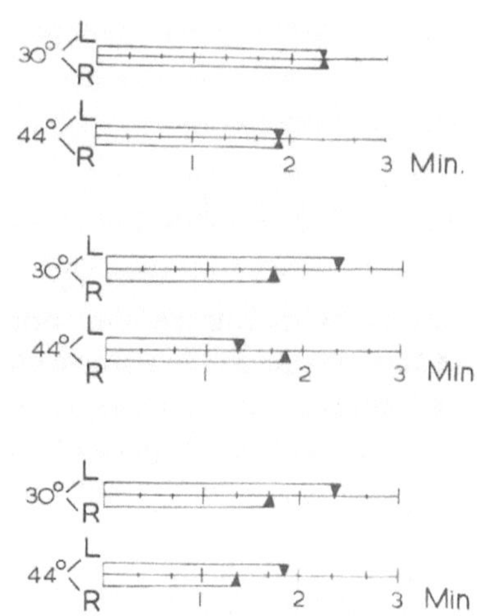

Figs. 6 and 7. Normal calorigram
Directional preponderance
Labyrinth preponderance

The physician in his office can perform a good caloric test. For every examination of the caloric responses, some rules are of great importance. The patient should be examined while lying on his back, his head raised on a pillow at an angle of about 30°. In that way the semicircular canals are in a vertical position and their reaction to the change of temperature provoked by caloric stimuli will be optimal. The patient is left on the couch for some minutes before starting the test, in order to let the effect of preceding vestibular stimuli pass and to give the patient time to quiet down. Nervous tension may have a strong influence on the results of the test. Irrigations (Fig. 6) are then given in a constant sequence: left cold, right cold, left warm, right warm with an ample interval between two irrigations (preferably 30 minutes but at least seven minutes) in order not to stimulate the vestibular system again while the effect of the preceding stimulus has not quieted down enough to give the right, uninfluenced answer upon the next one. The temperature of warm and cold water should be equidistant from body temperature, usually temperatures of 30 and 44° C are used, since they give the best results, without too many disagreeable side effects (vomiting and nausea). The use of an ear syringe, as used for washing out ear wax, is useful.

The number of parameters which the examiner can handle properly without the use of ENG is limited: they include duration of the postcaloric nystagmus and frequency to this nystagmus. The former is not easy to measure and too often the results are influeced by the anticipation of the examiner, since the endpoint of nystagmus is not very clearly discernible. Therefore the decision as to whether a nystagmus beat is the last one is rather arbitrary. The frequency is a much easier parameter to measure. The most efficient way is to count the number of nystagmus beats in the period between 50 and 60 seconds after the end of the irrigation. These results will be hardly influenced by expectation: they are clear.

Electronystagmograph is not necessary either for the determination of the size of either a directional preponderance (Fig. 7) or a preponderance of one of the labyrinths, since there is a formula that can be used for any parameter of the caloric nystagmus-duration, speed of the slow phase or all kind of combinations.

Labyrinth preponderance

$$\frac{(1+3)-(2+4)}{1+2+3+4}\times 100=\%\text{LP}$$

Directional preponderance

$$\frac{(1+4)-(3+2)}{1+2+3+4}\times 100=\%\text{DP}$$

I am sure many of you use this formula, which is, may be, not perfect but extremely practical, if at least the borders of normality of the examined parameter in the examined population with the used technique of calorization are known. They usually vary between 15 and 30 percent. Not very precise! So, do not be tempted to draw conclusions from a small difference in the answers of both ears or both directions of nystagmus.

What can the caloric test give the examiner of the vestibular system? Nothing, if the caloric test is not carried out in accordance with the rules. If the test is performed with water of only one temperature (Fig. 8) it cannot even always indicate with certainty that the labyrinth is either dead or alive. In the presence of a subliminal spontaneous nystagmus (as for instance after labyrinthine destruction or in case

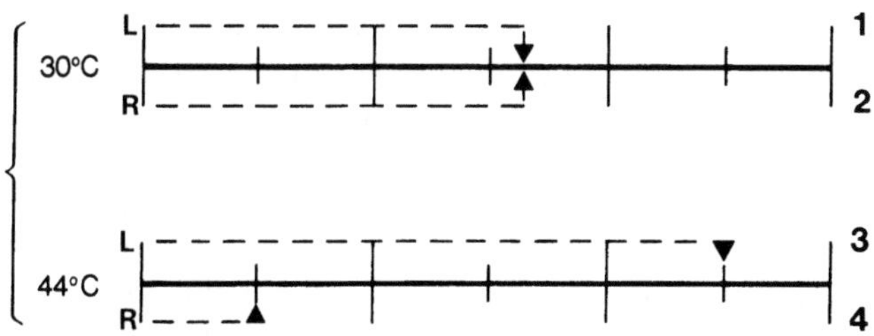

$$\frac{(100 + 150) - (100 + 30)}{100 + 150 + 100 + 30} \times 100 = 30\% \quad R < L$$

$$\frac{(100 + 30) - (100 + 150)}{100 + 150 + 100 + 30} \times 100 = 30\% \longrightarrow L$$

Fig. 8. Cold caloric test on both sides equal reactions. Hot test shows a great difference of the two reactions caused by a summation of directional and labyrinth preponderance

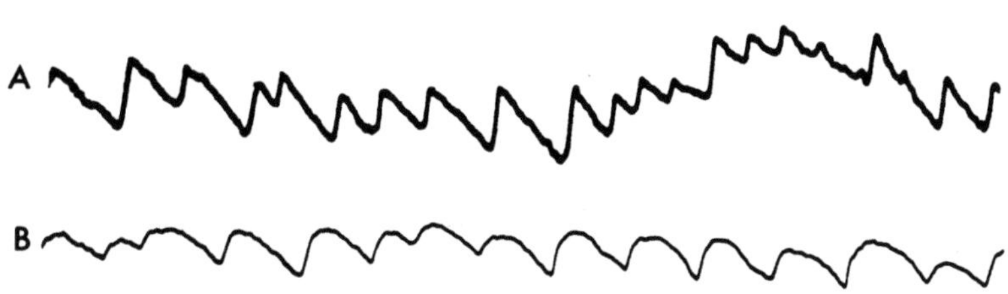

Fig. 9. **A** 'Saw tooth' labyrinthine nystagmus. **B** Congenital central nystagmus

of a tumor of the eighth nerve), the caloric stimulus can provoke a simulated caloric vestibular eye nystagmus by enhancing the subliminal nystagmus into a visible one. Only if the nystagmus has the direction that matches with each of the two opposite temperature stimuli, has the labyrinth proved that it is alive. It is also impossible to state that the two labyrinths react with equal strength if the two labyrinths yield equal direction upon stimulation with one temperature only. And a difference of the reactions of the two labyrinths cannot be explained if we do not know the reactions with the opposite temperature. Only the bithermal bilateral test gives the answers with any amount of probability. It is better not to perform a caloric test than to do it the easy way viz. only one temperature, or taking too little time between the various irrigations.

The practitioner can do excellent work as long as he does not think that he can make a shortcut anywhere in the time-consuming business of vestibular testing. He can make many diagnoses in his own office even without an E.N.G apparatus. However, it must be emphasized that electronystagmography is an interesting and important aid in other cases and also has important aspects from a general point of view.

The recording of nystagmus facilitates the evaluation of this passing and cursory phenomenon. It is indispensable if one wants to compare the situation at a certain moment with that of an earlier or later date. A nystagmogram is the most important record of facts if various clinicians want to discuss their data on a scientific and objective basis. Electronystagmography supplies us with tenable documents that also allow us a careful study of the form of a nystagmus beat (Fig. 9) and of non-nystagmic movements of the eye (Fig. 10). Nystagmography makes it possible to visualize many eye movements indistinguishable to the naked eye (its quantitative superiority).

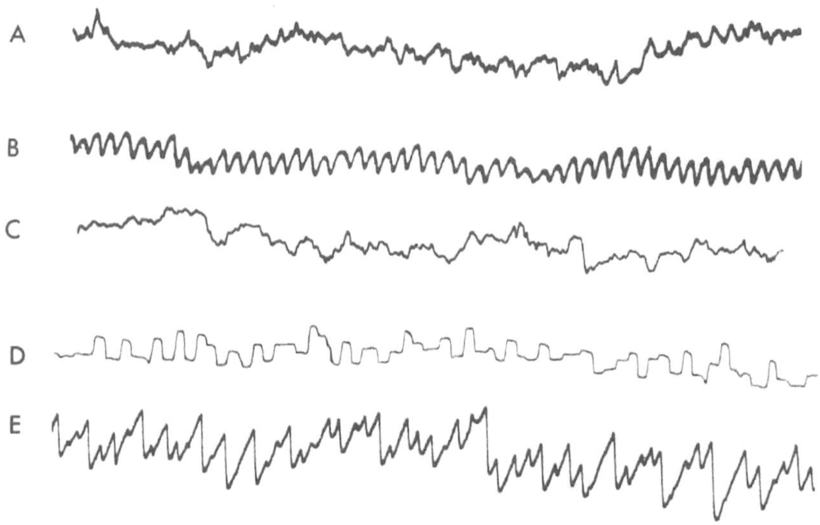

Fig. 10. Nystagmic and non-nystagmic movements. **A** Haemangioma cerebelli: atactical eye movements. **B** Tremor of the eye lid (cerebral arteriosclerosis). **C** Pethidine nystagmus. **D** Square wave pattern after head trauma. **E** Spontaneous nystagmus with hook pattern (crochetage)

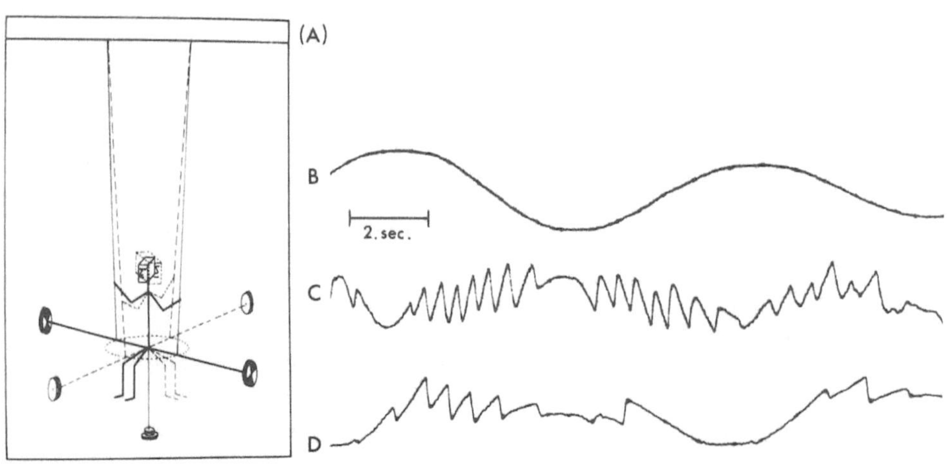

Fig. 11.

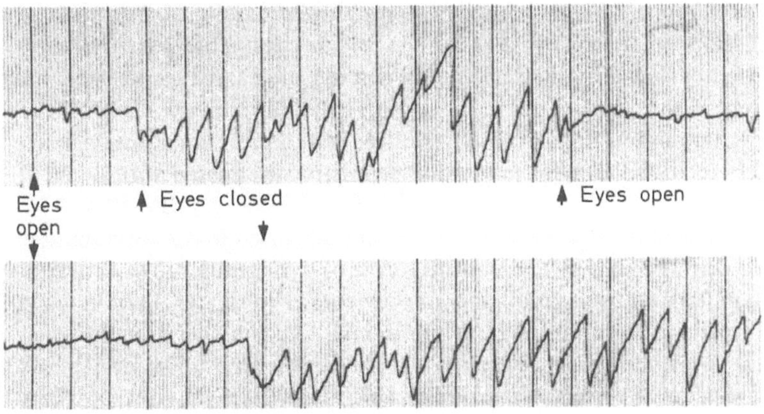

Fig. 12.

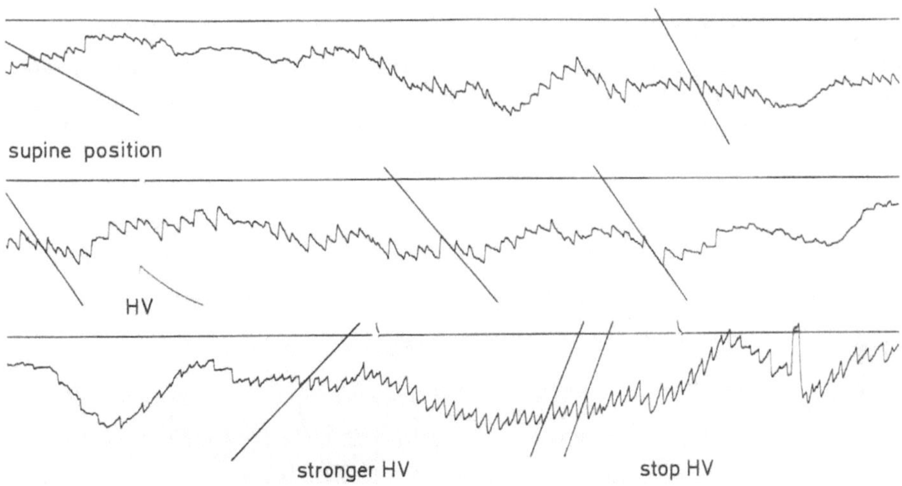

Fig. 13. The influence of hyperventilation (HV) on spontaneous nystagmus

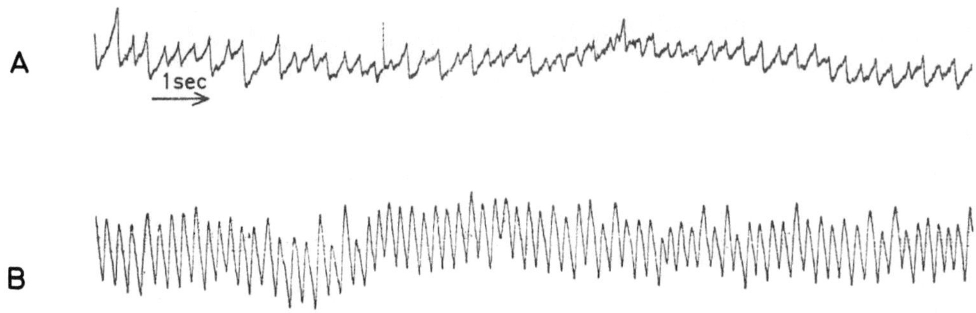

Fig. 14. Gaze nystagmus
A Looking to the left, nystagmus to the left
B Looking to the right, nystagmus to the right (clear preponderance)

The physician in the usual office cannot perform a great variety of tests such as rotatory tests on the torsion swing (Fig. 11), an eye tracking test, observation of nystagmus behind closed eyelids (Fig. 12); he cannot discern the variations in the form of the nystagmus that E.N.G. can visualise, he cannot even measure the speed of the slow phase of a nystagmus but he should realise that, with all the most modern instrument, computers included, a great many diagnoses are still missed with an electronystagmograph.

Nystagmus may be evaluated with both eyes open and closed to discover smaller nystagmus beats, to distinguish between various forms of nystagmus and to differentiate between nystagmus and nystagmoid eye movements. The E.N.G. may be used to examine more trustworthy parameters of nystagmus like the speed of the slow phase, and qualitative variations, to examine various influences upon nystagmus like hyperventilation (Fig. 13) or gaze nystagmus (Fig. 14). E.N.G. gives the examiner a chance to perform a rotatory test in a very short time, to investigate the effect of rotating the neck only (Fig. 15), in order to find cervical pathology. It makes it possible to perform tests about central vestibular function, like OK nystagmus (Fig. 16), or eye tracking (Fig. 17).

It is even possible to investigate the function of the otoliths on the parallel swing (Fig. 18). All together quite a wide horizon. But even in the most sophisticated and modern vestibular laboratory not all cases of giddiness are solved.

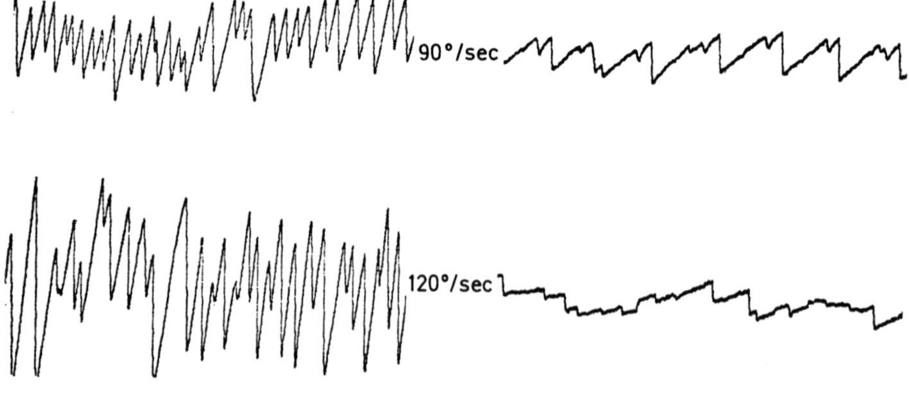

Fig. 15. O.K.N. 3 speeds

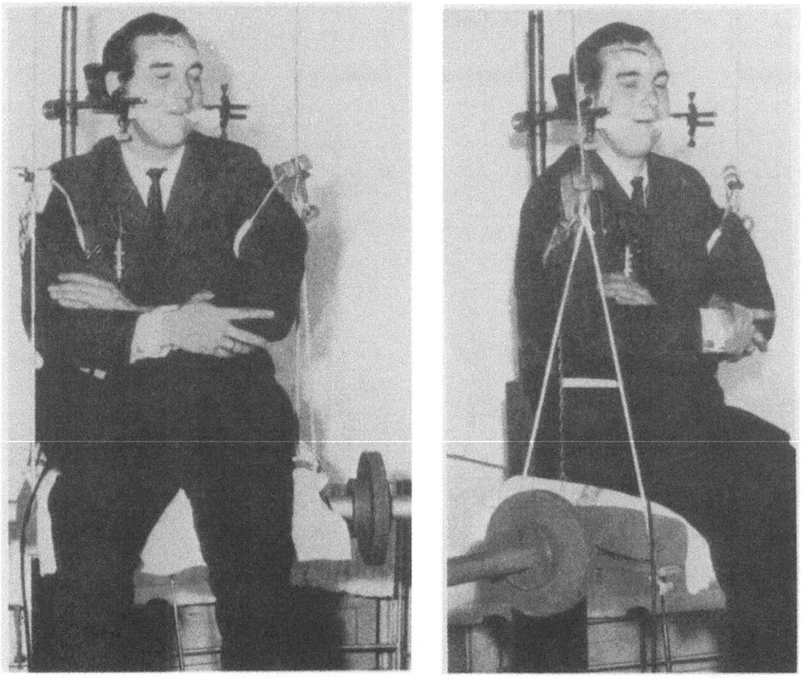

Fig. 16. Neck torsion test. The head of the patient is fixed. The chair rotates

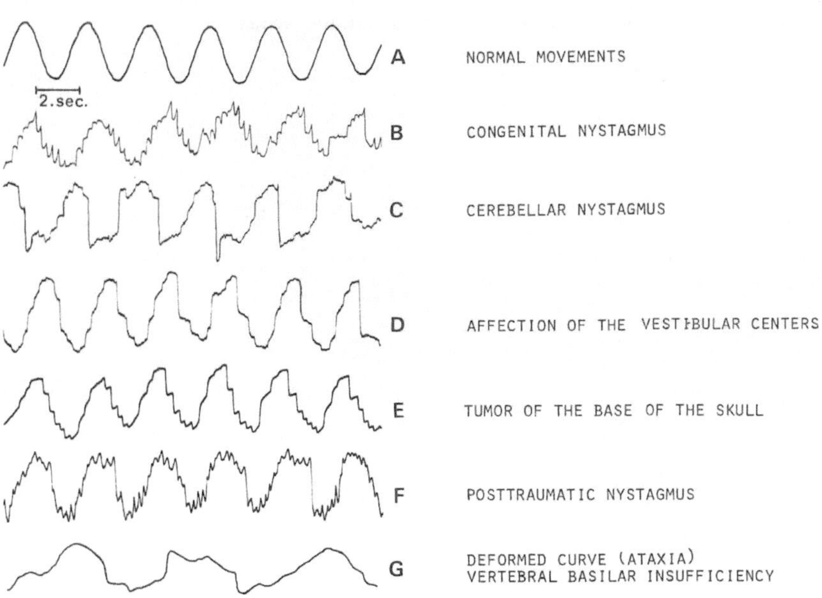

Fig. 17. Eye tracking test

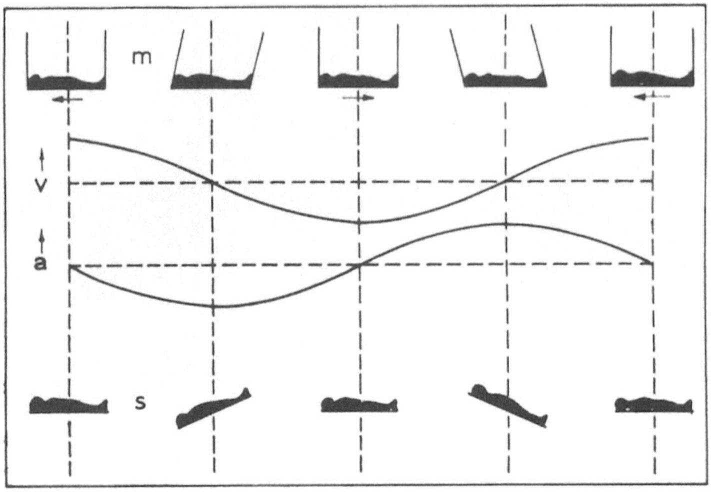

A

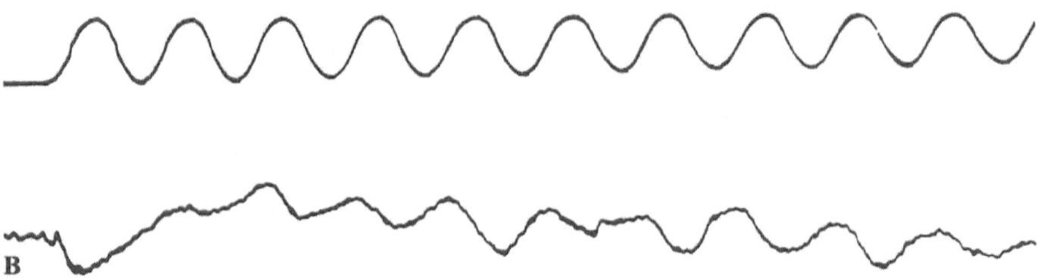

B

Fig. 18. A Scheme of place, movement and acceleration of the parallel swing, with the subjective position of the test subject. m = movement; s = sensation; v = velocity; a = acceleration. **B** Eye movements provoked by movements of the parallel swing

Early Diagnosis of Eighth Cranial Nerve Lesions by Positional Testing and Meatography

T. HAID, Erlangen-Nürnberg/FRG

Introduction

In diseases of the eighth cranial nerve, it is important to rule out a tumorous process in the internal auditory canal or cerebello-pontine angle. Neurinomas of the acoustic nerve are the most common lesions in this region. Audiological, radiographic and vestibular evidence of a tumour in the internal auditory canal or cerebello-pontine angle furnish the indication for cisternomeatography.

In vestibular testing, the quantifying positional test together with tone-threshold audiometry rather than the caloric testing, proved to be the most sensitive examination method in the early diagnosis of a space-occupying lesion of the internal auditory canal or the cerebello-pontine angle which has led to an injury of the eighth cranial nerve.

Materials and Methods

During the period from January, 1974 to March, 1980, 80 patients with a tumor of the internal auditory canal including the cerebello-pontine angle were studied (Table 1). Following evaluation of the ENT status, audiological and X-ray studies of the petrous bone, the positional test was carried out in the following manner:

The patient was first examined in the *head-down position.* He was then examined in the recumbent position with the *head turned to the right,* and then *to the left.* Subsequently, he was directed to *turn his body* at first *to the right,* thereafter *to the left* and finally he had to *rise quickly into the sitting position.*

The examination was performed with the aid of Frenzel spectacles, but an electronystagmogram (ENG) was also taken. The quantitatively measured nystagmus deflections were recorded in the so-called positiogram (Haid 1978, Fig. 1 d).

Cisternomeatography has been carried out in the clinic for 4 years. During this period, 170 examinations of this type were performed. During the first two years, we used Pantopaque as a contrast medium. Subsequently we switched over to Duroliopaque because of its lower viscosity and better flow velocity.

Table 1. Histological findings in tumors of the internal auditory canal and the cerebellopontine angle

Neurinoma	73 [a]	Epidermoid	1
Meningioma	4	Cholesteatoma	1
Hemangioma	1		

[a] 65 confirmed at surgery

Results

Between 1974 and 1980, at the Erlangen ENT Clinic, 80 patients, who underwent audiological and radiographic studies as well as vestibular tests, were found to have a tumor of the internal auditory canal or cerebello-pontine angle. This figure also includes those tumors in which cisternomeatography had not been used.

All patients with a tumour of the internal auditory canal or cerebello-pontine angle presented, with one exception, an abnormal tone threshold audiogram. Supraliminal audiometry used to identify a retrocochlear hearing impairment yielded conclusive findings only in roughly half of the cases. Moreover, many of our patients were deaf on the tumor side (41 percent). In such instances, supraliminal audiometry is no longer possible.

Table 2. Pathological findings dependent upon the size of tumors involving the internal auditory canal and the cerebello-pontine angle

	A	B, C, D	Total
Tone threshold audiogram	100%	98%	99%
Positional test	91%	91%	92%
Caloric test	73%	83%	82%
Tomography	67%	79%	76%
Stenvers projection	55%	59%	58%

Type A = small tumor ($n = 11$)
Type B = medium-sized tumor ($n = 19$)
Types C, D = large tumor ($n = 50$)

The radiographic visualization of the petrous bones and the internal auditory canals furnished less reliable clues than would be generally surmised. Stenvers projections identified a difference between the two sides in only six out of 11 intrameatal tumors (55 percent). Tomography increased the diagnostic yield slightly, to 67 percent.

In all patients afflicted by a tumor of the internal auditory canal or of the cerebello-pontine angle, it was possible to verify a pathological process of the vestibular nerve. The positional test proved to be the most sensitive, also with small tumors (Table 2). The use of the Frenzel spectacles helped to identify a positional or positioning nystagmus in 92 percent of the patients with a tumor in the internal auditory canal or the cerebello-pontine angle, while the same finding was obtained in 10 out of 11 patients suffering from small tumors. In 82 percent, a reduced caloric excitability existed on the tumor side, and in the case of small tumors, 73 percent (eighth out of 11 patients).

During the period from 1976 to March 1980, cisternomeatography helped to diagnose a space-occupying lesion in 39 out of 170 patients because of suspected neurinoma of the acoustic nerve (Table 3). Of these 39 tumors, 33 were confirmed at surgery. Five of them were small, i.e. still intrameatal, 11 were medium-sized, meaning that they reached beyond the porus acusticus internus by 1.5 cm and 17 were

Table 3. Results of 170 cisterno-meatographies

Lumbar contrast-medium injection	170
Cisterna filled with contrast-medium	161
Meatus filled, no evidence of tumor	122
Tumor suspected because of filling defect	39
Out of 39 radiologically suspect cases, operated on:	36
Operative findings:	
Large neurinoma	15
Large meningioma	2
Medium-sized neurinoma	11
Intrameatal neurinoma	4
Intrameatal haemangioma	1
Filling defect originating from arachnoiditis	1
False/positive findings	2
False/negative findings	0

large tumors. Three suspect cases, two small intrameatal tumors and a large tumor of the cerebello-pontine angle, have not yet been operated upon. In another patient with suspected tumor and presenting the symptoms of Menière's disease, the contrast-free niche in the X-ray, which was believed to be indicative of a tumor, originated from arachnoiditis. Neurectomy of the vestibular nerve liberated the patient from vertigo which had been resistant to conservative therapy. Operation produced evidence that two findings were false-positive. In both cases a small intrameatal tumor had been believed to exist.

Indications for Cisternomeatography

In light of our personal experience, we recommend cisternomeatography to rule out a tumor of the internal acoustic canal or the cerebello-pontine angle associated with a lesion of the eighth cranial nerve in any patient with unclarified, mainly unilateral sensori-neural hearing impairment, no matter whether audiometrically of the cochlear or retrocochlear type, when it is accompanied by a pathological vestibular diagnosis, such as positional or positioning nystagmus, independent of the X-ray view of the petrous bone (Table 4).

Table 4. Indications for cisterno-meatography in the early diagnosis of tumors affecting the internal auditory canal and the cerebello-pontine angle

In unclarified and unilateral sensori-neural hearing-loss

1. of progressive character or sign of a retrocochlear lesion
2. with a positional or positioning nystagmus
3. with a caloric hypoactivity
4. with a roentgenological difference of the internal auditory canal
5. with combinations of 1, 2, 3, and 4.

Materials

An example showing no radiological difference between the unaffected side and the lesion side is given to illustrate the diagnostic importance attaching to the tone-threshold audiometry and the vestibular test.

A 55 year old man became suddenly deaf in the right ear and experienced slight tinnitus and rotary vertigo with nausea. The audiogram (Fig. 1 a) demonstrated deafness in the right ear. Neither the Stenvers projections nor tomography of the petrous bones could establish a difference between the unaffected and lesion side of the internal acoustical meatus (Fig. 1 b, c). Vestibular testing demonstrated a striking positional nystagmus (Fig. 1 d) and the caloric test revealed lack of excitability on the right side (Fig. 1 e). At first, we assumed an acute hearing loss to exist in the right ear involving the vestibular nerve. When, during the clinical treatment of the acute hearing loss, the patient gradually developed a progredient paresis of the facial nerve on the right side, we decided to carry out cisternomeatography to rule out the presence of an intrameatal tumor. In the region of the right porus acusticus internus, a small recess not filled by contrast agent was present, indicating a tumor (Fig. 1 f).

Since the patient was deaf in his right ear, the translabyrinthine route was selected for surgery. A small tumor on the facial nerve, which proved histologically to be a hemangioma, was removed. Since the lesion had completely invaded the facial nerve, the nerve was deliberately severed. For plastic repair of the facial nerve, a transplant was interposed and fixed with fibrin glue. As this oparation was carried

Figs. 1 a–g. Small hemangioma of the facial nerve in the right internal auditory canal (K. Ch. 55 years old, male)

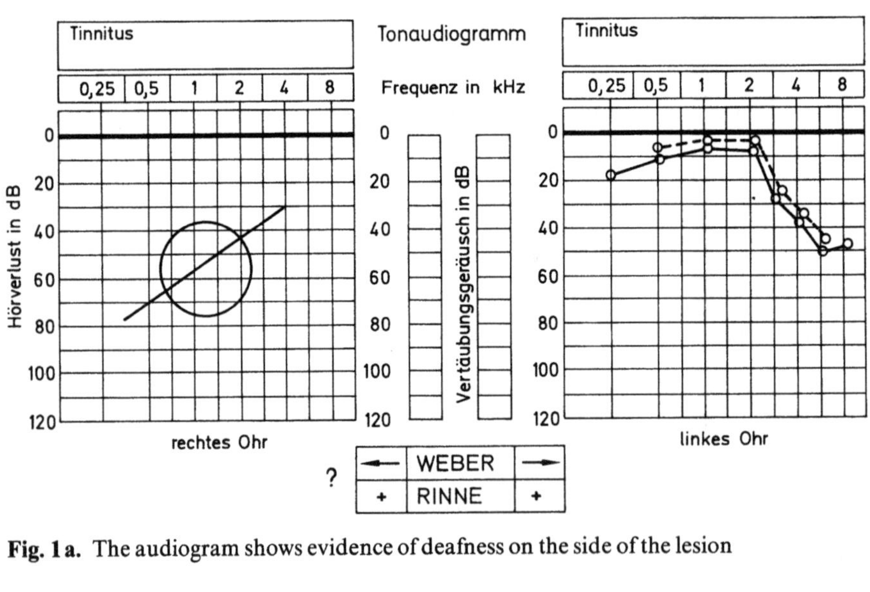

Fig. 1 a. The audiogram shows evidence of deafness on the side of the lesion

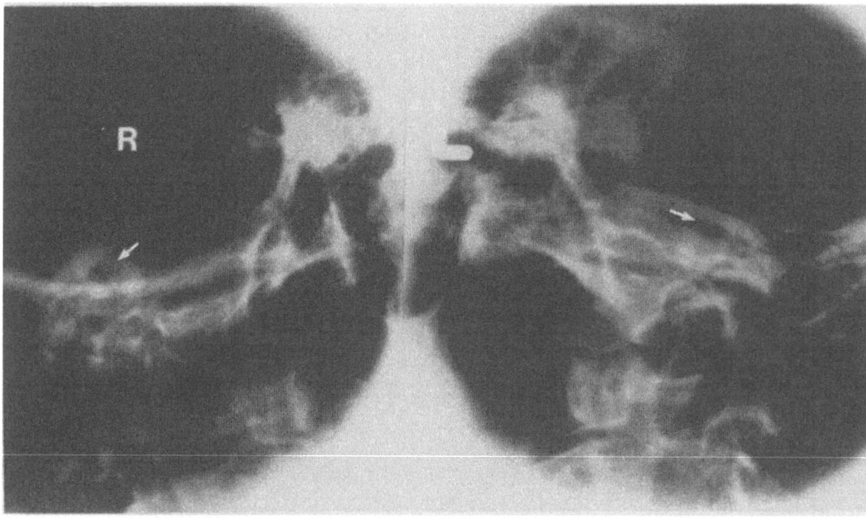

Fig. 1b. Same patient as in Fig. 1a. Stenvers projections reveal no difference between the two internal auditory canals (*arrows*)

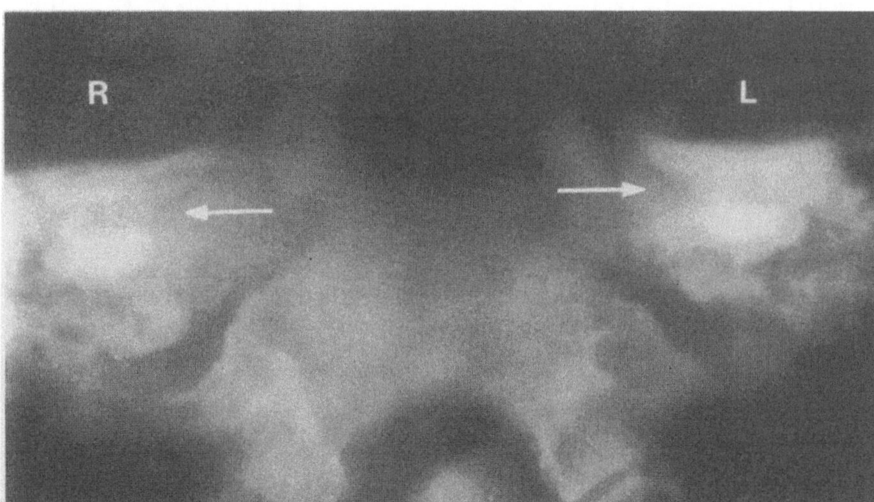

Fig. 1c. Same patient as in Figs. 1a, b. Tomography of the petrous bones does not demonstrate any difference between the two internal auditory canals

Fig. 1e. Same patient as in Figs. 1a–d.
The frequency calorigram, an analogous chart of the caloric reaction, reveals non-excitability on the side of the tumor. On the right side, the spontaneous nystagmus to the left, having 20 movements in 30 seconds, is not interrupted by the caloric stimulation. On the left side, the number of movements was 72 during 30 seconds in the case of hot-water syringing, and 42 movements were recorded in the case of cold-water syringing. The light-shaded and dark-shaded fields furnish information as to the values found in the standard collective. Values ranging between 25 and 80 during the culmination time of 30 seconds can be found in the standard collective at almost 90 percent

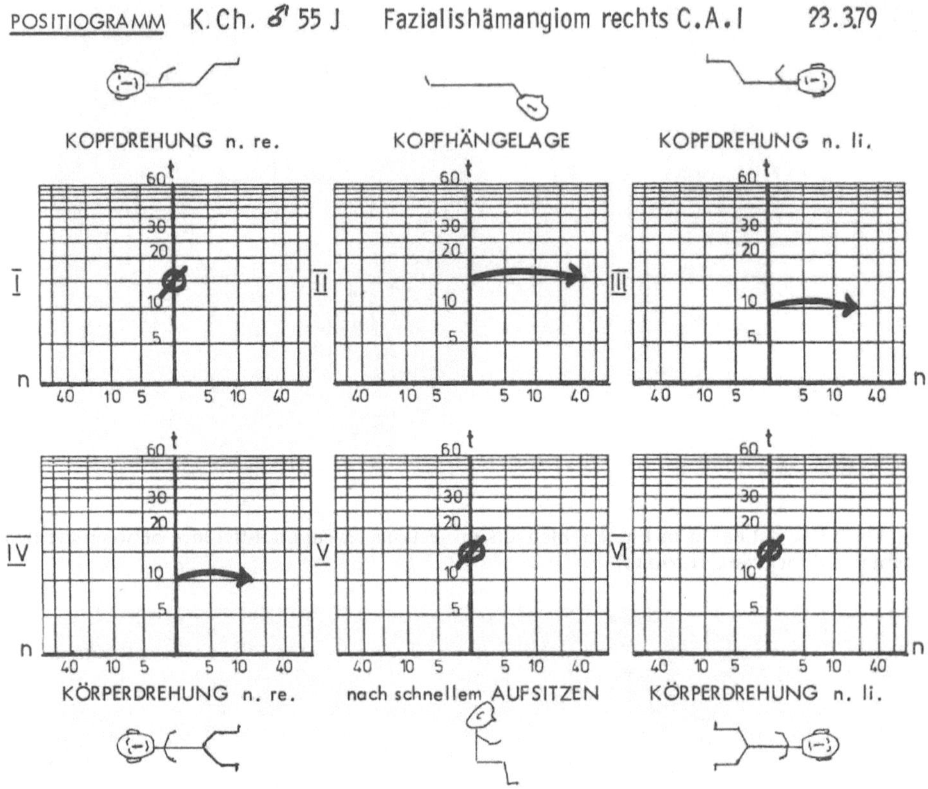

Fig. 1d. Same patient as in Figs. 1a–c. In the positiogram, a quantitative record of the positional test, a positional nystagmus is discernible. In the head-down position, there is a horizontal rotatory nystagmus to the left with 40 movements and a duration of 15 seconds.
When the head is turned to the left and the body to the right, there is a nystagmus to the left with 20 and 15 movements, respectively, having an identical duration of 10 seconds. In the remaining three positions, no nystagmus was elicited

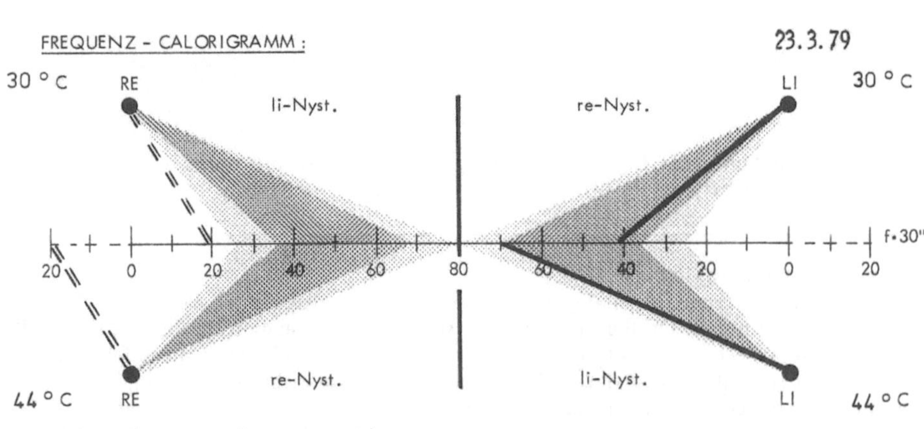

Fig. 1e (Caption see page 543)

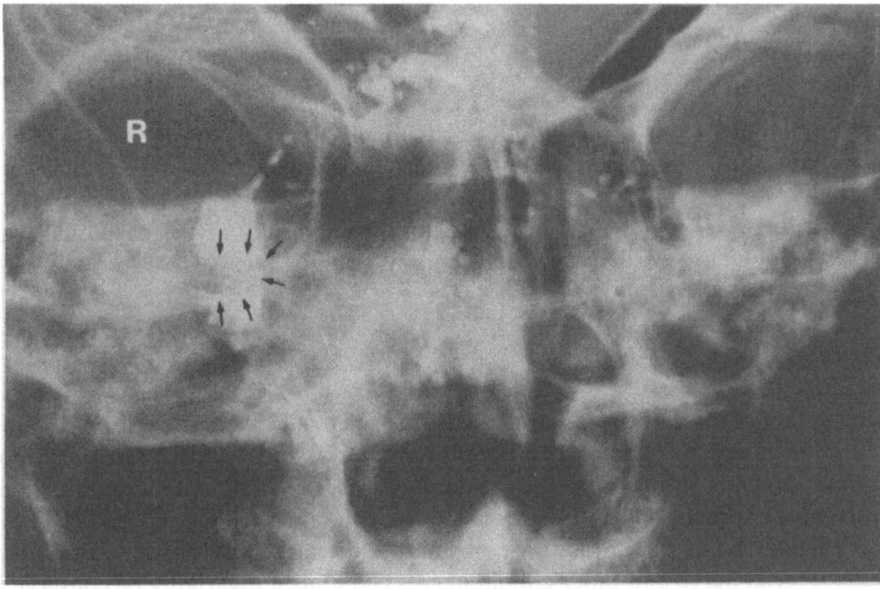

Fig. 1 f. Same patient as in Figs. 1 a–e.
Cisterno-meatography reveals a small filling defect in front of the porus acusticus internus, on the right side (*arrows*)

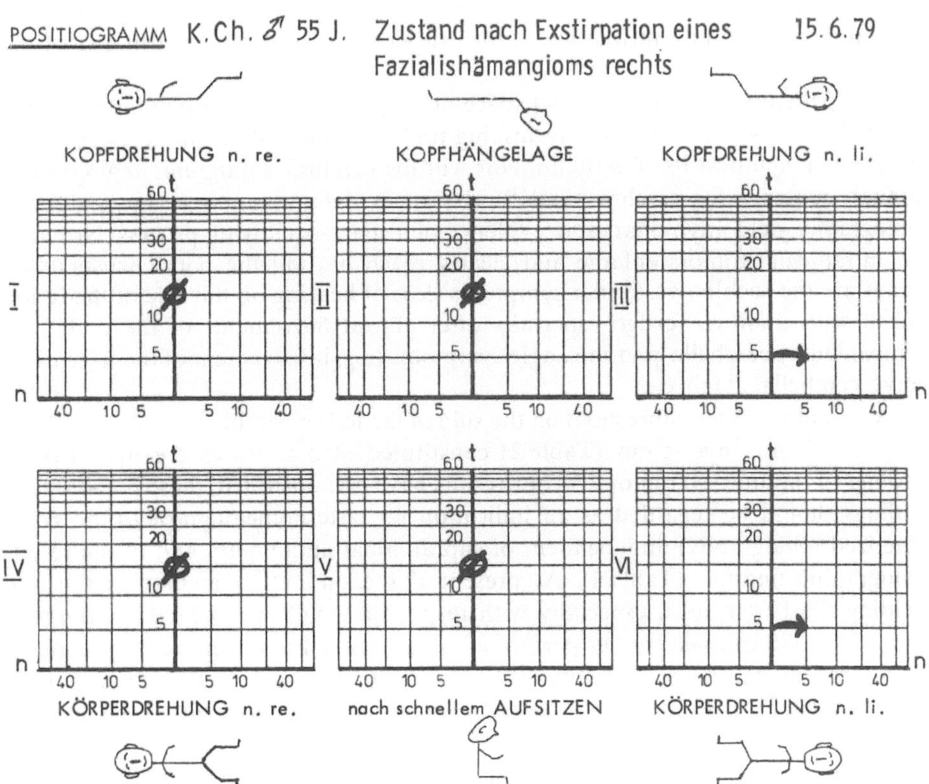

Fig. 1 g. Same patient as in Figs. 1 a–f.
Result of the positional test three months following extirpation of a small hemangioma in the right internal auditory canal. The intensity of the nystagmus has clearly abated. Only when the head and body are turned to the left, is a nystagmus to the left elicited, with only 5 movements in each case and a duration of 5 seconds

out nine months ago, it is too early to pass final opinion as to the success of the neuroplasty. During the last follow-up check, the EMG revealed voluntary innervation.

As was expected, after the tumor excision, the intensity of the positional nystagmus was found to have decreased considerably (Fig. 1 g).

Discussion

When a lesion of the eighth cranial nerve is suspected, all diagnostic efforts must be aimed at the timely recognition of a tumor, however small it may be. The success of operation depends on the size of the tumor. The mortality rate subsequent to microsurgery is practically zero percent (House, 1968; Fisch, 1978; Glasscock et al., 1978; Wigand et al., 1980) in the case of small, especially intrameatal, tumors. The ipsilateral facial nerve and other cranial nerves can almost invariably be conserved. Total excision of the tumor is practically always achieved.

In our patients we succeeded in saving hearing on the operative side in five out of ten small tumors which were operated upon. We have had one fatality among our 53 patients who underwent otomicrosurgery for intrameatal tumors including tumors affecting the cerebello-pontine angle. One very obese woman died of massive pulmonary embolism one week after surgical removal of a neurinoma of the acoustic nerve.

In a patient with an intrameatal space-occupying lesion, examination of the trigeminal nerve will not furnish any striking findings, and seldom will a lesion of the facial nerve manifest itself early on. Nor will the cerebral scintigram, angiography, lumbar puncture for cerebrospinal fluid protein determination or computerized tomography yield any remarkable evidence of a space-occupying process. Not until the intrameatal tumors enlarge and clearly reach beyond the porus acusticus internus are the cochleo-vestibular symptoms (loss of hearing on the side of the lesion linked with tinnitus, vertigo especially after abrupt movements of the body) accompanied by cerebello-pontine angle symptoms (e.g. involvement of the trigeminal nerve, cerebellar ataxia etc).

A pathological tone threshold on the side of the lesion combined with a positional or positioning nystagmus (Table 2) constituted in most cases the first striking findings of intrameatal tumors. As our results have demonstrated, these pathological findings should be regarded as an indication for cisternomeatography (and computerized tomography), independent of supraliminal audiometry and of the roentgenographic findings (Table 4). At present this examination method is the one yielding the best results, especially with respect to small intrameatal tumours. In view of the 170 contrast studies performed, it has proved to be an excellent complication-free diagnostic tool. Every fifth examination revealed the presence of a tumor (Table 3). Histologically, the lesion was usually a neurinoma of the acoustic nerve.

In the literature only reduced caloric excitability on the side of the lesion is advanced as vestibular indication for cisternomeatography (House, 1968; Sheehy, 1968; Fisch and Wegmüller, 1974). The positional test proved in our hands to be even more responsive than the caloric test, both in the early diagnosis of intrameatal tumors and in the identification of tumors affecting the eighth cranial nerve in cerebello-pontine angle. Ninety-two percent of the patients examined had a positional or positioning nystagmus. Needless to say, reduced caloric excitability on the side of the lesion together with a sensori-neural hearing impairment are indications for a neuroradiological examination. However, our results have shown that in these tumor patients the reduced caloric excitability is always accompanied by a positional or positioning nystagmus ascertained during the positional testing. This test represents a minimum stimulus and can stimulate all three semicircular canals, the otolith system and the higher centers of the vestibular nerve; while the caloric test provides a maximum stimulus and thus practically stimulates the horizontal semicircular canal only. This may serve as an explanation for the higher sensitivity of the positional test observed by us.

The quantitative evaluation of the results gained from positional testing is of great importance if progressiveness, constancy or remission are to be identified. With acute loss of hearing with involvement of the vestibular nerve, with vestibular neuronitis or Menière's disease, progressive pathological results gained from the follow-up checks of the positional testing, or lack of improvements over a longer period of time, constitute definite indications for neuroradiological examination. Audiometry is required in every patient complaining of unilateral hearing loss. If unilateral sensory-neural deafness is ascertained, an equilibrium test must be carried out. In this context the positional test together with tone-threshold determination have proved to be very sensitive examination methods in the early diagnosis of a still intrameatal tumor.

Summary

Because most of the intrameatal tumors with a lesion of the eighth cranial nerve are only belatedly diagnosed as tumors affecting the cerebello-pontine angle and considering that such large lesions are associated with a relatively high operative complication rate, the indications for cisternomeatography are justly given with a certain generosity in our ENT clinic:

Any unclear, prevailingly unilateral sensory-neural hearing impairment combined solely with a positional or positioning nystagmus may point to an intrameatal tumor, independent of the result obtained from supraliminal audiometry and the X-ray views of the petrous bones. In 170 complication-free contrast studies, 36 tumors were found to involve the internal auditory canal and the cerebello-pontine angle.

References

Fisch U, Wegmüller A (1974) Early diagnosis of acoustic neuromas. ORL 36: 129

Fisch U (1978) Otomikrochirurgische Behandlung des Akustikusneurinoms In: Plester, Wende, Nakayama (eds) Kleinhirnbrückenwinkeltumoren, Diagnostik und Therapie. Springer, Berlin Heidelberg New York

Glasscock ME, Hays JW, Jackson CG, Steenerson RL (1978) A onestage combined approach for the management of large cerebello-pontine angle tumors. Laryngoscope 10: 1563

Haid T, Berg M (1978) Zisterno-Meatografie mit Pantopaque zur neurotologischen Differentialdiagnose des Akustikusneurinoms. Fortschr Neurol Psychiatr 46: 579

Haid T (1979) Das Positiogramm, eine Aufzeichnungsmethode der Lageprüfung in der Neurotologie. Laryngol Rhinol Otol (Stuttgart) 58: 443

House WF (1968) Acoustic Neuroma. Arch Otolaryngol 88: 6

House WF, Luetje CM (1979) Acoustic tumors, vol II. Management. University Park Press, Baltimore

Sheehy JL (1978) The neuro-otologic evaluation. Arch Otolaryngol 88: 44

Wigand ME, Haid T, Berg M, Rettinger G (April 1980) Early diagnosis and transtemporal removal of small nerve VII and VIII tumors. Vortrag auf der ORL-Tagung in Bordeaux

Neurectomy of the Vestibular Nerve for Menière's Disease

J. Helms*, E. Steinbach**, and M. Galic**

Research to explain the etiology of Menière's disease is still in progress. Hydrops of the endolymphatic system (Hallpike and Cairns, 1938 [6]; Schuknecht, 1974 [17]) in the inner ear has frequently been observed and is the only generally accepted pathological finding in this disease. Since we began performing neurectomy of the vestibular ganglion (Scarpae) in order to stop the most annoying symptom, the attacks of vertigo, we have observed another constant pathological finding in Menière's disease.

Materials and Methods

Patients with the classical symptoms of Menière's disease are treated conservatively as long as hearing remains good in the main speech frequencies. When a pronounced fluctuation or a constant decrease is observed and when the patient suffers from a feeling of fullness in the ear, a saccotomy [14, 15, 16] is carried out. If the inner ear hearing loss proceeds quickly or the feeling of fullness is less pronounced, we perform a vestibular neurectomy. This is done with the technique of Fisch [2], a modification of technique of House [11]. Other authors follow the same principles [1, 5, 18]. As long as hearing is worth saving, a transtemporal neurectomy is carried out. When the ear is completely deaf, the inner auditory canal is reached by the translabyrinthine route.

The vestibular nerve is cut laterally and medially from Scarpa's ganglion, which is thereby removed. This procedure was performed in 91 patients. The number of cases histologically examined is now 51. The resected tissue was prepared for light- or electron-microscopy. For comparison vestibular nerves were removed from 54 non-Menière cadavers and prepared for light microscopical examination in the same way.

Results

When compared with the non-Menière nerves we found an increase in the connective tissue in all cases with Menière's disease. This was controlled in a double blind study. The histological slides were separated according to the amount of connective tissue present. A clear separation between the Menière- and the non-Menière group of tissues was achieved. The amount of connective tissue in the

* Mainz/FRG
** Tübingen/FRG

Menière group varied considerably but in all samples was considered to be pathological. The cellular elements of the connective tissue seemed to be reduced in the majority of cases.

A definite correlation between the duration of the disease and the amount of connective tissue formed in the vestibular nerves could not be seen. The samples of a group of 11 patients with a saccotomy performed one half to three years before the vestibular neurectomy resembled the findings in the group with neurectomy only. Of the first 39 cases, seven had a slight increase of connective tissue. A moderate surplus was observed in 21 cases and a fibrosis-like amount of connective tissue in 11 cases. We were unable to count the neuroms in our resection material due to injury to the nerve bundles during surgical removal.

Electronmicroscopical examination revealed an increase in lipofuscin formation. The amount exceeded the aging processes by far. In addition the overproduction of connective tissue was found in more detail. Vascular changes were also seen. These examinations were carried out mainly by Galic of Plester's clinic [4]. Out of the same clinic Steinbach earlier reported on the vascular changes [9].

Discussion

Earlier findings [7, 8, 9] had demonstrated that the vestibular nerve reacts sensitively to a mechanical trauma of the labyrinth such as labyrinthectomy, fracture or ultra-sound. In all these cases a bone-like material was observed in the surrounding area of the vestibular ganglion, combined with a considerable increase in connective tissue formation. A similar alteration in the composition of the vestibular nerve but without bone-like material, was observed in Menière's disease [10] in our series and in the material of Hildmann [11], whereas Ylikoski and co-workers did not see these changes [19].

It is not yet known whether the increase in connective tissue formation, the deposition of excess lipofuscin and the vascular changes as seen in our series are caused by a labyrinthine alteration or whether they cause the labyrinthine disease. The pathological changes in Scarpa's ganglion might contribute to the clinical symptoms in a long lasting Menière's disease. This part of the nerve should therefore be removed in appropriate cases.

Summary

In 51 patients with Menière's disease an increase in connective tissue formation in the vestibular nerve was found combined with the deposition of excess lipofuscin and vascular changes. The patients were treated with a transtemporal or translabyrinthine vestibular neurectomy. The excision material including Scarpa's ganglion was histologically examined and showed the pathological changes in all cases proven in a double blind study.

References

1. Bryan V, Bucy PC (1973) Vestibular nerve section for Menière's. Arch Otolaryngol 97:115
2. Fisch U (1969) Die transtemporale, extralabyrinthäre Chirurgie des inneren Gehörgangs. Arch Klin Exp Ohr-Nas-Kehlk Heilk 194:232
3. Fisch U (1972) Pers. comm. Second. internat. course in transtemporal microsurgery of the internal auditory canal, Zürich
4. Galic M, Helms J (1977) Elektronenmikroskopische Untersuchungen über die Häufigkeit, Verteilung und Struktur des Lipofuscins im Ganglion vestibuli bei Morbus Menière. INSERM (Les Colleques de l'Institut National de la Santé et de la Recherche Médicale) 68:243–261
5. Glasscock ME (1973) Vestibular nerve section. Middle fossa and translabyrinthine. Arch Otolaryngol 97:112
6. Hallpike CS, Cairns H (1938) Observation on the pathology of Menière's syndrome. J Laryngol Otol 53:625
7. Helms J (1973) Labyrinthectomy as a therapy for Menière's disease. Proc. X. World Congr. Otolaryng., Venice (in press)
8. Helms J (1974) Labyrinthectomy for Menière's disease. Proc. Barany Society Meeting, Los Angeles (in press)
9. Helms J, Steinbach E (1974) Ungewöhnliche Befunde bei Operationen am inneren Gehörgang. Arch Klin Exp Ohr-Nas-Kehlk Heilk 207:495
10. Helms J, Steinbach E (1974) Umbauprozesse im Nervus vestibularis nach Labyrinthschädigung und beim Morbus Menière. 11. Internat. Tagung über Biologie des Innenohres, Würzburg 4.–7.9.
11. Hildmann H Pers. communication.
12. House WF (1961) Surgical exposure of the internal auditory canal and its contents through the middle, cranial fossa. Laryngoscope 71:1363
13. Plester D (1970) Pers. communication.
14. Plester D (1970) Die chirurgische Behandlung des Morbus Menière. HNO 18:205
15. Portmann G (1927) The saccus endolymphaticus and an operation for draining the same for the relief of vertigo. J Laryngol Otol 42:809
16. Pulec JL (1970) The surgical treatment of vertigo. Rev Laryngol Otol Rhinol (Bord) 91:41
17. Schuknecht HF (1974) The histopathology of Menière's disease. Proc. Barany Society Meeting, Los Angeles (in press)
18. Silverstein H, Makimoto K (1973) Superior vestibular and 'singular nerve' section. Laryngoscope 83:1414
19. Ylikoski J, Collan Y, Palva T (1979) Menière's disease: Morphological findings in eighth nerve and vestibular end organs. ORL 41:26–32

Neurovascular Cross-Compression of the Eighth Cranial Nerve in Patients With Vertigo and Tinnitus

P. J. JANNETTA, Pittsburgh, PA/USA

The eighth (stato-acoustic) cranial nerve, like the trigeminal, facial, and glossopharyngeal nerves, is subject to symptoms of disordered hyperactivity which may be gradually accompanied by progressive loss of function. The hyperactive symptoms in this special sensory nerve which carries hearing (cochlear nerve) and balance (superior and inferior vestibular nerves) functions consist of a caricature of these normal functions of the nerve, just as the hyperactive symptoms in a somatic sensory nerve include pain (i.e. trigeminal neuralgia, N V) and in a somatic motor nerve, abnormal muscular movements or twitching (hemifacial spasm – N VII). Patients may first have symptoms of cochlear and/or vestibular nerve involvement. Symptoms which may include tinnitus, hyperacusis, diplacusis, hearing loss and vertigo, may vary in time and intensity. Symptoms may develop in one branch of the eighth cranial nerve and then gradually involve the other. Operative treatment over the years has generally consisted of peripheral denervation. This has indeed been the best available treatment for patients with intractable symptoms. The results regarding quality of life have not been excellent. Replacing one symptom with another has not proven to be a superior method of treatment.

The present series is based upon the continued extrapolation of the findings by the author in trigeminal neuralgia and hemifacial spasm: i.e. as abnormalities of the root entry zones of these nerves, usually vascular cross compression were found and mobilized away from the nerve as definitive microsurgical therapy of the hyperactive symptoms, usually with improvements of the accompanying decreased function (numbness, weakness, etc.). It seemed reasonable that the same should be true in the eighth cranial nerve. Therefore, starting in December 1972, a series of patients with disabling symptoms of hyperactive > hypoactive eighth nerve dysfunction underwent microsurgical exploration of the nerve throughout its intracranial course in the cerebellopontine angle [1, 2, 3].

Patient Population

The series consisted of 38 patients, 25 females and 13 males, whose symptoms were on the right side in 17 and on the left in 21. The age at onset of their symptoms was from 15 to 59 years. Three had begun in the second decade, five in the third, seven in the fourth, 12 in the fifth and 10 in the sixth. The age of onset was unknown in one patient who simply could not remember when the symptoms had started except that they had been present for many years.

Symptoms consisted of vertigo alone in seven patients. Twenty patients had vertigo and tinnitus, frequently with hearing loss. Eleven patients had tinnitus alone.

All but two of the latter patients (tinnitus alone) had incidental evaluation of their eighth nerve during a retromastoid craniectomy done primarily to relieve vascular compression in trigeminal neuralgia or hemifacial spasm.

Preoperative Evaluation

The patients in this series fell into three groups: 1. Disabling vertigo with or without tinnitus, 2. Incidental tinnitus in a patient operated upon for another cranial nerve problem in the same cerebellopontine angle, 3. Tinnitus alone (two patients) without other cranial nerve symptoms.

In addition to the usual basic workup including skull and chest roentgenograms, electrocardiography, blood count, and urinalysis, etc., all patients underwent tomography of the petrous bone, computerized tomography with and without contrast, and complete otovestibular testing. Recent patients have had brain stem evoked potentials as part of the routine. A broad spectrum of various types of hearing loss and vestibular dysfunction was noted in these patients.

Operative Techniques, Findings, and Results

The operative technique is essentially the same as that performed for hemifacial spasm (chapter 62) with the exception that the root entry zone of the eighth nerve must be gently dissected free from its caudal contact with the flocculus of the cerebellum more medially than in the hemifacial spasm operation if one is to see clearly the veins at the brain stem which may be causal of the symptoms.

Operative findings are tabulated in Table 1. It should be noted that all patients had obvious, though frequently subtle, vascular cross-compression of the eighth nerve and with a clear clinical-pathological correlation: cross-compression of the vestibular portion of the nerve was associated with vertigo, of the cochlear portion with tinnitus, of both portions of the nerve with both vertigo and tinnitus. Vertigo

Table 1. Operative findings in eighth cranial nerve dysfunction. (From: Jannetta PJ (1980) Annals of Surgery 192:518 – 525)

Offending vessel				
Artery				26
Cochlear	6	Cochlear + AICA	1	
AICA	5	Vertebral	2	
PICA	5	Superior cerebellar	2	
Unidentified artery	4	AICA + PICA	1	
Vein				8
Artery and vein				4
				Total 38

AICA = Anterior Inferior Cerebellar Artery
PICA = Posterior Inferior Cerebellar Artery

Table 2. Results of operation in eighth cranial nerve dysfunction (From: Jannetta PJ (1980) Annals of Surgery, 192:518 – 525)

Symptoms	Relieved	Mild improvement	Recurred or no relief	Worse
Vertigo and tinnitus	13		6	1
Vertigo	6	1		
Tinnitus	5		6	

Table 3. Complications in eighth cranial nerve dysfunction. (From: Jannetta PJ (1980) Annals of Surgery, 192:518 – 525)

Temporary	– Epidural hematoma postoperative and n. VI paresis	1
	– X cranial nerve paresis	1
	– aseptic meningitis	1
	– urinary tract infection	1
Permanent	– internuclear ophthmoplegia and worsening of vertigo	1
	– deterioration of hearing	3

was always associated with cross-compression located at the brain stem. In patients with tinnitus without vertigo but with decreased vestibular function on testing, compression was quite lateral and was caused by an anterior inferior cerebellar artery loop coursing horizontally under the internal auditory meatus and giving a branch to the canal from the apex of the loop. This is extremely difficult to treat.

The results of operation are tabulated in Table 2. It should be noted that we have had progressively better success as our experience has grown. Relief of vertigo is much more satisfactory than of tinnitus. The use of shredded teflon felt as the implant has improved the results greatly. The postoperative course is variable but of interest is the fact that improvement in both symptoms and in testing of function is gradual postoperatively, often taking weeks to months for maximum improvement.

Complications of operation are tabulated in Table 3. One patient developed an epidural hematoma in the immediate postoperative period, was initially quite ill, recovered completely but has had recurrence of her vertigo. One older woman developed a presumed small brain stem infarction on her second postoperative day and has residual internuclear ophthalmoplegia and worse vertigo than she had preoperatively. Although hearing was made worse in three patients, more recently we have noted gradual postoperative hearing improvement in the majority of patients.

Discussion

The techniques of microvascular decompression of the eighth nerve are still in development. It would appear that combinations of arteriosclerotic elongation of the arteries of the cerebellopontine angle, as has been found in a large series of patients with trigeminal neuralgia, hemifacial spasm and glossopharyngeal neuralgia, occasionally in combination with sagging of the hindbrain as is found in the older population, are the apparent contributory factors to these symptom complexes [3]. The procedure of microvascular decompression appears to be definitive and to reverse both disordered hyperfunction and hypofunction. The extensive studies of pathological changes in cranial nerves V, VII, IX, X, due to vascular cross-compression, must be extented to the acoustic nerve. The author awaites publication of verifying work by others who have performed microvascular compression for eighth nerves disfunction.

References

1. Jannetta PJ (1975) Neurovascular cross-compression in patients with hyperactive dysfunction symptoms of the eighth cranial nerve. Surg Forum 26:467–469
2. Jannetta PJ (1977) Observations on the etiology of trigeminal neuralgia, hemifacial spasm, acoustic nerve dysfunction and glossopharyngeal neuralgia. Definitive microsurgical treatment and results in 117 patients. Neurochirurgia (Stuttg) 20:145–154
3. Jannetta PJ (1980) Neurovascular compression in cranial nerve and systemic disease. Ann Surg 192:518–525

Early Experiences in Vascular Decompression for Vestibulo-Cochlear Malfunction

M. Samii and A. Ohlemutz, Hannover/FRG

During the last seven years our experiences with vascular decompression in cases of hemifacial spasm and trigeminal neuralgia showed very good results. In accordance with these results and the suggestions by Jannetta we decided to perform vascular decompression on vestibulo-cochlear malfunction, such as tinnitus, sudden hearing loss and vertigo, when all other conservative treatments had failed.

At this stage we are able to report on four cases, the follow-up from immediately after the operation, to four months (Table 1).

Table 1. Preliminary results of vascular decompression in vestibulo-cochlear dysfunction

Patient	Principal symptoms preop.	Side	Subject feeling	Vestib. function	Cochl. function	Tinnitus	Follow up (month)
1 T.S. ♂ 18. 11. 25	tinnitus hearing decrease vertigo	right	better	↓	↑	Φ	3
2 S.R. ♀ 10. 9. 54	tinnitus hearing decrease	left	slightly better	↓	↓	(+)-Φ	3
3 G.F. ♂ 23. 10. 25	tinnitus hearing decrease facial spasm	right	better	(↓)	(↑)	Φ	2
4 C.H. ♀ 14. 3. 23	tinnitus vertigo	left	slightly better	Φ	↓	Φ	2 weeks post op.

First case:

A 54 year old man, who 20 years ago first suffered from sudden loss of hearing in the left ear and became deaf within a few years. In 1978 he developed sudden loss of hearing in the right ear and was treated with Novocaine infusions, with the result of hearing increase for a few weeks, after which sudden hearing loss again occured. Meanwhile, vertigo and a very disturbing tinnitus appeared. Diverse treatments brought no evident improvement, and when his hearing worsened in December, 1979, we decided to perform a vascular decompression. In January, 1980 suboccipital craniotomy was performed and a compression of the eighth nerve by the inferior anterior cerebellar artery was found. A piece of muscle was interposed at the exit zone of the nerve at the brain stem, and the artery thereby dislocated (Figs. 1 and 2).

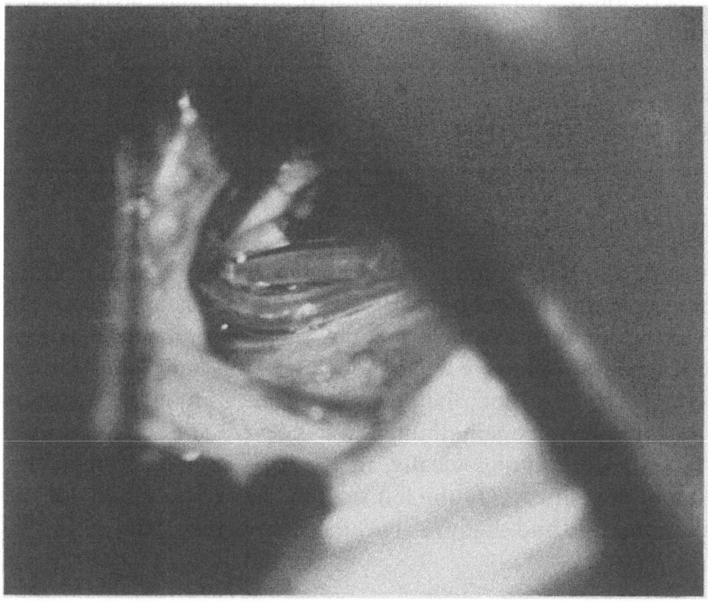

Fig. 1. Lateral suboccipital exposure of the cerebellopontine angle on the right side. VIIth and VIIIth nerves are elevated. The anterior inferior cerebellar artery compressing the brain stem is demonstrated

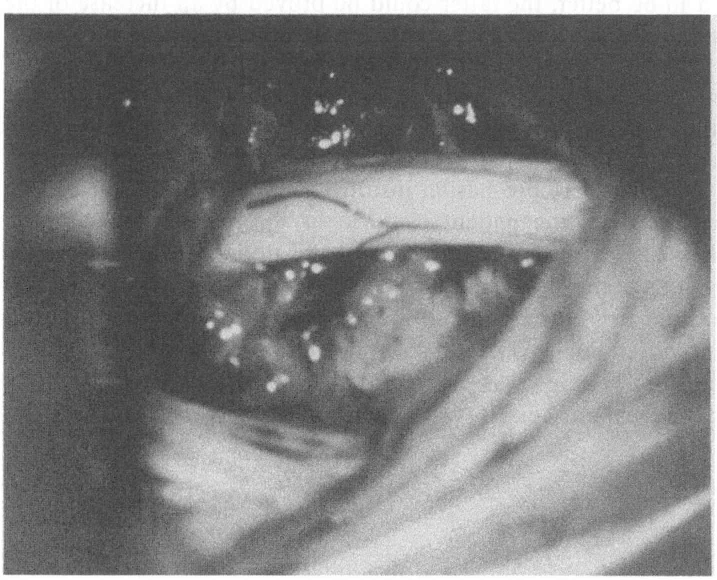

Fig. 2. The same case as Fig. 1. Interposition of a piece of muscle between the nerves and the artery at the brain stem

Directly after the operation the tinnitus had vanished. Recent audiological control showed no alteration of the hearing threshold in the lower frequencies, but a slight increase of the higher frequencies. Attacks of vertigo were no longer reported. Vestibulometry still showed the same low excitibility as before. Since the disturbing tinnitus was no longer present, the patient felt very content with the result of the operation.

Second case:

A 25 year old woman suffered from childhood on from progressive loss of hearing function, as well as increasing tinnitus in both ears. The tinnitus became unbearable during recent years. Various kinds of treatment, among them vasodilatation as well as tranquilizers, proved ineffective. Thus we felt that operation was indicated.

Directly after vascular decompression, the patient was free of tinnitus, but soon after, a remittent sound could be felt again, though not as severe as before and only after having used a hearing aid. Audiologically, the hearing showed a slight decrease of 10 dB function of the left ear. On the left side the lack of excitibility of the vestibular system had not changed and slight vertigo attacks were reported.

Third case:

Tinnitus, facial spasm, and hearing decrease on the right side were the main symptoms in the following patient, a 54 year old man. Since various kinds of conservative therapy had failed, we suggested vascular decompression, which was performed on the right side in March, 1980. The anterior inferior cerebellar artery, the compressing vessel, could be found and repositioned in the before mentioned technique. After the operation the patient was very content as the facial spasm had vanished and the hearing was reported to be better, the latter could be proved by an increase of the tone threshold. Tinnitus was no longer reported. The vestibulogram showed slight loss of excitability.

To conclude, we report on the fourth patient, a 57 year old woman, who suffered from left sided tinnitus and vertigo beginning in 1960. A progressive hearing loss was also present. For a long time the patient had been treated with the diagnosis of 'vegetative dystony' as well as vertebro-basilar insufficiency. With the suspicion of a tumor which was not verified, the patient came to us for treatment. Otological examination now showed hearing loss, especially in the upper frequencies and a high-grade functional loss of the left vestibular system. Vascular decompression was suggested and performed in February, 1980. Directly after the operation tinnitus was no longer present, but otological examination showed nearly complete deafness and no vestibular function. Vertigo was not reported, whereas, walking instability could be recognized. The patient herself was content, since the very disturbing tinnitus had ceased.

Combination of Hearing Loss and Blindness

L. Osterwald, Hannover/FRG

My study deals with a group of 24 patients who lost their eyesight and hearing ability or lost hearing alone; both due to war effects. In many patients remaining hearing ability could not be evaluated by the usual methods of audiological examinations. However, a surprisingly productive communication was made possible through hearing-aids. Since the method of lip-reading did not apply to any of my blind patients, I asked myself whether the gained hearing impressions could not only be supplemented but even be replaced by sensitive perception. A blind person is especially suited for the clarification of these issues, because the other senses are further developed after loss of eyesight. I can show two patients where after long years of complete deafness, solely by the reconstruction of the eardrum membrane as well as the sound conduction, verbal communication was made possible. Yet, most intensive hearing exercises, first with the physician, later with their wives, or using tape recorders, and naturally an especially developed mechanical acoustic amplification device, were necessary.

I will now demonstrate our patient M. F. and his audiogram (Fig. 1). Sensitivity is more strongly developed in blind people. As an example a young American girl who had been blind from birth. From the information transmitted to a seismograph on tape she can forecast earthquakes more accurately and earlier than the most complicated computer. Also Helen Keller, who was deaf-blind, as is commonly known, wrote in her book 'The Story of my life': 'I do not feel each letter any more than you see each letter seperately, when you read.'

I cannot yet tell whether the utilization of sensitivity as a supplement to the remaining hearing ability, or maybe even as a replacement of the hearing itself, will also be possible in the same mode for seeing people. The seeing person would hardly take the trouble of the necessary intensive learning process. Instead he would turn to lip-reading. Besides, his sensitivity is less pronounced and he also receives much more distracting information by his eyesight. It will all depend on the success with which mechanical aids for the utilization of sensitivity will be further developed.

A last comment on the Cochlea-Implants: they concern, as you will know, the attempt of achieving a hearing impression by direct stimulation of the hearing nerve. The results are so bad that there is doubt whether genuine hearing impressions exist.

Possibly sensitive factors have a large impact on the recorded hearing results in these cases, too. It also must be doubted whether the hearing with cochlea-implants or the hearing of deaf-blind patients has any qualitative simularity to normal hearing at all. I believe that only fragments of signals reach the central nerve system and that most of the hearing of the blind is made up of very tiny bits of information. These are transformed into hearing through great energy which I have very often come to observe in blind people.

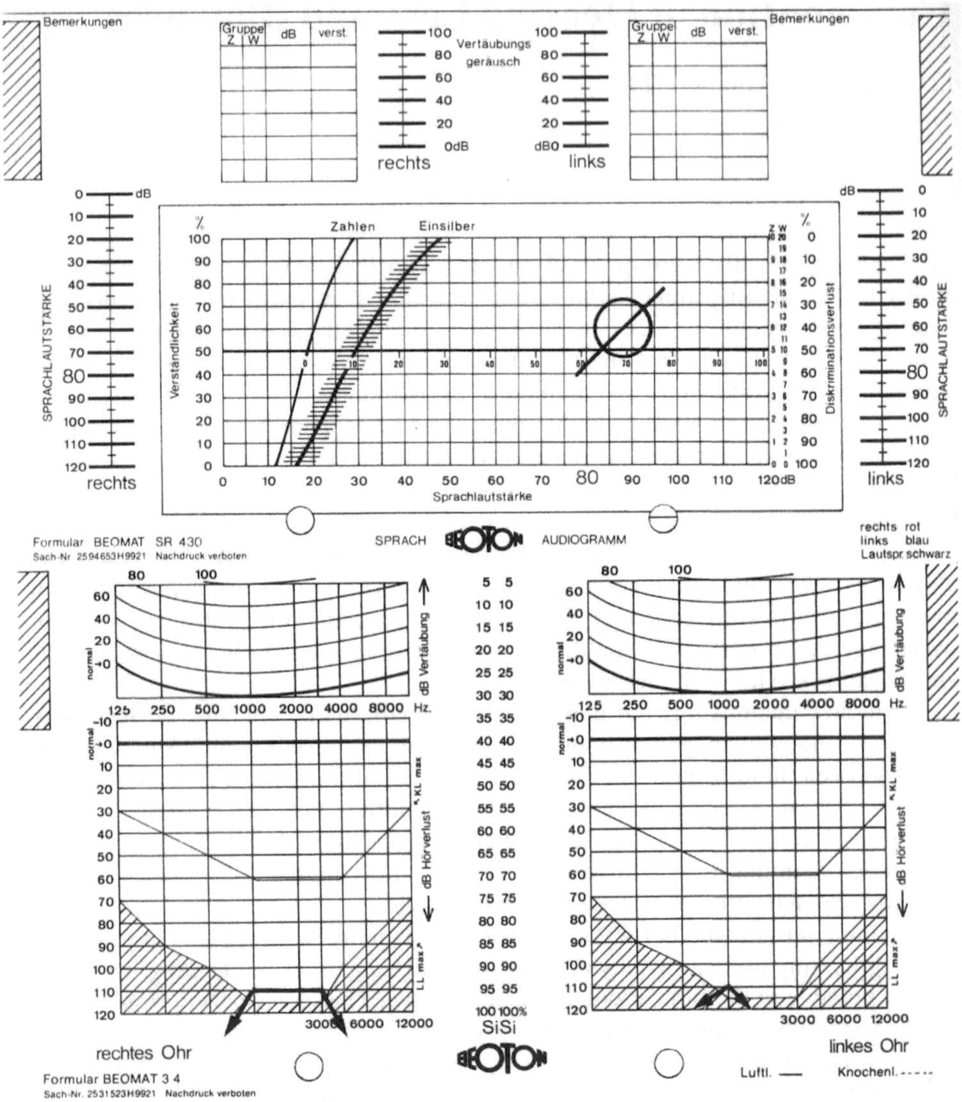

Bemerkungen
Gruppe Z W
dB
verst.
Vertäubungs geräusch
rechts
links
SPRACHLAUTSTÄRKE
Verständlichkeit
Zahlen
Einsilber
Diskriminationsverlust
Sprachlautstärke
Formular BEOMAT SR 430
Sach-Nr. 2594653H9921 Nachdruck verboten
SPRACH
AUDIOGRAMM
rechts rot
links blau
Lautspr. schwarz
dB Vertäubung
normal
dB Hörverlust
KL max
LL max
125 250 500 1000 2000 4000 8000 Hz.
3000 6000 12000
SiSi
rechtes Ohr
linkes Ohr
Formular BEOMAT 3 4
Sach-Nr. 2531523H9921 Nachdruck verboten
Luftl. ——
Knochenl. -----

Fig. 1

Preservation of Hearing in Acoustic Neurinoma Surgery

N. L. Cohen and J. Ransohoff, New York/USA

Introduction

During the past two decades, the surgical treatment of acoustic neurinoma has improved enormously, so that the goals of total tumor removal, acceptable morbidity, low mortality and preservation of facial nerve function are routinely achieved.

Ideally, in the patient with serviceable hearing, an additional goal should be the preservation of hearing. Since 1974, we have been attempting to preserve the cochlear nerve and internal auditory vessels when operating on reasonably small extracanalicular tumors with good hearing.

Material

From 1973 through 1979, a total of 50 patients have been operated upon, jointly by the departments of otolaryngology and neurosurgery. Not included are those patients (mostly old with very large tumors) who were operated upon solely by neurosurgery. Of these, 15 had serviceable hearing, defined by a speech discrimination score of 60 percent. For a variety of reasons it was elected to attempt to save hearing in nine of these patients. The most common reasons for sacrificing hearing were: large tumors, significant medical problems, leading us to limit the duration of operation and selection of the translabyrinthine approach by the patient with the associated loss of inner ear function.

Table 1. Population. Total cases 1973 – 1979

Total cases	50	Male	26
Acoustic neuroma	48	Female	24
Ganglioneuroma	1	Age range	16 – 68
Facial neuroma	1	Median	44.9

The type of tumor, age and sex distribution are listed in Table 1. As expected, the great majority of tumors were acoustic neurinomas. All patients had unilateral tumors. There were 25 right- and 25 left-sided tumors. The median age was 44.9 years, with a range of 16 to 68 years.

Our diagnostic record is outlined in Table 2. Briefly, all patients with a unilateral sensori-neural hearing loss were subjected to the non-invasive portion of the work-up. Those with a retrocochlear pattern of hearing loss, decreased vestibular response on bithermal caloric testing monitored by electronystagmography, or a wide

Table 2. Diagnostic protocol. Unilateral sensorineural hearing loss

Calorics	IAC		
1. Normal and normal → 6 month follow-up unless SOL retrocochlear			
2. DVR and/or wide CAT scan			
Negative	Positive	PEG Air CT cisternogram Angiogram?	
1. old, sick patient		6 month follow-up	
2. Healthy patient		Pantopaque fossagram	
Normal IAC		Pantopaque fossagram	
Wide IAC		Acoustic PEG	Air CT cisternogram

Table 3. Qutpatient test results

	Abnormal	Normal
Audiogram	42	8
Vestibulars	48	2
Polytomes	43	7
CT [a] Scan	23	20

[a] Negative CT becoming less common with increasing sophistication of CT equipment

Table 4. CT scan and tumor size

Size	Positive	Negative
14 Less than 2 cm	0	14
13 2–4 cm	8	5
15 More than 4 cm	14	1
42	22	20

Table 5. Size of tumor and approach

	Middle fossa	Trans-labyrinthine	Suboccipital
2 Intracanalicular	1	1	–
16 Less than 2 cm	–	7	9
14 2–4 cm (2 2-stage)	–	6	10
18 More than 4 cm (4 2-stage)	–	4	18
50	1	18	37

internal auditory canal on polytomography, were admitted for definitive x-ray study. For most of this period, the study consisted of a small volume pneumoencephalogram with polytomography, followed by Pantopaque if needed. During the past two years, we have been using air with the CT scan, as described by Kritcheff et al. (1979), Fig. 1. This is followed by a small volume Pantopaque cisternogram only if filling of the canal is not obvious with the air. Recently, we have been able to demonstrate even a small intracanalicular tumor with air alone.

The results of the non-invasive studies are shown in Table 3. Although all patients had a unilateral sensori-neural hearing loss, in eight the hearing had either returned to normal following a sudden loss (three cases) or the hearing in the affected ear was only mildly disturbed (PTA $\leqq$ 25 dB with good speech discrimination).

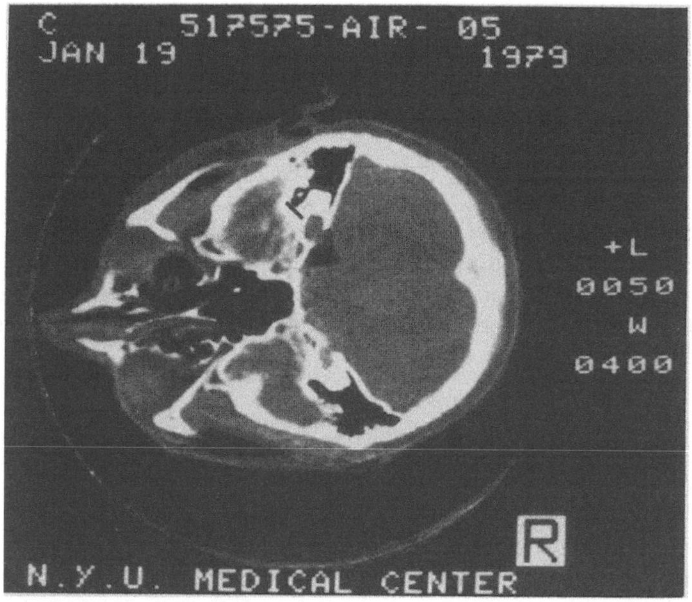

Fig. 1. Air-CT Cisternogram showing tumor bulging into CPA. Internal auditory canal is bulbous

The most sensitive test was the caloric, since all but two patients had a decreased vestibular response greater than 20 percent in the affected ear.

Normal internal auditory canals were noted on polytomography in seven patients, and twenty of the 43 patients who underwent CT scanning showed no tumor. The breakdown of these results is shown in Table 4. It is to be expected that many tumors less than two cm in size will not visualize on CT scanning, but unfortunately six of the 28 larger masses also did not. This is less of a problem with newer scanners. During the past year, only one out of eight larger tumors (2.5 cm) were not recognized on CT scan.

Our operative approach was determined by three main factors: the patient's age and general condition; size of tumor; and state of hearing. This is summarized in Table 5. Of the patients in whom an attempt was made to preserve hearing, one was a middle-fossa approach for an intra-canalicular tumor, while the remaining eight were suboccipital for extracanalicular tumors. One of these was slightly more than two cm in size; the remainder were two cm or less. There were six two-stage operations, in which the translabyrinthine portion followed the suboccipital in four patients.

The patients chosen for the suboccipital approach are operated upon in the seated position, with appropriate safeguards, monitoring, and medications (Table 6). The procedure is carried out jointly, with the Neurosurgeon performing the craniotomy, retracting the cerebellum, freeing the tumor from the brainstem if necessary, identifying nerve VII inferiomedially at the brainstem and, if needed, debulking the posterior portion of the mass. The Otologist then drills away the posterior wall of the internal auditory canal, identifies the facial nerve at the lateral end

Table 6. Suboccipital craniectomy

Sitting position	Foley Catheter
Monitoring – Doppler	Steroids
– Arterial	Antibiotics
– Central venous	Mannitol

of the IAC and removes the tumor either piecemeal or intact, with or without preservation of the cochlear nerve. A free muscle graft is then placed in the bone defect of the IAC to prevent leak of cerebrospinal fluid. The craniotomy is closed by the neurosurgical team. Corticosteroids and antibiotics are continued for several days post-operatively.

Results

Hearing was preserved at the preoperative level in the one intra-canalicular tumor approached via the middle fossa.

Of the eight cases in which the suboccipital approach was used for extra-canalicular tumors, hearing was preserved in four (Table 7). Pre- and post-operative audiograms of the patients with good hearing are seen in Figs. 2 to 5. There has been no deterioration during a follow-up period from one to five years.

Tumors were totally removed in 27 of 32 patients with small and medium tumors and in 11 of 18 large tumors.

Complications have, in the main, been related to tumor size. Facial nerve palsy has been transient in three of 18 small and six of 14 medium-sized tumors. No permanent facial paralysis occurred in any of these patients. In the 18 large tumors, there were four transient and four permanent facial palsies. This indicated an overall incidence of eight percent. There have been no deaths, but several of our patients with large tumors had protracted and complicated post-operative courses.

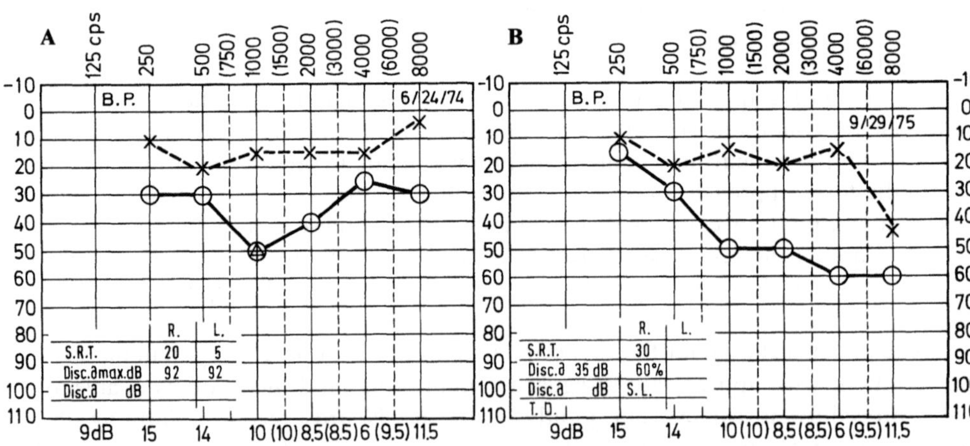

Fig. 2A. Patient B.P. Pre-operative audiogram. **B** Patient B.P. Post-operative audiogram 16 months later

Figures 2, 3 and 4 reproduced by permission of The Laryngoscope, Vol. LXXXIX, No. 6, pp. 886–896, June 1979

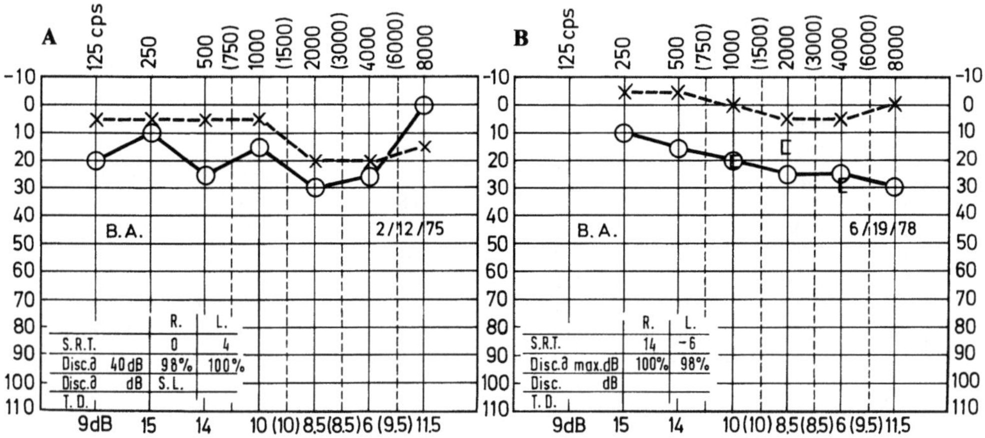

Fig. 3A. Patient B.A. Pre-operative audiogram. **B** Patient B.A. Audiogram 40 months post-operative

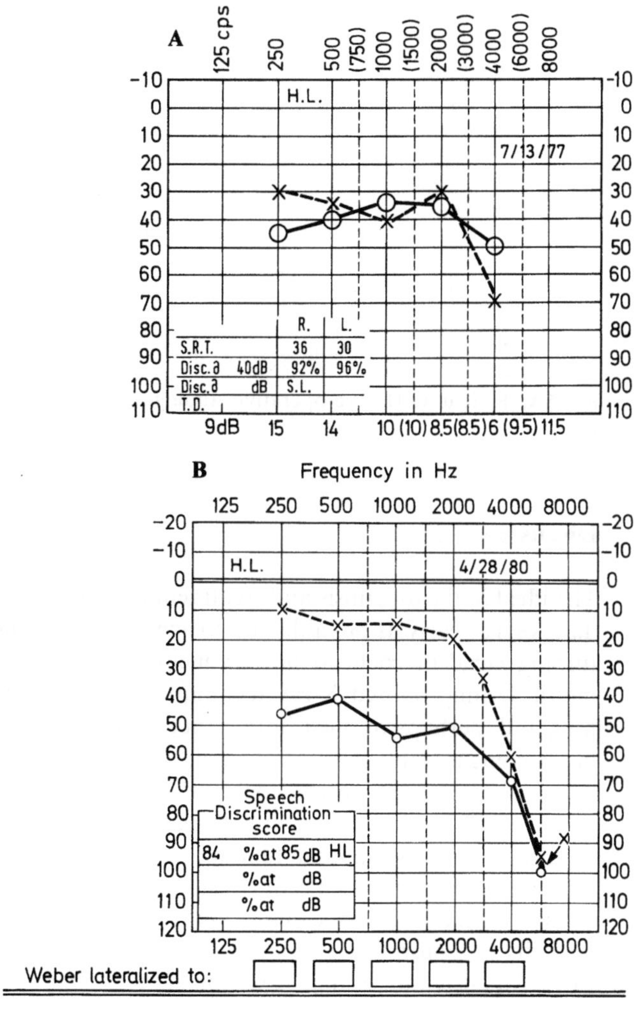

Fig. 4A. Patient H.L. Pre-operative audiogram. **B** Patient H.L. Post-operative 33 months

Table 7. Preservation of cochlear nerve, with hearing results

Date	Patient	Size	Route	PTA Pre/Post	Speech	Follow-Up
7/74	B.P.	1.5 cm	SO	40/43	92/60	16 mos.
9/74	D.H.	1.0 cm	SO	38/NR	100/NR	–
2/75	B.A.	1.5 cm	SO	23/20	98/100	60 mos.
6/76	A.B.	1.5 cm	SO	18/NR	96/NR	–
6/77	R.T.	1.5 cm	SO	55/82	66/NR	–
7/77	H.L.	1.0 cm	SO	23/48	92/92	30 mos.
11/77	D.W.	I.C.	MF	25/33	80/72	24 mos.
1/79	T.A.	3.0 cm	SO	30/NR	60/NR	–
4/79	G.H.	1.5 cm	SO	28/8	100/92	13 mos.

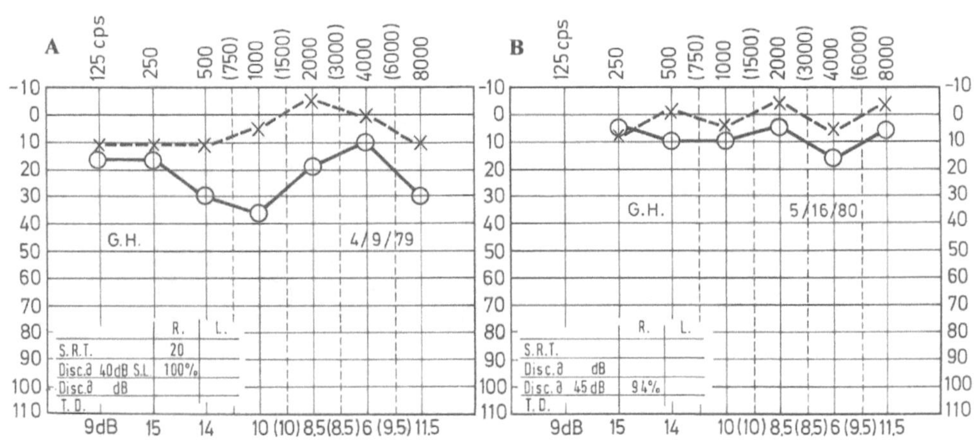

Fig. 5A. Patient G.H. Pre-operative audiogram. **B** Patient G.H. Post-operative 12 months later

Discussion

The ideal in the diagnosis and treatment of acoustic neuromas would be to make the diagnosis as early as possible and to achieve total removal of the tumor without disturbing facial or cochlear nerve function. With the help of vestibular and audiometric testing, refined X-ray techniques including polytomography and CT scanning and, perhaps of most importance, a high index of suspicion, earlier diagnosis has become possible, but still many lesions elude us. It is not unusual for an acoustic neuroma to present with a 'cochlear' site of lesion location by the testing battery, and there is an increasing experience with normal hearing despite subsequently verified tumors. Vestibular function, as measured by caloric testing, may also be normal. Acoustic neuromas of considerable size may not cause substantial widening of the internal auditory canal. Finally, the CT scan consistently fails to reveal the majority of tumors of less than two cm in diameter. All of these factors tend to delay early diagnosis and resultant excision at the smallest possible size.

In regard to preservation of hearing, the difficulty of early diagnosis certainly plays a role, but so do other factors. Among these are the not uncommon lack of correlation between tumor size and level of hearing, and the occurrence of a sudden hearing loss during the normally slow growth of the tumor.

When it has been possible to make the diagnosis of an acoustic neuroma while the hearing is still serviceable, we as otologists must ask whether the tumor can be removed without sacrifice of hearing. In order to answer this question, we must know the size of the tumor, the level of hearing, whether there is a technique available to preserve the hearing without increasing the risk to the patient substantially, and what the chances are of success. House (1964) and others have shown that hearing can be preserved in a significant percentage of intracanalicular tumors, via the middle cranial fossa approach. Although by up to 50 percent of patients hearing may be preserved, the technique is difficult, the risk to the facial nerve is greater than by other approaches, and operation deaths have been reported (Harker and McCabe, 1978). Tumors protruding more than a few millimeters into the cerebellopontine angle cannot be removed via the middle fossa route. These larger tumors are approached very well via the translabyrinthine route, but this necessitates the sacrifice of hearing. The logical alternative is the suboccipital approach, a well proved neurosurgical route. Several variations have been described (Rand and Kurze, 1968; Smith et al., 1977; Rhoton, 1977), all having in common the posterior approach to the internal auditory canal, drilling away of the posterior wall, identification of the facial and cochlear nerves, and removal of tumor by microsurgical techniques which have become commonly accepted by the neurosurgeon as well as the otologic surgeon.

Three surgical approaches are utilized:

The intracanalicular tumor with good hearing is removed via the middle fossa, with preservation of the cochlar nerve and vasculature within the canal.

The translabyrinthine route is used for intracanalicular tumors with poor hearing, as well as for small (less than two cm) and some medium-sized (two to four cm) extracanalicular tumors with poor hearing.

If the posterior fossa study shows that the tumor has reached the brain stem, we feel that it is safer approached via the suboccipital route. This approach is also used for smaller extracanalicular tumors with good hearing.

Using these three approaches, we feel that we have the best chance of removing acoustic neuromas of all sizes, while attempting to spare the facial nerve in all cases, preserving the cochlear nerve where appropriate, and lessening the risk to the patient by utilizing the wide, neurosurgical, suboccipital approach to those tumors which are at or adherent to the pons.

Conclusions

Using the diagnostic criteria and surgical techniques described, we have identified and operated upon 50 patients with acoustic neurinoma between 1973 and 1979. In nine of these patients, an attempt was made to preserve hearing, and was successful in five. We feel that this approach is sound, the complications acceptable, and the results satisfactory. It is possible to remove some extra-canalicular acoustic neurinomas measuring less than two cm in diameter, and preserve normal hearing.

References

Harker LA, McCabe BF (1978) Iowa results of acoustic neuroma operations. Laryngoscope 88:1904

House WF (1964) Microsurgical removal of acoustic neuromas. Arch Otolaryngol 80:599

Kricheff II, Pinto RS, Bergeron RT, Cohen NL (1980) Air-CT cisternography and canalography for small acoustic neuromas. Am J Neuroradiology 1:57

Rand RW, Kurze T (1968) Preservation of vestibular, cochlear, and facial nerves during microsurgical removal of acoustic tumors: report of two cases. J Neurosurg 28:158

Rhoton Al Jr (1977) Suboccipital microsurgical approach to acoustic neuromas. In: Silverstein J, Norrell H (eds) Neurological surgery of the ear, Aesculapius Publishing Co., Birmingham, Alabama, p 220–234

Smith MFW, Clancy TP, Lang JS (1977) Conservation of hearing in acoustic neurilemmoma excision. Trans Am Acad Ophthalmol Otolaryngol 84:704

Early Diagnosis and Transtemporal Removal of Small Nerve VII and VIII Tumors

M. E. Wigand, T. Haid, M. Berg, and G. Rettinger, Erlangen/FRG

When, in 1961 and 1964, William F. House and his associates published their new techniques of removing the acoustic neuroma by either the transtemporal or the translybyrinthine approach, this was a great step forward with regard to survival rate and to facial nerve function. Furthermore, the interest of this type of microsurgery was focussed on the attempt of preservation of hearing during recent years, when eradicating the disease from the internal auditory canal or from the cerebello-pontine angle (Glasscock et al., 1978; House, 1961, 1964; Wiegand, 1976; Cohen, 1979).

All of us know that the prognosis of the auditory function would improve considerably if the neuroma could be diagnosed earlier; but, unfortunately, most of the tumors are detected not before having reached medium or large size, giving rise to severe oto-neurological symptoms. Therefore, all efforts should be undertaken to make early diagnosis possible.

Table 1. The size of 67 tumors of the internal auditory canal, confirmed by surgery.
A = Limited to the internal auditory canal
B = Extending into the c.p.a. = 1.5 cm
C = Larger tumors than B
D = Invading tumors

Size A	10
Size B	14
Size C	36
Size D	7
Total	67

Table 2. Presenting symptoms by early C.A.I.-Tumors ($n = 10$)

Progressive unilateral hearing loss	7
Fluctuating hearing loss	1
Sudden hearing drop	2
Tinnitus	6
Vertigo, dizziness	8
Facial paralysis	3
Head ache	4

In our own series of 67 tumors, related to the internal auditory canal, and confirmed by surgery, only 10 (= 15%) could be detected in an early stage of growth, that is the size A, according to Fisch and Wegmüller (1978) (Table 1). When we evaluated our case histories, no characteristical patterns of presenting symptoms could be found. Table 2 shows that deafness was the most common complaint of our patients, but its appearance varied from sudden hearing drop to fluctuating deafness, and even to total deafness. On the other hand, normal hearing was present in one advanced tumor case.

Also with regard to vertigo and facial paralysis we had to state that there was no typical symptomatology of the growing acoustic neuroma. This was the reason why in our department all suspicious cases of unilateral 'pyramidal irritation' were sub-

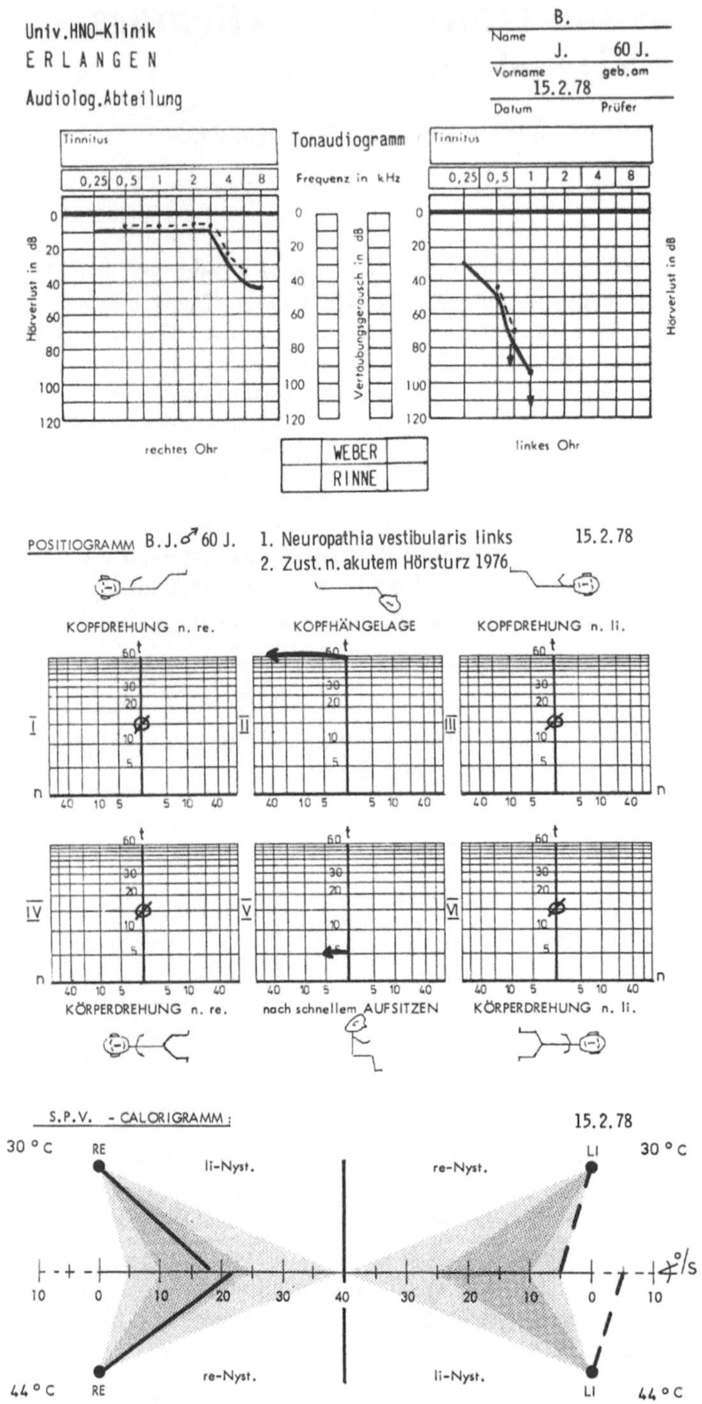

Fig. 1A

Fig. 1. Follow-up examination of positional nystagmus in a case of nerve VIII neurinoma. Intensity and excitability of the provoked nystagmus have increased within five months

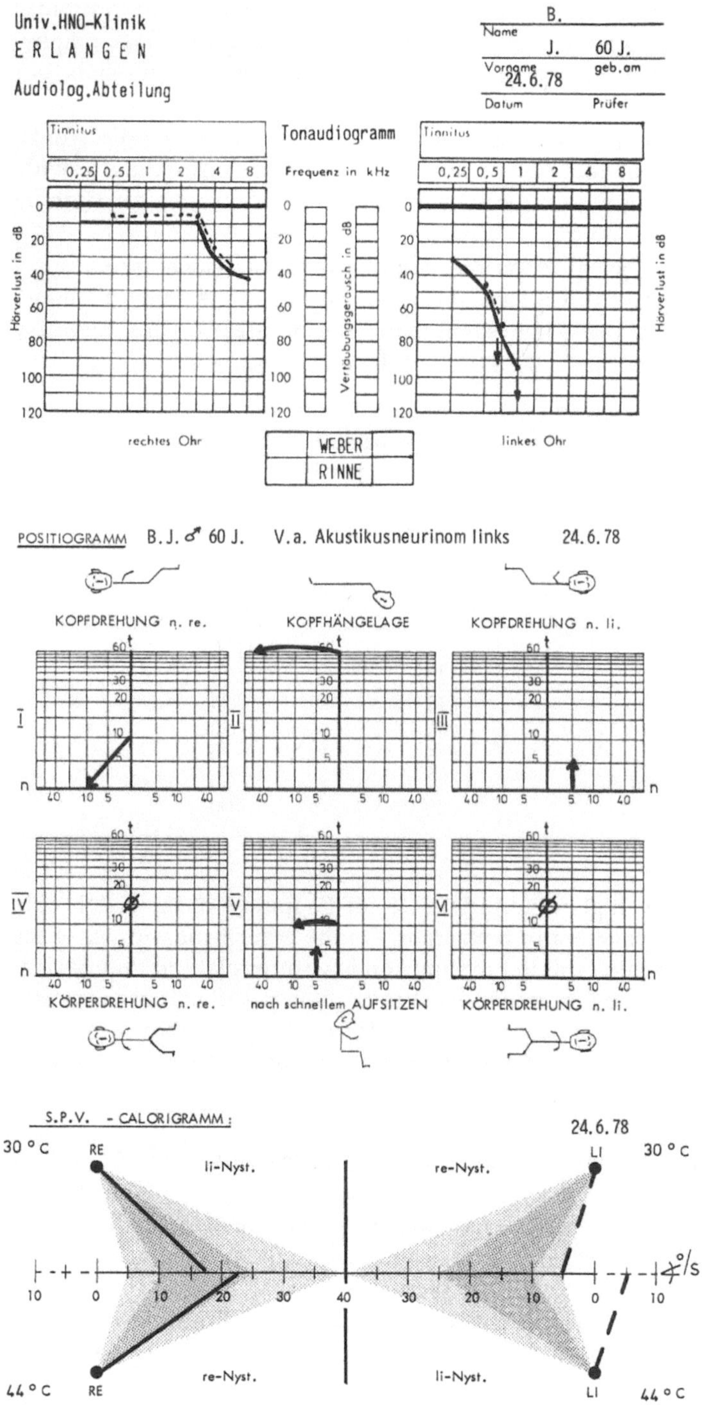
Univ.HNO-Klinik
ERLANGEN
Audiolog.Abteilung
B.
Name
J. 60 J.
Vorname geb.am
24.6.78
Datum Prüfer
Tinnitus
Tonaudiogramm
Tinnitus
0,25 0,5 1 2 4 8
Frequenz in kHz
Hörverlust in dB
Vertäubungsgeräusch in dB
rechtes Ohr
linkes Ohr
WEBER
RINNE
POSITIOGRAMM B.J. ♂ 60 J. V.a. Akustikusneurinom links 24.6.78
KOPFDREHUNG n. re.
KOPFHÄNGELAGE
KOPFDREHUNG n. li.
KÖRPERDREHUNG n. re.
nach schnellem AUFSITZEN
KÖRPERDREHUNG n. li.
S.P.V. - CALORIGRAMM:
24.6.78
30 °C
RE
li-Nyst.
re-Nyst.
LI
°/s
44 °C
re-Nyst.
li-Nyst.

Fig. 1B

mitted to a diagnostical regimen, which consisted of audiological and vestibular tests, X-ray examinations, computer-tomography (C.T), and cisterno-meatography. Other tests were also performed, such as Sisi, v. Bekesy audiometry and others, but were cancelled from the scope because of minor reliability.

The retrospective evaluation of all 67 tumors reveiled that there was no typical pattern of test reactions, but that the battery of tests would consistantly provide pathological results, pointing to a retrocochlear lesion with or without labyrinthine involvement (Table 3).

How can the great number of suspicious cases be reduced, which are to be referred to C.T. and meatography, what are expensive and time consuming methods? In our experience a refined vestibular examination can be used for this necessary selection of cases: Especially the combination of the caloric test with a quantitative

Table 3. Pathological test results in 73 C.A.I.-tumors (in percent of examined cases)

	A	B, C, D
Pure tone threshold	100	98
Stapedial reflex	66	64
Carhart	40	65
Speech discrimination	50	83
B.E.R.A.	?	(100)
Calorigram	70	88
Positiogram	90	94
Stenvers	60	62
Spiral tomography	75	80
Computer tomography (without gas)	25	89
Cisterno-meatography	90	100

positional testing (Fig. 1) is highly indicative. Out of 67 tumors of the C.A.I. only two percent had a normal function in both trials. On the other hand, not all of the many patients with positional vestibular dysfunction have a retrolabyrinthine lesion. The sophisticated method of quantitative evaluation of the positional reactions, designed by Haid, allows exact follow-up controls. He could show, that in cases of neuroma there is a time course of the intensity of the vestibular dysfunction, entirely different from that in other diseases, such as Menière's disease or vestibular neuronitis.

In all suspicious cases computer tomography and the cisternomeatography were carried out. These procedures convey the highest accuracy of direct tumor tracing. Figure 2 shows an example of computer tomography, visualizing a small acoustic neuroma at the porus of the internal auditory canal, the contrast being enhanced by filling the cerebello-pontine angle with air. We have observed only one case with a false positive C.T. picture. In spite of a spherical increase of density at the cerebello-pontine angle the internal auditory canal could be filled with pantopaque. When we opened both the internal auditory canal and the c.p.a. by the translabyrinthine route, both were empty, but a small neurinoma could be found within the vestibule and the semicircular canals. This is the first case of a purely intralabyrinthine neurinoma, what was not described in the literature until now.

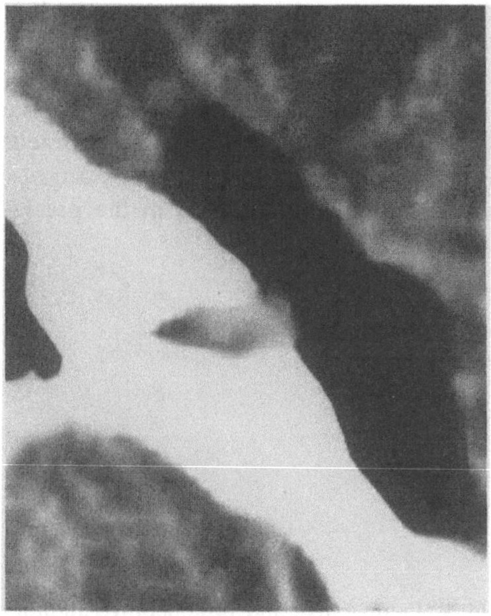

Fig. 2. A small nerve VIII neurinoma visualized by computer tomography of the left cerebello-pontine angle, which is filled with air. Density increment of the tumor enhanced by contrast medium

On the basis of our diagnostical schedule it was possible to detect 10 small tumors (size A) of the internal auditory canal out of a total of 67 tumors (sizes A + B + C + D), that are 15%. This is a higher incidence than was reported in the literature.

Table 4 shows our results of oto-microsurgery. All cases were operated by one of the authors (M.E.W.). A complete tumor removal was possible in all 10 A-cases, operated either transtemporally or by the translabyrinthine approach. Among them are three tumors of the facial nerve. There was no or only transitional facial paralysis in seven cases. In the three cases with the facial nerve tumor, facial paralysis was unavoidable. Immediate nerve grafting could be performed in two of these cases, using fibrin glue for the fixation of the graft, with good functional result after more than nine months. The third case of severe facial paralysis was rehabilitated by muscular facial plastic surgery.

Table 4. Results of oto-microsurgery for C.A.I.-tumors ($n = 53$)

	A	B, C, D
Complete transtemporal removal	6	4
Complete translabyrinthine removal	4	20
2 nd neurosurgical intervention	0	19
Death from oto-microsurgery	0	0
No or transitory facial paralysis	7	36
Facial nerve reconstruction	3	4
Cochlear nerve preserved	5	5
Total	10	43

No patient of the 53 A + B + C + D-cases, operated in our department, died in direct relation to the operation. One died a week later, walking around, from massive lung embolization.

In 5 of 9 operated small tumors, operated transtemporally, the cochlear nerve could be preserved. It might be of interest, that it was possible even in some size B tumors, that is extending by less than 1.5 cm into the c.p.a., to advance by a transtemporal approach, and to save the cochlear nerve, what resulted in the preservation of hearing (Fig. 3).

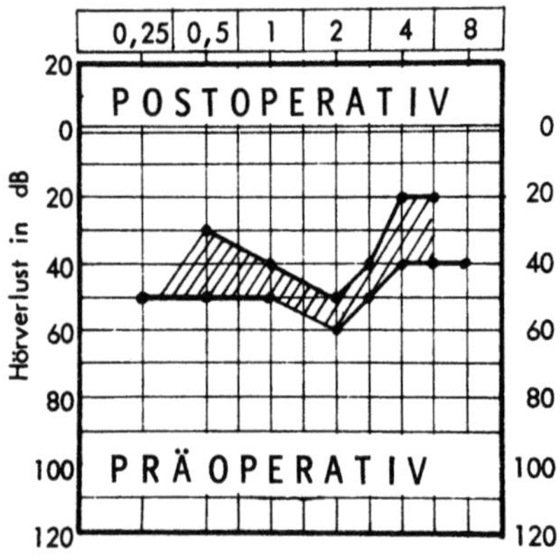

Fig. 3. Preoperative and postoperative auditory thresholds in a case of nerve VIII neurinoma of the size B, removed by the transtemporal approach

In larger tumors (size C) we nowadays follow the concept of a two-stage procedure: Transtemporal cleaning of the C.A.I. and porus in a first session, and tumor removal from the c.p.a. by a neurosurgical suboccipital approach with microdissection of both, the facial and the cochlear nerve, if possible, in a second session. I have to thank Prof. Samii from Hannover for collaboration in this program.

Finally, I would like to comment on the suboccipital technique, which is recommended by neurosurgeons as a one stage procedure. In our own series we could observe five cases of intralabyrinthine invasion of the neurinoma. On these cases a suboccipital approach alone certainly would have failed to detect the tumor borders within the petrous bone, and a recurrence would have to be expected. Therefore, in our opinion a safe exposure of the meatal bottom and the control of the vestibular nerve canals, performed by the oto-microsurgeon, seems always to be advisable.

References

Cohen NL (1979) Acoustic neuroma surgery with emphasis on preservation of hearing. Laryngoscope 89:886–896

Fisch U, Wegmüller A (1974) Early Diagnosis of Acoustic Neuromas. ORL 36:129–140

Glasscock ME, Hays JW, Miller GW, Drake FD, Kanok MM (1978) Preservation of hearing in tumors of the internal auditory canal and cerebello-pontine angle. Laryngoscope 88:43–55

House WF (1961) Surgical exposure of the internal auditory canal and its contents through the middle cranial fossa. Laryngoscope 71:1363–1385

House WF (ed), Monograph (1964) Transtemporal bone microsurgical removal of acoustic neuromas. Arch Otolaryngol 80:597–756

Wigand ME (1976) Schwindel, ein Leitsymptom der Felsenbeinneurinome. Neurol Psychiatr (Bucur) 2:307–313

Reversible Functional Damage of VIIIth Cranial Nerve in Arachnopathia Pontocerebellaris

K. Ehrenberger, Wien/Austria

Introduction

Functional damage to the acoustic nerve in arachnopathia pontocerebellaris is not necessarily irreversible in all cases. In the case of postarachnitic strangulation where only circumscript myelin sheath damage is present in the sense of a neurapraxia, functional integrety can be achieved with surgical decompression of the nerve. With the aid of various neuro-otological examination methods such as cisternoscopy, electrocochleography, and brain stem audiometry, we are now able to exactly differentiate and diagnose arachnopathia from an expansive process in the pontine angle (i.e. acoustic neurinoma) as well as reversible postarachnitic neuropraxia of the acoustic nerve from an irreversible nerve damage such as axonotmesis and neurotmesis (Ehrenberger et al., 1977).

Cisternoscopy

This method allows direct endoscopy of the pontine angle and permits accurate topodiagnosis and pathodiagnosis with the possibility of biopsy. This method is only indicated when all other diagnostic possibilities have been exhausted and the suspicion of an arachnitic or expansive process of the posterior cranial fossa can neither be confirmed nor ruled out. Correspondingly, cisternoscopy is therefore rarely performed. In any case, it is preferable to neurosurgical diagnostic transoccipital craniotomy, since the latter must be considered a severe intervention in comparison with cisternoscopy. After preparation of Trautmann's triangle in the mastoid bone, the dura mater of the posterior cranial fossa is opened precisely only to the extent necessary to introduce an endoscope (diameter 2.7–3.5 mm) for direct observation of pontine angle (Fig. 2). This method allows the differentiation of arachnitic adhesions from tumors (Ehrenberger, 1978).

Electrocochleography and Brain Stem Audiometry

Both of these methods help to detect a reversible neural damage of VIIIth cranial nerve. In electrocochleography, compound acoustic action potentials from the first neuron are recorded from the promontorium with stainless steel needles and averaged (Aran, 1971). In brain stem audiometry the action potentials from the first and following neurons are recorded from the vertex (Jewett and Williston, 1971). Normal action potentials presuppose normal function of receptor cells and first neurons. If there is a positive response from the first neuron in electrocochleography or brain stem audiometry in a case of subjective deafness, the receptor cells and generators of the first neurons must be intact. However, if other diagnostic methods indicate a lesion of the VIIIth cranial nerve, the same first neuron is damaged centrally from the generators to the extent that the sensory function fails due to blockage, without degeneration of the entire neuron. However, this is only the case in circumscript damage of the myeline sheath. The damage of the myelin sheath is reversible after removal of the causative agent. On the other hand degeneration of the nerve itself is irreversible because it affects the entire neuron (Spoendlin, 1971) including the generators of the electroacoustic potentials. Degeneration causes the extinction of all potentials in cochleography and brain stem audiometry. To present, we have examined 14 patients with definite electrophysiological signs indicating circumscript damage of the acoustic nerve myelin sheath in the pontine angle whereby a tumor was definitely excluded. Because of our rigorous criteria regarding indications for operation, we performed an acoustic nerve decompression in only three patients.

Indications for Acoustic Nerve Decompression

An existing arachnopathia is not an indication for operation as long as it does not present repairable damage, because arachnopathia is not a progressive and expansive process, as for example an acoustic neurinoma. The proof of an existing repairable nerve damage in arachnopathia is for us only a relative indication for surgery. In the case of unilateral deafness with positive neural response and a normally functioning opposite ear we are in principle against a transoccipital operation to decompress the nerve because of the risks involved. We are motivated to operate only for the following reasons: 1. deafness on both sides. 2. one sided deafness: when the patient is dependent on binaural hearing for social (schooling) or professional reasons, or when the patient absolutely wishes the operation in spite of the risk, or when other nerves are affected as for example the trigeminal nerve which can also exhibit reversible functional damage (see case report).

Case Report

(Patient K. K., 59 years old)
Summary: progressive sensoneural deafness in the left ear leading to complete left sided deafness within a few weeks. Ipsilateral hypaesthesia of the trigeminal nerve developed simultaneously. Pure tone audiometry: deafness left, age-normal threshold right (Fig. 1 A). Electrocochleogram: nearly normal threshold of acoustically evoked potentials over a wide range of frequencies (Fig. 1 A). Electronystagmography: age-normal symmetric functioning of vestibular nerve. Facial nerve: normal function on both sides. X-rays: no excavation of the left internal auditory canal. Computer tomography: no indication of a tumor. Angle myelogram: complete filling of the left internal auditory canal, whereas on the pyramidal tip a filling defect constant in all positions is found. Cisternoscopy: numerous connective tissue scars visibly sheath the Vth and VIIIth cranial nerves (Fig. 2). Clinical history: one

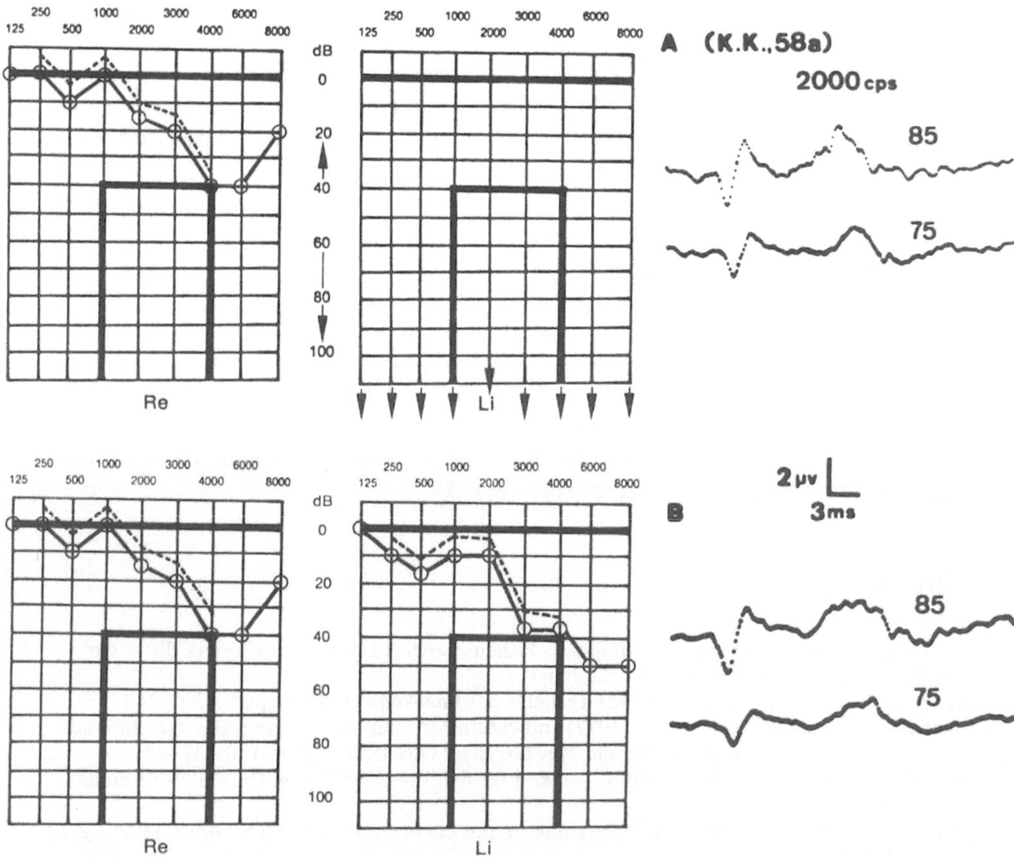

Fig. 1 A, B. Patient K. K. **A** Preoperatively: unilateral deafness in the pure tone audiogram with positive electrocochleogram in the left side (tone bursts 2000 cps, 85 dB and 75 dB HL). **B** Postoperatively: age-normal auditory functions in pure tone audiogram and electrocochleogram

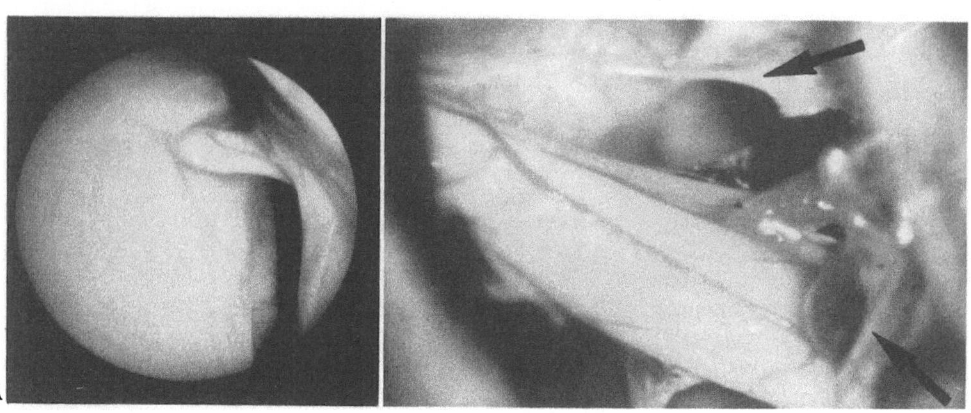

A B

Fig. 2 A, B. Patient K. K. Cisternoscopic aspect of the left cerebellopontine angle: post-arachnitic scar tissue is covering the brain stem and especially the entering of the VIIIth cranial nerve. **A** General endoscopic view. **B** Higher amplification: arrows indicating the sails of scars. Star: strangulation mark week after neurosurgical decompression of the nerves, the expected return of function occurs. After another week, and to present, the patient has shown age-normal hearing function (Fig. 1 B), and the trigeminal hypaesthesia has disappeared. The other two patients exhibited partial functional integrity postoperatively.

Conclusions

For the first time, we are now in a good position to provide an indication for craniotomy in case of arachnitic adhesions: proof of reversible neural damage, furnished by means of electro-acoustic test methods. This predictibility distinguishes decompression of the acoustic nerve from that of the optic nerve, where predictibility of success does not exist. Nevertheless, one must always primarily ponder the anticipated surgical results against the surgical risks.

References

Aran JM (1971) L'electrocochleogramme. I. Principe et technique. Les Cahiers de la Compagne Française d'Audiologie, Nr. 12, Paris

Ehrenberger K (1978) Endoscopy of the Cerebello-pontine Angle. Endoscopy 10:260–264

Ehrenberger K, Innitzer J, Koos W (1977) Indication for operation in cases of arachnitic adhesions of the cerebello-pontine angle. Rev Laryngol Otol Rhinol (Bord) 98:437–441

Jewett DL, Williston JS (1971) Auditory-evoked far fields averaged from the scalp of humans. Brain 94:681–696

Spoendlin H (1971) Degeneration behaviour of the cochlear nerve. Arch Otorhinolaryngol (NY) 200:275–283

Retro-Sigmoid Approach for Preservation of Hearing in Early Acoustic Neuroma Surgery

J. M. STERKERS, Paris/France

The diagnosis of acoustic tumor is now frequently made before major impairment of the hearing has developed. It is reasonable to try to maintain this function, as long as the other goals of the early surgery of the acoustic tumors have been attained, i.e. total removal of the tumor, no mortality, no ataxia and total preservation of facial function. Some results of preservation of hearing have already been reported (Pertuiset et al., 1966; Rand and Kurze, 1968; House, 1968; Sterkers and Billet, 1972; Smith and Clancy, 1973; Glasscock et al., 1978, Bremond G., 1979). These results encouraged us to try to save the hearing in such cases, and especially in bilateral tumors (Hitselberger and Hughes, 1968; Sterkers and Hamann, 1979). Therefore, since 1977 we have utilized the retro-sigmoid approach with an atraumatic technique, developed from our experience in transtemporal removal of acoustic neuromas.

Material and Approach

Over the last three years, 80 acoustic neuromas have been operated upon by a retro-sigmoid approach. The size of the tumor was less than 10 mm (intracanalar tumor) in nine patients, between 10 and 25 mm (middle size tumor) in 56 patients, and more than 25 mm in 15 cases, reaching 50 mm in greatest diameter (large size tumor). A total hearing loss was observed before the operation in six patients (four middle size and two large size tumors) which are not included in the results regarding preservation of hearing.

The retro-sigmoid approach is a personal modification of the lateral route, using the micro-surgical technique, the supine position, protection of the cerebellum by lyophilised dura and no self-retaining retractor.

Step I, Approach to the Angle

The patient is placed in a *supine* position, the head is rotated and fixed with adhesive. A vertical retro-mastoid *incision* ten centimeters long is made. A *craniotomy* of 3 cm in diameter is made behind the sigmoid sinus, between the linea nuchalis superior and inferior (Fig. 1). Two *incisions* of the dura are made, one vertical, and one horizontal, which divides in two triangular flaps the anterior area of the dura. Five hundred ml of Mannitol (25 per cent) are infused intra-veinously during the first step.

A sheet of *lyophilised dura* is inserted between the cerebellum and the medial wall of the petrous bone, and is pushed with a blunt dissector until the arachnoid of the lateral cisterna is reached and opened. Throughout the operation, the cerebellum is protected by the lyophilised dura. This technique provides a 'sort of extradural approach' and avoids any trauma, hemorrhage or edema of the cerebellum. No self-retaining retractor is used. No cottonoid is placed on the cerebellum. The surgical microscope is used from the time of the craniotomy to the last step of the operation.

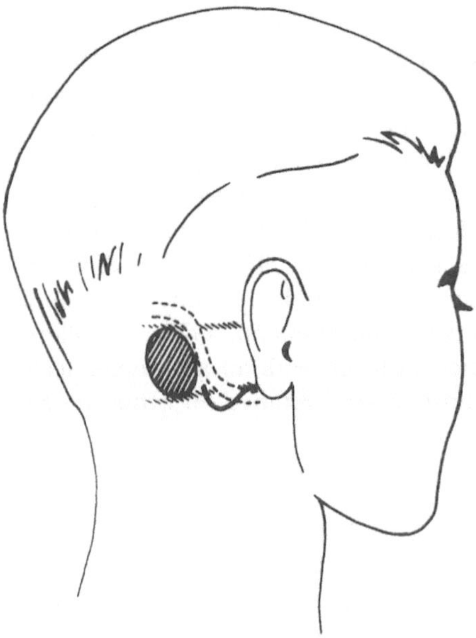

Fig. 1. The retrosigmoid craniotomy. Patient in supine position, head rotated. (From Neurological Surgery of the Ear II. Aesculapius pub. comp.)

Step II, Removal of the Acoustic Tumor

Electrical stimulation of the posterior pole of the tumor is performed to ensure that the Facial nerve is not displaced behind the tumor. This is exception (1 percent of our cases).

The porus and the posterior wall of the internal auditory canal are drilled for a distance of six to eight millimeters (Fig. 2). The Fundus is generally not exposed. The position of the jugular bulb and the posterior semi-circular canal has been located by a pre-operative roentgenogram (basal view).

The basis of preservation of facial and auditory nerve function is to decompress the nerve and its vascular supply by a subarachnoid removal of the tumor inside the meatus before removing the tumor in the angle. The intracanalicular part of the tumor is first removed. After incision of the dura, the tumor bulges outside the canal, it is removed piecemeal until the subarachnoid sheet which covers the Facial and Cochlear nerves is reached. Then, the Facial nerve is identified, first by electrical stimulation (using the Hilger apparatus) and secondly by direct visual identification. The Facial nerve is flattened against the anterior wall of the canal by the tumor. A straight arteriole follows the Facial nerve. It is a good landmark for recognition of the 7th nerve. A tongue of neuroma is frequently expanded between the Facial and Cochlear nerves. It is removed by light traction. The cochlear nerve lies against the inferior wall. All remnants of the root of the neuroma are removed with a perpendicular dissector which cleans the posterior part of the Fundus. When the fibers of the Vestibular nerves are visualized, one can be sure that all the root of the tumor has been removed.

The method of removing the tumor in the angle depends on the size of the tumor. When the tumor does not reach the brain stem, the nerves are identified medially; the Facial nerve is located first and then the eighth nerve. Dissection of the tumor is performed from the medial pole to the porus. As in the meatus, it is essential to keep intact the arachnoid sheath over the nerves and vessels to avoid any traction and devascularisation.

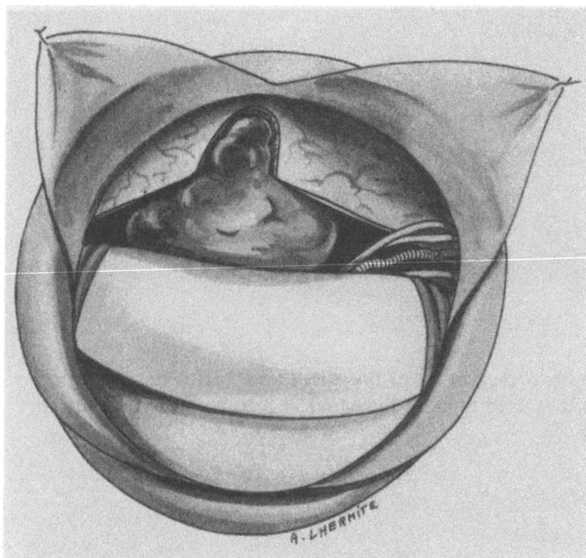

Fig. 2. The cerebellum is protected by sheets of lyophilised dura. The internal auditory canal is opened. Exposure of the tumor. (From Neurological Surgery of the Ear II. Aesculapius pub. comp.)

When the tumor reaches the brain stem, an intracapsular removal is first carried out; then the Facial nerve is identified in two places: near the porus and at its exit from the brain stem. A smooth dissection to the last parts of the tumor is done along the nerve, avoiding any traction and suction against the nerve. The same method of dissection is applied for preserving the cochlear nerve. The anterior and inferior cerebellar artery is always identified and preserved. The internal auditory arteries are exceptionally identified.

Step III, Closure

The internal auditory meatus is filled by a graft of free muscle or fat graft to close any potential opening of the petrous cells (Fig. 3). The posterior fossa dura is closed using a sheet of lyophilized dura, and a fascia graft (from the fascia lata). These grafts are sutured to the dura and then glued using Histoacryl; adipose or muscle free grafts are applied to fill the dead space under the muscle and subcutaneous sutures. The skin is closed using interrupted nylon sutures without any drainage.

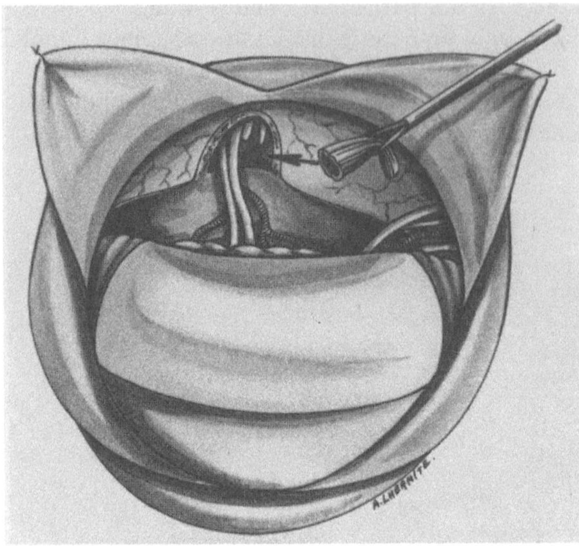

Fig. 3. After total removal of the tumor, preservation of the VIIth and VIIIth nerves with the vascular pedicles. A free graft of muscle is used to close the canal. (From Neurological Surgery of the Ear II. Aesculapius pub. comp.)

Results

The preservation of hearing was achieved in 23 cases (31%) out of 74 tumors with a pre-operatory hearing. Identical hearing function which means identical post-operatory tonal and speech audiometry tests was obtained in 13 cases. The hearing was worse than before the operation in 7 cases but with a tonal threshold or/and a percentage of discrimination which was still useful. The tonal threshold and the percentage of discrimination were improved in 3 cases (N° 15, 16, 22). In all of these cases, except two bilateral neuromas, total removal of the tumor was performed. A planned decompression of the acoustic nerve with partial removal of the tumor on the second ear was done in these two bilateral neuromas (N° 19 and 20). In Table 1 are shown the results of the pre-operatory and post-operatory audiometric tests.

Preservation of hearing was obtained in 67 percent of the intra-canalar tumors (six out of nine cases) and in 34 percent of the middle size tumors (17 out of 50 cases). When the tumor was larger than 25 mm, the hearing function has never been preserved. The preservation of facial nerve function has been already discussed in detail in another chapter, we will only report here that normal postoperative function was observed in 77.6 percent, a residual facial weakness in 20 percent and a permanent facial palsy in 2.5 percent. When the hearing function was preserved, the postoperative facial function was always normal.

Other complications are summarized in Table 2.

Table 1. Results of the pre-operative and post-operative tests in 23 acoustic tumors

Cases	Size of the tumor in mm	Pre-operative audiometric tests					Post-operative audiometric tests				
		Tonal audiometry				% Discrimination	Tonal audiometry				% Discrimination
		500 Hz	1000 Hz	2000 Hz	4000 Hz		500 Hz	1000 Hz	2000 Hz	4000 Hz	
1	15	40	70	85	100	0	40	70	–	100	0
2	10	10	80	75	70	60	20	70	70	60	60
3	20	10	10	70	75	90	10	10	65	–	90
4	20	25	45	65	85	30	60	60	70	–	0
5	14	40	50	60	70	100	80	75	70	70	0
6	15	35	35	80	55	100	30	40	90	–	100
7	10	50	60	70		50	50	55	55	80	60
8	15	15	60	45	35	100	25	50	50	50	100
9	8	30	35	40	50	10	90	90	80	90	0
10	15	20	20	60	70	90	80	60	60	65	20
11	20	50	85			0	50	85	–	–	0
12	22	50	60	95	105	ND	50	60	95	–	ND
13	15	20	40	60	50	0	25	40	75	75	0
14	10	35	45	65	85	100	60	85	80	100	ND
15	18	30	40	100	90	0	30	30	50	90	100
16	15	35	40	60	70	60	15	35	55	70	100
17	15	30	20	45	70	100	50	40	60	75	100
18	10	0	0	30	55	100	10	10	50	60	100
19	15	10	10	10	100	100	10	10	10	10	100
20	20	30	60	100	90	0	15	50	90	–	0
21	10	30	15	30	50	70	45	40	60	–	ND
22	20	30	30			0	30	30	40	50	100
23	13	15	25	30	50	100	15	30	45	60	100

Table 2. Complications of the retro-sigmoid approach in 80 patients

Meningitis	2
C.S.F. Leakage	7
Benign hydrocephaly	1
Reversible cerebellar ataxia	1
Reversible abducens palsy	3
Death	0

Discussion

Hearing preservation in acoustic neuroma surgery is in all cases a very rewarding goal; this is especially true when the hearing is not too badly affected by the tumor; but even in the other cases, retention of some hearing function might become of vital importance when the second ear in the future should be affected by another pathology (virus, infection, traumatism, sudden deafness, etc.).

Hearing preservation is a reasonable objective if the other purposes of early surgery of acoustic neuromas are achieved, especially facial nerve function and preservation of life. The choice of operation is between two approaches to preserve hearing: the middle fossa approach and the retro-sigmoid approach. We have a personal comparison between these two approaches (Table 3). Even in intracanalar tumors a better result was obtained by using the retro-sigmoid approach.

Table 3. Results of preservation of hearing in 94 acoustic neuromas. Comparison between middle-fossa (MFa) and retro-sigmoid approach (RSa)

	Hearing preservation, number of tumors		Intracanalar acoustic neuroma		Middle size acoustic neuroma		Large size acoustic neuroma	
	n	%	*n*	%	*n*	%	*n*	%
MFa	8/20	40	7/13	54	1/6	17	0/1	0
RSa	23/74	32	6/9	67	17/50	34	0/15	0

Conclusions

The retro-sigmoid approach, utilizing microsurgical techniques, supine position of the patient, and the cerebellum protected by lyophilized dura fulfills the conditions for total removal of small and middle size acoustic tumors, with an interesting rate of preservation of hearing function. This approach permits progress, as the cochlear function is not deliberately destroyed.

References

Bremond G (1979) Le problème de la conservation de l'audition au cours de l'exérèse des tumeurs de l'angle ponto-cérébelleux. Rev Laryngol Otol Rhinol (Bord) 100: 111–114

Glasscock ME, James WH, Miller GW, Drake FD, Kanock MM (1978) Preservation of hearing in tumors of the auditory canal and cerebello-pontine angle. Laryngoscope 88:43

Hitselberger WE, Hughes RL (1968) Bilateral acoustic tumors and neurofibromatosis. Arch Otolaryngol 88:700–711

House WF (1968) Monograph II Acoustic neuromas. Arch Otolaryngol 88:576–715

Pertuiset B et coll. (1966) La conservation des fonctions auditive et faciale au cours de l'exérèse totale des neurinomes de l'acoustique par voie sous-occipitale. Presse Med 74:2327–2330

Rand RW, Kurze T (1968) Preservation of vestibular, cochlear and facial nerves during microsurgical removal of acoustic tumors. J Neurosurg 28: 158–161

Smith MF, Clancy Th (1977) Conservation of hearing in acoustic neurilemoma excision. In: Neurological surgery of the Ear. Aesculapius pub. comp. Birmingham, Alabama, USA, p 261

Sterkers JM, Billet R (1972) Petites tumeurs de l'acoustique. Diagnostic et cure précoce. Ann Otolaryngol Chir Cervicofac 89:323–339

Sterkers JM (1979) Neurinomes de l'acoustique et autres tumeurs de l'angle et du conduit auditif interne. Résultats opératoires et choix de la voie d'abord (126 cas). Ann Otolaryngol Chir Cervicofac 96:373–386

Sterkers JM, Hamann KF (1979) Neurinomes de l'acoustique bilatéraux. Ann Otolaryngol Chir Cervicofac 96:623–635

Sterkers JM (1980) Removal of bilateral and unilateral acoustic tumors with preservation of hearing. In: Neurological Surgery of the Ear. II. Aesculapius pub. comp. Birmingham, Alabama, USA (to be published)

Preservation of Eighth Cranial Nerve in Cerebello-Pontine Angle Tumors

M. SAMII and A. OHLEMUTZ, Hannover/FRG

In eight patients with cerebello-pontine angle tumors, operated upon in the Neurosurgical Clinic, City of Hanover, from October 1977 through January, 1980, the eighth cranial nerve could be preserved. These patients, operated upon by the author using the same technique as in the Neurosurgical University Clinic of Mayence, have not been reported previously.

Seven of these tumors were neurinomas; one, an epidermoid. The size of the tumors varied mostly between four and five cm, only two were about two cm diameter. Compression of the brain stem and displacement of the fourth ventricle was found in all cases four cm diameter and larger. The symptoms caused by irritation of the eighth cranial nerve differed. In one case tinnitus was the only complaint, but most patients reported more or less intense diminution of hearing function, as well as vertigo attacks of different intensity. The lateral suboccipital approach was performed in all cases. The follow up varies from immediately after the operation in one patient, to thirty in another (Fig. 1).

PRESERVATION OF EIGHTH CRANIAL NERVE IN CEREBELLOPONTINE ANGLE TUMORS

Patient	kind of tumor	size cm	IV. ventr.	cochlear function pre op.	cochlear function post op.	vestib. function pre	vestib. function post	facial function pre	facial function post	follow up (month)
1) E.B. ♀ 15.06.46	neurinoma right	4	displacement	↓	no change	ø	(+)	+	+	< 1
2) J.E. ♂ 24.06.48	neurinoma left	2	ø	↓	↑	ø	(+)	+	+	10
3) P.A. ♂ 29.11.52	neurinoma r.+l.	l 4 r 5	displacement displacement	l ↓↓ r ø	l ø r ø	l (+) r ø	l (+) r ø	l + r +	l (+) r (+)	1 8
4) U.S. ♀ 17.08.41	neurinoma right	4	displacement	↓	↑	(+)	(+)	+	+	< 1
5) K.F. ♂ 08.02.46	epidermoid left	5	displacement	↓	↑	(+)	+	+	+	30
6) V.P. ♀ 20.03.39	neurinoma right	4	displacement	(↓)	↓	(+)	(+)	+	+	4
7) R.G.M. ♂ 14.04.44	neurinoma right	2	ø	normal tinnitus ++	↓ ø tinnitus	+	(+)	+	+	6
8) P.S. ♂ 19.05.53	neurinoma right	5	ø	↓↓	ø	ø	ø	(+)	(+)	7

Symbols: ↑ increase; (↓) slight decrease; ↓ " "; ↓↓ high " "; + function; (+) lower function; ø no " "

Fig. 1. Table of cases and results

The results of technique of preservation of the nerve were encouraging. In three patients we could find an increase in hearing function (see Figs. 2–4). In one, no alteration could be recognized (preoperatively a middle-grade hearing loss existed). Two patients showed a decrease in hearing function, but not to a great extent. In one of them an intense and disturbing tinnitus ceased, so that a subjective feeling of improvement was finally described. Two other patients showed deafness after the operation. In one of these, the preoperative hearing function was near to total deafness, and in the other a trans-temporal attempt to remove the tumor had been preceded in another clinic with the result of near deafness. It should be mentioned that this patient suffered from multiple neurinomas, and that other intracranial operations had already been performed. The postoperative evaluation of vestibular function showed similarly good results. In one patient equal excitibility of both vestibular systems without vertigo and spontaneous nystagmus was found, whereas preoperatively lower excitibility of the left side was ascertained. In two patients the function increased from non-excitibility to a well releasable caloric excitibility, though still different to the other side. Three patients showed no change in comparison to the preoperative findings, but vertigo was clearly less intense. Among them was one patient suffering from deafness after the operation. However, the other procedure which resulted in complete deafness showed no excitibility of the vestibular system. To conclude, it can be stated that preservation of the eighth cranial nerve during cerebello-pontine angle tumor operations shows hopeful results, so that every attempt to preserve the nerve should be made, even in middle and large size acoustic neurinomas. It is of great importance that not only the preoperative level of function of the eighth cranial nerve could be preserved, but that an improvement in the preoperative status could be achieved in some patients.

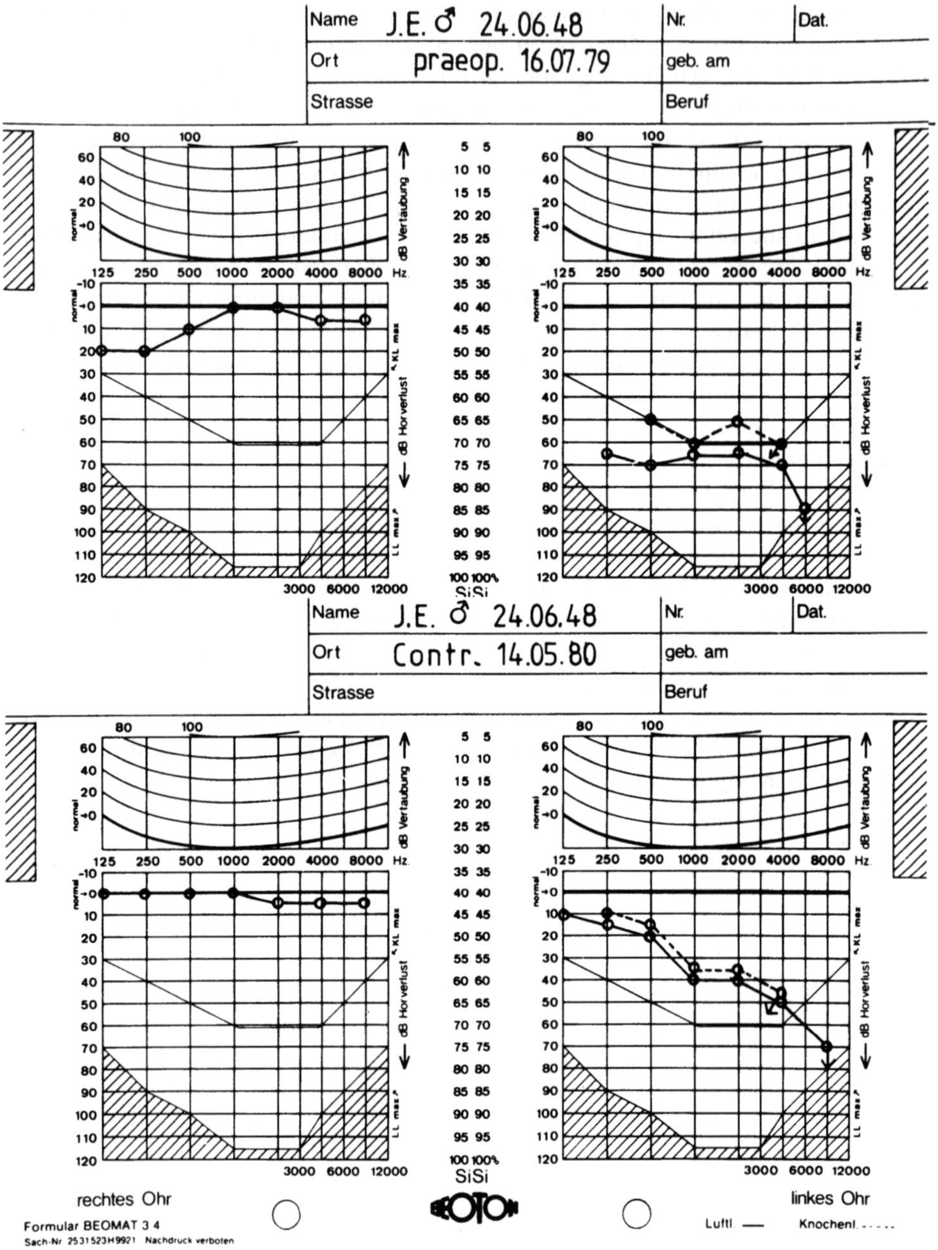

Fig. 2. Pre- and postoperative audiograms in case two. A left sided neurinoma of two cm diameter was removed. Principle symptoms, preoperatively, were hearing decrease, tinnitus, and vertigo. Vestibular function returned after 10 months. Tinnitus was no longer reported

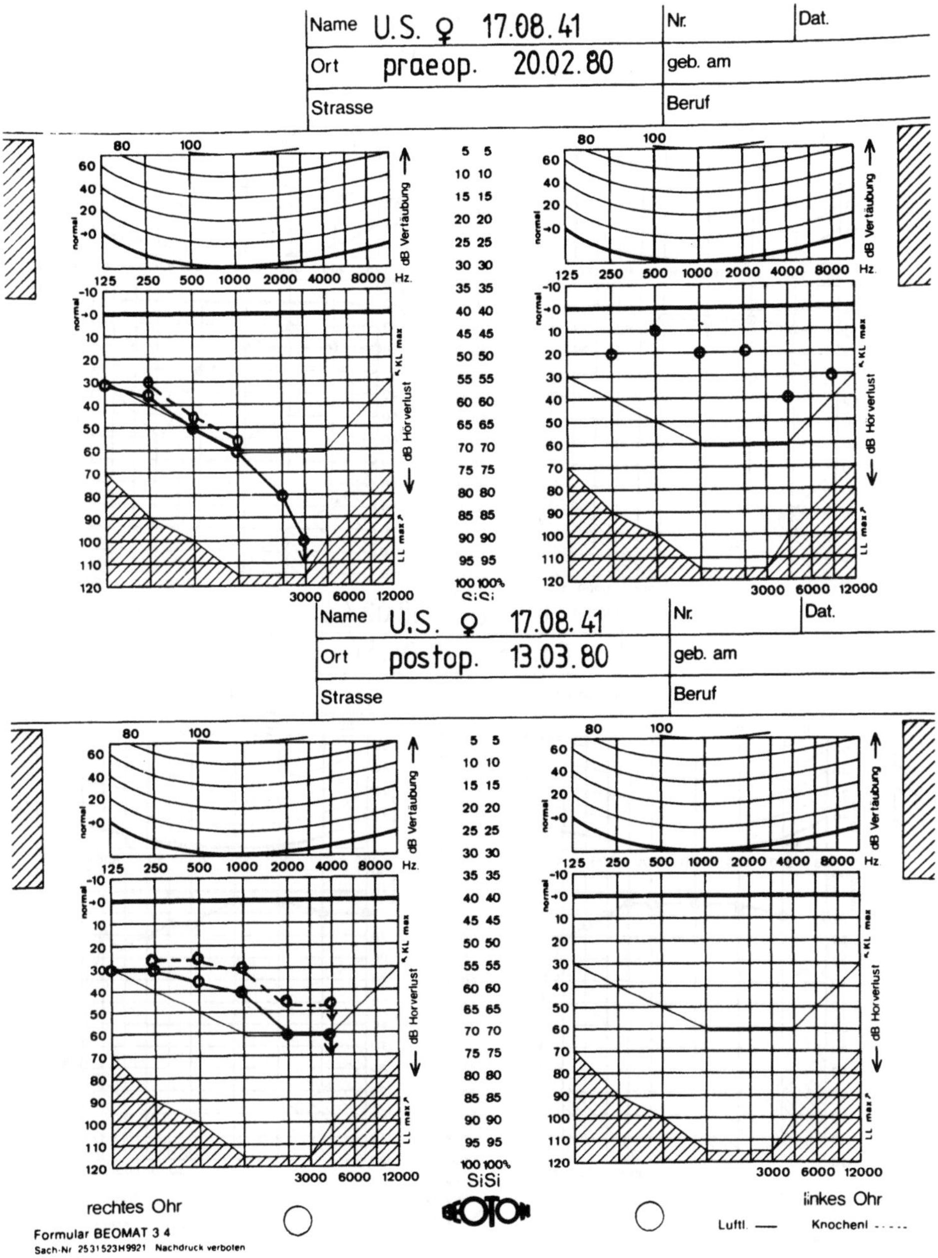

Fig. 3. Pre- and postoperative audiograms of case four. A 38 year old woman, suffering since 1975 from vertigo hypacousis and tinnitus. Later on, trigeminal irritation was found as well. During the operation a four cm diameter tumor compressing the brain stem and displacing the fourth ventricle was found

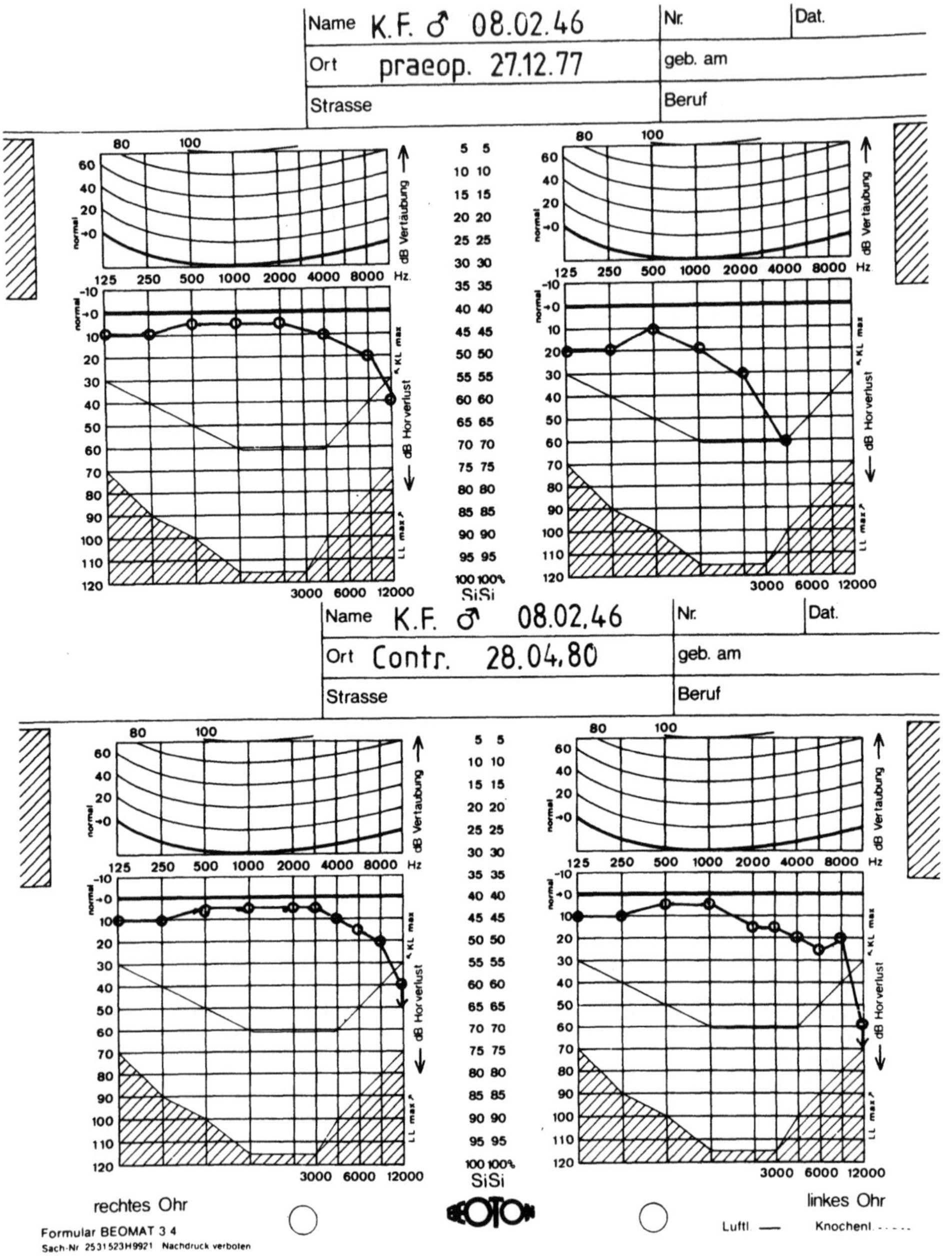

Fig. 4. Pre- and postoperative audiograms of case five. Here a five cm diameter epidermoid with compression of the brain stem and the fourth ventricle could be removed. The patient suffered for 10 years from progressive hearing loss and sudden vertigo. Vestibular function became normal

Caudal Cranial Nerves

Neurological Diagnosis of Caudal Cranial Nerves Lesions

M. Mumenthaler, Bern/Switzerland

1. Introduction

The ninth, tenth, eleventh, and twelfth cranial nerve are called caudal cranial nerves. The anatomical characteristics of these nerves have been reviewed in this volume by Sir Sidney Sunderland. The following chapter will just describe the typical clinical aspects and the diagnostic tests, which allow the diagnosis of lesion of one of these cranial nerves.

2. The Diagnosis of Glossopharyngeal Nerve Lesions

The ninth nerve contains motor fibers to the stylomastoid muscle, sensory fibers from the soft palate, the pharynx, the fauces, the posterior third of the tongue, the tonsils and the tympanic cavity, special visceral afferents from the taste buds of the posterior third of the tongue and parasympathetic fibers to the parotis gland as well as fibers from the receptors of carotid sinus. An isolated lesion of this nerve is rare and generally combined with a lesion of the vagus nerve.

In unilateral lesion of glossopharyngeal nerve one finds:

- a slight dysphagia
- a loss of the gag reflex (which, however, shows quite important individual differences)
- a deviation of the uvula to the opposite side
- In a co-operative patient one can make evident the difference of sensation of the soft palate and the pharynx between the side of the lesion and the well one
- The loss of taste in the posterior third of the tongue is very difficult to demonstrate (easiest with better material, e.g. chininum sulfuricum)
- If the plexus tympanicus has also been involved, there is a diminution of the saliva secretion in the parotid gland and when the carotid sinus reflex is eliminated, there may be acceleration of heart rate.

The easiest way to demonstrate a paralysis of glossopharyngeal nerve is to show the deviation of the uvula to the opposite side with phonation ('ah') (see also Fig. 1). A bilateral glossopharyngeal paralysis produces an important disturbance of speach (rhinolalia aperta) due to the bilateral palsy of the soft palate.

3. The diagnosis of Paralysis of the Vagus Nerve

The tenth cranial nerve is responsible for the motor innervation of the soft palate, the pharynx and most muscles responsible for swallowing. The recurrent branches innervate the larynx muscles. It also contains sensory fibers from the larynx (nervus laryngicus superior), the external ear and the posterior fossa. Through the vagus parasympathetic fibers reach the organs of the thoracic and abdominal cavity.

A paralysis of vagus is characterized by:

- hoarseness (test singing!)
- dysphagia (slowing of swallowing and coughing)
- the most clear-cut sign is the unilateral paralysis of pharyngeal muscles: due to the loss of constriction on the pathologic side, the raphe in the mid-line is deviated to the well side (side-scenes phenomenon) (Fig. 1)
- paralysis of vocal cord can be seen at the laryngoscopic examination
- One has to look for the sensory loss in the external auditive canal and part of the concha auriculae
- The loss of parasympathetic innervation causes an acceleration of heart beat, which does not respond to carotid sinus compression or to the oculo-cardiac reflex.

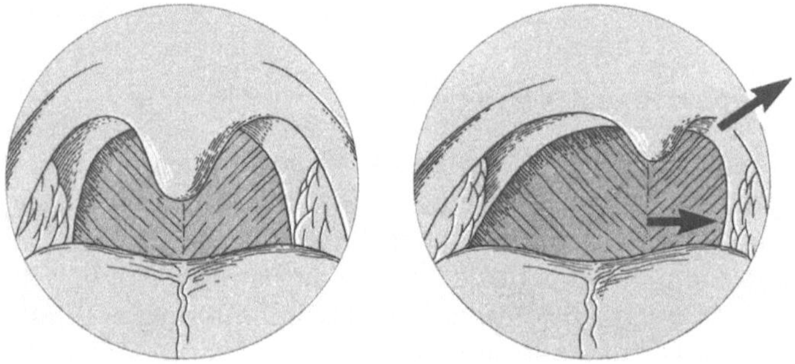

Fig. 1. 'Side-scenes phenomenon' in a right sided paralysis of the vagus. (From Mumenthaler, Neurologie, 6th edit., Thieme Stuttgart 1979)

4. The Diagnosis of Paralysis of the Accessory Nerve

The fibers of the internal or medullary branches of the eleventh cranial nerve join those of the external branch, the spinal one, within the jugular foramen. The medullary branch joins the vagus, the spinal branch reaches the sternocleidomastoid muscle and then the cranial part of the trapezius muscle. This is also innervated in a variable amount by direct branches from the first couple of spinal nerves, which reach the muscle either directly or by anastomosis between the cervical plexus and the accessory nerve.

The most frequent site of a lesion of the accessory nerve is the lateral part of the neck. This is the reason why the sternocleidomastoid muscle, which lies proximal to the site of lesion, remains intact. Paralysis of the cranial portion of the trapezius muscle causes:

- a lowering of the shoulder. The scapula stays somewhat more lateral than usual, the lateral angle is lower and therefore the scapula seems slightly rotated. The upper line of the shoulder does not show the usual harmonic aspect, but seems somewhat angled.
- There is weakness in elevating the shoulder against resistance and the elevation of the arm to the side is weak because of insufficient fixation of the scapula to the thorax.

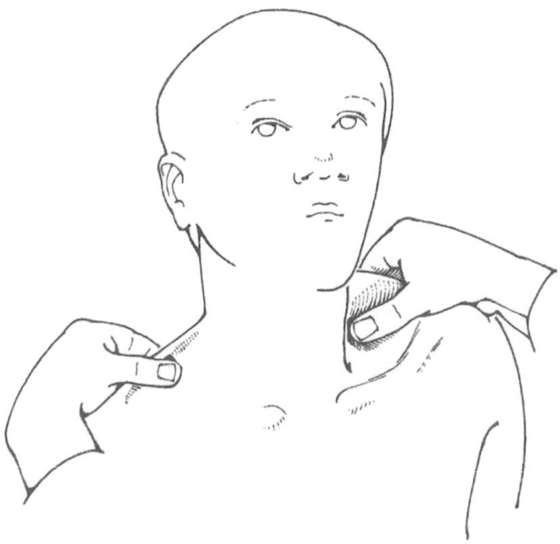

Fig. 2. How to test the strength of the upper trapezius-portion. Paralysis on the right side. (From Mumenthaler: Der Schulter-Arm-Schmerz, Huber Berne 1980)

- The most impressive sign is paralysis of the cranial portion of the trapezius muscle. This is best shown, when the examiner stands in front of the patient, puts his hands on both acromia and holds the angle of the trapezius between his thumb and index finger when the patient tries to lift the shoulders (Fig. 2).

In a proximal lesion of the accessory nerve the *sternocleidomastoid muscle* is also paralysed.

- It seems less prominent when the patient pushes his head strongly against the examiner's hand.
- If one wants to test just one of the two muscles, the patient is asked to turn his head to the opposite side, whilst the examiner holds his hand against the patient's chin and his second hand palpates the muscle belly (Fig. 3).

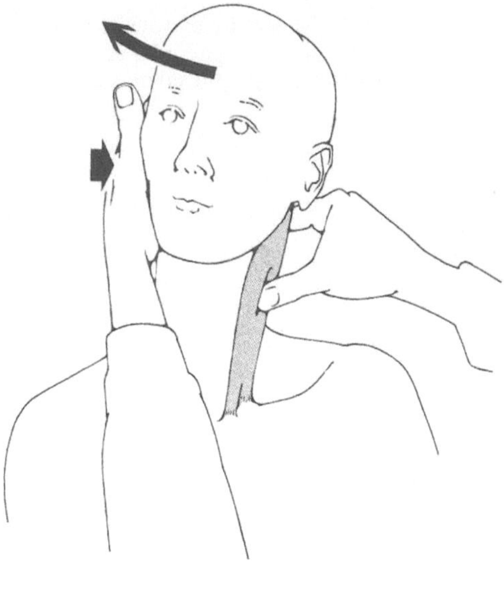

Fig. 3. How to test the strength of the sternocleidomastoid muscle. (From Mumenthaler, Neurologischer Untersuchungskurs, Deutsches Aerzteblatt *71,* 3475 (1974)

5. The Diagnosis of Paralysis of the Hypoglossal Nerve

The twelfth cranial nerve has only motor fibers for the tongue muscles. In a *unilateral* paralysis:

- initially, a slight impairment of speach and of swallowing appears, which however is rapidly compensated
- inspection shows a hemiatrophy of the tongue by two weeks after injury, which seems thinner on the paralysed side and shows folds on the edge
- when the tongue is actively pushed out of the mouth, it deviates towards the paretic side (Fig. 4)
- the protruded tongue can hardly be moved towards the well side and pushes a spatula less strongly to the healthy side
- when the patient keeps his tongue in the mouth and tries to push the cheek from the inside, the examiner can feel the weakness on the paralysed side, if he puts his fingers on the patient's cheeks.

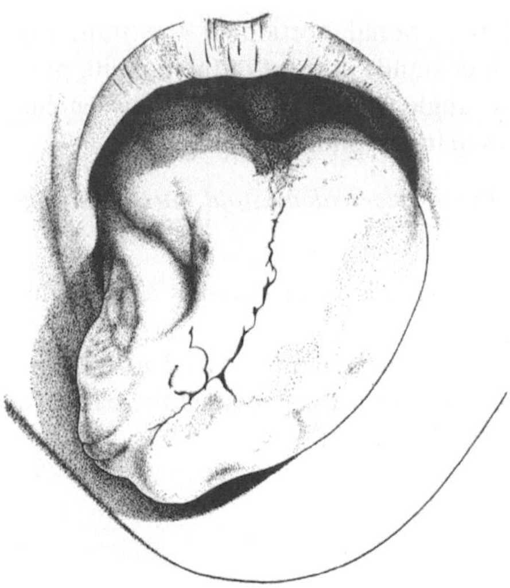

Fig. 4. Deviation of the protruded tongue to the right in a right sided paralysis of hypoglossal nerve

A *bilateral* paralysis of the hypoglossal nerve produces:

- a total paralysis of the tongue with atrophy and
- a profound disturbance of chewing and swallowing (the food cannot be moved around inside the mouth)
- as well as a slurred and deformed speach.

6. Summary

The clinical signs of paralysis of the glossopharyngeal, vagus, accessorius and hypoglossal nerve are described. The technical procedure for demonstrating these paralyses is shown.

Endoscopic Electromyography and Neurography

(Examination of the Inferior Cranial Motor Nerves: Nn. IX, X, XI, XII)

W. THUMFART, Erlangen/FRG

I. Electromyography of the Larynx

Introduction

Vital functions such as breathing and swallowing, as well as speaking, are coordinated by the inferior cranial nerves: The ninth, tenth, and twelfth nerves. Their lesions therefore require an exact diagnosis and treatment, often of an emergency nature. Electrophysiological techniques, the best tools for the prediction of the course of motor nerve paralysis, however, are difficult in the hidden muscles of the hypopharynx and larynx (Buchthal 1959, Faaborg-Andersen 1965).

The laryngeal muscles are supplied by the tenth cranial nerve, especially by the recurrent laryngeal nerve with one exception, the cricothyroid muscle, which is innervated by the upper laryngeal nerve. Bilateral immobilization of the vocal cords induces asphyxia, and a tracheostomy is often necessary.

Since one muscle, the posterior crico-arytenoid muscle, is responsible for the inspiratory opening mechanism of the glottis, the predominant diagnostic interest is always focussed on this muscle ('M. posticus'). The other intrinsic laryngeal muscles are involved in the closure of the glottis, they are responsible for the phonatory activity of the larynx. Both groups of muscles, abductors and adductors of the glottis, should be examined in case of recurrent nerve paralysis. Electromyography of the laryngeal muscles has, to present, been of minor importance, because the transcutaneous, blind insertion of needle electrodes (Hirano, 1961; Satoh, 1978) could not provide selective records of muscle activity, while the controlled placement of the electrodes during general anesthesia (Dedo, 1970; Kotby, 1970) prevented the recording of voluntary activity.

We, therefore, have tried a new access to electromyography of the larynx in the awake patient, when v. Stuckradt (1975) developed a new zoom-lens endoscope, which has proved very convenient for the precise examination of the endolarynx.

Technique

The endoscope (Fig. 1) is a one-piece instrument incorporating a 90° endoscope, an antifog air channel and fiber optic bundle for illumination. It provides a superior and comprehensive view of the entire hypopharynx and larynx in one field without any other auxiliary instruments. An integrated sliding-lens system permits an up to five fold magnification, without additional optical aids which allows a more close inspection of the vocal cords (Steiner, 1978).

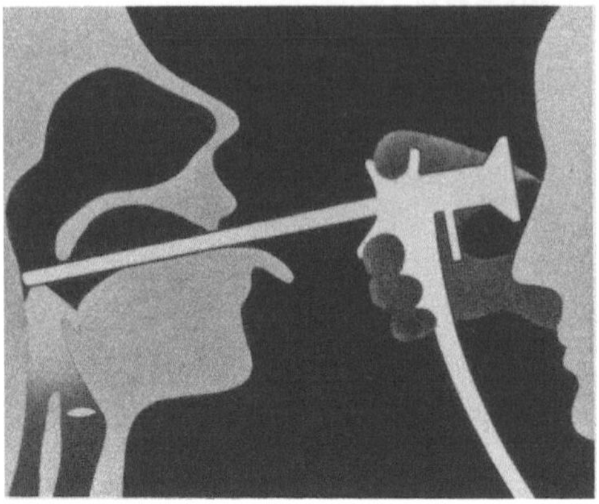

Fig. 1. Endoscopy of the larynx using the zoom-endoscope after v. Stuckradt (schematic drawing)

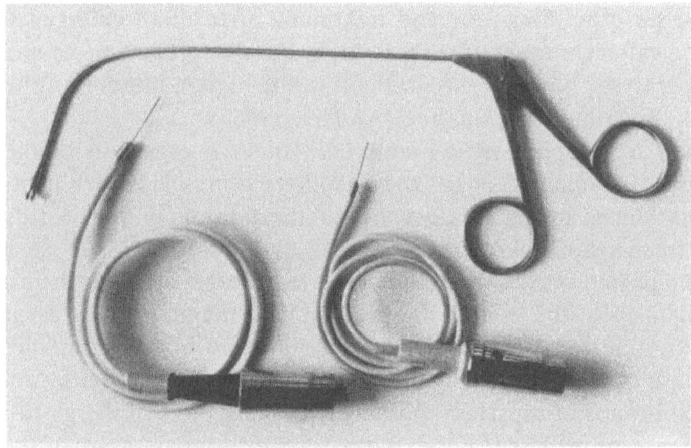

Fig. 2. Bipolar needle electrodes and electrode applicator

The application of needle electrodes is performed after superficial spray anesthesia of the pharynx and larynx with the aid of a special needle applicator (Fig. 2).

A model demonstrates the method of application: The needle electrode can be transorally applied exactly into any muscle of the larynx under optimal optic control (Fig. 3). The arytenoid cartilage is used for orientation. If the mucosal layer is removed in an anatomical preparation, the right position in the posterior crico-arytenoid muscle is apparent (Fig. 4). In the same manner muscle activity potentials can be derived from any muscle of the larynx, even simultaneously (Fig. 5).

If an EMG measurement over more than a few minutes is wanted, the so called 'hooked-wire' electrode (Hirano, 1961) is placed into the intrinsic laryngeal muscles. It consists out of two copperwires with 80 μ in diameter, which are placed into the muscle with a cannula. The patient is very well able to inspire, phonate, and even to sing. Simultaneous recording of the patient's voice with the microphone allows correlation of special muscle activities to inspiration or phonation.

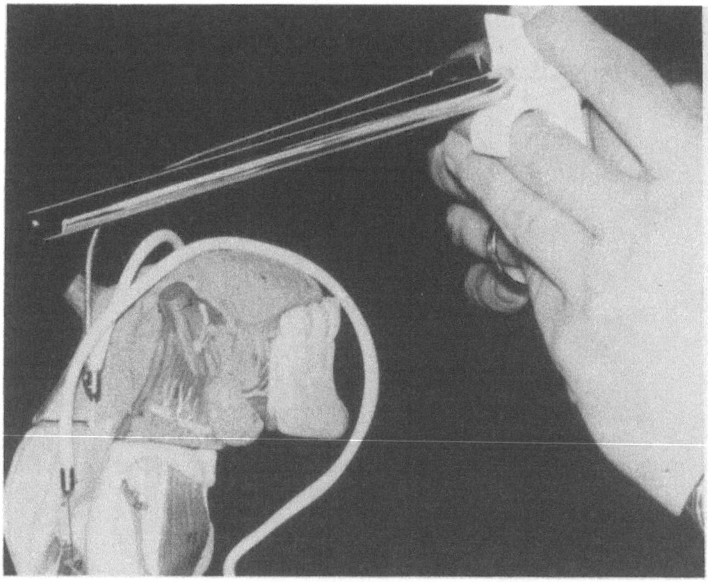

Fig. 3. Model of electrode application into the laryngeal muscles under zoom-endoscopic control

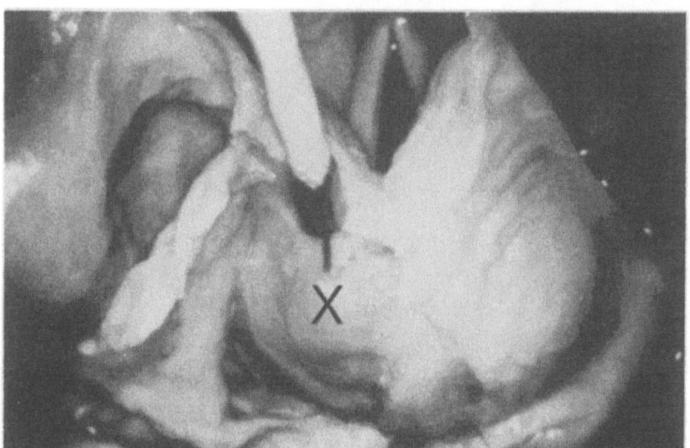

Fig. 4. Zoom-endoscopic view of electrode placement in the posterior cricoarytenoid muscle (*X*, anatomical preparation)

Results

The intact laryngeal muscles have a typical pattern of voluntary activity in the electromyogram: Figure 6 demonstrates an intact posterior cricoarytenoid with only some basic activity during phonation, but an increase of both frequency and amplitude during inspiration. The paralytic larnygeal muscle of the contralateral side shows only the basic activity. A reverse activity is recorded from the vocal muscle,

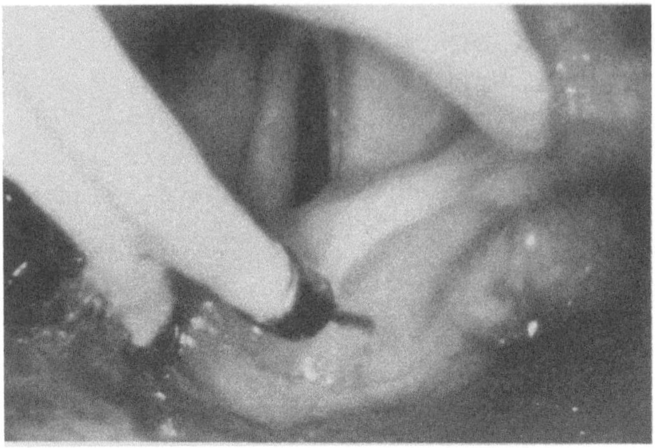

Fig. 5. Simultaneous electrode insertion in the posterior cricoarytenoid muscle of an awake patient

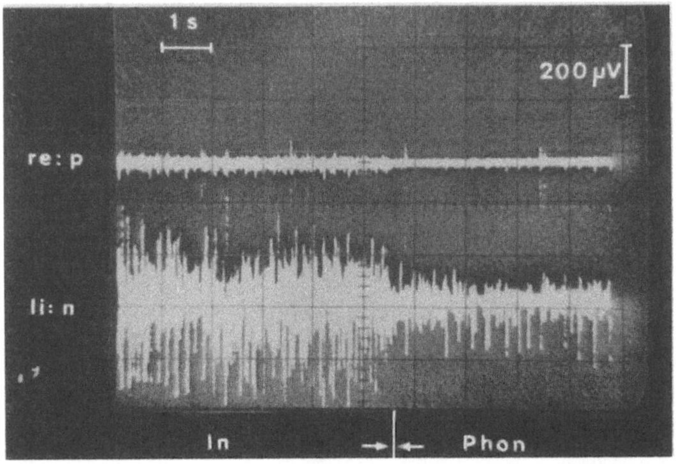

Fig. 6. Electromyogram of a paretic (*right*) and intact (*left*) posterior cricoarytenoid muscle during inspiration and phonation

the background activity being subscribed to the constrictor muscles of the larynx. About 350 ms before the onset of voice, voluntary activity starts in this muscle, if it is unimpaired (Fig. 7).

In cases of degeneration of the laryngeal nerves the occurrence of pathological spontaneous activity, for instance positive sharp waves or fibrillation potentials may be observed (Fig. 8). The early diagnosis of the initial signs of beginning denervation of the larynx is of primary interest for the indication of immediate surgical interventions.

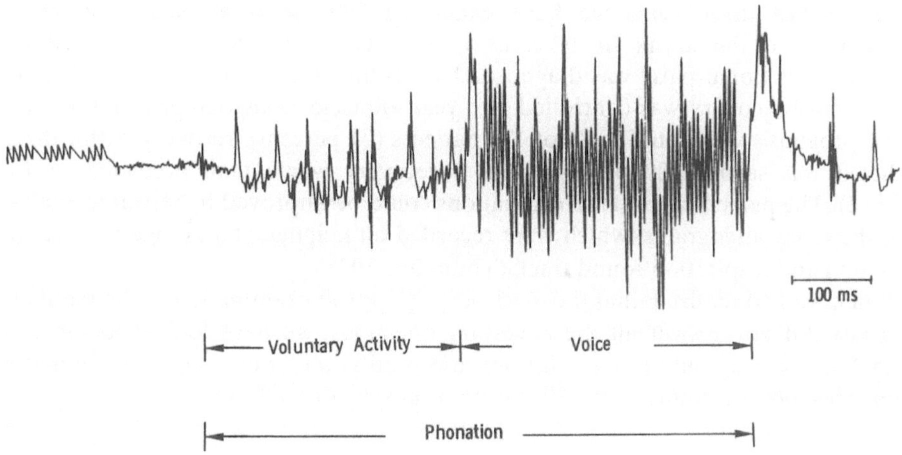

Fig. 7. Electromyogram of the intact vocal muscle

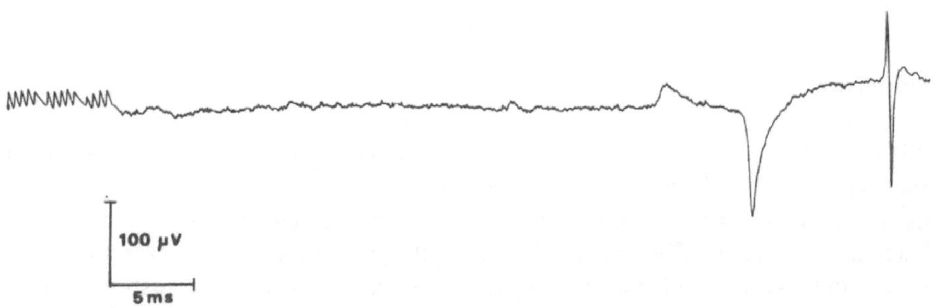

Fig. 8. Spontaneous activity in the vocal muscle with recurrent nerve paralysis

Table 1. Endoscopical EMG examination of the larynx (1976–79) $n=299$

Unilateral palsy	173
Bilateral palsy	63
Degenerative palsies	191
Neurapraxia	108

Table 2. EMG prognosis of laryngeal palsy in correlation with clinical course (1 year follow up; $n=114$)

Adequate prognosis	81 (71%)
Recovery better than predicted	20 (17%)
Recovery worse than predicted	13 (11%)

In the last three years we have examined 299 laryngeal palsies by electromyography of the larynx. In 191 cases signs of denervation could be observed. In 108 only a functional palsy was diagnosed by this method (Table 1). The prediction of vocal cord recovery was controlled one year after electromyography and an adequate prognosis was found in 81 of 114 patients (71 percent), recovery better than predicted was seen in 20 patients, and a recovery worse than predicted in 13 (Table 2). The percentage of false evaluations could be improved by repeated analysis of the electromyograms, which were recorded on magnetic tapes together with a phonation and inspiration sound track (Thumfart, 1978).

When we had realized, that the electromyographical examination of the paralyzed larynx did not answer all the necessary questions, we have looked for an additional test, which could provide further information about the outcome of a nerve lesion. This tool was found in the Electroneurography of the larynx.

II. Electroneurography of the Larynx

Introduction

By this term the recording of summating muscle action potentials of the laryngeal muscles after electrical stimulation of the laryngeal mixed nerves is understood, similar to the 'Electroneurography' of the facial muscles, described by Esslen (1973).

Two answers have to be expected: One is the indirect muscle contraction (first response), the second one is the synchroneous reflex activity (second response), provoked by the afferent excitation of the laryngeal nerves (similar to reflex). First essays of a stimulated EMG of the larynx were reported by Satoh (1978).

Technique and Material

By stimulation of the upper laryngeal nerve in the region of its penetration through the hypothyroid membrane with surface electrodes (Fig. 9, 10) a first potential can be induced in the cricothyroid muscle after 4 to 6 ms as a stimulated electromyogram. In the other laryngeal muscles this potential can be recorded after stimulation of the vagus or recurrent laryngeal nerves. Intraoperative direct nerve stimulation of the superior laryngeal nerve provoked a second answer, which could be observed only after stimulation of this nerve. This second or reflectory potential is seen 16–18 ms after onset of stimulation by 0.5 ms impulses (Fig. 11). After stimulation of the superior laryngeal nerve a second potential can be measured also in the posterior cricoarytenoid or vocal muscle with a longer latency. On the left side, reaction can be recorded after 24 ms, on the right side, according to the shorter course of the recurrent laryngeal nerve, after 22 ms (Fig. 12) (Thumfart, 1979).

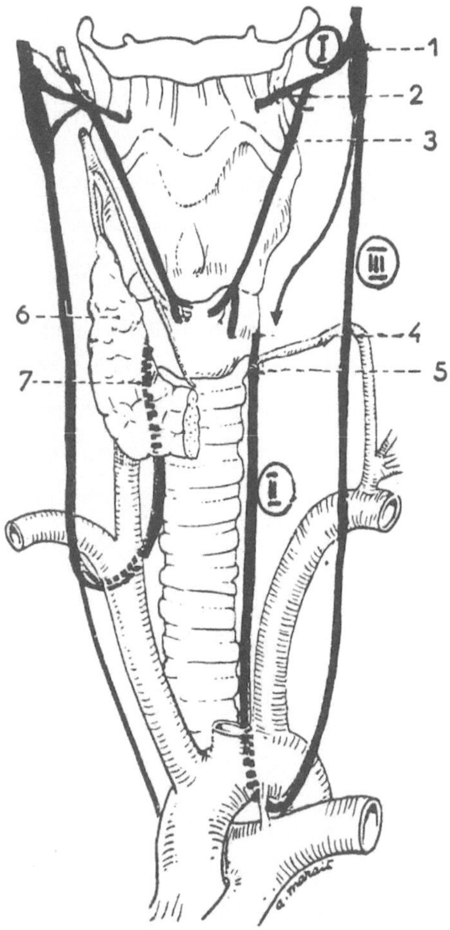

Fig. 9. Innervation and reflex pathways after stimulation (*I–III*) of the laryngeal nerves

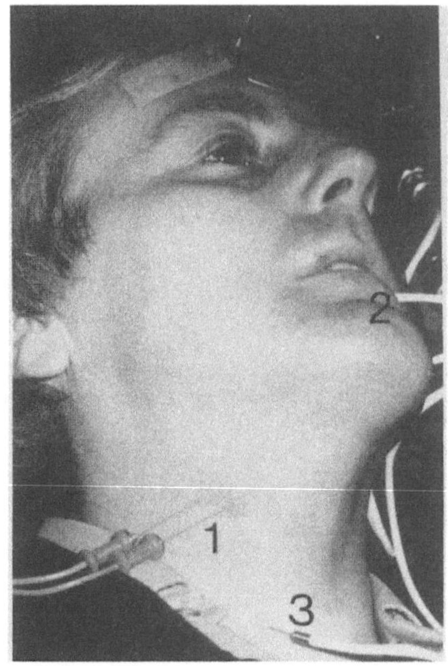

Fig. 10. Electroneurography of the larynx in the awake patient (*1* = stimulation electrodes; *2* = recording electrode in the vocal muscle; *3* = recording electrode in the cricothyroid muscle)

Results

Sixty patients with vocal cord paralysis were examined with this method. The findings were controlled one year after onset of the paralysis. In a first group of 12 patients initial neurography reveiled time intervals of about 6 ms or 18–22 ms, respectively, for the first and second answer. Ten of these 12 palsies recovered completely without signs of denervation or regeneration. They, therefore, were labelled as 'neurapraxia' or functional lesions. Two other showed no return of voluntary movements.

In 48 of the 60 cases of laryngeal palsy no electrical reflex activity could be observed in the first trial. At the second examination, one year later, there still were no reflex responses in 45, while three showed positive reflex activity with normal time intervals. The later patients had recurrence of glottic mobility, while the group of 45 palsies showed no improvement of laryngeal function.

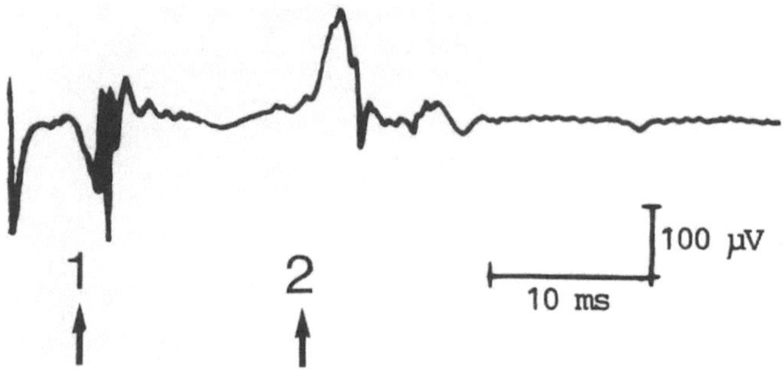

Fig. 11. Electroneurography of the cricothyroid muscle after stimulation of the superior laryngeal nerve (*1* = first response; *2* = second response)

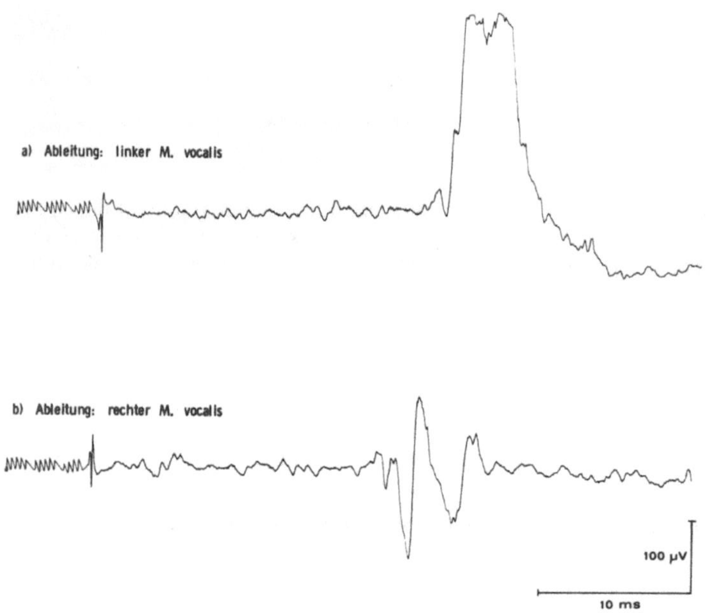

Fig. 12. Reflexactivity in the left and right vocal muscle after stimulation of the left superior laryngeal nerve

Discussion

From these experiments it may be concluded that electroneurography provides valuable additional help for the prediction of the spontaneous recovery of laryngeal nerve function.

As to the correlation between the regular EMG examination and electroneurography, Table 3 shows the figures of both, agreement (92 percent) and disagreement (8 percent) of these tests. Our material is still too limited to allow definite conclusion, but from these preliminary results it may be inferred that electrophysiological test procedures allow a representative prediction of the nerve lesion at a very early state. If you reconsider the fast process of muscular atropy after denervation (8 to 12 weeks after onset of the palsy), this early diagnosis provides better chances for functional nerve repair (Miehlke, 1974; Tucker, 1976; Wigand et al., 1969), than the traditional attitude of expecting control, which up to now has been the consequence of the laryngologist's lack of appropriate test procedures.

Table 3. Prognosis of neurography in laryngeal nerve palsy (1978/1979)

Functional palsies (concordant with EMG)	10 (17%)
Degenerative palsies (concordant with EMG)	45 (75%)
Functional palsies (discordant with EMG)	3 (5%)
Functional palsies (discordant with EMG and neurography)	2 (3%)
Total amount	60 (100%)

Summary

For the exact evaluation of a motor nerve dysfunction there is no better technique than electromyography and electroneurography. The development of new endoscopes has enabled the laryngologist to control the oropharyngeal and endolaryngeal muscles with direct inspection. The combination of the zoom-endoscope with needle electromyography now allows the separate investigation of the muscular agonists and antagonists in the awake patient. Both, spontaneous and voluntary activity, may be recorded.

Further, with electroneurography it has become possible to test the reflex pathway in order to localize the site of a lesion of the recurrent laryngeal nerve.

In a very similar way electrodiagnosis can be done in diseases of the glossopharyngeal, accessory and hypoglossal nerves.

References

Buchthal F (1959) Electromyography of Intrinsic Laryngeal Muscles. Q J Exp Physiol 44:137–144

Esslen E (1973) Electrodiagnosis of Facial Palsy. In: Surgery of the Facial Nerve. Urban-Schwarzenberg, München

Faaborg-Andersen K (1965) Electromyography of the Laryngeal Muscles in Humans. Technics and Results. Karger, Basel

Hirano O, Ohala J (1961) Use of Hooked-wire Electrodes for Electromyography of the Intrinsic Laryngeal Muscles. J Speech Hear Res 12:362–373

Miehlke A (1974) Rehabilitation of Vocal Cord Paralysis. Arch Otolaryngol 100:431–441

Satoh I (1978) Evoked Electromyography Test applied for Recurrent Laryngeal Nerve Paralysis. Laryngoscope 88:2022–2031

Steiner W (1978) Zoom-endoscopy of the Larynx. Endoscopy 1:148

v. Stuckradt H, Lakatos I (1975) Über ein neues Lupenendoskop (Pharyngoskop). Laryngol Rhinol Otol (Stuttg) 54:336–340

Thumfart W, Steiner W, Jaumann MP (1978) Lupenendoskopische Elektromyografie des M. crico-arythenoideus dorsalis (Posticus) am wachen Patienten. Arch Otorhinolaryngol (NY) 219:492

Thumfart W, Gschwandtner R (1979) Elektroneurografie des Nervus recurrens mittels lupenendoskopischer EMG-Ableitung aus dem Kehlkopf des wachen Patienten. Arch Otorhinolaryngol (NY) 223:281–283

Tucker HM (1976) Human laryngeal Reinnervation. Laryngoscope 86:769–779

Wigand ME, Naumann C, Hölldobler E (1969) Versuche zur Reinnervation des Abductormuskels nach Recurrenslähmung durch Einpflanzen freier Nerventransplantate zum N. phrenicus. Arch Otorhinolaryngol (NY) 194:372–376

Surgical Management of the Caudal Cranial Nerves

W. Draf, Fulda, and M. Samii, Hannover/FRG

Tumors of the petrous bone and the lateral posterior and middle skull base may involve the caudal cranial nerves primarily, also there is some risk to these important structures at operation. Pioneers of the field of extracranial surgery of the middle and hind skull base are Arena (1974), Conley (1965, 1970), Grunert (1894), House (1964, 1968), Rehn (1919), Zehm (1969) and others. Denecke (1953, 1959, 1960, 1969) has published many important surgical details. In 1967 Wullstein and Wullstein gave an excellent survey concerning the surgery of tumors of the ear.

Symptoms and Diagnosis (Table 1)

Benign and malignant tumors in this region can grow to a remarkable size without any clinical signs. Tumors around the jugular foramen quite often may present us with a unilateral paralysis of the vocal cords. Therefore it is useful to examine the vagus and recurrent nerves along their entire length during diagnostic working. In large tumors one can find disturbances of swallowing with deviation of the soft palate to the unaffected side as consequence of paralysis of the glossopharyngeal and vagus nerve.

Table 1. Tumors of the lateral posterior skull base symptoms

1. Jugular foramen syndromes (IX, X, XI)	4. Vestibular symptoms
2. Hypoglossal nerve paralysis	5. Facial nerve paralysis
3. Hearing loss, tinnitus	

In our experience patients can compensate for such a paralysis to a certain degree, if this develops slowly and is unilateral. Otherwise, we have seen severe problems due to aspiration in patients with sudden paralysis of the IXth and Xth nerve after cerebral vascular accident or a trauma. This was the same in patients with bilateral damage to the caudal nerves. Occasionally one can see an additional lesion of the spinal accesory nerve and the hypoglossal nerve causing speech problems. If the mastoid and petrous bones are involved by the tumor, the patient may suffer from hearing loss, tinnitus, vestibular symptoms, and paralysis of the facial nerve. Quite often one cannot decide if the tumor is localized extra- or intradurally or how extensive is an infiltration of the dura, which makes at least partial resection necessary. Therefore interdisciplinary teamwork of ENT- and neurosurgeons is advisable preoperatively and occasionally at operation.

Principles of Operative Technique

Benign tumors are exposed step by step. The resection of surrounding tissue should be done only as far as necessary for tumor removal and as sparingly as possible.

The first step is (Fig. 1) the exposure of important landmarks in the neck region: the internal jugular vein, the carotid artery and the caudal cranial nerves IX to XII. Depending on the size of the tumor it is possible to widen the surgical field by dissection of the sternocleidomastoid and the digastric muscle, and by resection of the styloid process and the mastoid. Sometimes it is necessary to remove the jugular bulb for a wider access to the anterior nervous part of the jugular foramen (Fig. 2). The facial nerve can be preserved after mobilizing it from the osseus channel.

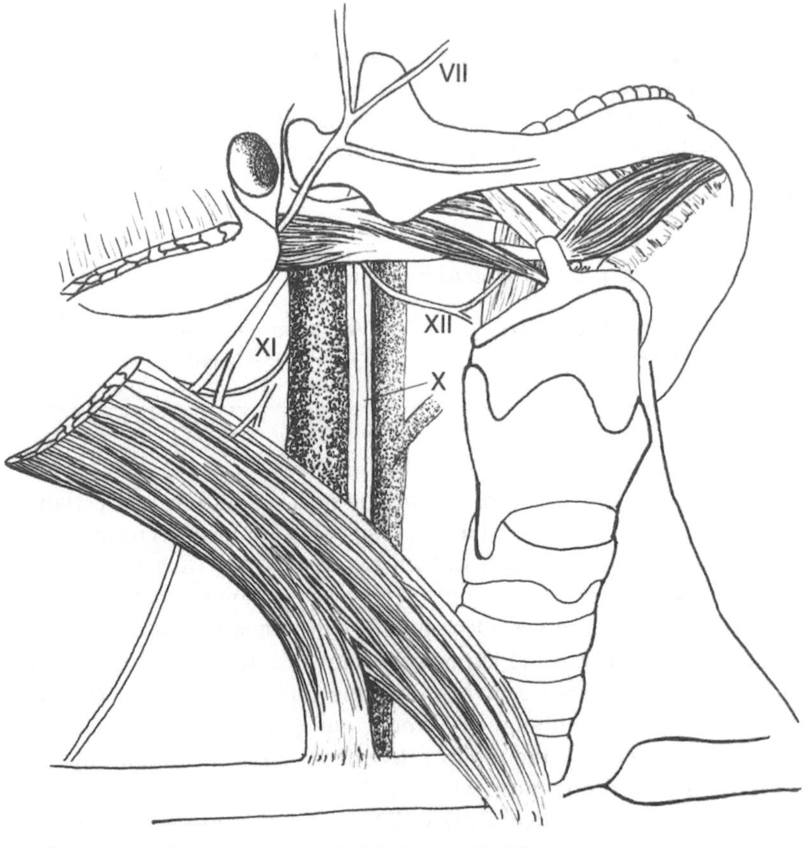

Fig. 1. Landmarks for tumor removal of the lateral skull base

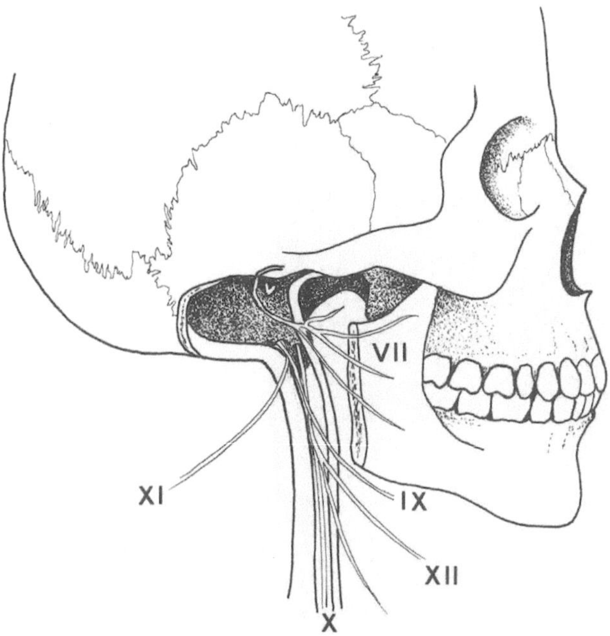

Fig. 2. Surgical field after partial resection of the temporal bone, exposure of the jugular bulb

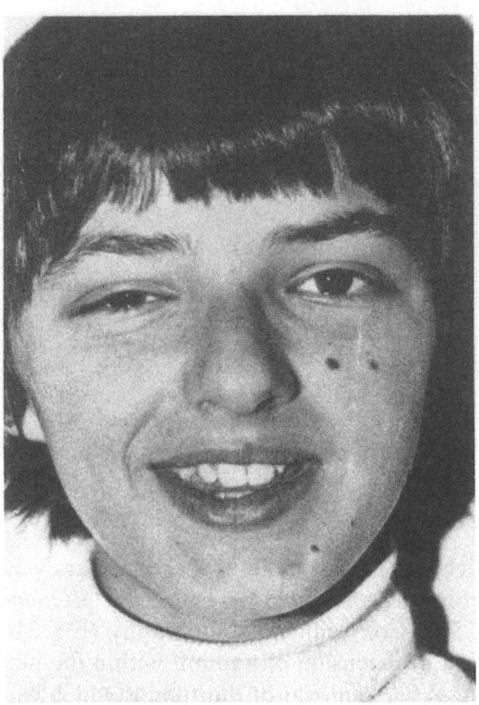

a

Fig. 3a–d. Large neurinoma of the left jugular foramen in a 15 year old boy. **a** Preoperatively, the paresis of the left mandibular branch of the facial nerve is visible. **b** X-ray-tomogramm: the *arrows* show the big osseus defect at the lateral skull base. **c** CT scan showing the tumor involving the left cerebellopontine angle. **d** The boy six weeks postoperatively. (For Fig. 3b and 3c we are grateful to Prof. Dr. S. F. Wende, Department of Neuroradiology of Mainz University Clinic)

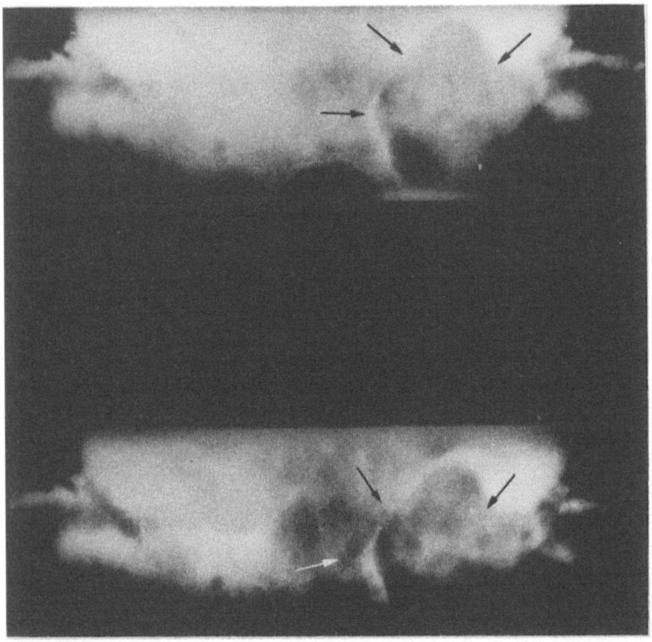

Fig. 3 b

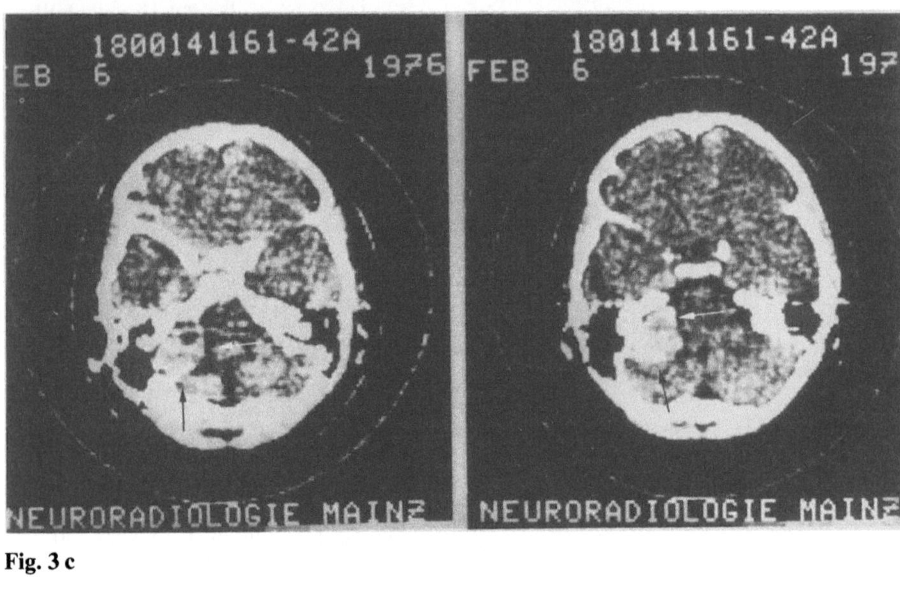

Fig. 3 c

Case Report

A 15 year old boy noticed hoarseness which was caused by left vocal cord paralysis. Three years later he developed deafness, tinnitus, and slight paresis of the left mandibular branch of the facial nerve (Fig. 3a). Conventional tomography (Fig. 3b) and the CT scan (Fig. 3c) demonstrated major extension of a tumor within the petrous bone and the cerebellopontine angle. After removal of the tumor, which was

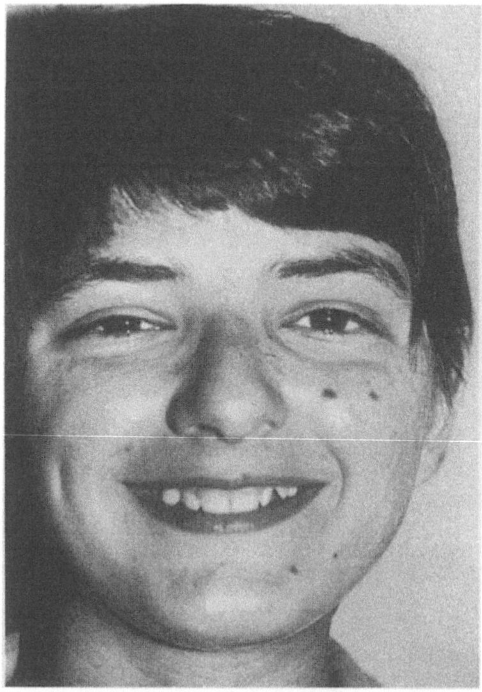

Fig. 3 d

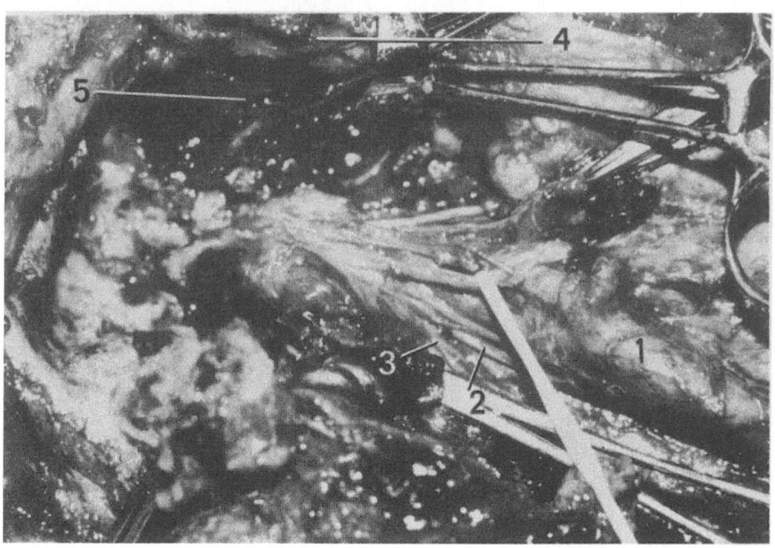

a

Fig. 4 a–d. Carcinoma of the right auditory channel. Block resection, including the petrous bone, radical parotidectomy and radical neck dissection **a** The tumor is outlined, the caudal cranial nerves and the vascular structures of the neck region are exposed (*1* = carotid artery, *2* = vagus nerve, *3* = accessory nerve, *4* = parotid gland, *5* = tumor region) **b** The tumor is removed and facial nerve grafting performed (*arrow*). 1 shows a flap of the temporal muscle to fill the cavity **c/d** The result one and a half years postoperatively

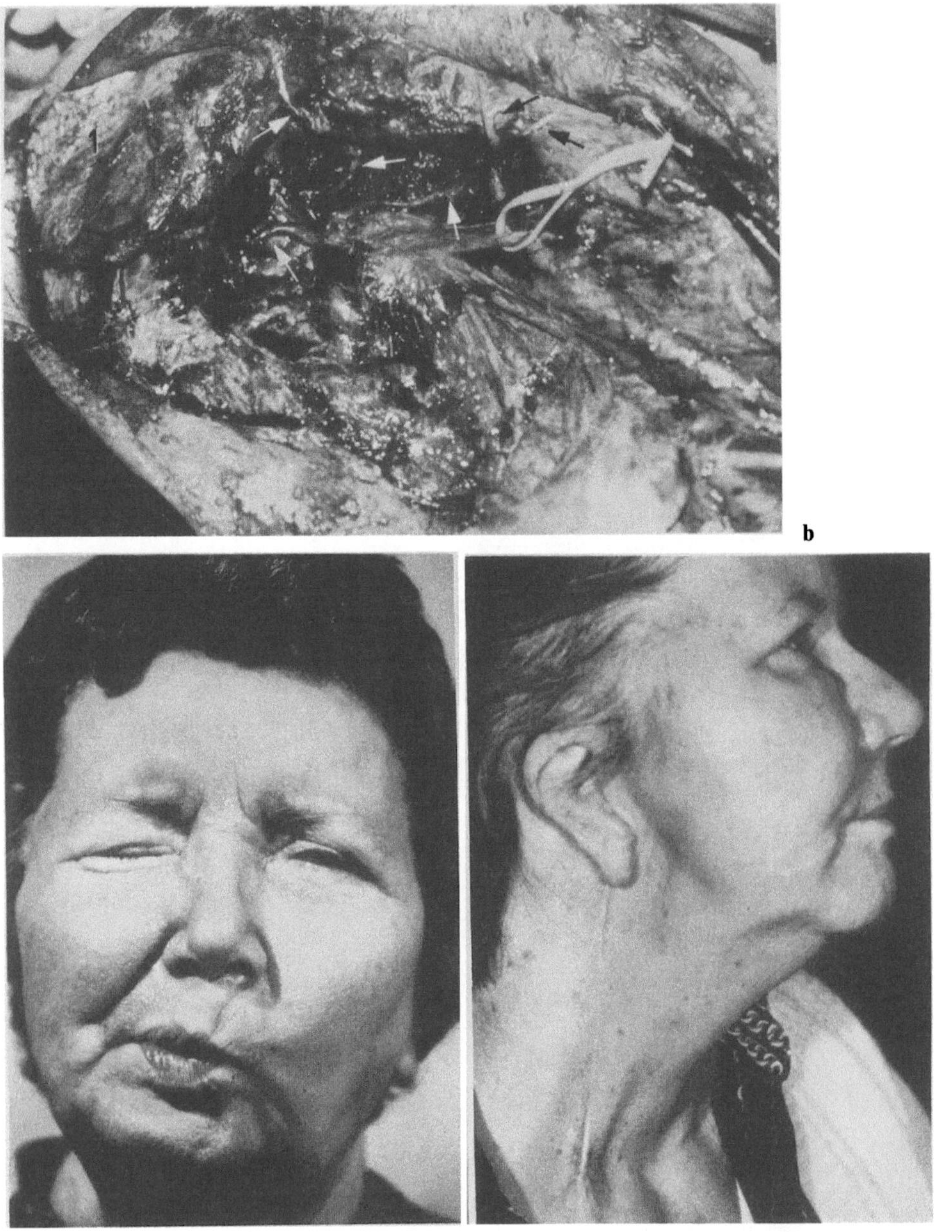

Fig. 4b–d

localized only extradurally and was diagnosed histologically as a neurinoma, the facial paresis disappeared (Fig. 3). The hearing loss and the paralysis of the vagus nerve remained unchanged. Pre- and postoperatively there was no disturbance of swallowing.

Radical removal of malignant tumors of this region (Fig. 4a/b) is justified if preservation of the internal carotid artery is expected.

Case Report

A woman suffered from a carcinoma of the right external auditory canal. A block-resection was performed which included the petrous bone and radical parotidectomy with resection of the facial nerve from the geniculate ganglion to its peripheral branches. The caudal cranial nerves were saved by careful partially microsurgical dissection. The facial nerve was reconstructed using a transplant from the cervical plexus.

One and a half years after operation the functional (Fig. 4c) and the esthetic result (Fig. 4d) were satisfactory. The caudal cranial nerves functioned normally.

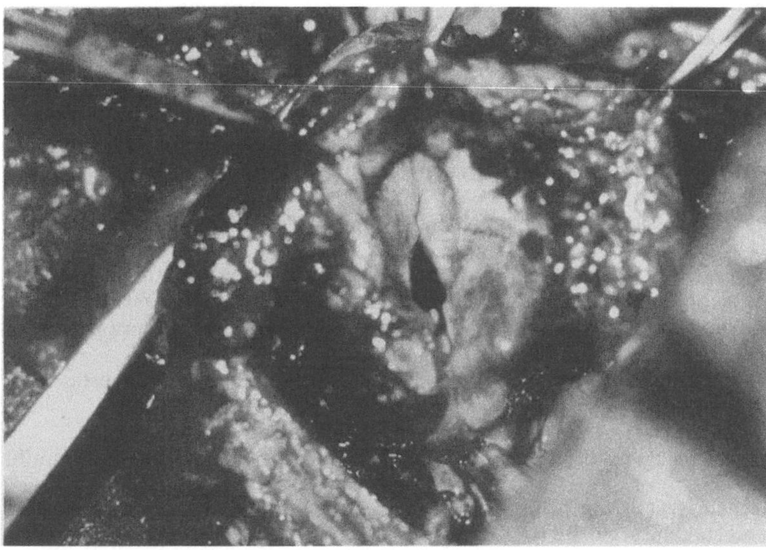

Fig. 5. Partial closure of the glottis in a patient with bilateral paralysis of the caudal cranial nerves

In the very rare cases of bilateral paralysis of the caudal cranial nerves with permanent danger of pneumonia caused by aspiration, the ENT-surgeon can improve the quality of life for the patient by performing a partial closure of the glottis. Thus aspiration is decreased remarkably and speaking is still possible when the tracheostomy is closed with a finger (Fig. 5).

For cases of sudden, unilateral paralysis of the caudal cranial nerves without spontaneous recovery of swallowing, Prof. Denecke developed a special surgical strategy. This is discussed below.

From our experiences we come to the following conclusions:

1. By using microsurgical techniques it is often possible to save the caudal cranial nerves during tumor surgery of the lateral skull base.
2. If the function of the vagus nerve was lost prior to surgery, we never achieved a recovery, although the nerve could be preserved structurally.

3. Permanent disturbances of swallowing were seen only after *sudden* lesions of the caudal cranial nerves, whereas the patients could always compensate a *slowly* developing paralysis.
4. The capacity of regeneration seems to be greater in paresis of the facial and the accessory nerve, compared to the vagus nerve.

References

Arena S (1974) Tumor Surgery of the Temporal Bone. Laryngoscope 84:645

Conley JJ, Novack AJ (1960) The surgical treatment of malignant tumors of the ear and temporal bone. Arch Otolaryngol 71:635–652

Conley JJ (1964) Tumors of the infratemporal fossa. Arch Otolaryngol 79:498

Conley JJ (1974) Cancer of the middle ear. In: Barbosa, Fairbanks J (eds). Surgical treatment of Head and Neck Tumors. Grune & Stratton, New York

Denecke HJ (1953) Die oto-rhino-laryngologischen Operationen. In: Kirschner v M (Hrsg) Allgemeine und spezielle Operationslehre, Bd V. Springer, Berlin Heidelberg New York

Denecke HJ (1959/60) Operationstechnische Probleme bei der Entfernung großer Neurinome im Bereich von Felsenbeinpyramide, N. facialis, Pharynx, Gefäßscheide, Ösophagusmund und Zunge. HNO 8:343

Denecke HJ (1969) Diskussionsbemerkung Nobel Symposium 10 Almquist and Wiksell, Stockholm

Fisch U (1976) Chirurgie im inneren Gehörgang und an benachbarten Strukturen. In: Naumann HH (Hrsg) Kopf- und Halschirurgie, Bd. III: Ohrregion. Thieme, Stuttgart

Grunert KA (1894) Die operative Ausräumung des Bulbus venae jugularis (Bulbusoperation). Arch Ohrenheilk 36:71

House WF (1964) Monograph I: Trans-temporal bone microsurgical removal of acoustic neuromas. Arch Otolaryngol 80:597

House WF (1968) Monograph II: Acoustic neuroma. Arch Otolaryngol 88:576

Rehn ED (1919) Die Freilegung der A. carotis interna in ihrem oberen Halsteil. Zentralbl Chir 17

Wullstein HL, Wullstein SR (1976) Chirurgie der Tumoren des Mittelohres. In: Naumann HH (Hrsg) Kopf- und Halschirurgie. Bd III: Ohrregion. Thieme, Stuttgart

Zehm S (1969) The surgical approach to the external part of the base of the skull related to the anterior and medial cranial fossa. Nobel Symposium 10. Almquist and Wiksell, Stockholm

On the Pathogenesis, Treatment and Prognosis of Lesions of the Vagus Nerve

J. Menzel and H. J. Denecke, Heidelberg/FRG

Lesions of the vagus nerve have devastating effects on the vital functions of coughing, swallowing, and phonation. Therefore, early diagnosis and appropriate treatment are important to the otolaryngologist as to the neurosurgeon. As in other central nervous system disorders, the anatomic defects can be divided into supranuclear, nuclear, and peripheral vagal lesions. The aim of the present paper is to demonstrate the consequences of nuclear and peripheral vagal lesions.

The distribution of the vagal nuclei in the brainstem is demonstrated in the first Figure (Fig. 1). The most important causes of vagal lesions in this area are represented in Table 1. For the neurosurgeon, tumors involving the lower brainstem occur most frequently. Signs and symptoms of nuclear vagal lesions are listed in Table 2. Dysphonia is caused by unilateral vocal cord paralysis. Coughing is diminished and associated with the danger of aspiration. Swallowing is complicated or impossible.

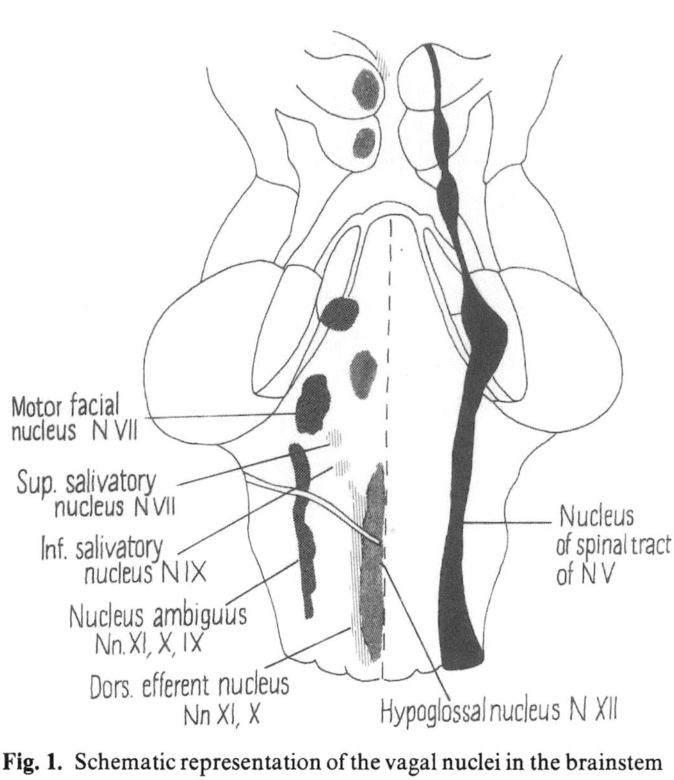

Fig. 1. Schematic representation of the vagal nuclei in the brainstem

We have analyzed a group of six patients with tumors arising from the floor of the fourth ventricle or from the lower brainstem: three ependymomas, two epidermoids, and one arterio-venous malformation. In all patients radical tumor extirpation was attempted, and in all cases nuclear vagal nerve lesions occured postoperatively in spite of microsurgical technique. All patients died within two to eight weeks after the operation. Cause of death was severe pneumonia after aspiration in four cases. Two patients died of central cardiac dysregulation.

The course of the peripheral part of the vagus nerve is demonstrated in Figure 2. The etiology[1] is listed in Table 3. We have to differentiate those that are high and those that are low, relative to the take off of the pharyngeal and superior laryngeal nerves. For the neurosurgeon, tumors in the jugular foramen are the most frequent and the most important causes of peripheral vagal lesions. Signs and symptoms are listed in Table 4. Ineffective coughing associated with aspiration is life threatening. We have analyzed a series of 22 patients with peripheral vagal nerve lesions (Table 5). Among 12 patients with extensive glomus jugulare tumors (Fig. 3) seven had signs of unilateral vagal nerve lesion before the intervention. Symptoms were aggravated in all cases postoperatively and surgical repair was necessary in five patients. All patients with neuroma of the jugular foramen (Fig. 4) had signs of vagal

1 = of peripheral vagal lesions

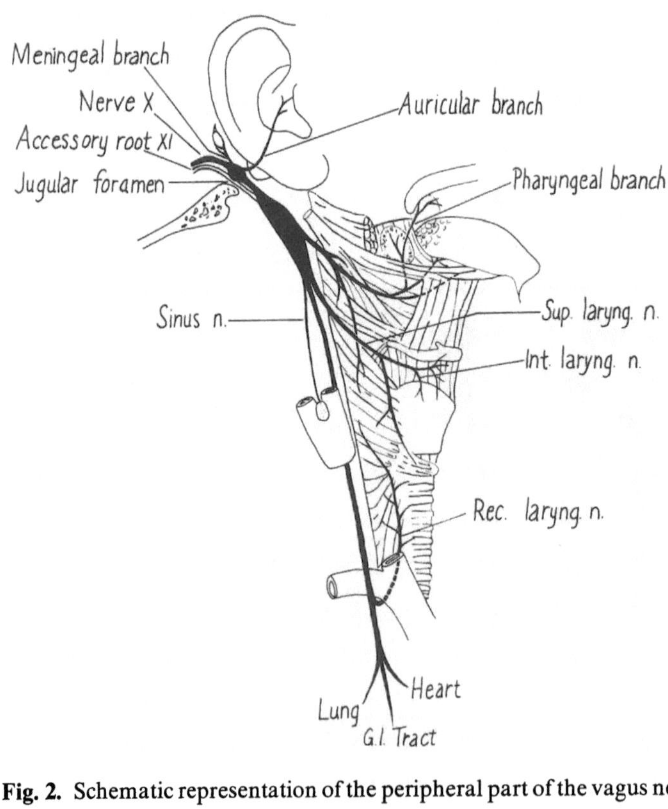

Fig. 2. Schematic representation of the peripheral part of the vagus nerve

nerve lesion preoperatively. Surgical therapy became indispensable after the extirpation of the tumor in all cases. In a case of angioma of the jugular foramen (Fig. 5) vagal nerve palsy disappeared two months after the operation. In three patients with extensive acoustic neuroma (Fig. 6) operative repair was necessary.

The surgical therapy begins with tracheostomy immediately after tumor extirpation when the inability of swallowing and coughing is clear. We prefer the

Table 1. Etiology of nuclear vagal lesions

Inflammatory:	Poliomyelitis, Guillain-Barré, diphteria tabes dorsalis, MS
Vascular:	Thrombosis, hemorrhage, angioma
Trauma	
Neoplasms:	Primary, metastatic
Congenital:	Arnold-Chiari, Klippel-Feil, Dandy-Walker
Progressive bulbar palsy	

Table 2. Signs and symptoms in nuclear vagal lesions

Voice:	Dysphonia secondary to unilateral cord paralysis
Cough:	Diminished effectiveness with aspiration
Swallowing:	Dysphagia
Other:	Hearing loss, vertigo, nystagmus, ataxia, paresis

Table 3. Etiology of peripheral vagal lesions

Inflammatory:	Meningitis, polyneuritis, diphteria
Vascular:	Hemorrhage, aneurysm
Trauma:	Skull fractures
Neoplasms:	Foraminal neoplasia: meningioma, neuroma, glomus jugulare tumor
Toxic causes	

Table 4. Signs and symptoms in peripheral vagal lesions

Voice:	Unilateral vocal cord paralysis
Cough:	Ineffective and associated with aspiration
Swallowing:	Dysphagia
Other:	Hypoglossal nerve paralysis, palatal paralysis, Horner's syndrome

Table 5. Etiology of peripheral vagal lesions

		Op. after Denecke
Glomus jugulare tumor:	12	5
Neuroma of the jugular foramen:	3	3
Angioma of the jugular foramen:	1	–
Extensive acoustic neuroma:	6	3

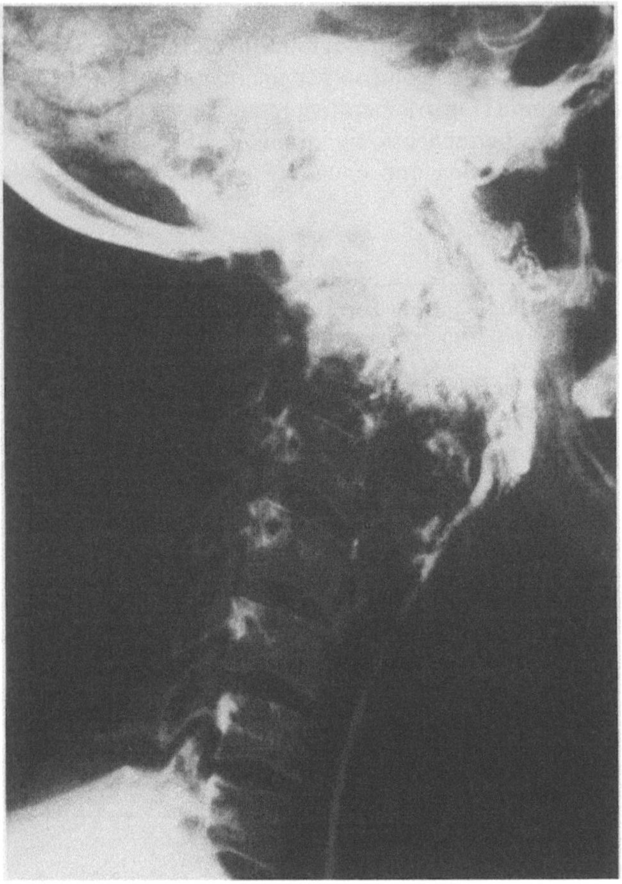

Fig. 3. Angiographic representation of an extensive glomus jugulare tumor

epithelized tracheostoma following the rules of plastic surgery. According to Soerensen (1930) the entire tracheostoma is lined with skin. Denecke (1977) modified and improved the technique using skin from the anterior thoracic wall. This procedure prevents complications such as tracheal stenosis and hemorrhage.

The recovery of coughing, swallowing and phonation is performed in four steps:

1. First, myotomy of the pars fundiformis of the cricopharyngeal muscle and division of the circular muscle fibers of the cervical esophagus are performed.
2. The second step consists of glottal repair with insertion of a cartilage implant into the paralyzed vocal cord and rotation of the arytenoid cartilage to attain a midline position of the vocal cord.
3. In the third step the atrophic pharyngeal wall is resected from the introitus of the esophagus up to the tonsil and the pharyngeal defect is sutured.
4. The final step is the fixation of the velum palatini to the posterior pharyngeal wall.

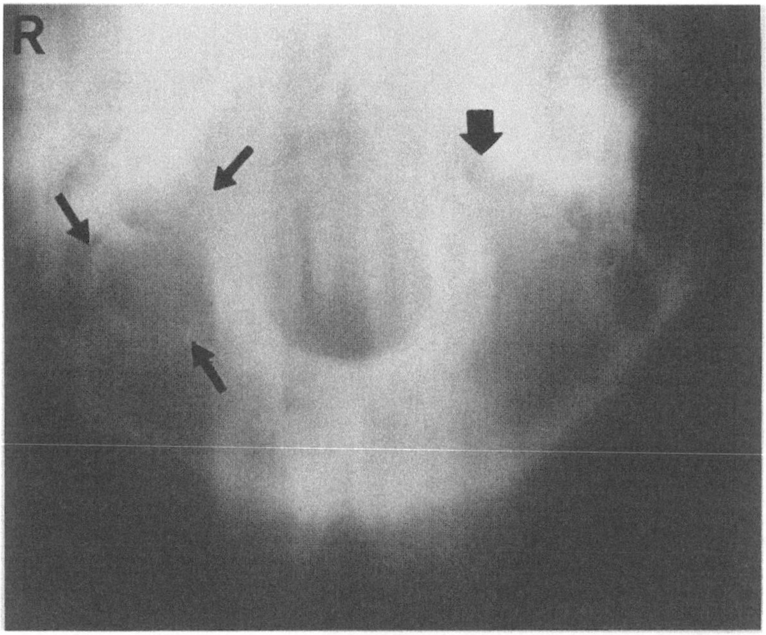

Fig. 4. Neuroma of the right jugular foramen (*small arrows*); normal size of the left jugular foramen (*big arrow*)

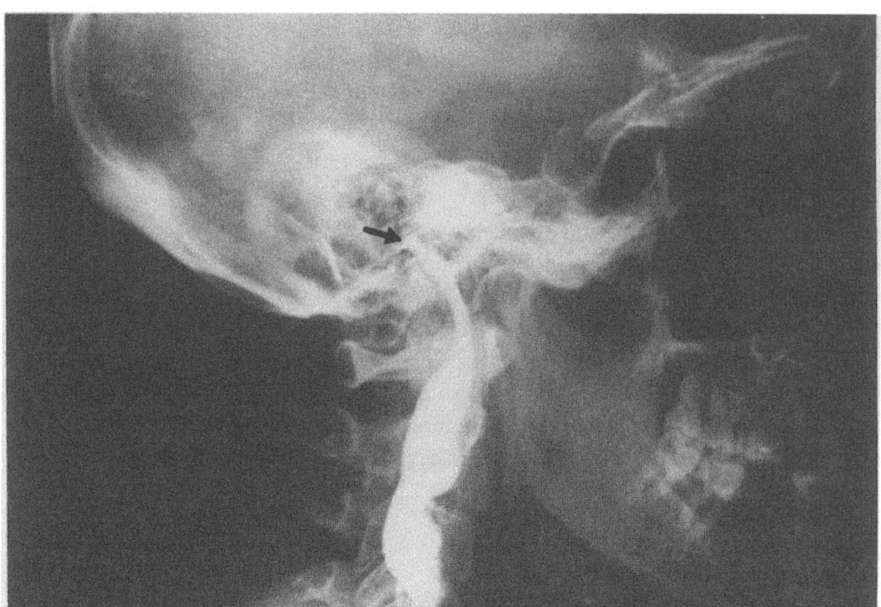

Fig. 5. Angioma of the right jugular foramen with occlusion of the internal jugular vein

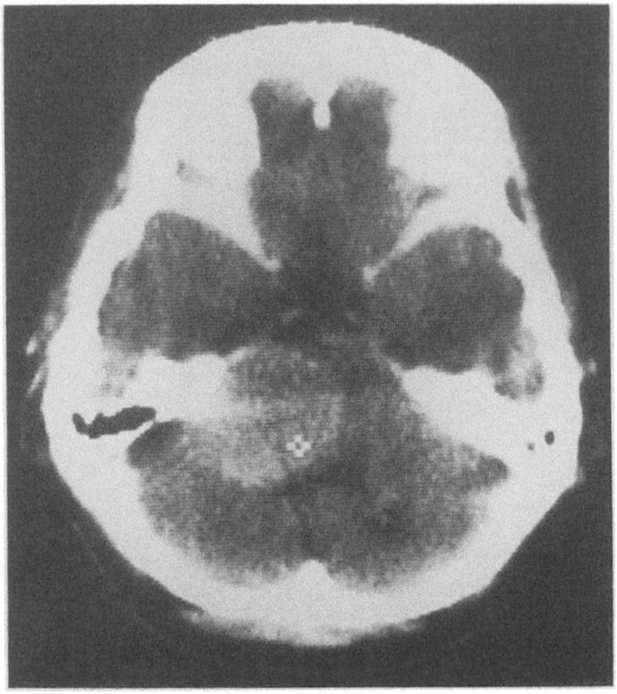

Fig. 6. Extensive acoustic neuroma

We have operated upon 12 patients in the described manner. We had no mortality. Eight patients are able to practice their former occupation. Three patients had to change their profession, but they are able to work. Phonation is good in all cases. No recurrence of the basic disease was observed to present.

In conclusion we can say:

1. Nuclear vagal lesions of tumor origin have a poor prognosis. In our series of six patients, all died after radical tumor extirpation. Therefore, we recommend subtotal extirpation with subsequent CSF shunt and/or irradiation.
2. Peripheral unilateral vagal lesions have a better prognosis. They must be diagnosed as early as possible and treated in the described manner. In our series of 12 patients we had no mortality. Longterm follow up demonstrates excellent results.
3. Neurosurgical-otolaryngeal teamwork is the basis for operative treatment of extensive tumors in the posterior fossa and especially in the jugular foramen.

References

Denecke HJ (1977) Plastische Korrektur des Schluckaktes und der Stimme bei Vaguslähmung HNO 25: 140–143

Soerensen J (1930) Die Mund- und Halsoperationen. Urban und Schwarzenberg, Berlin, Wien

Percutaneous and Selective Radiofrequency Thermocoagulation of Essential Glossopharyngeal Neuralgia

F. ISAMAT and E. FERRAN, Barcelona/Spain

Since the introduction by Sweet [4] of radiofrequency percutaneous, selective, and differential thermocoagulation of the gasserian ganglion as a neurosurgical treatment for trigeminal neuralgia, this technique has been successfully used in hundreds of patients.

Essential glossopharyngeal neuralgia is another extremely painful syndrome, although not as common as trigeminal neuralgia [2]. One glossopharyngeal neuralgia was considered to come in every 500 trigeminal neuralgias, but the special interest in the treatment of facial pain in certain neurosurgical clinics has led to the more realistic ratio of one in every 70 in the series of Tew [5]; and 1 in 100 in our own clinic.

Due to the lack of morbidity, good tolerance and satisfactory results obtained with RF thermocoagulation in our cases of trigeminal neuralgias we decided to use this technique in essential glossopharyngeal neuralgias, finding out only afterwards that Tew [5] had had the same idea. Since then Broggi and Siegfried [1] and Lazorthes [3] have also reported their own experiences. Nonetheless the cases published by all these authors (6, 2 and 12 respectively) were all, but for three, facial pain with glossopharyngeal nerve involvement due to cancer of the oropharynx or the base of the skull. And in the only three reported cases of real glossopharyngeal neuralgia – 2 of Tew [5] and one of Lazorthes [3] – although the operation was succesful regarding pain, deglutition and phonation deteriorated due to injury of the vagus nerve; and this to an extent that Tew stated that 'this procedure should be reserved for patients with pain of neoplasmic origin'. We think this an important point and in our opinion a questionable one. A selective and an isolated glossopharyngeal lesion in the petrous ganglion of Andersh at the exit of the jugular foramen without involvement of the vagus nerve was obtained in our cases where this technique was applied.

Three patients with essentially idiopathic glossopharyngeal neuralgia have been operated upon in our clinic using RF thermocoagulation. All of them were screened

Table 1. Case 1

- Female
- 52 years
- 6 months of neuralgic pain in left pharynx and external auditory canal
- Trigger with swallowing (acids)
- Positive initial response to Tegretol ineffective for the last 3 months
- Parenteral feeding 1 month

Table 2. Case 2

- Female
- 61 years
- 4 years: First isolated neuralgic pain in left pharynx
- 3½ years: Repeated mild neuralgic pain in left pharynx and external auditory canal during 6 months. Swallowing as trigger
- 1 year: Severe neuralgic pain with loss of consciousness. Tegretol
- 6 months: 'Continuous' painful crisis in left pharynx. Tegretol ineffective

Table 3. Case 3

- Male
- 58 years
- 15 years: Neuralgic periodical pain in left pharynx, tonsil, and external auditory canal. Swallowing as trigger. Tegretol
- 3 years: Microsurgical cerebello-pontine angle exploration and reported fiber section. No sensory loss. Some improvement but with mild crisis. Tegretol
- 2 years: Periodical severe neuralgic pain besides Tegretol
- 5 months: 'Continuous' painful crisis in left pharynx, tonsil, and external auditory canal. Tegretol ineffective

in order to rule out a secondary etiology by neurological examination, plain and tomographic X-ray, computerized tomography, ENT and cavum examinations, and EKG studies. All of the patients were treated previously by Tegretol with a positive response at the beginning, but without effect later on. And in the most recent case a cerebellopontine surgical exploration with nerve decompression and reported fibers section had been previously performed in another European hospital, without solution of the pain. The summaries of their histories are presented in Tables 1, 2, and 3.

Technique

Percutaneous and selective radiofrequency thermocoagulation of the petrous ganglion is performed with the patients placed in the supine position on the Mimer III X-ray table, taking advantage the mobility of the tube and the incorporated image amplifier (Fig. 1). The patient is monitorized, with constant recording of the electrocardiogram, and of the intra-arterial blood pressure by means of a Statham P-23, during the whole procedure. This monitoring is essential for a selective glossopharyngeal lesion, since any current spreading to the other jugular foramen structures, and particularly any possible interference with the vagus nerve, will be rapidly detected by bradycardia and hypotension (Figs. 2–3). Propanid is used for short lasting anesthesia during the painful moments of the operation.

A 7.0 mm active surface electrode is introduced by a puncture placed 35 mm lateral and 0.5 mm below the labial angle. The electrode is directed, with the help of the operator's finger and located into the patient's mouth, at the pterigoid fossa, some 20 degrees more posteriorly than for a gasserian puncture, with the external targets being the pupil and the external auditory meatus planes. Following this introduction and upon obtaining a bony resistance, lateral and oblique X-rays pictures are indispensable. For the oblique projection the X-ray beam is centered fol-

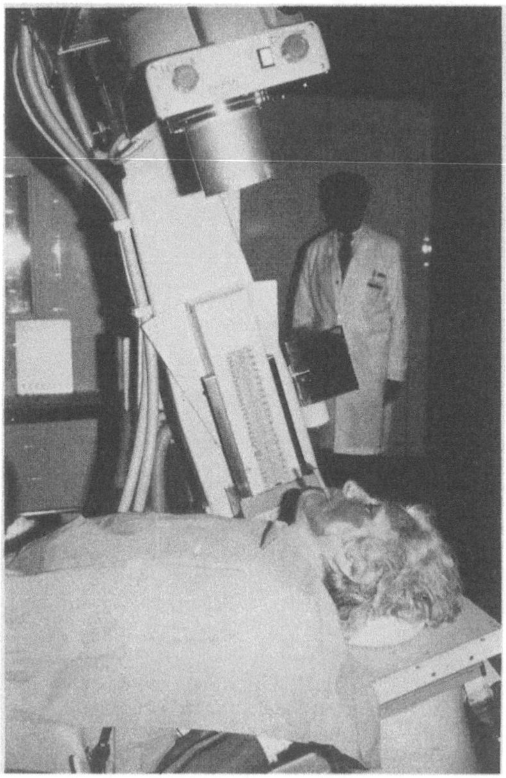

Fig. 1. Situation of the patient for RF thermocoagulation at the Mimer III X-ray

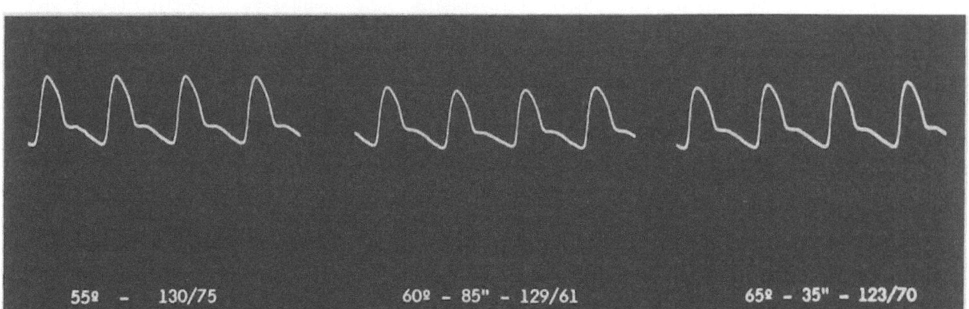

Fig. 2. Selective glossopharyngeal lesion. No vagal response

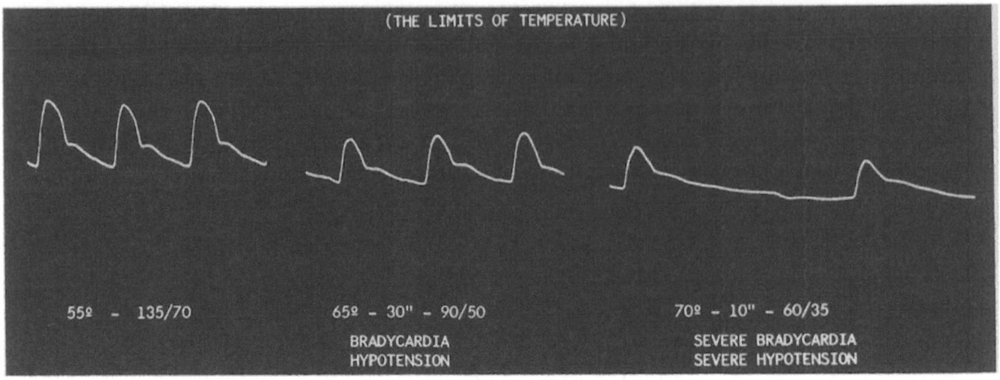

Fig. 3. Vagal interference during the heating pretest for thermocoagulation of the petrous ganglion

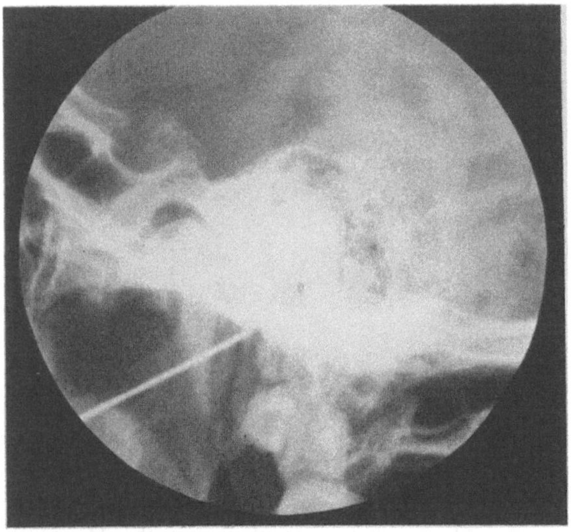

Fig. 4. Lateral projection with the electrode's tip at the jugular foramen

lowing the electrode axis. The jugular foramen is visualized and the pertinent corrections of the electrode, in order to place the tip at the part nervosa of the foramen, are done under fluroscopy with the image amplifier and a set of new radiograms (Figs. 4–5).

At this point physiological control of the positioning of the electrode must take place. For this we first use low voltage stimulation followed by a thermocoagulation pretest (Radionics, RFG-5, Burlington, Mass.). Stimulation with 0.1 to 0.3 volts should induce localized dypesthesias in hemipharynx, tonsil, and external auditory canal. There should not be spinal accessory motor response nor alterations in blood pressure or EKG recordings. The electrode is modified if needed until the above physiological parameters are obtained.

Prior to the definitive RF lesion a thermocoagulation pretest is performed with the patients fully awake to check for spread of heat and involvement of the vagus nerve. This point is of vital importance. A slow continuous rise in temperature is conducted, and if no modifications in blood pressure and heart rate is recorded up to 65–70 degrees the chances for an isolated selective glossopharyngeal lesion should be adequate. But if vagal response is elicited (bradycardia – hypotension) the test is stopped at once. The highest temperature just before the onset of the vagal effect will be the one to use, to avoid postoperative vagal response.

For a definitive RF thermocoagulation we have used a temperature from 65° C to 70° C for 60 seconds in the cases with no vagal response. And since the highest temperature just prior to the vagal response was 60° C in one patient, this temperature, plus prolongation of the time to 90 seconds, was sufficient for an adequate result.

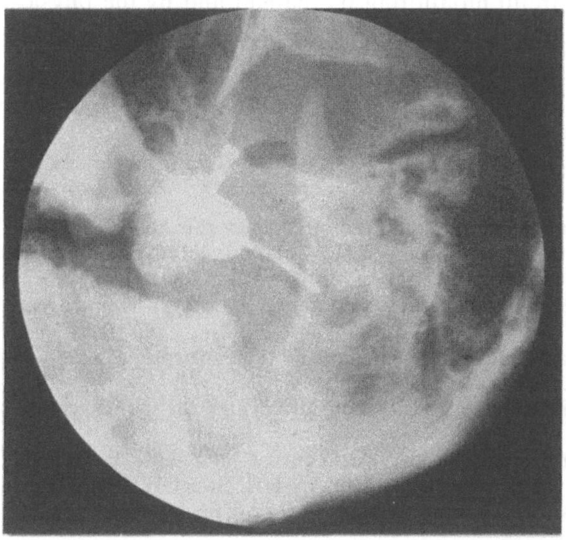

Fig. 5. Oblique projection: Electrode at pars nervosa of the jugular foramen

Conclusions

The three patients treated by this technique obtained a complete disappearance of the neuralgic pain, maintaining normal deglutition and phonation. In two patients a slight hypoalgesia of the external auditory canal and tragus was present postoperatively. No complications were encountered, and the patients have been free from pain and without medication for 18, six and two months respectively (Table 4).

Radiofrequency thermocoagulation of the petrous ganglion has been demonstrated to be of value in secondary glossopharyngeal neuralgias due to cancer of the oral cavity and base of the skull [1, 3, 5]. Essential glossopharyngeal neuralgias can also be treated by this technique, a non-aggressive, non-open neurosurgical pro-

Table 4

Case no	Pretest for vagal response	Final RF lesion	Results			Follow up
			Sensory loss	Compli-cations	9th pain free	Months
1	no	65 °C – 60 s 70 °C – 60 s	Ext. audit. canal	no	complete	18
2	yes at 65 °C	60 °C – 90 s	ext. audit. canal	no	complete	6
3	no	70 °C – 60 s	no	no	complete	2

cedure. The problem of interference during thermocoagulation of the petrous ganglion of the neighbouring structures at the jugular foramen, particulary the vagus nerve, can be avoided by careful monitoring the patient and by the physiological control and surgical technique described above. A painfree patient without side-effects can be the result of this operation.

References

1. Broggi G, Siegfried J (1979) Percutaneous differential radiofrequency rhizotomy of glossopharyngeal nerve in facial pain due to cancer. In: Bonica JJ, Ventafidda V (eds) Advances in Pain Research and Therapy, vol 2, New York, Raven Press, pp 469–473
2. Dandy WE (1927) Glossopharyngeal neuralgia (tic douloureux): Its diagnosis and treatment. Arch Surg 15: 198–214
3. Lazorthes Y, Verdie JC (1979) Radiofrequency coagulation of the petrous ganglion in glossopharyngeal neuralgia. Neurosurgery 4: 512–516
4. Sweet WH (1976) Treatment of facial pain by percutaneous differential thermal trigeminal rhizotomy. Prog Neurol Surg 7: 153–179
5. Tew JM Jr (1977) Percutaneous rhizotomy in the treatment of intractable facial pain (trigeminal, glossopharyngeal, and vagus nerves). In: Scmidek HH, Sweet WH (eds) Current Techniques in Operative Neurosurgery. Grune Stratton, New York pp 409–426

Shunt-Operations for the Recurrent Laryngeal Nerve

A. Miehlke and R. Arold, Göttingen/FRG

I would like to point out from the very beginning that we are with this work in the status nascendi, so to speak, and so I cannot tell if the whole concept can be accepted. But this is the fate of every new idea.

Reconstruction of the served recurrent laryngeal nerve has become possible in the era of microsurgery. These operations may become a task of the near future. When dealing with them we enter new ground on which there is as yet very little experience. Experimental and clinical research is of utmost importance in this field, since we know that the recurrent laryngeal nerve is damaged by the surgeon during 0.3 to 9.4 percent of all thyroidectomies especially in reoperations. This nerve is also increasingly often severed in traffic accidents.

In my discusion I shall present the experimental steps of research for the development of a new type of microsurgical technique at the peripheral vagus-recurrent-neuron. I shall describe how this surgical technique was finally applied in man, and I shall call your attention to success and draw-backs in the first operated patient. You will hear how these draw-backs can be overcome.

In 1967, I conducted, together with my collaborators Dal Ri, Schmidt, Haubrich, and Schätzle, for the first time animal experiments concerning the reconstitution of recurrent nerve function. Experiments in dogs had the aim to isolate from the medial segment of the vagus trunk the recurrent nerve which is already preformed and well recognizable at the level of the larynx, and to anastomose it with the recurrent nerve stump near the larynx. In eight out of 10 dogs, reinnervation of the vocal cord could be demonstrated by electrophysiological studies as well as by histological and histochemical findings.

The following restrictions had to be made concerning the possible utilization of this vagus-recurrent nerve shunt developed by me, as far as its application in rehabilitation surgery in man was concerned:

The experimental studies do not indicate whether the various types of recurrent nerve fibers which are different for glottis opening and glottis closing can correctly find their appropriate neuromuscular connections during regeneration. It had rather to be assumed that, due to undirected reinnervation, the complicated cooperations of the inner larynx musculature during respiration and phonation could not be regained by this vagus-recurrent nerve shunt. Therefore the next logical step had to be to achieve simultaneously the denervation of all glottis-closing muscles and controlled reinnervation of the only glottis opener, that is, of the posticus muscle.

On this basis the vagus-recurrent shunt was further developed by anastomosing exclusively to the posterior branch of the recurrent nerve with simultaneous elimination of all other recurrent nerve fibers. We called this more sophisticated operation principle 'the vagus-recurrent nerve plasty, type ramus posterior shunt'. In 1973 I employed this technique in a patient for the first time. Concerning functional

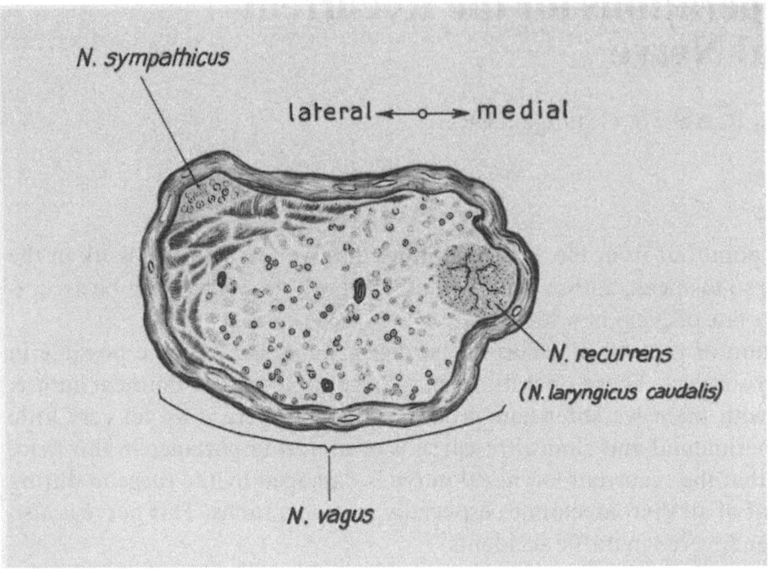

Fig. 1. Cross-section through the dog vagus nerve at the level of the larynx (From Chase and Ranson 1940)

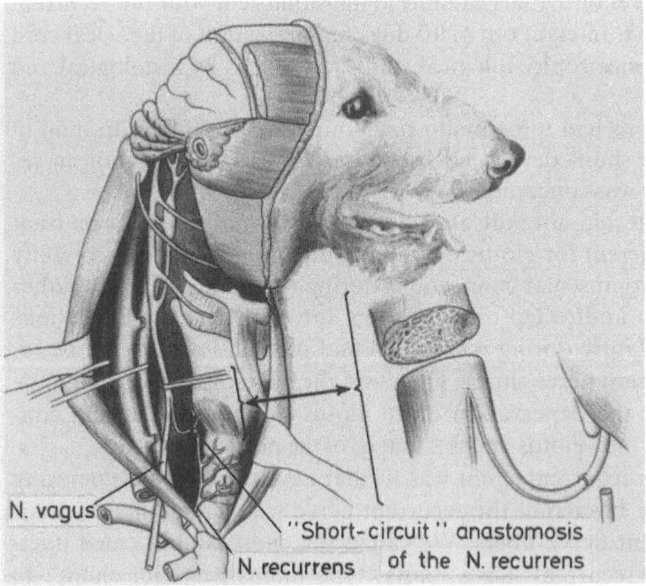

Fig. 2. Vagus recurrent nerve plasty (recurrent bypass anastomosis). (From Miehlke 1967)

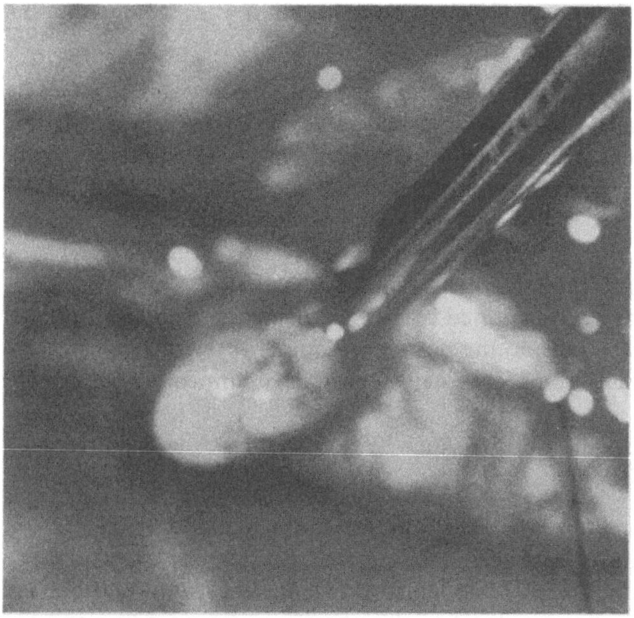

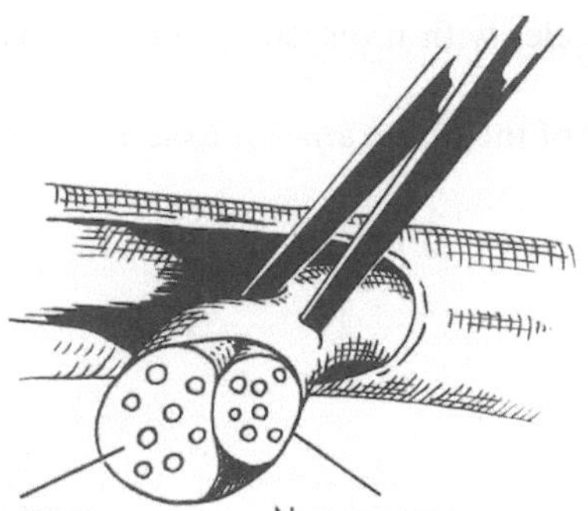

Fig. 3. Transection of the Vagus Nerve in a human being. Note the separate fascicles of the recurrent laryngeal nerve

recovery, however, only partial success was achieved. Not only clinical experience, but also findings from animal experiments showed that an isolated reinnervation of only the abductory larynx musculature does not at all result in satisfactory adduction of the arytenoid cartilage, by contractive action at the intact cricothyreoid muscle via ramus externis, the prerequisite of phonation. The functional outcome of a recurrent nerve plasty of the ramus posterior shunt type therefore approximately equals that which is to be expected after latero-fixation operations of the vocal cord.

On the basis of these findings, my collaborator R. Arold started another series of animal experiments together with his colleagues Schmidt and Dal Ri (Göttingen), with the aim of achieving separate reinnervation of the abductory as well as the adductory musculature. I wish to report here briefly on the results of these studies.

After transection of the recurrent nerve in dogs, reconstruction was performed in the following different ways:

1. Phrenic-recurrent nerve plasty, the so-called 'type ramus posterior shunt'. The phrenic nerve was extralaryngeally anastomosed to the recurrent trunk. The adductor-innervating terminal branch of the recurrent nerve was intralaryngeally exposed and cut through, so that regeneration at the axons of the phrenic nerve could proceed selectively into the posticus muscle, via the recurrent trunk and the posterior ramus.
2. Vagus-recurrent nerve plasty, the so-called 'type ramus anterior shunt'. Selective reinnervation of adductors was performed by anastomosing the recurrent portion, prepared from the cervical vagus, to the peripheric stump of the intralaryngeally transected adductory branch of the recurrent nerve (anterior ramus).

Investigations on the reinnervation of the inner laryngeal muscles were performed after 16 to 21 months in the following way:

1. Direct laryngoscopy of vocal cord movements at respiration and phonation.
2. Electromyography of the inner laryngeal muscles.
3. Electrical stimulation of the vagus proximal to the vagus-recurrent anastomosis and the ascending recurrent nerve distal to the phrenic-recurrent nerve anastomosis.
4. Electromyography of the inner laryngeal muscles with transection of the afferent nerves.
5. Histological and histochemical investigations of the nerve anastomosis and of the inner laryngeal musculature.

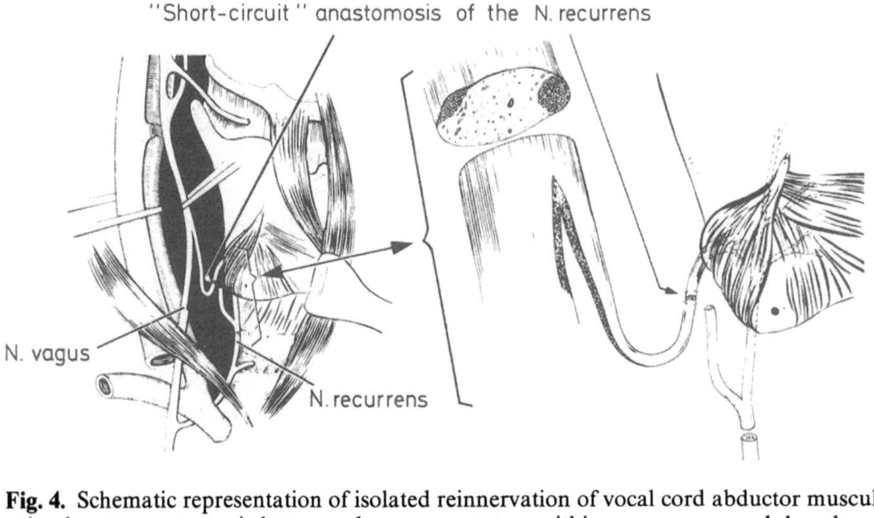

Fig. 4. Schematic representation of isolated reinnervation of vocal cord abductor musculature, using bypass anastomosis between the recurrent stem within vagus nerve and dorsal ramus of the caudal laryngeal nerve. (From Miehlke 1974)

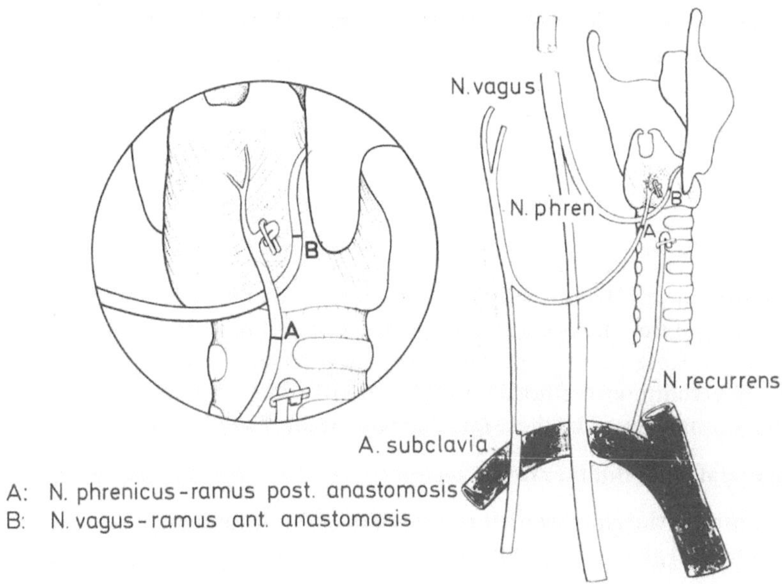

Fig. 5. Combined Phrenicus – Ramus post – Anastomose with Vagus – Ramus ant. – Anastomose. Diversification-technique (From Arold 1980) (for explanation see text)

The reconstitution of conductivity of the phrenic-recurrent nerve anastomosis with selective reinnervation of the posticus muscle could be demonstrated in all animals. This could also be achieved in the same way with the vagus-recurrent nerve anastomosis for the specific adductors.

Despite the demonstrated reinnervation of the inner laryngeal musculature, the extent of adductory and abductory movements was different and dependent upon intensity of phonation and respiration, so that in most cases opening and closing movement identical to the unimpaired vocal cord was observed only during forced respiration and phonation. In some animals it was possible to demonstrate only an increased resting tone of the inner laryngeal muscles, but unequivocal return of adductory or abductory function. The experimental results show clearly that reinnervation of abductor and adductors can be achieved using the vagus nerve, on the one hand, and the phrenic nerve on the other, and that this reinnervation can also be sufficiently controlled in respect to phase-synchronicity.

We call this experimentally developed operation-technique 'the diversification method' because we are working diversifying with two donor nerves. This method is now ready for clinical application.

Functional Rehabilitation of the Denervated Larynx; Concept and Consequence

M. E. WIGAND, Erlangen/FRG

While unilateral recurrent nerve paralysis does not offer severe problems to the patient but a hoarse voice, bilateral palsy of the vocal cords requires definite and often immediate surgical treatment because of obstruction of the glottic air way. For those cases with irreversible nerve impairment the surgical laterofixation of one or both vocal cords is a common method, but phonation is deteriorated to the same degree as inspiration is improved by these mutilating procedures.

An ideal functional rehabilitation would restore:

- automatical opening of the glottis with the onset of inspiration, and
- adequate closure of the glottis during the phase of phonation.

All types of surgical repair of the recurrent nerve, such as neurolysis, nerve suture, nerve grafting, have up to now failed to show this synchronization of muscle activity, while auxiliary neuro-muscular interventions, including the Tucker operation, have not provided automatic activity, but require voluntary muscle action. Our own results (Eitschberger, Thumfart) with 6 cases of the Tucker operation were hardly satisfactory in this respect.

According to the concept of a self-regulating glottic activity only the phrenic motor nerve offers the properties of an ideal timer of glottic abduction, because its automatic inspiratory impulses are absolutely coincident with the automatic activity in the glottic abductor muscle (Fig. 1).

In a series of experiments we have severed the recurrent nerve of rabbits and dogs, and have selectively reinnervated the posticus abductor muscle by implantation of the phrenic nerve or by grafts sutured to the phrenic nerve. Positive functional and histological results were reported earlier (Wigand, Naumann, Hölldobler). An example is shown in Fig. 2.

When we tried this procedure for the treatment of human laryngeal palsy, however, we failed in almost all of our eight cases. This negative outcome may be explained by the fact that all cases suffered from the palsy for more than two years, and we know that muscular degeneration starts already after a denervation time of eight weeks (Thormann).

This situation has stimulated us to look for an early diagnosis of recurrent nerve degeneration in order to indicate such nerve implantations in patients at an earlier date, when muscle atrophy has not yet taken place. I am delighted, therefore, that the endoscopical electromyography of Thumfart apparently provides the means of exact prediction of laryngeal palsies, so that we may reassess the phrenic nerve grafting to the laryngeal abductor muscle in the near future. May be, that combinations with selective reinnervation after the principles of diversification of Miehlke may be helpful.

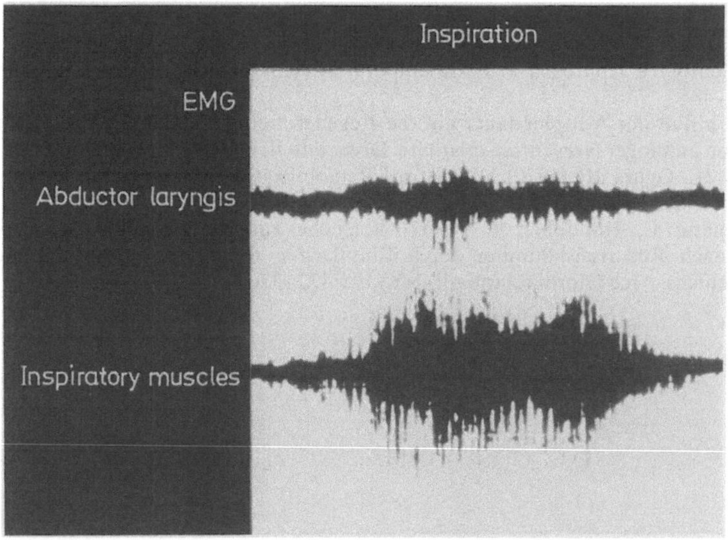

Fig. 1. Synchronous electrical activity in the abductor laryngis muscle (*uper track*) and in the diaphragm (*lower track*) at the onset of inspiration. EMG recordings from a human patient in general anesthesia

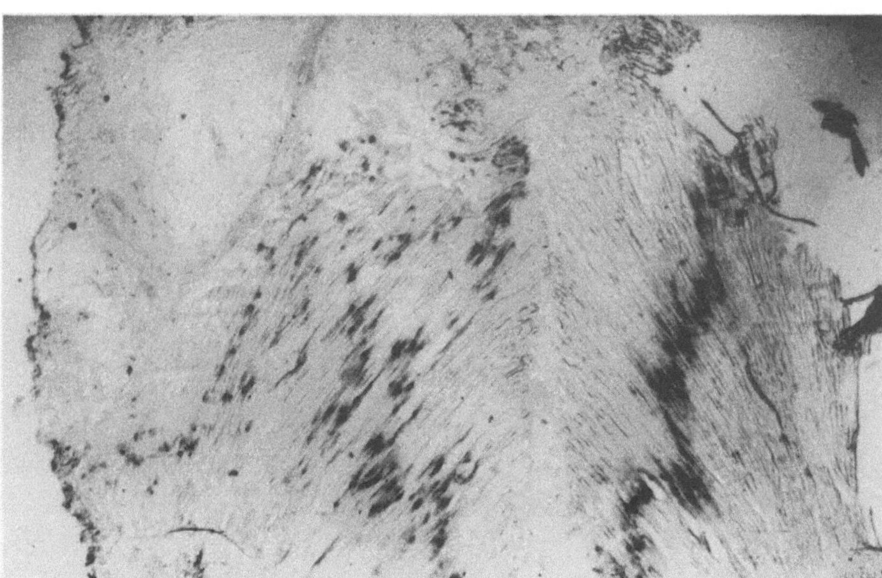

Fig. 2. New motor end plates in the abductor laryngis muscle of a rabbit six months after the implantation of a free nerve graft with nerve synthesis to the phrenic nerve. While on the left side, the motor end plate zone is compact, the new end plates (right abductor muscle) are disseminated

References

Stennert E (1979) Combined Approach in Extratemporal Facial Nerve Reconstruction. Clin Plast Surg 6:471–486

Thomann J (1972) Einfluß der Atrophiedauer auf die Regeneration denervierter Muskulatur nach Implantation autologer Nerventransplantate. Dissertation, Universität Würzburg

Tucker HM, Harvey JE, Ogura JH (1970) Vocal Cord Remobilization in the Canine Larynx. Arch Otolaryngol (Stockh) 92:530–533

Wigand ME, Naumann C, Hölldobler G (1969) Versuche zur Reinnervation des Abduktormuskels nach Recurrenslähmung durch Einpflanzen freier Nerventransplantate zum Nervus phrenicus. Arch Otorhinolaringol (NY) 194:372–376

Operative Treatment of Accessory Nerve Lesions

M. Samii, Hannover/FRG

Neurological deficit of the accessory nerve has serious clinical impact. Preservation of function or reconstruction of the accessory nerve is very important. Patients suffering complete loss of function of this nerve with paralysis of the trapezius muscle are no longer in a position to practise professions demanding strenouous physical activity. Damage to the accessory nerve due to accidents is relatively rare, even though the nerve lies in the lateral neck triangle close under the skin. However, the accessory nerve may frequently be damaged during extirpation of a tumor or of a lymphatic gland lateral to the posterior border of the sternocleidomastoid muscle (Fig. 1 a).

Excision of lymphatic glands and small tumors in this region must be performed very carefully. During such an intervention the accessory nerve in this area should always be exposed at the posterior border of the sternocleidomastoid muscle. Subsequently, the removal of a tumor or the lymphatic gland may be executed. If postoperative paralysis occurs, the accessory nerve must be operated as soon as pos-

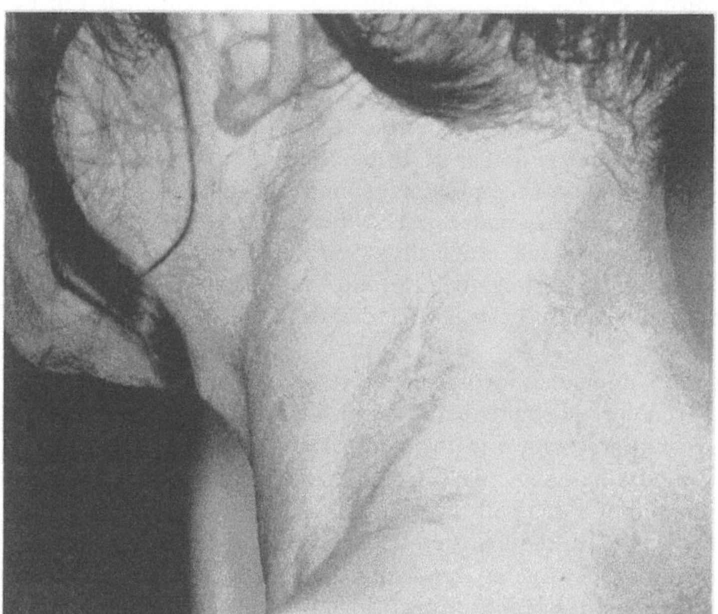

Fig. 1 a. Typical Skin scar to the lateral border of the sternocleidomastoid muscle after removal of a lymph node with injury to the accessory nerve

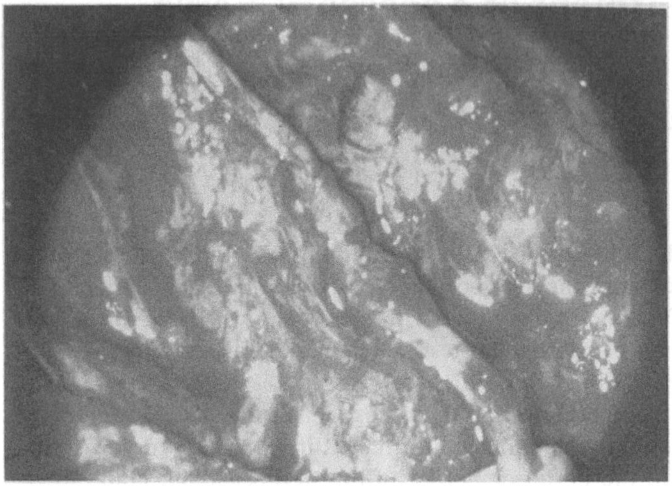

Fig. 1b. Exposure of the accessory nerve at the lateral border of the sternocleidomastoid muscle. The continuity of the accessory nerve is preserved. One can observe a thickening of a nerve trunk

sible, by means of neurolysis, nerve suture, or nerve grafting. When exposing the nerve, one must avoid the scar in the area of the lesion and start with exposure in the healthy part of the nerve at the posterior margin of the sternocleidomastoid muscle. If the continuity is evident macroscopically a fascicular neurolysis can be performed using the microscope. In some cases there may be only a serious fibrosis with compression of the nerve, requiring the removal of the fibrotically changed epineurium (Fig. 1b–d). In the case of neuromatous change of the fascicles, even if continuity is preserved, the neuroma should be resected and an end-to-end anastomosis or nerve grafting performed (Fig. 2a–d). If the accessory nerve is interrupted in its continuity and the neuroma of the proximal stump is located in scar with no relation to the distal stump, one must endeavour to trace the accessory nerve distal to the nerve lesion. Extensive damage, especially when the lesion is located over a distance, may cause difficulties with regard to the exposure of the distal stump, as the nerve at this point soon begins to branch off and ends in the anterior segment of the trapezius muscle.

Benign and malignant tumors that involve the accessory nerve and cases that demand radical neck dissection require preoperative consideration of accessory nerve reconstruction. Biopsy of a large tumor in the sternocleidomastoid muscle in a 17 year old girl demonstrated a hemangioma (Fig. 3a–b). Together with Doctor Osterwald we removed the tumor along with the sternocleidomastoid muscle and had to sacrifice the accessory nerve. In the first step the acessory nerve was exposed distal to the tumor. The tumor then was separated and the accessory nerve transected proximally. The eight cm long nerve defect was bridged by means of a sural nerve graft (Fig. 3c and d).

Encouraged by the excellent results of nerve grafts, together with Professor Scheunemann and his team, in 1971 we started to develop indications for the re-

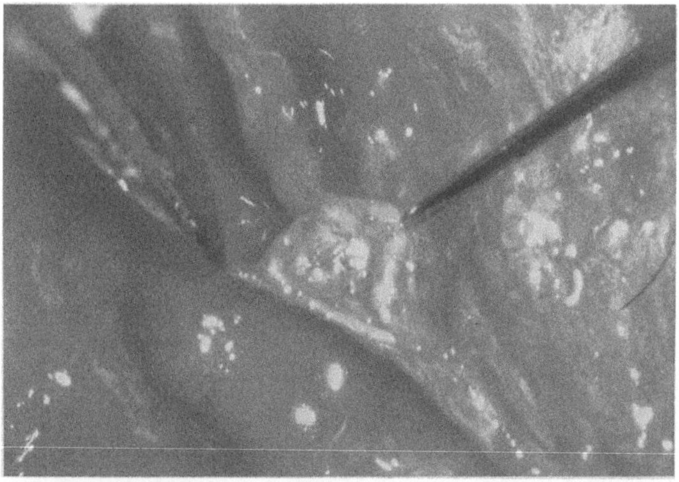

c

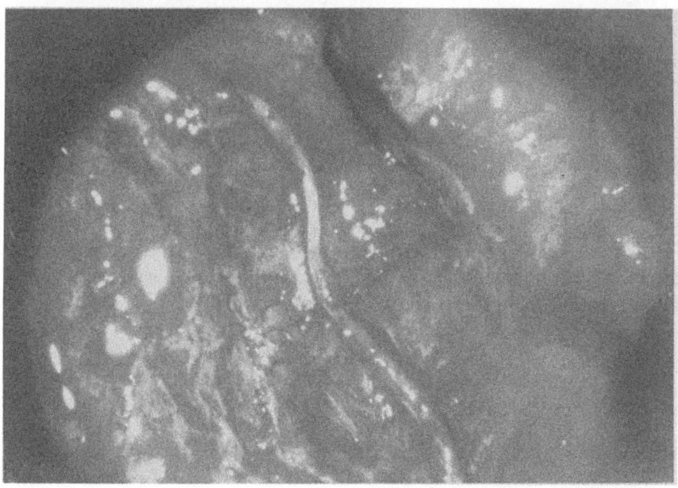

d

Fig. 1 c, d. The same case as Fig. 1 a and b. Microsurgical opening of fibrotically changed epineurium. The fascicle of the nerve is exposed (**c**). A fascicular neurolysis has been performed. The fascicle is preserved in its continuity (**d**)

construction of the accessory nerve in malignant tumors of the head and neck when performing neck dissections. As soon as the skin flap is prepared for neck dissection, the central portion of the accessory nerve distal to the jugular foramen is marked and sectioned. The distal part is traced out and sectioned before its entrance into the trapezius muscle (Fig. 4a). After neck dissection, the existing defect can be bridged by a graft from the sural nerve approximately 12 cm long (Fig. 4b). An example of a combined reconstruction of facial and accessory nerve in case of a large tumor of the middle and posterior skull base is demonstrated in Fig. 5. The dura defect is closed by lyophilised dura and the facial and the accessory nerve are reconstructed by means of a sural nerve graft.

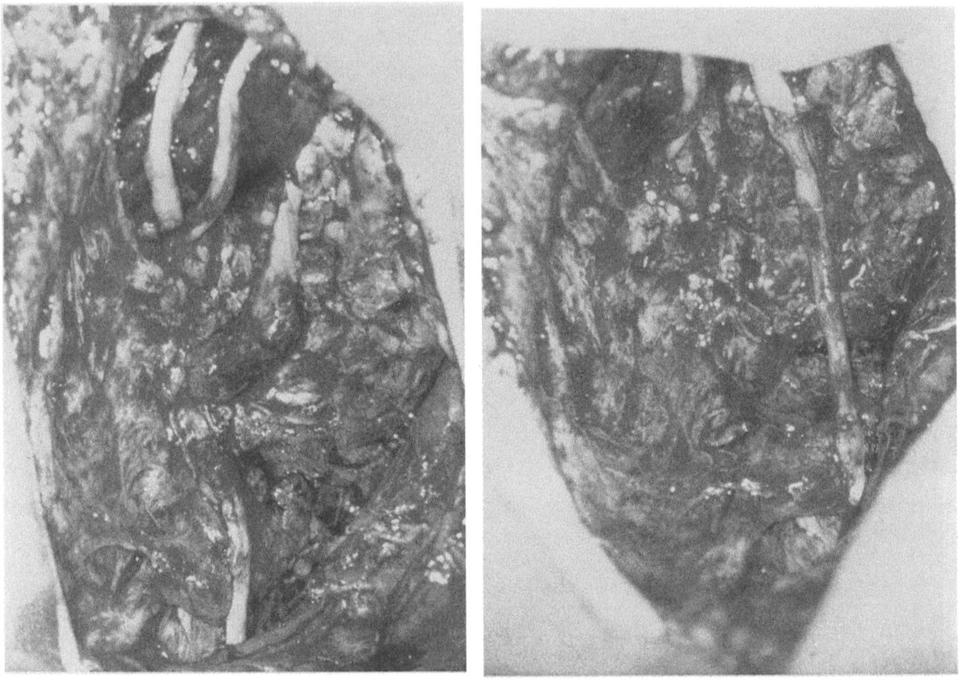

a b

Fig. 2a, b. Total interruption of the accessory nerve with development of a large neuroma at the proximal stump (**a**). After resection of the neuroma and the scar, the 4 cm nerve defects in length is bridged by means of a nerve graft from the auricular magnus nerve (**b**)

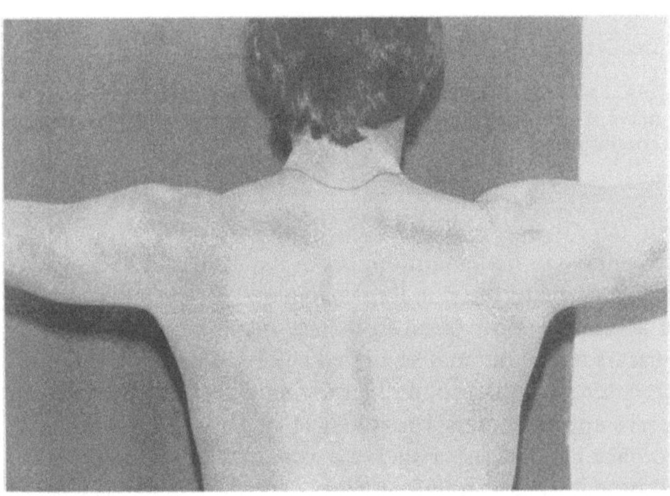

c

Fig. 2c, d. The same case as Fig. 2a and b. Postoperative result 18 months after the operation. The restoration of the trapezius muscle is visible and the function improved

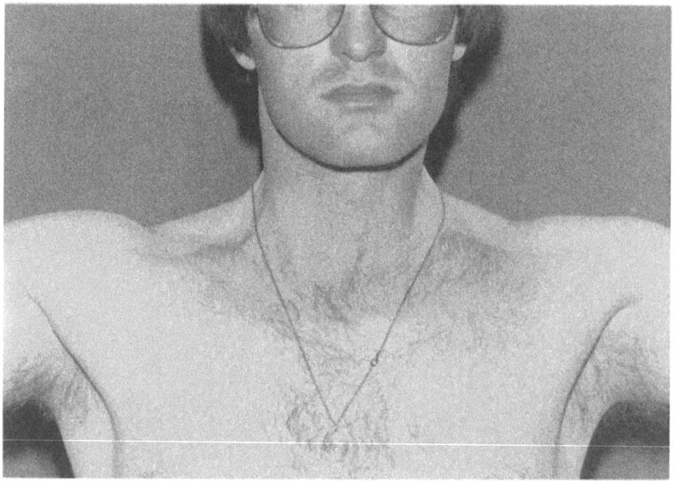

Fig. 2 d

Summary

From 1970 to 1980 we had the opportunity of microsurgical treatment of the accessory nerve in 40 patients (Table 1).

Table 1. Neurolysis, nerve suture, nerve grafting in forty cases of accessory nerve lesion

Tumors of jugular foramen	12
Neck dissection in malignant tumors	15
Lesion during excision of lymphatic node	9
Lesion through accident	4

In 12 patients we were dealing with benign tumors, including neurinomas, meningeomas and glomus tumors in the craniocervical region with overlapping of the jugular foramen. In 14 patients with neck dissection necessitated by malignant tumors, reconstruction of the accessory nerve was achieved at the same time by means of a free nerve graft. In malignant tumors, reconstruction of the accessory nerve was achieved at the same time by means of a free nerve graft. In malignant tumors follow up was not possible, as most patients died within a relatively short period after tumor therapy. Therefore the indications for accessory nerve reconstruction in malignant head and neck tumors are limited. In nine patients the accessory nerve had been damaged during removal of a lymphatic node in the lateral triangle of the neck. In four patients the lesion was caused by an accident. Among the traumatic injuries of the accessory nerve, three neurolysis, two end-to-end-sutures and eight nerve grafts were performed. In only one patient we were not successful. All the others showed satisfactory results.

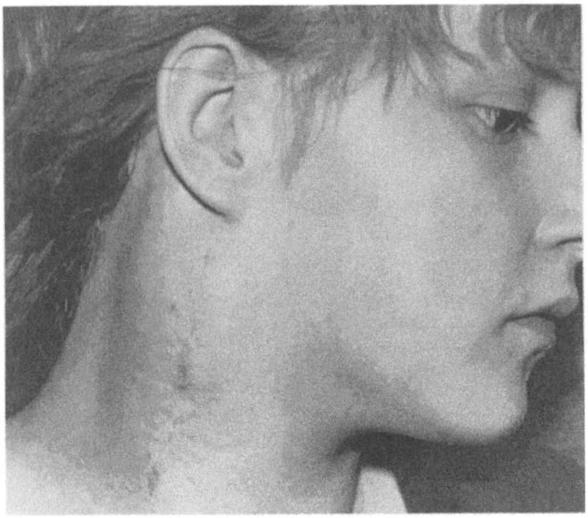

a

Fig. 3a, b. A biopsy of the large tumor in the sternocleidomastoid muscle resulted in this 17 year old girl a hemangioma (a). The angiography shows the extension of the tumor (b)

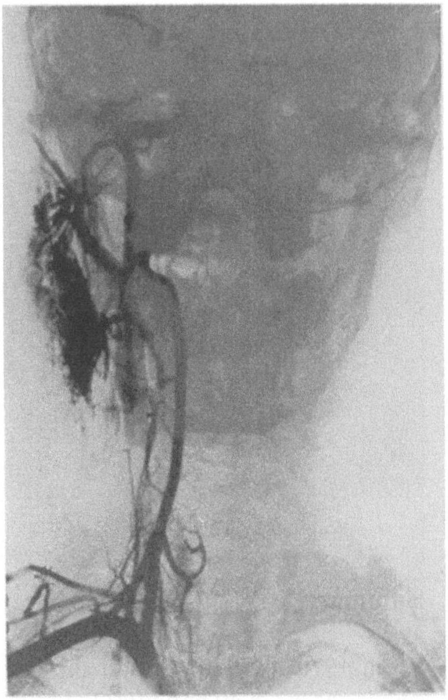

b

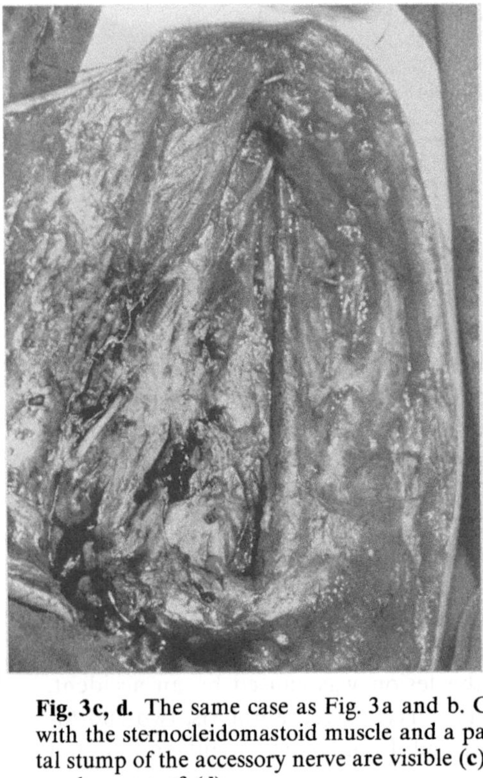

c

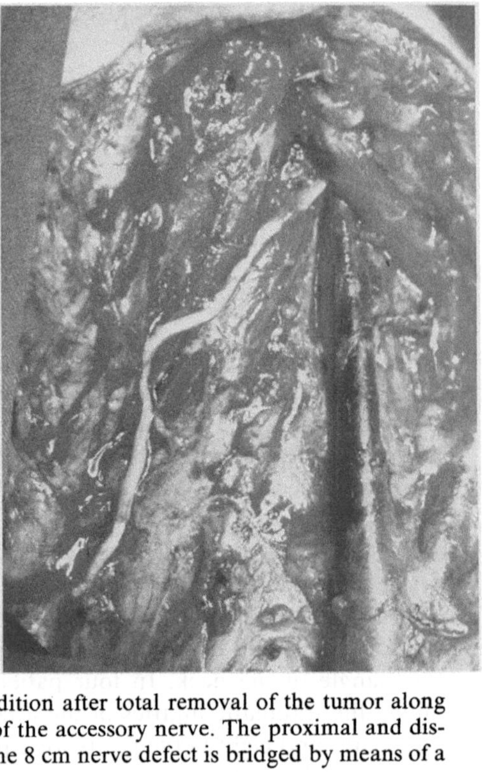

d

Fig. 3c, d. The same case as Fig. 3a and b. Condition after total removal of the tumor along with the sternocleidomastoid muscle and a part of the accessory nerve. The proximal and distal stump of the accessory nerve are visible (c). The 8 cm nerve defect is bridged by means of a sural nerve graft (d)

Résumé and Future Perspectives of Surgery on Cranial Nerves

K. SCHÜRMANN, Mainz/FRG

The symposium draws to a close, but our work is not at an end. I believe that all participants have been very impressed and stimulated by this unusual way of exchanging knowledge, ideas and – as Jongkees put it – of presenting speculations. Of course, one has to start with speculations and new ideas for finding out in the future what really happens. This symposium has shown us that we are reurged to proceed in a more scientific manner in the future in preparing the next step forward. However, we may be optimistic with regard to future advances.

It is impossible to summarize all important points of this meeting. Some questions were answered, but still more questions remain open.

The following questions ran like a red thread through the congress:

1. Are there differences in regeneration from one cranial nerve to another?
2. How do we preserve nerve elements during surgery?
3. How do we repair damaged nerve structures?
4. How do we manage plastic reconstructions?

On the one hand, we were fascinated by the excellent anatomical pictures presented by Lang and Rabischong. On the other hand, we were reminded of the need for all surgeons to study microanatomy and topographical anatomy intensively. The very close juxtaposition of the cranial nerves to the main feeding vessels and brain stem underscores the high surgical risk, especially in space occupying lesions in the deep middle and posterior fossa. Possibly, more attention should have been paid to the central nuclei of cranial nerves and intracerebral connections so as to enable the function to be better understood.

A wide gap in our knowledge about the regeneration of both central nerves, – the olfactory and the optic nerve – has become evident. The origin of these two nerves from cerebral tissue could not be described any better than by Lang: the first and second cranial nerves are not 'nerves'! It is clear that future research on regeneration of the olfactory and optic nerve is urgently needed. Sir Sidney Sunderland may perhaps be prompted to carry out further investigations in this field, especially since he was able to demonstrate so well the different kinds of nerve regeneration after stretching and compression of peripheral nerves, even with respect to degree of lesion and time factors.

Kreuzberg could demonstrate very nicely the high growth capacity of axons as early as 11 to 12 hours after nerve section: intracellular energy metabolism increased by nearly 100 percent.

Of course, it is not possible to give a survey dealing with all cranial nerves, although it would be very attractive. Nervetheless, a few remarks on some essentials should be ventured.

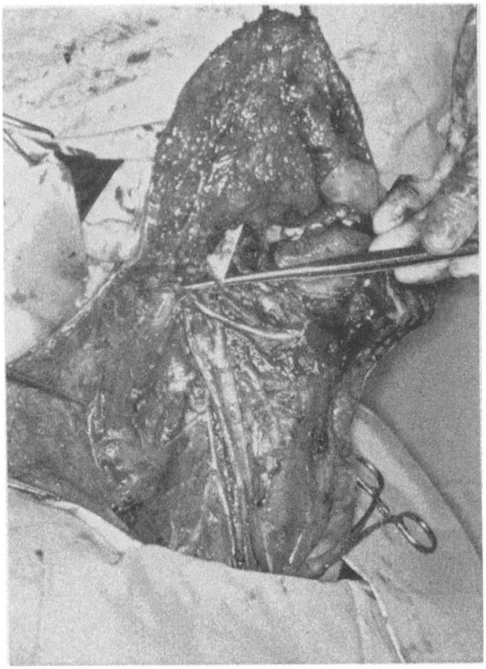
a

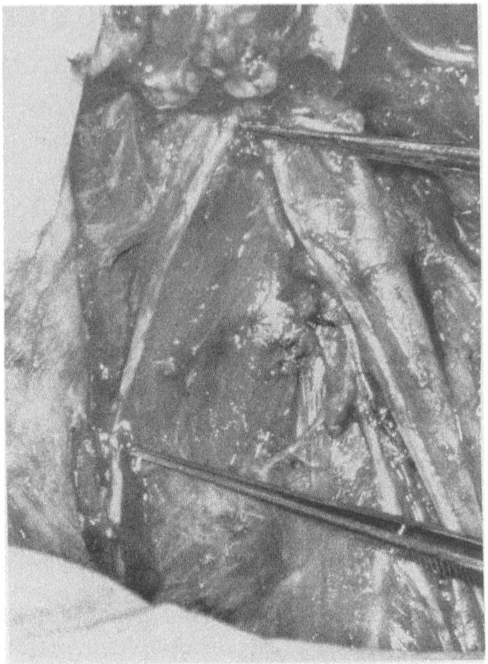
b

Fig. 4 a, b. Operative field following neck dissection including the resection of the accessory nerve in a case of a malignant tumor. Exposure of the distal and central stumps (**a**). Bridging of the nerve defect by means of a 12 cm nerve graft (**b**)

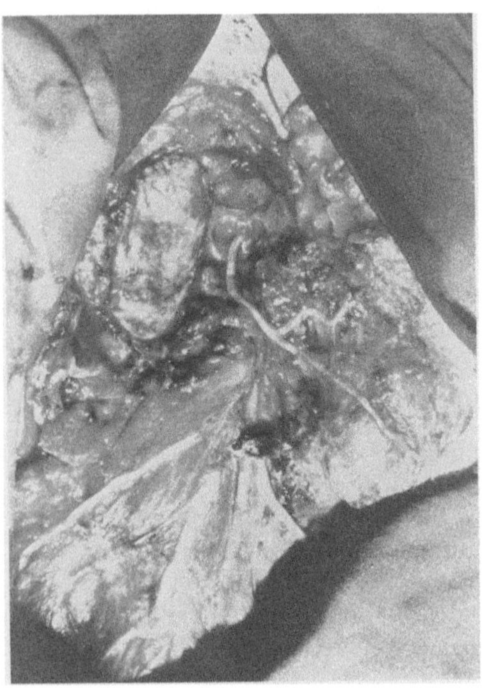

Fig. 5. An example of a combined reconstruction of facial and accessory nerve in case of a large tumor of the middle and posterior skull base. The dura defect is closed by lyophilised dura and the facial and accessory nerve are reconstructed by means of sural nerve grafts

With regard to preservation of olfactory sense, it was pointed out by our Japanese colleagues Suzuki and others that in certain cases of fronto-basal CSF fistulae and anterior communicating aneurysm surgery, an approach between the fronto-basal brain and the olfactory tracts of bulbs can be aimed for. Surely one cannot preserve the olfactory sense in every case but an attempt for preservation should be made.

In optic nerve lesions, it was demonstrated that the development of the latest computer tomograph generation by Newton and Meyer and intradural application of metrizamide has enabled the optic nerve sheath to be visualized. This optic nerve tecography will, without doubt, be of importance in the diagnosis of optic nerve lesions in the future.

The controversy about the indication for optic nerve decompression operations after traumatic optic nerve lesions persists. However, if an operation is indicated, the transethmoidal approach would involve lower risks.

Visual function recovery in pituitary tumor surgery was better in transphenoidal than in transcranial operations, as Fahlbusch illustrated with his large series. However, it should be borne in mind that a few transcranially removed tumors were larger in size.

In a series of 231 tumors of the orbit, there were 37 meningiomas. The meningiomas of the anterior part of the orbit, which only produced a secondary compression of the optic nerve, showed a very good recovery of visual function disturbances. The optic nerve sheath meningeomas, however, had a bad prognosis of visual function recovery, as presented in my own contribution.

A new aspect of intracranial optic nerve or chiasm compression syndrome resulting from vascular variations (carotid artery and ophthalmic artery near the intradural optic nerve channel) or compression by dorsum sellae in case of low located optic chiasm could be demonstrated by Samii.

In disturbances of cranial nerves III, IV and VI, it was demonstrated by Newton that the intracranial part of the oculomotor nerve could also be visualized by special computer tomographic techniques. Furthermore, with a fine superselective angiographic subtraction technique Lasjaunias demonstrated the intracavernous arterial supply of the cranial nerves III, IV, V and VI. In consequence, intracavernous vascular lesions may be better controlled in the future.

The electrophysiological differentiation of ocular muscle palsy or nerve palsy had reached a high standard, as shown by Struppler and Heuser.

It is significant that the oculomotor nerve paresis caused by supraclinoidal aneurysms had a better prognosis if patients were operated upon within the first two weeks after hemorhage (Suzuki).

As demonstrated by Schürmann, CN III, IV and VI pareses in intraorbital lesions are mainly caused by tumors in the posterior orbital tip. The functional recovery is better in tumors which cause a displacement of the tendinous circle in the posterior tip of the orbit than when the lesion has invaded the posterior muscle cone.

It is understandable that nothing has been mentioned about intracavernous nerve repair, but it is surprising that there have been no reports on intracranial nerve repair or nerve reconstruction of cranial nerves III, IV, VI outside the cavernous sinus.

Naturally, facial pain was at the center of discussion on the Vth cranial nerve.

However, it could be demonstrated by the group of Struppler and coworkers that evoked potentials of the trigeminal nerve in man enabled a close differentiation between peripheral and pontine lesions. A long discussion arose about Jannetta's hypothesis that the pathophysiology of the 'idiopathic' trigeminal neuralgia results from arterial compression of the nerve root within the posterior fossa. Logically, his concept for treatment is to decompress the trigeminal root approaching the posterior fossa microsurgically.

Perhaps sufficient experience will be gained in the next decade to allow a judgement. One of the critical aspects has to be mentioned, i.e. that many anatomical variations with relation to the cranial nerves have been demonstrated by anatomists in which the case history, particularly in respect of pain attacks, is unknown. This is a stimulus to further investigations in the future.

There is no great difference between the thermo-coagulation and the controlled and selective electrocoagulation in respect to the high effectiveness in the treatment of tic douloureux, as it could also be shown by Penzholz and Schürmann. However, it was stressed by Jannetta that a 'symptom' is treated with the coagulation techniques, but that the 'cause' would be treated with his method of vascular decompression. He believes in a peripheral cause but central mechanism. What does this mean? The surgeon has to make his own decision in respect to the surgical risk on the one hand and the effect on the other hand, particularly in elderly patients. Pathogenesis, treatment and recurrences of facial pain will still concern us in the future. Are there biochemical or mechanical changes within the nerve and/or central nuclei? Do we change or reduce the input of pathological stimuli? Our knowledge is appallingly scanty!

Lesions of the VIIth cranial nerve were of utmost interest to all participants. Besides the important anatomical and topographical variations of the course of the facial nerve in its intracranial, intrapetrosal and extracranial portion (Lang, Helms), the intraneural topography of the fascicle groups in the peripheral branches (Millesi), and the number of fibers (Søgard) found great interest in relation to surgical nerve repair. On the other hand, nothing could be said about the function of various anastomoses between the cranial nerves VII and VIII or between VII and V, which were seen by the anatomists.

With respect to clinical experience with facial nerve lesions, such as Bell's palsy as well as hemifacial spasm, there were controversial standpoints. Some special features are to be reported. Jongkees expressed regret about the large gap in knowledge concerning the origin of Bell's palsy. He asked Jannetta, who wished to explain the origin of some cases of Bell's palsy by vessel loop compression of the facial nerve in the posterior fossa, how the sudden onset of Bell's palsy might be accounted for, since the vessel loops have been there for a long time? A contradiction remains here.

Increasing caution was noticeable with regard to the indication for surgery, because the mostly incomplete pareses have a very good prognosis in more than 90 percent when treated conservatively. On the other hand, a complete palsy has a bad prognosis, whether treated conservatively or surgically. The indication for surgery should be decided in accordance with Stennert's score (principles of investigation). On the basis of Stennert's score, the indication for surgery could be reduced to about eight percent of cases. There was a tendency to minimize the extent of intrapetrosal facial nerve decompression by an approach through the external acoustic meatus and no longer by the sub- and transtemporal approach (Helms). In cases of Bell's palsy in which there was no recovery of nerve function, various techniques of nerve substitution and plastic repair were intensively discussed. There remains competition between the two techniques facial-hypoglossal nerve anastomosis and facio-facial crossface anastomosis, as shown by the respectable results obtained with both techniques in some cases in recent years. In crossface anastomosis, frontal grafting above the eyebrows can be dispensed with, since it never produces functional results. Two anastomoses between the buccal branches and the zygomatic branches are sufficient (Millesi, Samii). This confirms the findings of Søgard et al., who found that of the 6,000 to 7,000 fibers of the main stem of facial nerve only 18 percent distribute to the frontal branches, but about 30 percent to the zygomatic and 30 percent to the buccal branches. In the 'hopeless cases' of Bell's palsy, plastic muscle grafting with free three muscle transfer and microvascular anastomoses (donator muscles are the M. gracilis and M. latissimus dorsi) seems to be preferable (Harii).

In the treatment of hemifacial spasm, the partial section of the three peripheral branches of the facial nerve (50 percent section each) gave rise to disappointing results: more than 50 percent recurrences arose after one year follow up, and spasm recurred after some years in nearly all patients (Miehlke, Samii). Fisch (quoted by Miehlke) has therefore sectioned 90 percent of the peripheral facial nerve branches in his recent series. However, the results are still unknown at the time of writing. On the other hand, Jannetta's pioneer work in this disease of so far unknown origin is to be emphasized. Jannetta found a vascular compression of the facial nerve in the posterior fossa near the brain stem in his 229 surgically treated cases of hemifacial spasm, and he concluded a possibly nuclear dysfunction caused by the vessel loop in the disease. Nevertheless, the facial spasm disappeared after surgical decompression of the nerve in 201 cases, and after a repeated operation in 12 further cases. The good results have now lasted over some years. As a technical note, Samii commented that he preferred to separate the nerve from the vessel loop by a muscle piece instead of fibrin sponge and confirmed the good results with reference to six cases, as did Kondo in 71 cases, too. It is hoped for that the future will provide answers to the following questions:

Is there nuclear compression near the brain stem?
Do emotional influences act in addition?
Does the duration of the spasm have an influence, because of growing emotional reaction?

In contrast to Jannetta, Struppler postulates a peripheral origin, because of his findings that the examination of the M. orbicularis oculi reflex (as a central reflex) was negative in his cases of hemifacial spasm. The confusion in the controversy between central (nuclear) or peripheral origin of hemifacial spasm has been complicated by Jongkees' panel remark that he has not seen any hemifacial spasm in the Netherlands, but has seen more than 100 cases in Mexico.

Turning now to the eighth cranial nerve, the technological development of CT scanning has proved to have great diagnostic significance. It enables the intracranial course of the facial and acoustic nerves to be visualized and allows early diagnosis even of small tumors in the cerebellopontine angle. Early diagnosis with clinical methods will continue to dominate in the future, since a 'suspicion' is necessary to prompt further investigations. The functional tests of cochlear and vestibular functions were intensively discussed by the ENT surgeons and neurologists (Wigand, Plester, Kornhuber, Jongkees). These tests do not enable definitive diagnosis, but result in a high level of suspicion.

In the treatment of acoustic neurinomas, Pulec and Sterkers had an opportunity to present their special techniques from the ENT viewpoint and to report their results with transtemporal, translabyrinthal and retrosigmoidal approaches. The discussion was completed by comments on experience with the neurosurgical suboccipitoretrosigmoidal approach (Kurze, Samii, Schürmann). The essential topic of the discussion was not only the preservation and repair of the facial nerve, but also the possibility and benefit of preserving the cochlear position of the eighth cranial nerve (Helms, Pulec, Samii, Schürmann, Sterkers, Wigand). The aim of preserving as much function as possible in the future is undisputed. However, there was not yet a clear consensus about the 'usefulness' of a residual but not serviceable hearing function. This may be combined with severe tinnitus, which may disappear after a certain time. Moreover, in recent years, the scope for closer cooperation between ENT surgeons and Neurosurgeons with a view to preserving auditory function even in large acoustic neurinomas has opened up (Helms, Samii, Schürmann, Wigand).

With respect to the caudal cranial nerve group (CN IX to XII) some points of special significance are to be emphasized. A very interesting review on the anatomical and physiological connections of the intramedullary nuclei and the interrelations between motor and sensory functions of the cranial nerves IX to XII was presented by Sunderland. A comprehensive general survey on dysfunction and neurological diseases affecting this important CN group was given by Mumenthaler. Thumfart's endoscopic electromyography (EMG) and neuronography with insertion of a needle electrode into the pharynx for differentiating laryngeal muscle lesions following vagal nerve damage in laryngeal surgery deserves special attention. During the ensueing panel discussion, Miehlke and Wigand had the opportunity to present their new techniques of recurrens nerve repair after laryngectomy. Thumfart's intralaryngeal EMG findings enable more precise application of these techniques. The recent advances in restoring a certain function by means of nerve-nerve anastomoses, nerve-muscle anastomoses and muscle-muscle anastomoses could be explained very concisely.

Rather fascinating was the assertion of Jannetta that a left-sided arterial compression of the medulla at the level of vagal nerve nuclei causes a systemic arterial hypertension. Jannetta's statement was based primarily on the clinical observation that in his series of 11 patients with a glossopharyngeal neuralgia caused by vascular compression of the IXth CN in the posterior fossa, a severe hypertensive crisis was to be seen in two patients (one patient died). In these two cases, he observed a vascular compression of the CN IX and X near the brain stem. Jannetta performed animal experiments in cats and baboons to confirm this clinical observation. By insertion of a balloon to the lateral wall of the medulla near the vagus nerve an increase of blood pressure from 90 to 160 mmHg could be produced by balloon inflation. It seems to be of importance that the hypertensive reaction could be obtained in acute as well as in chronic experiments (of about four weeks duration). Blood pressure decreased only when the balloon was deflated or removed. Jannetta believes that some cases of 'essential hypertension' in man are caused by vessel loop compression of cranial nerve X near brain stem on the left side, since he observed this in a series of 28 patients (in 23 patients on the left and only in five patients on the right side). His therapeutic conception is of course to effect surgical vascular decompression by separation of vessel and vagus nerve near brain stem. Jannetta's daring hypothesis does not remain uncontradicted, especially by Kurze, who reminded us of the historical observations by Claude Bernard, of stereotactic damage to certain brain structures. Kurze also recalled Wilder Penfield's observations in epileptic foci studies, and reminded of the well-known clinical observations in acoustic neurinomas with arterial hypertension and blood pressure decrease after tumor removal. Kurze also pointed out that many other intracranial lesions can cause hypertension. This does not seem to be a specific reaction. One should therefore be cautious with too far-reaching interpretations.

The almost artistic superselective angiographic investigations of CN IX to XII presented by Lasjaunias will provide stimuli for more precise diagnostic vascular investigation in the future. They will also have some therapeutic consequences for application of carefully directed embolization in certain selected cases.

In the last panel, surgical management of manifold affections of the caudal CN IX to XII were discussed comprehensively. Besides the microsurgical vascular decompression of the IXth CN in patients with glossopharyngeal neuralgia mentioned above by Jannetta, a new and simple percutaneous technique for selective thermocoagulation of cranial nerve IX was presented by Isamat. Although only a small number of patients were treated by this method, it seems to be effective and has the advantage of practically zero risk, analogous to the similar technique in trigeminal neuralgia.

Much attention was accorded to diagnostic measures and surgical strategy in jugular foramen tumors, especially in glomus tumors (Denecke, Draf, Helms, Menzel, Samii, Schürmann, Wigand). Although not all problems of this difficult field of surgery could be covered, it was to be seen that especially here very close cooperation between experienced ENT surgeons and neurosurgeons enables a successful total removal in one step in most circumstances. On the other hand, efforts to facilitate surgery by preoperative selective embolization remain controversial, with the possible exception that surgery must be performed directly after embolization to diminish the risk of hemorrhage in these highly vascularized tumors. However, pretreatment with full tumor radiation in glomus tumors was recommended only by Wigand. In a critical summing-up, it was evident even in view of the limited experience of each surgeon that the better the topographical exposure of tumor, both extracranially and intracranially, with as extensive a bone resection around the skull base as possible, the more radical the removal of tumor masses which could be attained. This extensive extracranial and intracranial exposure also enables more certain isolation and preservation of the internal carotid artery as well as of the nerve elements.

All in all, this exchange of ideas and experience has been enriching for all of us. There is a wise old saying: the better the preoperative information, the more precise the planning of surgery, the safer its performance. The more profound the theoretical background, the better the concepts of therapy. All surgeons must bear in mind:

preservation of function is, of course, in any case preferable to repair or reconstruction. Our goal must be to minimize the risks of surgery with the aim of achieving the greatest possible effectiveness. Moreover, it was evident that progress in this wide field of surgery will proceed very fast in the near future, to the benefit of our patients as well as ourselves.

Subject Index

Computed Tomography in Intracranial Tumors – Clinical Aspects and Differential Diagnosis

Edited by: E. Kazner, S. Wende, Th. Grumme, W. Lanksch, O. Stochdorph

In Preparation
ISBN 3-540-10815-7

This textbook and atlas is the first comprehensive and systematic presentation dealing with the diagnosis of brain tumors, including lesions in the orbits and at the base of the skull, using computed tomography. Special emphasis has been placed on clinical aspects and differential diagnosis. The work is the result of a co-operative effort involving three leading German university hospitals and is based on CT studies in more than 5000 patients with verified intracranial space-occupying lesions and orbital diseases.

The extensive illustrative material demonstrates the most common brain tumors by means of typical computed tomograms as well as rare histological entities and atypical sites. In some cases plain skull films, angiograms or post-mortem studies complement the computed tomograms. Each histological tumor group is described individually, using a system related to the new WHO brain tumor classification.

Separate chapters are devoted to processes at the base of the skull and in the vault as well as orbital lesions causing proptosis. The discussion of possible differential diagnoses covers all non-neoplastic space-occupying intracranial lesions and includes inflammatory diseases, acute demyelinating processes, granulomas, cysts, parasites, hemorrhages, vascular anomalies and brain infarctions.

Springer-Verlag
Berlin
Heidelberg
New York

MIX
Papier aus verantwortungsvollen Quellen
Paper from responsible sources
FSC® C105338

If you have any concerns about our products,
you can contact us on
ProductSafety@springernature.com

In case Publisher is established outside the EU,
the EU authorized representative is:
Springer Nature Customer Service Center GmbH
Europaplatz 3, 69115 Heidelberg, Germany

Printed by Libri Plureos GmbH
in Hamburg, Germany